Brief Contents

Documentation for Medical Practices

Cheryl Gregg Fahrenholz, RHIA, CCS-P

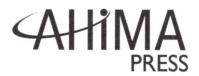

AHIMA
PRESS

ISBN: 978-1-58426-228-2
AHIMA Product No.: AB101509

AHIMA Staff:
Claire Blondeau, MBA, Senior Editor
Angela Dinh, MHA, RHIA, Reviewer
Cynthia Douglas, Developmental Editor
Katie Greenock, Editorial and Production Coordinator
Ashley Sullivan, Assistant Editor
Ken Zielske, Director of Publications

All information contained within this book, including Web sites and regulatory information, was current and valid as of the date of publication. However, Web page addresses and the information on them may change or disappear at any time and for any number of reasons. The user is encouraged to perform his or her own general Web searches to locate any site addresses listed here that are no longer valid.

All products mentioned in this book are either trademarks of the companies referenced in this book, registered trademarks of the companies of the companies referenced in this book, or neither.

American Health Information Management Association
233 North Michigan Avenue, 21st Floor
Chicago, Illinois 60601-5809
ahima.org

Contents

About the Author and Contributors

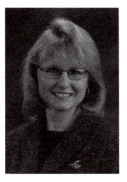**Cheryl Gregg Fahrenholz, RHIA, CCS-P,** is the president of Preferred Healthcare Solutions, LLC, and has more than 25 years of experience working with healthcare facilities, providers, and their staff. Her consulting services include revenue cycle performance improvement, documentation and coding audits, operational assessments, charge description master reviews, coding seminars for physician and staff, denial audits, risk and sanction analysis, compliance plan evaluations, electronic health record selection and implementation, expert testimony and defense work, along with interim and retainer professional support and customized project work.

Before establishing her own consulting firm in 1998, Gregg Fahrenholz served as the Director of Documentation, Coding, and Reimbursement at the Primary Care Networks of Premier Health Network and as the Manager of Information Management at Miami Valley Hospital.

Gregg Fahrenholz holds a BS in health information management (HIM) from Bowling Green State University. She is a nationally recognized speaker on the topics of revenue cycle, documentation, coding, and compliance. She has many publications at the national level.

Highlights from her involvement with the American Health Information Management Association (AHIMA) are: Discovery Triumph Award Recipient, Delegate, Nominating Committee, member; Physician Practice Council, chair; Program Committee, member; Communities of Practice Advisory Task Force, member; Compliance Task Force, member; Ambulatory Care Section, chair; and Release of Information Task Force, member. She has served for numerous years on the Board of Directors for the Ohio Health Information Management Association and received their Distinguished Member Award. The Miami Valley Health Information Management Association also awarded her as their Distinguished Member. She has served on many other boards and committees to include the Miami Valley Medical Group Management Association, Sinclair Community College, and the Ohio Association of Advanced Practice Nurses.

Gregg Fahrenholz served on the Centers for Medicare and Medicaid Services' (CMS) Technical Working Group for the Provider Education Project, which was responsible for conducting the needs assessment and development of the educational rollout for proper claims processing and reimbursement. She also served as the coding expert on the CMS's Negotiated Rulemaking Committee for National Laboratory Coverage Policies. This committee's work resulted in many National Coverage Determinations.

The author may be contacted at cheryl@phs4you.com.

Margret K. Amatayakul, MBA, RHIA, CHPS, CPHIT, CPEHR, CPHIE, FHIMSS, has more than 40 years of experience in HIM. She is a leading authority on electronic health record (EHR) strategies for healthcare organizations and has extensive experience in EHR selection and project management.

Before forming her own consulting firm, Margret\A Consulting, LLC, in 1999, Amatayakul served as director of medical record services at the Illinois Eye and Ear Infirmary, associate professor at the University of Illinois at the Medical Center, associate executive director of AHIMA, and executive director of the Computer-based Patient Record Institute. She provides information systems consulting services, freelance writing, and educational programming to the healthcare industry.

Amatayakul earned her bachelor's degree from the University of Illinois at the Medical Center and her master's in business administration, with concentrations in marketing and finance, from the University of Illinois at Chicago. She is a sought-after speaker, has published extensively, and has an impressive list of professional service awards to her credit. She is active in national policy setting and standards initiatives, has served on the board of directors of the Healthcare Information and Management Systems Society (HIMSS), is on the faculty and board of examiners of Health IT Certification, and continues to serve the health informatics community as adjunct faculty of the College of St. Scholastica.

She can be contacted at margret@margret-a.com.

Carolyn Buppert, JD, NP, (Law Office of Carolyn Buppert, P.C., Bethesda, MD) specializes in the legal issues affecting medical practices and nurse practitioners. Her clients include hospitals, health systems, physician and nurse practitioner practices, visiting nurse agencies, nursing homes, hospices, schools of nursing, and a certification organization. She is a frequent contributor to *The American Journal for Nurse Practitioners*, *The Journal for Nurse Practitioners,* and *Dermatology Nursing*. Her articles appear on Medscape.com, and she is on Medscape's nursing editorial board. She lectures extensively on avoiding malpractice, legal issues regarding scope of practice, prescribing and reimbursement, and negotiating terms of employment. She is the author of eight books and an instructional CD. Her Web site is http://www.buppert.com.

Susan Grennan, RHIA, is the director of medical records and privacy officer at the Boys Town National Research Hospital in Omaha, NE. The hospital has been internationally recognized as a leader in clinical and research programs focusing on childhood deafness, visual impairment, and related communication disorders. The hospital also offers a broad range of clinical services.

As a member of the Nebraska Health Information Management Association (NHIMA), Susan has represented NHIMA on a committee for Ambulatory Care Standards and Verbal Orders for the Nebraska Health Department. She was the chair and editor of the *Nebraska Legal Guide for Health Data* in 1999. Between 1995 and 1999, she testified on behalf of NHIMA in the Nebraska Legislature on a number of bills related to medical records and patient access to records. In 1999, NHIMA named her as their Distinguished Member. Susan has chaired numerous state committees, and in 1987 to 1988 was the president of NHIMA.

As a member of AHIMA, Susan wrote chapters for the *Ambulatory Handbook* in 1985, 1995, and 2000. She was the Secretary of the Ambulatory Care Section of AHIMA in 1999 and delegate to the AHIMA National Meetings in 1987 and 1988.

Bryon D. Pickard, MBA, RHIA, is director of business office operations for the 1,500-member Vanderbilt Medical Group, the faculty practice plan at Vanderbilt University Medical

Center in Nashville, TN. Pickard has spent 25 years in the healthcare industry and has worked in a variety of professional leadership capacities. Prior to joining Vanderbilt, Pickard was director of patient financial and information services for a large Midwest integrated delivery system and has held positions at both the University of Illinois and University of Florida. Pickard holds a BS in HIM and a master's of business administration from the University of Central Florida. He has taught courses in healthcare finance and reimbursement, co-authored numerous textbooks, and is a frequent speaker on such topics as revenue cycle operations and health information management. Pickard has also testified before Congress, served on several national professional boards, and is past president and board chairman of AHIMA.

Laurie A. Rinehart-Thompson, JD, RHIA, CHP, is an associate professor of clinical allied medicine in the Health Information Management & Systems program at The Ohio State University in Columbus, OH. She earned both her Bachelor of Science degree in medical record administration and her Juris Doctor degree from The Ohio State University. Her professional experience spans the behavioral health, home health, and acute care arenas. She has served as an expert witness in civil litigation, testifying as to the privacy and confidentiality of health information. She has served on the AHIMA CHP Exam Construction, Advocacy & Policy, and Education Strategy committees, the Release of Information Task Force, and is currently a member of the AHIMA Privacy and Security Practice Council. She has served twice on the Board of Directors of the Ohio Health Information Management Association. A frequent speaker on the HIPAA Privacy Rule, she is also a co-editor of and contributing author to AHIMA's *Fundamentals of Law for Health Informatics and Information Management* (2009), and a contributing author to *Ethical Challenges in the Management of Health Information* (2006, co-published by AHIMA and Jones and Bartlett), AHIMA's *Health Information Management Technology: An Applied Approach* (2010), and the *Journal of AHIMA*.

Acknowledgments

The author wishes to thank the expert contributors for sharing their professional knowledge to enhance the comprehensiveness of this book.

Margret Amatayakul, MBA, RHIA, CHPS, CPHIT, CPEHR, CPHIE, FHIMSS

Carolyn Buppert, JD, NP

Susan Grennan, RHIA

Bryon D. Pickard, MBA, RHIA

Laurie A. Rinehart-Thompson, JD, RHIA, CHP

In addition, the author is grateful to Angela Dinh, MHA, RHIA (Manager, Professional Practice Resources, AHIMA) for her content review of the chapters and Cynthia Douglas (Developmental Editor, AHIMA) for her detailed eye and continued guidance with this publication.

A special thanks from Cheryl to her husband, Mark, and mother, Pat, for their never-ending support in making this book a reality. With all of the challenges of balancing professional and family life, they have made this journey successful.

Chapter 1

Content and Format of Medical Practice Health Records

Cheryl Gregg Fahrenholz, RHIA, CCS-P

Learning Objectives

- Understand the general content and format of medical practice health records

- Gain a comprehension of the different purposes of each electronic or paper-based form in the health record

- Recognize the documentation requirements for different portions of the health record

- Learn to acknowledge the differences between and similarities across documentation for sample specialties

- Identify resources to assist medical practices with content, format, and documentation of health records

Key Terms

Abbreviations
Accreditation
Accreditation Association for Ambulatory Health Care (AAAHC)
Accreditation organization
Accreditation standards
Acute
Acute subluxation
Ambulatory care
American Chiropractic Association (ACA)
American College of Obstetricians and Gynecologists (ACOG)
American Medical Association (AMA)
American Physical Therapy Association (APTA)

American Society of Anesthesiologists (ASA)
Ancillary services
Anesthesia report
Appeal
Assessment
Authentication
Best practice
Carrier
Centers for Medicare and Medicaid Services (CMS)
Certified registered nurse anesthetist (CRNA)
Charge ticket
Chief complaint
Chronic
Chronic subluxation
Chronological order
Claim
Clinical guidelines/protocols

Clinical practice standards
CMS-1450
CMS-1500
Consent
Consultation report
Credentialing
Database
Discharge
Documentation
Documentation guideline (DG)
Electronic health record (EHR)
Encounter
Episode of care
e-Prescribing (e-Rx)
Evaluation and management (E/M) codes
Evaluation and management (E/M) services

Examination
Fiscal intermediary (FI)
Free text data
General consent to treatment
General health record documentation policy
Group practice
Growth chart
Guidelines
Healthcare provider
Health history
Health record
History and physical (H&P)
Hybrid health record
Implied consent
Informed consent
Integrated health record
Joint Commission
Legal health record
Local coverage determination (LCD)
Medical history
Medical necessity
Medicare Part B

Medication list
MMR vaccine
Multispecialty medical practice
National Committee for Quality Assurance (NCQA)
National Coverage Determination (NCD)
NPO (nothing by mouth)
Office of the National Coordinator for Health Information Technology (ONC)
Operative report
Orders
Paper-based health record
Past, family, and/or social history (PFSH)
Pathology report
Patient
Patient history questionnaire
Personal health record (PHR)
Physical examination

Physical therapy (PT)
Policies
Preoperative evaluation
Primary care provider (PCP)
Problem list
Problem-oriented medical record (POMR)
Progress note
Registration record
Reimbursement
Reverse chronological order
Review of systems (ROS)
Secure messaging systems
Source-oriented health record
Standing orders
Structured text data
Telephone contact record
Unique identifier
Urgent care medicine
Vaccination
Visit

Introduction

The health record is a compilation of identifying information about the patient including pertinent facts about his or her current health status and medical history. Provided by the healthcare professionals who participate in the patient's care, the information in the health record is used in planning and managing care, evaluating its appropriateness and medical necessity compliance, substantiating reimbursement claims, and protecting the legal interests of both the patient and his or her healthcare providers. Moreover, the health record is a tool for communication among the patient's providers along the continuum of care. Finally, it is used for education, quality outcomes, research, and public health, as well as medical practice organizational management areas such as performance improvement, risk management, and strategic planning.

A paper-based health record that incorporates well-designed forms makes data collection easy and guarantees that all of the information needed to fulfill documentation requirements is up-to-date. Forms and checklists arranged in a logical sequence enable providers to document care completely without having to prepare separate reports.

Effective forms design also is critical to the successful implementation of electronic health record (EHR) systems. Carefully planned input screens and data-entry fields make the process of loading information from paper records efficient and reliable. The system of organized paper-based health records also can be used as a template for determining EHR access categories and assigning responsibility for updating the various types of information in the electronic health record. During the transition from a paper-based health record to an EHR, a medical practice may have a hybrid health record that is a combination of paper-based and electronic health records. For example, a medical practice may have a paper-based health record, yet have laboratory and pathology records housed electronically.

This chapter identifies the different formats of health records and discusses their advantages and disadvantages. It also describes in detail the elements that make up the basic content of every type of health record. Separate sections discuss the content of urgent care records and health records for specialty care such as surgery, obstetrics and gynecology, pediatrics, chiropractic, and physical therapy. Finally, this chapter explains the practice of obtaining consent forms.

Quality of Documentation

The provider of each service is responsible for thoroughly documenting the care provided. The provider of record or billing provider is responsible for the care performed on a single date of service as submitted on the appropriate claim form.

Along with all entries being legible, there are general documentation guidelines that should be followed by any professional documenting in the medical practice health record (LaTour and Eichenwald Maki 2010; Odom-Welsey et al. 2009). Figure 1.1 illustrates these guidelines.

Figure 1.1. Guidelines for documenting in the medical practice health record

1. Policies should be based upon all applicable standards, including accreditation standards, state and local licensure requirements, federal and state regulations, reimbursement requirements, professional practice standards, along with unique needs for the medical practice.

2. All entries in the health record must be legible and authenticated to identify the author (name and professional status) as well as dated. Such entries should only be documented by authorized professionals as defined in the medical practice's policies and procedures.

3. Format and content of health records should be uniform.

4. No erasures or deletions should be made in the health record.

5. All entries in the paper-based health record should be in ink. Photocopying or scanning should be considered when colored ink or colored forms are used because some colors do not reproduce well.

6. Only approved abbreviations should be documented in the health record. Each medical practice should have an approved abbreviation listing.

7. Entries should be made at the time of service or immediately after the service. An entry should not be documented in advance.

8. Blank spaces should not be left on forms, including consent forms. If blanks are left, they should be marked out with an X so that additional information cannot be inserted.

9. If a correction must be made in the paper-based health record, then one line should be neatly drawn through the error, leaving the incorrect text legible. The error should be initialed and dated so that it is obvious that it is a corrected mistake. Corrections in the EHR should be made according to the medical practice's documentation policy.

10. Medical practice policies should address how the patient or patient's representative may request corrections and amendments to the health record. The amendment should refer back to the information questioned and include date and time. At no time should the documentation in question be removed from the health record or destroyed in any way. The patient cannot require that information in the health record be removed or deleted.

11. Clinicians should indicate that they have reviewed diagnostic reports by signing/initialing and dating each report and in the case of abnormal findings, document a plan of care for the patient that addresses the abnormal findings.

12. The original report should always be maintained in the health record. Cumulative reports, such as laboratory reports, may be replaced with the latest cumulative report. Faxed copies of reports, such as a preoperative history and physical report, may be used as originals in the health record.

13. Chart folder labeling, dotting, or other methods of identifying at a glance a particular type of patient, such as one with a drug or alcohol diagnosis or HIV-positive status, should be discouraged to prevent inadvertent breaches of patient confidentiality.

Health Record Format

For documentation in the medical practice health record to be meaningful, the information must be arranged in a predefined format. This requirement is especially important when multiple providers use the same record. The record can be arranged according to one of three formats: the source-oriented record, the integrated record, or the problem-oriented record. Although these formats are widely used in a paper-based health record, the format of the EHR systems may vary based upon the vendor. Further considerations for EHR models may be found in chapter 5.

The advantages and disadvantages of each of these formats must be weighed against the needs of the providers using the health record. For example, because it was developed to enhance comprehensive patient care, the problem-oriented record system is especially appropriate for medical practices where a team of professionals offers total patient care. Different practitioners then can easily identify existing conditions and current treatments as well as adjust their own treatment strategies accordingly. In an urgent care setting, however, an integrated record system may be more suitable owing to the episodic nature of urgent care. Urgent care patients usually present for treatment of a single acute problem and then return to their primary care physician for follow-up care. Of course, the record formats also can be combined. The only requirement is that the resulting record contains sufficient information to identify the patient and to support the diagnosis and plan of treatment for each episode of care.

Source-oriented Health Records

As the name implies, source-oriented health records are organized into sections according to the source of information. One section contains physician notes, another contains laboratory results, and a third contains radiology results. Large multispecialty medical practices frequently label sections for each specialty department—obstetrics, orthopedics, ophthalmology, and so on—with dividers separating the sections. In turn, each section is arranged in a logical order. For example, laboratory reports may be filed together by type of examination (urinalysis, microbiology, cytology) or by report date.

The source-oriented record format enables users to quickly determine the diagnosis and treatment for a particular organ system. One drawback to this health record format is that all of the documentation within each specialty area must be reviewed to arrive at an accurate assessment of the patient's overall health status. The more specialties within the medical practice, the more sections the source-oriented health record may have for review.

Integrated Health Records

The order in which the episodes of care occurred determines how integrated health records are arranged, with all documentation and diagnostic reports for each episode filed together. This format grouping may be in chronological or reverse chronological order. Although it is easy to assess the diagnosis and treatment for a single episode of care, it is more difficult to compare test results or results of treatment over a longer period of time. All reports generated for a particular episode of care are filed in the record as a unit rather than being incorporated with similar reports.

Problem-oriented Health Records

Introduced in the 1960s by Dr. Lawrence L. Weed, the problem-oriented medical record (POMR) reflects a comprehensive approach to patient care management. The POMR consists of four basic elements: the database, the problem list, the initial plan, and the progress notes.

The *database* consists of the information that typically is collected for every patient encounter, including:

- *Chief complaint:* A statement of the patient's present signs and symptoms

- *Present illness:* A description of the events leading up to the patient's current status

- *Social history:* Nonmedical information that may have an effect on the patient's health, such as family environment; childhood events; education; occupation; social activities; eating, sleeping, and exercise habits; foreign travel; and financial status

- *Medical history:* A summary of childhood and adult illnesses, operations, accidents, hospitalizations, drug sensitivities, and current medications

- *Physical examination:* The provider's review of the patient's body structure and function to determine signs of illness

- *Baseline laboratory data:* Diagnostic tests to assist in establishing an accurate diagnosis

The *problem list* is a permanent, itemized list arranged on a single form or viewing screen to show all of the patient's past and present social, psychological, economic, and medical problems. When providers consistently refer to the unique number assigned to each problem, the problem list serves as an index to the entire record.

Developed and documented for each problem, the *initial plan* may include information on diagnostic workups, therapy, consultations, or patient education.

The *progress notes,* written by healthcare providers, document changes that occur as a result of treatment and any alterations to the initial plan. For example, one practice in streamlined documentation is writing a number beside each problem documented in the progress note. This number must correspond with the number listed on the problem list. This type of documentation links the itemized problem on the problem list to the documented care provided in the progress note.

Basic Health Record Content

Several basic components are required in every medical practice health record. These include:

- The registration record, which documents demographic information about the patient

- The problem list, which summarizes all of the medical and surgical problems that have long-term clinical significance for the patient's care

- The medication list, which lists pertinent information about the medications the patient is taking

- The patient history questionnaire, which asks the patient for information about his or her current and past medical condition

- The medical history report, which documents the provider's findings on the patient's health status

- The physical examination report, which contains the provider's findings upon examination of the patient

- Immunization and injection records, which chronicle the patient's vaccinations

- Progress notes, which provide a chronological summary of the patient's illness and treatment at each encounter

- Orders, which document the physician's instructions to other parties involved in providing the patient's care

- Ancillary testing results, such as laboratory, radiology, pathology, cytology, and audiology studies

- Consultation reports, which describe the findings and recommendations of consultants

In addition, the following items are recommended:

- Patient instructions, which document the instructions the provider gave to the patient regarding follow-up care

- The failed appointment form, which documents patient noncompliance with recommendations for follow-up appointments with the provider

- Flow sheets, which can be used to document treatment between patient visits

- Telephone contact records, which document telephone communications between the patient and his or her healthcare providers

Registration Record

The registration record documents the basic demographic data collected before or during the initial patient visit. This information is maintained and updated, as needed, on subsequent visits. Because it defines the data elements that medical practices are required to collect for billing and reporting purposes, the Uniform Ambulatory Care Data Set (UACDS) usually is used as baseline data.

Individual facilities must determine what additional data they need to perform various internal activities such as research, utilization management, Physician Quality Reporting Initiative reporting, planning, and marketing. For example, an analysis of basic demographic data might provide answers to questions about the need to hire additional staff or to open medical practices in different locations. The goals and objectives of a medical practice also play a role in determining what data should be collected. For example, practices featuring family-centered care may collect basic demographic data on all of the patient's family members.

In general, the following data elements are collected and maintained for every patient:

- Surname, first name, and middle name or initial

- Unique identifying number

- Residence address

- Telephone numbers for home, work, and cellular phones

- Date of birth

- Gender

- Marital status

- Race or ethnic origin

- Medicare, Medicaid, or insurance group number

- Insurance company, address, and name of subscriber

- Guarantor, if applicable

- Name of insured

- Patient relationship to insured

- Employer

- Occupation

- Business address and telephone number

- Name, relation, address, and telephone number of emergency contact

- Any other emergency contact

- Primary care physician

- Referring physician/address, if applicable

In many medical practices, registration (demographic) information is maintained on the practice management or billing software. It is a best practice to offer the medical practice's registration form online. Patients may complete this form online and submit it electronically. In some medical practices, the registration form is offered electronically in the EHR or on the medical practice's Web site, but must be printed, completed, then brought to the medical practice at the time of the patient's appointment. For paper-based or hybrid health records, a copy may be printed and placed in the patient's record. This copy may contain only limited data elements. A new registration record may be printed and placed in the patient's record whenever the registration information changes. It is a common practice to review registration form information at each visit—especially the payer data, which affects reimbursement.

For marketing purposes, some medical practices also collect from the patient how he or she heard about the medical practice, such as Internet, telephone book, hospital help-line, family, friend, neighbor, and so forth.

For greater efficiency, an identifying number unique to each patient should be assigned. Additional information on unique identifiers may be found in chapter 4. (Examples of registration forms are provided in the Sample Forms folder on the CD-ROM accompanying this book.)

Problem List

According to the Joint Commission's *Comprehensive Accreditation Manual for Ambulatory Health Care (CAMAC),* section RC.02.01.01, the clinical record should contain the patient's initial diagnosis, diagnostic impression(s), or condition(s), as well as any diagnoses or conditions established during the patient's course of care, treatment, or services (Joint Commission 2009). This list is sometimes referred to as a summary list and may additionally include medications, allergies, and procedures, along with updates to each of the listings.

The problem list or summary list is a valuable tool in patient care management and should always be visible and easy to read. A single page summarizes all of the major medical and surgical problems that have long-term clinical significance for the patient, including social and psychiatric problems. The dates of onset and resolution are recorded for each problem. The healthcare provider can use the problem list to determine at a glance which problems are active or resolved and can adjust treatment plans accordingly.

As a communication tool, the problem list helps specialty physicians make evaluation and treatment decisions about the patients referred to them for care; having this information often eliminates the need to duplicate costly tests. Each provider documents his or her care of the patient on the same list, thereby creating a comprehensive overview of the patient's medical status. For consistency and clarity, medical practices should develop guidelines for recording several key elements in the problem list, including problems, dates of onset, active versus inactive status, and resolution dates.

Significant problems include both chronic and acute conditions that affect patient management. For example, both hypercholesterolemia and status postcholecystectomy would be included on the problem list. Although the cholecystectomy occurred in the past, knowledge of this major surgical event could prove valuable in future clinical evaluations. Abnormal signs and symptoms that have the potential to become significant problems also are recorded, but short-term illnesses that were resolved quickly and "ruled-out" conditions are not. Including ruled-out conditions would defeat the list's purpose, which is to provide a quick reference to the patient's confirmed conditions and his or her management status.

The problem list also records social situations that may have a significant impact on clinical management (for example, the fact that the patient lives alone or has a history of child abuse), risk factors (smoking, alcohol and drug usage, and personal and family history of conditions such as cancer, diabetes, or heart disease), and allergies. Every provider involved in a patient's care should have information on these factors. The National Committee for Quality Assurance (NCQA) requires notation on the use of cigarettes, alcohol, and substances for all patients over 14 years of age. Frequently, this information is included on the problem list (NCQA 2009).

Moreover, the date of onset for each problem should be documented. Guidelines should specify which date should be used; that is, the date the patient reported first noting the condition or the date the provider confirmed the condition. Consistency in documentation is important for interpretation and use in evaluation.

Each problem should be labeled as active or inactive so that providers can determine treatment priorities quickly and develop a treatment plan. Resolved or inactive problems may still be relevant to management of the patient. When its cause is confirmed, the symptom is not erased but, rather, is linked to the new diagnosis. The resolution date is important as an indicator of problems that have been resolved and as a means for monitoring recurrences. (Examples of a paper-based problem list and an EHR integrated problem list are included in the Sample Forms folder on the CD-ROM accompanying this book.)

Medication List

The medication history is a delineation of the drugs used by an individual (both past and present), including prescribed and unprescribed drugs and alcohol, along with any unusual reactions to those drugs (Joint Commission 2009). In section RC.02.01.07 of the Joint Commission's *Accreditation Requirements*, it states that the clinical record contains a summary list for each patient who receives continuing ambulatory services. Figure 1.2 illustrates these requirements, which include medications.

Key data elements include:

- Names of medications
- Dosages and amounts dispensed
- Dispensing instructions (with signature)
- Prescription dates and discontinued dates

Organizations may decide to omit medications prescribed for a single, short-term course of therapy, such as an antibiotic prescribed for an infection. In pediatric patients, however,

Figure 1.2.   The Joint Commission RC.02.01.07: The organization maintains complete and accurate clinical records

1	A summary list is initiated for the patient by his or her third visit.
2	The patient's summary list contains the following information: • Any significant medical diagnoses and conditions • Any significant operative and invasive procedures • Any adverse or allergic drug reactions • Any current medications, over-the-counter medications, and herbal preparations
3	The patient's summary list is updated whenever there is a change in diagnoses, medications, or allergies to medications, and whenever a procedure is performed.
4	The summary list is readily available to practitioners who need access to the information of patients who receive continuing ambulatory care services in order to provide care, treatment, or services.

Source: Joint Commission 2009.

even short-term medications should be included. Many pediatric illnesses (for example, otitis media) are recurrent in nature, and so the physician needs a record that shows which medications were effective in past episodes of the illness.

Dates of medication refills often are charted on the medication list as well. The medication list is an acceptable location for documentation of patient allergies. However, this information should be documented in only one specific location of the paper-based health record to ensure its completeness and consistency. In the EHR, the patient allergies may be entered once, but appear in multiple screens. The patient's current medications and allergies should be verified during each patient visit and the health record updated appropriately.

When consistent, accurate, and properly updated, the medication list serves multiple purposes. The medication list (whether electronic or hard-copy format) alerts the provider to drug sensitivities and allergies. The medication list is often utilized in conjunction with other portions of the health record, such as the problem list, to coordinate care and justify the clinical necessity of medications. For those cases in which patients are taking several medications or seeing several providers, the medication list helps providers evaluate and adjust the drug regimen appropriately by taking into account potential incompatibilities or interactions. (An example of a medication list is provided in the Sample Forms folder on the CD-ROM accompanying this book.)

With the acceleration of e-prescribing, medical errors have been reduced and proper medication information is recorded in the EHR (IOM 2007).

As patients are more involved with their healthcare and their own prevention of medication errors, many have personal health records (PHRs) in electronic or paper-based format. More detailed information on PHRs may be found in chapter 10. However, medications are one of the health information facts commonly recorded by patients. The Massachusetts Coalition for the Prevention of Medical Errors publishes online a sample medication list that may be maintained by patients. This form may be found at http://www.macoalition.org/Initiatives/docs/AmbulatoryTestTrackingLog.doc.

Patient History Questionnaire

The patient history questionnaire is structured to prompt the patient to provide certain items of information, including the presence or absence of significant conditions that may represent potential medical problems. The responses to specific questions not only provide information but also serve as starting points for the provider who must gather additional historical data.

The patient should be asked to complete a new history questionnaire periodically. Placing an updated patient questionnaire in the health record makes it possible to keep a complete, current history in one place and frees providers from reading through multiple progress notes in the paper-based health record or multiple screens in the EHR. (Examples of patient history questionnaires in the form of an adult health questionnaire, pediatric family history, neurology medical review of systems, and initial visit for cardiology are provided in the Sample Forms folder on the CD-ROM accompanying this book.)

Medical History

A comprehensive medical history should be obtained periodically from the patient or his or her representative. Frequency depends on the patient's age and health status. Often the initial medical history is obtained by questioning patients in detail about their health history. Specialists may utilize short history forms to supplement and expand the information provided on the patient's general health history questionnaire. Updates to the history often are included in the progress note made during the patient visit.

A complete medical history establishes the foundation for comprehensive care by documenting current complaints and symptoms in addition to past medical, personal, and family history. It should include pertinent aspects of basic physiological systems as well. The medical histories obtained by specialists such as gynecologists, cardiologists, and gastroenterologists are comprehensive for the particular organ system involved.

Health Information Management (LaTour and Eichenwald Maki 2010) suggests that the information shown in figure 1.3 be included in a complete medical history (the second element—present illness—may not be included in a primary care health record when the patient presents for preventive care or health maintenance).

Physical Examination Report

The health history is a record of subjective statements made by the patient; the physical examination is a record of the provider's assessment of the patient's current health status. Information on vital signs and all of the major organ systems should be documented in the physical examination report and should include the information as detailed in figure 1.4 (AMA 1999). (An example of a vital signs flow sheet and samples of preparticipation (sports) physical examination forms may be found in the Sample Forms folder on the CD-ROM accompanying this book.)

Immunization and Injection Records

The health records of patients who receive immunizations or injections of medication should include the date(s) of administration; information on the manufacturer and lot number, drug, dosage, and route of administration; and the signature of the person administering the vaccine. Often a consent form for the vaccination is incorporated into the same record. (An example of an immunization record used for patients receiving a series of injections is provided in the Sample Forms folder on the CD-ROM accompanying this book.)

Progress Notes

Progress notes provide a chronological summary of the patient's status and treatment at each encounter. They can be either source oriented, with each specialty recording its notes on a separate form, or integrated, with each specialty using the same form.

When the initials of the provider are used, the medical practice must maintain a key listing of initials and a corresponding full signature.

In addition, the NCQA requires a notation, where indicated, regarding follow-up care, telephone calls, or visits. The specific time of return is to be noted in weeks or months, or as needed.

Figure 1.3.   Information usually included in a complete medical history

Components of the History	Complaints and Symptoms
Chief complaint	Nature and duration of the symptoms that caused the patient to seek medical attention as stated in his or her own words
Present illness	Detailed chronological description of the development of the patient's illness, from the appearance of the first symptom to the present situation
Past medical history	Summary of childhood and adult illnesses and conditions, such as infectious diseases, pregnancies, allergies and drug sensitivities, accidents, operations, hospitalizations, and current medications
Social and personal history	Marital status; dietary, sleep, and exercise patterns; use of coffee, tobacco, alcohol, and other drugs; occupation; home environment; daily routine; and so on
Family medical history	Diseases among relatives in which heredity or contact might play a role, such as allergies, cancer, and infectious, psychiatric, metabolic, endocrine, cardiovascular, and renal diseases; health status or cause and age at death for immediate relatives
Review of systems	Systemic inventory designed to uncover current or past subjective symptoms that includes the following types of data: • *General*: Usual weight, recent weight changes, fever, weakness, fatigue • *Skin*: Rashes, eruptions, dryness, cyanosis, jaundice; changes in skin, hair, or nails • *Head*: Headache (duration, severity, character, location) • *Eyes*: Glasses or contact lenses, last eye examination, glaucoma, cataracts, eyestrain, pain, diplopia, redness, lacrimation, inflammation, blurring • *Ears*: Hearing, discharge, tinnitus, dizziness, pain • *Noise*: Head colds, epistaxis, discharges, obstruction, postnasal drip, sinus pain • *Mouth and throat*: Condition of teeth and gums, last dental examination, soreness, redness, hoarseness, difficulty in swallowing • *Respiratory system*: Chest pain, wheezing, cough, dyspnea, sputum (color and quantity), hemoptysis, asthma, bronchitis, emphysema, pneumonia, tuberculosis, pleurisy, last chest x-ray • *Neurological system*: Fainting, blackouts, seizures, paralysis, tingling, tremors, memory loss • *Musculoskeletal system*: Joint pain or stiffness, arthritis, gout, backache, muscle pain, cramps, swelling, redness, limitation in motor activity • *Cardiovascular system*: Chest pain, rheumatic fever, tachycardia, palpitation, high blood pressure, edema, vertigo, faintness, varicose veins, thrombophlebitis • *Gastrointestinal system*: Appetite, thirst, nausea, vomiting, hematemesis, rectal bleeding, change in bowel habits, diarrhea, constipation, indigestion, food intolerance, flatus, hemorrhoids, jaundice • *Urinary system*: Frequent or painful urination, nocturia, pyuria, hematuria, incontinence, urinary infections • *Genitoreproductive system*: Male—venereal disease, sores, discharge from penis, hernias, testicular pain, or masses; female—age at menarche, frequency and duration of menstruation, dysmenorrhea, menorrhagia, symptoms of menopause, contraception, pregnancies, deliveries, abortions, last Pap smear • *Endocrine system*: Thyroid disease; heat or cold intolerance; excessive sweating, thirst, hunger, or urination • *Hematologic system*: Anemia, easy bruising or bleeding, past transfusions • *Psychiatric disorders*: Insomnia, headache, nightmares, personality disorders, anxiety disorders, mood disorders

Source: LaTour and Eichenwald Maki 2010, 196.

Figure 1.4. Components included in a multisystem physical examination

Constitutional—Vital Signs and Measurements
Measurement of **any three of the following ten** vital signs (may be measured and recorded by ancillary staff): 1) sitting blood pressure, 2) standing blood pressure, 3) supine blood pressure, 4) heart rate and regularity, 5) respiratory rate, 6) temperature, 7) weight, 8) height, 9) head circumference, 10) body mass index
General appearance (includes development, nutrition, growth, color, body habitus, deformities, attention to grooming, Cushingoid features, acromegalic features)
Assessment of ability to communicate

Head, Face, and Neck	
Examination Item	**Examples**
Inspection of head and/or face	Overall appearance, scars, lesions, masses
Examination of neck	Overall appearance, scars, masses, torticollis, webbing, symmetry Inspect/palpate for tracheal deviation
Palpation and/or percussion of face	Presence or absence of sinus tenderness
Examination of salivary glands	Masses, tenderness
Examination of thyroid	Goiter, nodule, tenderness
Examination of fontanels	Presence or absence of fullness
Examination of cranial bones and sutures	Swelling, open/closed sutures
Examination of jugular veins	Distention
Examination of carotid arteries	Presence or absence of bruit
Examination of cervical lymphatics	Enlargement of nodes in the anterior/posterior triangle, submental, supraclavicular

Eyes	
Examination Item	**Examples**
Inspection of conjunctivae, globe, and/or lids	Erythema, sty, chalazion, ectropion, ptosis, xanthelsama, proptosis
Inspection of sclera	
Measurement for exophthalmus	Measure forward protrusion
Test visual acuity (not including determination of refractive error)	Snellen chart
Gross visual field testing including primary gaze and alignment	Nystagmus, strabismus
Examination of lacrimal glands, lacrimal drainage, and/or orbits	Swelling
Examination of pupils	Reaction to light, myosis, mydriasas, anisocoria, equality
Examination of iris/irides	Reaction to light, accommodation, size, and symmetry
Measurement of intraocular pressure	
Ophthalmoscopic examination of optic discs and posterior segment through undilated pupils	Retinal hemorrhages, exudates, cotton-wool patches, pigmentation C/D ratio, size, atrophy, tumor, elevations
Ophthalmoscopic examination of optic discs and posterior segment through dilated pupils	Retinal hemorrhages, exudates, cotton-wool patches, pigmentation C/D ratio, size, atrophy, tumor, elevations
Slit lamp examination of the cornea(s) including epithelium, stroma, endothelium, and tear film	Bowman's membrane, Decemet's membrane
Slit lamp examination of the lenses including clarity, anterior and posterior capsule, cortex, and nucleus	
Slit lamp examination of the anterior chambers including depth, cells, and flare	

Figure 1.4. Components included in a multisystem physical examination *(continued)*

Ear, Nose, Mouth, and Throat	
Examination Item	**Examples**
Examination of external ears (auricles)	Overall appearance, scars, lesions, masses
Otoscopic examination of external auditory canal and/or tympanic membranes	Otitis externa, otitis media
Pneumo-otoscopy	Mobility of tympanic membranes
Assessment of hearing and/or clinical speech reception thresholds	Whispered voice, finger rub, tuning fork, acoustic blink reflex
Examination of external nose, nasal mucosa, septum and/or turbinate(s)	Swelling, redness, pallor, polyps, deviation, perforation
Examination of teeth and/or gums	Dental caries, tooth loss, gingivitis, periodontal disease
Examination of lips and/or oral mucosa	Cyanosis, pallor
Examination of oropharynx (hard and soft palates, tongue, tonsils, and/or posterior pharynx)	Lesions, torii, glossitis, symmetry, pharyngitis
Examination by mirror of larynx, including epiglottis, pharyngeal walls and/or pyriform sinuses, false vocal cords, true vocal cords, and/or mobility of larynx	
Examination by mirror, of nasopharynx (including appearance of the mucosa, adenoids, posterior choanae and eustachian tubes)	
Assessment of suck reflex in infants	

Respiratory	
Examination Item	**Examples**
Inspection of chest	Shape, symmetry, expansion, intercostal retractions, use of accessory muscles, diaphragmatic movement Assessment of respiratory effort
Percussion of chest	Dullness, flatness, hyperresonance
Palpation of chest	Tenderness, masses, tactile fremitus
Ausculation of lungs	Breath sounds, adventitious sounds, rubs, rales, rhonchi

Cardiovascular	
Examination Item	**Examples**
Palpation of heart	Location, size, forcefulness of the point of maximal impact, thrills, lifts, palpable S3 or S4
Ausculation of heart	Abnormal sounds, murmurs
Examination of carotid arteries	Waveform, pulse amplitude, bruits, apical-carotid delay
Examination of abdominal aorta	Size, bruits
Auscultation of renal arteries	Pulse amplitude, bruits
Examination of femoral arteries	Pulse amplitude, bruits
Examination of popliteal arteries	
Examination of pedal pulses	
Examination of peripheral venous system by observation and/or palpation	Swelling, varicosities, suitability of lower extremity veins for use as conduit
Examination of jugular veins	Distention (JVD), A, V or cannon A waves
Examination of peripheral hemodialysis, A-V fistula	Patency, status of insertion site
Measurement of ankle—brachial index	

(continued on next page)

Figure 1.4.   Components included in a multisystem physical examination *(continued)*

Breasts (Chest)	
Examination Item	**Examples**
Inspection of breasts (chest)	Contour, symmetry, nipple discharge, inversion, retraction, Tanner stage, males—gynecomastia
Palpation of breasts	Masses or lumps, tenderness

Lymphatic	
Examination Item	**Examples**
Palpate lymph nodes in neck	Lymphadenopathy Submental, cervical (anterior/posterior), supraclavicular
Palpate lymph nodes in axillae	Lymphadenopathy
Palpate lymph nodes in groin	Lymphadenopathy
Palpate lymph nodes of each additional lymph node area	Lymphadenopathy epitrochlear, popliteal

Gastrointestinal (Abdomen)	
Examination Item	**Examples**
Inspection of abdomen	Obesity, distention, scars
Palpation of abdomen	Masses, guarding, tenderness, presence or absences of ascites
Percussion of abdomen	
Palpation of liver and/or spleen	Hepatomegaly, size, tenderness, edge Splenomegaly
Palpation of kidney	Enlargement
Examination for hernia(s)	
Digital anorectal examination	Hemorrhoids, rectal masses, sphincter tone (including obtaining stool sample for occult blood)
Inspection of anus and perineum	Condyloma, skin tags
Auscultate abdomen	Bowel sounds

Genitourinary (Female)	
Examination Item	**Examples**
Examination (with or without specimen collection for smears and cultures) of external genitalia	General appearance, estrogen effect, discharge, lesion(s)
Examination (with or without specimen collection for smears and cultures) of urethra and/or urethral meatus	Size, location, lesions, discharge, prolapse (masses, tenderness, scarring)
Examination of bladder	Fullness, masses, tenderness
Examination (with or without specimen collection for smears and cultures) of vagina	General appearance, estrogen effect, discharge, lesion(s)
Examination (with or without specimen collection for smears and cultures) of cervix	General appearance, lesion(s), discharge
Examination of uterus	Size, contour, position, mobility, tenderness, consistency, descent or support
Examination of adnexa/parametria	Masses, tenderness, organomegaly, nodularity
Examination of pelvic support assessment	Cystocele, rectocele, enterocele

Genitourinary (Male)	
Examination Item	**Examples**
Examination (with or without specimen collection for smears and cultures) of penis	Lesion(s), presence or absence of foreskin, plaque, masses, deformity(s), discharge
Examination (with or without specimen collection for smears and cultures) of scrotum	Lesion(s), cyst(s), rashes, hydrocele

Figure 1.4.   Components included in a multisystem physical examination *(continued)*

Genitourinary (Male) *(continued)*	
Examination Item	**Examples**
Examination of epididymides	Size, symmetry, masses
Examination of testes	Size, symmetry, masses, varicocele
Examination (with or without specimen collection for smears and cultures) of urethra and/or urethral meatus	Size, location, lesions, hypospadias, masses, tenderness, scarring
Digital rectal examination of prostate	Hyperplasia, enlargement, tenderness
Examination of bladder	Fullness, masses, tenderness

Integumentary	
Examination Item	**Examples**
Examination of hair of scalp, eyebrows, face, chest, pubic area (when indicated) and extremities	Hair quantity, texture, scalp, lesion(s), lump(s)
Examination of skin and subcutaneous tissues of the head and face	Color, texture, lesion(s), mole(s), birthmark(s), hair distribution Hyperhidrosis, chromhidroses, bromhidrosis
Examination of skin and subcutaneous tissues of chest, including breast axillae	Color, texture, lesion(s), mole(s), birthmark(s), hair distribution Hyperhidrosis, chromhidroses, bromhidrosis
Examination of skin and subcutaneous tissues of abdomen	Color, texture, lesion(s), mole(s), birthmark(s), hair distribution Hyperhidrosis, chromhidroses, bromhidrosis
Examination of skin and subcutaneous tissues of genitalia, groin, buttocks	Color, texture, lesion(s), mole(s), birthmark(s), hair distribution Hyperhidrosis, chromhidroses, bromhidrosis
Examination of skin and subcutaneous tissues of back	Color, texture, lesion(s), mole(s), birthmark(s), hair distribution Hyperhidrosis, chromhidroses, bromhidrosis
Examination of skin and subcutaneous tissues of right upper extremity	Color, texture, lesion(s), mole(s), birthmark(s), hair distribution Hyperhidrosis, chromhidroses, bromhidrosis
Examination of skin and subcutaneous tissues of left upper extremity	Color, texture, lesion(s), mole(s), birthmark(s), hair distribution Hyperhidrosis, chromhidroses, bromhidrosis
Examination of skin and subcutaneous tissues of right lower extremity	Color, texture, lesion(s), mole(s), birthmark(s), hair distribution Hyperhidrosis, chromhidroses, bromhidrosis
Examination of skin and subcutaneous tissues of left lower extremity	Color, texture, lesion(s), mole(s), birthmark(s), hair distribution Hyperhidrosis, chromhidroses, bromhidrosis
Inspection and palpation of fingernails and/or toenails	Dystrophies, mycosis, subungual tumor, infection, hematoma, psorriasis, abnormal curvature, separation or splitting

Musculoskeletal (Lower Extremity) (Hip, Pelvis, Knee, Ankle, Foot)	
Examination Item	**Examples**
Examination of hip and/or pelvis	Scars, deformity, immobility Range of motion (internal, external rotation, adduction, abduction, for example, Patrick's maneuver, muscle spasm) Swelling, tenderness, decreased motion in hip joint
Examination of leg	Overall appearance, masses, gross deformity, scars, trophic changes, atrophy Absence or presence of weakness in muscles, coordination, gait and station Range of motion (internal, external rotation, supination, pronation at joints) Assessment of muscle strength and tone Absence or presence of tenderness, swelling, misalignment, crepitation, inflammation, effusion Absence or presence (decreased), pulses (femoral, popliteal, dorsalis pedis, posterior tibial) Assessment of temperature

(continued on next page)

15

Figure 1.4. Components included in a multisystem physical examination *(continued)*

Musculoskeletal (Lower Extremity) (Hip, Pelvis, Knee, Ankle, Foot) *(continued)*	
Examination Item	**Examples**
Examination of knee	Swelling, scars, decreased motion, inflammation, effusion, deformity (varus or valgus) Range of motion, flexion, extension Absence or presence of instability (ligamentous, tendinous, cartilaginous) Tenderness, pain (patellofemoral joint, suprapatellar, prepatellar bursa)
Examination of ankle	Swelling, scars, growth(s) (corns, callouses), deformity (hallux valgus), masses Absence or presence of instability (ligamentous, tendinous) Range of motion, dorsiflexion, plantar flexion, inversion, eversion Tenderness over fibular/tibial, tarsal, metatarsal joints Absence or presence pain (ligamentous, tendinous, fibular/tibial, tarsal, metatarsal joints
Examination of foot	Assessment of tendons Range of motion of joints of the foot (for example, meta-tarsophalangeal, proximal phalangeal, interphalangeal, distal phalangeal joints, toes) Absence or presence of cyanosis, swelling, deformity (hammertoe, bunion), masses, inflammation Absence of presence of tenderness over (any) calcaneous, tarsal, metatarsal, metarsophalangeal, proximal phalangeal, interphalangeal, distal phalangeal joints of the foot, toes

Musculoskeletal (Spine) (Cervical, Thoracic, Lumbar, Sacrum)	
Examination Item	**Examples**
Examination of cervical spine	Overall appearance, alignment, gross deformity (kyphosis, lordosis, scoliosis), immobility, torticollis Range of motion (rotation, lateral bending, flexion, extension), muscle spasm, trigger point(s) Swelling, masses, tenderness, decreased motion (for example, arthritis), decreased sensation, triggering, spasm
Examination of thoracic spine	Overall appearance, list, masses, stature, gait, gross deformity (kyphosis, lordosis, scoliosis), immobility Absence or presence of weakness in spinal/peripherally innervated muscles Range of motion (rotation, lateral bending, flexion, extension), muscle spam, trigger point(s) Swelling, masses, tenderness, decreased motion (for example, arthritis), decreased sensation, triggering, spasm Assessment of spinous processes, paravertebral muscles
Examination of lumbar spine	Overall appearance, list, alignment, gait, gross deformity (kyphosis, lordosis, scoliosis), immobility Assessment of spinous processes, paravertebral muscles Range of motion (rotation, forward and lateral bending, side-to-side bending, flexion, extension) Straight-leg testing Swelling, masses, tenderness, decreased motion (for example, arthritis), decreased sensation, triggering, spasm

Figure 1.4. **Components included in a multisystem physical examination** *(continued)*

Musculoskeletal (Upper Extremity) (Neck, Shoulder, Elbow, Wrist, Hand)	
Examination Item	**Examples**
Examination of arm	Overall appearance, gross deformity, scars, trophic changes, atrophy Absence or presence in radially innervated muscles Absence or presence of tenderness over radial nerve (radial tunnel or arcade of Frohse) Tinel's sign over median nerve, antecubital fossa or forearm
Examination of shoulder	Symmetry, atrophy of trapezius, supraspinatous or infraspinatous, symmetry of deltoid muscle bulk Active and passive abduction, adduction and extension Shoulder instability (anterior, posterior, or inferior) Assessment of strength (forward flexion, abduction, or extension) Absence or presence of distal paresthesias (Adson's or Wright's maneuver, Roos test) Absence or presence of tenderness of the levator, scapula, or acromioclavicular joint, brachial plexus, subacromial region (anteriorly, posteriorly and laterally), and proximal biceps
Examination of elbow	Swelling, decreased motion Range of motion, flexion, extension, supination, pronation Absence or presence of instability (medial/lateral) epicondylitis Tenderness (radiocapitellar joint, olecranon bursa)
Examination of wrist	Swelling, deformity, masses Absence or presence of instability pisotriquetral, carpi ulnaris, hook of the hamate, midcarpal, or capitolunate Range of motion right and left dorsiflexion, palmar flexion, radial deviation, ulnar deviation, pronation, supination Tenderness in snuffbox or radioscaphoid, scapholunate, or radiolunate joints, ulnocarpal or distal radioulnar joints, hook of the hamate, extensor tendons Absence or presence of pain at lunatotriquetral or midcarpal region
Examination of hand	Absence or presence of cyanosis, swelling, deformity, masses, inflammation Assessment of tendons (flexor digitorum superficialis and profundus to all fingers, flexor pollicis lungus, extensors of thumb and fingers Absence or presence of instability of the thumb or index, long, ring, or small finger Range of motion of joints of the thumb and fingers (abduction, adduction, metacarpophalangeal, proximal interphalangeal, distal interphalangeal) Allen test (radial/ulnar arteries), capillary refill (fingers and thumbs) Absence or presence of tenderness over (any) of joints of thumb or index, long, ring, or small fingers Absence or presence of triggering

(continued on next page)

Figure 1.4. **Components included in a multisystem physical examination** *(continued)*

Neurologic	
Examination Item	**Examples**
Evaluation of higher integrative function (including level of consciousness)	Orientation of time, place, recent and remote memory, attention span and concentration, language, fund of knowledge
Test cerebellar function	Finger/nose, heel/knee/shin, rapid alternating movements, evaluation of fine motor coordination in children, nystagmus
Test 1st cranial nerve	
Test 2nd cranial nerve (count either as neurologic or eye, not both)	Visual acuity, fields, fundi
Test 3rd, 4th, and 6th cranial nerves (count either as neurologic or eye, not both)	
Test 5th cranial nerve	Facial sensation, corneal reflex
Test 7th cranial nerve	Facial symmetry, strength
Test 8th cranial nerve (count as ear or neurologic, not both)	Hearing with tuning fork, whispered voice
Test 9th cranial nerve	Gag reflex, reflex palatal movement
Test 10th cranial nerve	Voluntary movement of soft palate or vocal cord function
Test 11th cranial nerve	Shoulder shrug strength
Test 12th cranial nerve	Tongue protrusion
Evaluation for motor function	Strength, muscle tone, atrophy, fasciculations
Examination of sensation	Touch, pin, vibration, proprioception
Examination of deep tendon reflexes	
Evaluation for abnormal and/or superficial reflexes	Babinski, abdominal
Evaluation of peripheral nerves	Tinel's sign, Phalen sign
Provocative testing	Adson maneuver, Lasegue maneuver
Evaluation of autonomic nervous system	Bowel, bladder control
Evaluation of gait	

Psychiatric	
Examination Item	**Examples**
Description of speech	Rate, volume, articulation, coherence and spontaneity
Language assessment (count as neurologic or psychiatric, not both)	Naming objects, repeating phrases
Assessment of thought process	Rate of thoughts, content of thoughts (logical tangential, computation)
Assessment of abstract reasoning	
Assessment of association	Loose, tangential, circumstantial, intact
Assessment of abnormal or psychotic thoughts	Hallucinations, delusions, preoccupations with violence, homicidal or suicidal ideation, obsessions
Assessment of mood and affect (count as neurologic or psychiatric, not both)	Depression, anxiety, agitation hypomania, lability
Assessment of orientation	Time, place, person
Assessment of memory (count as neurologic or psychiatric, not both)	Recent/remote
Assessment of concentration	
Assessment of attention span	Span
Assessment of fund of knowledge (count as neurologic or psychiatric, not both)	Awareness of current events, past history, vocabulary

To prove useful to other reviewers of the health record, progress notes may be structured or narrative, but must remain legible and uniform.

The best example of a structured progress note lies in the SOAP format, commonly used with the problem-oriented health record format. In this format, the note itself is divided into four parts, each identified as:

- *Subjective:* Patient's complaints and comments

- *Objective:* Physical findings and laboratory data

- *Assessment:* Diagnosis and impression

- *Plan:* Medication, therapy, referral, consultation, and patient education

Every note need not contain documentation for every part. Under *subjective* information, the patient's statement of the reason for the visit is commonly recorded in quotes. Refrain from the common "no complaint" statement, and instead use more descriptive findings such as "patient feels better, pain is reduced from 6 to a 4." If the patient has had any treatment, this is the area the patient's response to treatment may be documented. *Objective* data consist of medical facts established during physical examinations and diagnostic workups. Avoid statements such as "no change." Rather, documentation should state the patient's current status. The documentation must be understood not only at the time of the current visit, but also a year from the visit. *Assessment* is the documentation of a diagnosis or status of an identified problem. Under *plan,* the provider records the steps that will be taken to manage the condition. This plan should correspond to the subjective, objective, and assessment documented for a given visit.

The SOAP format helps the provider to structure his or her decision-making process and produces notes that are complete and coherent. Each note contains a number that matches its corresponding number on the problem list. Using the problem numbers makes it easier to assess the progress on a particular problem. Moreover, because each note is uniform and concise, individual providers can review previous patient complaints, diagnoses, and treatments at a glance; and consultants or specialists can provide continuity of care without duplicating costly tests. Such complete information makes it easy to compare the actual care provided against acceptable standards, which helps third parties such as attorneys and insurers to determine accurate reimbursement or to build stronger legal defenses for the patient and/or the provider. (An example of a progress note from Greenway's electronic health record system may be found in the Sample Forms folder on the CD-ROM accompanying this book.)

Orders

Orders are the instructions the provider of service gives to other parties to complete specific medications, services, diagnostic tests, or treatments to a particular patient. Given the nature of care in the medical practice, patients may need to visit another site for the orders to be carried out; for example, they must go to the pharmacy to have a prescription filled or the laboratory to have blood drawn for testing. Orders for medication are written on prescription forms and presented to the pharmacy or provided electronically through e-Prescribing software. Orders for diagnostic tests are written on requisition or referral forms that the patient may or may not receive, yet are forwarded electronically or via fax directly to the performing laboratory. To comply with accreditation standards requiring that information on all studies, tests, and treatments be entered into the patient's health record at each visit, these orders at times are documented in the progress note. The orders must be written legibly and accompanied with the date and the provider's signature.

Standing orders are those which an individual provider has established as routine care for a specific diagnosis or procedure. Usually, standing orders are preprinted on a single sheet of paper and, like other orders, must be signed, dated, and filed in the individual patient's health record. (An example of an orders template is provided in the Sample Forms folder on the CD-ROM accompanying this book.)

Ancillary Testing Results, Such as Laboratory, Radiology, Pathology, Cytology, and Audiology Studies

Ancillary testing in the medical practice requires an order for the medically necessary tests. There is a variety of ancillary tests that may be performed in the medical practice setting.

Laboratory and cytology testing may be completed in the medical practice or at a laboratory facility. Some medical practices are certified to perform specific tests onsite through the Clinical Laboratory Improvement Amendments (CLIA), which regulate the quality of laboratory testing. Each state is regulated by a different organization for CLIA certification. The agency list may be found in appendix B and at http://www.cms.hhs.gov/CLIA/downloads/CLIA.SA.pdf. Routine laboratory test results contain the following information and may be available in paper or electronic format:

- Patient identification, including name and unique identifier

- Name of laboratory test performed

- Date that the laboratory test was drawn and performed

- Signature of the professional performing the laboratory test, such as laboratory technologist or registered nurse

- Name of the laboratory completing the test

- Results of the laboratory test

Radiology test results are documented for scans and x-rays taken of different parts of the body. Some of these tests are performed at the medical practice, whereas other tests may be performed at an outpatient imaging facility, such as CT and MRI scans. The American College of Radiology (ACR) published documentation guidelines for diagnostic imaging findings, which can be found in figure 1.5.

The ACR also published practice guidelines and technical standards for many of the imaging tests performed in this specialty. The detailed list of these standards, which includes documentation requirements for each test, may be found at http://www.acr.org/Secondary MainMenuCategories/quality_safety/guidelines/toc.aspx.

Consultation Reports, Which Describe the Findings and Recommendations of Consultants

Consultation reports are documented for medically necessary services provided to a patient that were ordered by a physician or other qualified healthcare professional. A consultation is offered when another provider is seeking an opinion or advice for the care of the patient. The requesting provider must document the request for the consultation in the patient's health

Figure 1.5.   Components of the diagnostic imaging report

1. Demographics

   a. The facility or location where the study was performed.

   b. Name of patient and another identifier.

   c. Name(s) of referring physician(s) or other healthcare provider(s). If the patient is self referred, that should be stated.

   d. Name or type of examination.

   e. Date of the examination.

   f. Time of the examination, if relevant (for example, for patients who are likely to have more than one of a given examination per day).

   g. Inclusion of the following additional items is encouraged:

      i. Date of dictation

      ii. Date and time of transcription

      iii. Birth date or age

      iv. Gender

2. Relevant clinical information and ICD-9 code as available

3. Body of the report

   a. Procedures and materials

      The report should include a description of the studies and/or procedures performed and any contrast media (including concentration, volume, and route of administration when applicable), medications, catheters, or devices used, if not recorded elsewhere. Any known significant patient reaction or complication should be recorded.

   b. Findings

      The report should use appropriate anatomic, pathologic, and radiologic terminology to describe the findings.

   c. Potential limitations

      The report should, when appropriate, identify factors that may compromise the sensitivity and specificity of the examination.

   d. Clinical issues

      The report should address or answer any specific clinical questions. If there are factors that prevent answering of the clinical question, this should be stated explicitly.

   e. Comparison studies and reports

      Comparison with relevant examinations and reports should be part of the radiologic consultation and report when appropriate and available.

4. Impression (conclusion or diagnosis)

   a. Unless the report is brief, each report should contain an "impression" section.

   b. A precise diagnosis should be given when possible.

   c. A differential diagnosis should be rendered when appropriate.

   d. Follow-up or additional diagnostic studies to clarify or confirm the impression should be suggested when appropriate.

   e. Any significant patient reaction should be reported.

5. Standardized computer-generated template reports

   Standardized computer-generated template reports that satisfy the above criteria are considered to conform to these guidelines.

record. The consultant must document the order for the services, the care provided, and proof that the communication of the opinion or advice occurred back to the ordering provider. (An example of a Consultation Verification Form is provided in the Sample Forms folder on the CD-ROM accompanying this book.) The documentation of a consultation may occur in a progress note, through the completion of a form supplied by the ordering provider or a written report (handwritten, transcribed, or electronic format). Consultation reports typically contain the following information:

- Name of the provider who requested the consultation, along with the reason for the consultation

- Date the consultation was completed by the consultant

- Patient identification, including name and unique identifier

- Pertinent findings of the history and examination

- Consultant's opinion of diagnoses or impressions

- Recommendations or advice on potential treatment options or diagnostic tests

- Signature, credentials, and specialty of the consultant

Patient Instructions

Unlike the hospital setting, where a healthcare team (headed by a physician) is responsible for all patient care, the medical practice setting leaves aftercare in the patient's hands. Therefore, it is essential that the patient be given clear, concise instructions. The Joint Commission's *Ambulatory Accreditation Requirements* (Joint Commission 2009) requires that conclusions reached at the termination of care, treatment, or services—including the patient's final disposition, condition, and instructions given for follow-up care, treatment, or services—be recorded in the health record. Additionally, a copy must be made available to the provider or medical organization providing follow-up care, treatment, or services.

Ideally, instructions to the patient should be communicated both verbally and in writing, with a copy of the documented instructions in the health record. When a group or individual other than the patient has assumed responsibility for the patient's aftercare, the record should indicate that the instructions were given to that group or individual. The healthcare professional should sign the record to indicate that he or she issued the verbal instructions, and the person receiving the instructions should sign the record to verify that understanding. Moreover, patient comments or questions should be documented, along with the clarifications the healthcare professional offered in response. Documentation of patient education during office visits may be accomplished by using forms or electronic screens that prompt the person providing instruction to cover important information. (An example of a patient instructions form is provided in the Sample Forms folder on the CD-ROM accompanying this book.)

Failed Appointment Forms

In medical practices, patients assume responsibility for much of their own healthcare. For example, they have their prescriptions filled and take their medications as prescribed, follow a prescribed diet, report to the laboratory to have diagnostic tests performed, or schedule follow-up appointments as their provider advises. By using a simple form, stamp, or electronic entry to note when the patient fails to keep such appointments, the provider can protect the medical practice in case of litigation by demonstrating compliance with clinical practice standards and offering evidence of the quality of care provided. It is important that the provider review the reason the patient was scheduled for an office visit and determine whether the patient should be contacted to reschedule. Attempts to contact the patient, and the advice given, also should be documented. (An example of a failed appointment record form is provided in the Sample Forms folder on the CD-ROM accompanying this book.)

Flow Sheets

Flow sheets can be an effective way to display information about the patient's treatment from episode to episode. This type of documentation makes it visually easy to identify abnormal results and patterns. Common subjects for flow sheets include chemotherapy, Coumadin therapy, blood glucose results, and vital signs taken during a visit. Another useful flow sheet documents the healthcare maintenance provided and serves to remind the provider when tests or exams are due. (Examples of vital signs flow sheets and age specific preventative care flow sheets may be found in the Sample Forms folder on the CD-ROM accompanying this book.)

Some patients complete flow sheets at home and bring the completed flow sheet to the medical practice for the next patient appointment. This commonly occurs with diabetic patients who frequently monitor blood glucose levels. These patient-documented flow sheets may be in paper or electronic format and also may be part of the patient's PHR.

Telephone Contact Records

From a risk management perspective, as well as a patient care perspective, it is critical to document any advice (instructions, prescriptions, orders, medication changes, and such) or patient follow-up that is communicated by telephone. Documentation should include the date and time of the call, the caller's name and telephone number, the patient's name and identifying information, the reason for the call, the date and time of the response (or attempts to return the call), the response given, and the signature of the person returning the call. Because the message may be relayed among several people, use of a standard form or electronic template to record important information should be encouraged. Telephone contacts are easily documented and tracked in an EHR system.

E-mail Contact Records

Enhanced patient–clinician communications and effective management of chronic care conditions may be promoted by e-mail communications. Patients may also benefit from message-based prompts initiated by clinicians and their staff to remind patients and their surrogates of recommended events and activities that are important to maintaining and improving health. According to the Office of the National Coordinator for Health Information Technology (ONC), the exchange of secure messages may occur in two scenarios.

- **Patient-to-Clinician Communication.** This scenario is focused on the patient's ability to use computerized technologies that are readily available, such as secure Web access, to communicate with clinicians using unstructured and structured messaging capabilities.

- **Clinician-to-Patient Communication.** This scenario includes the ability of clinicians to initiate communications to the patient and respond to their communications. This scenario also includes the ability of a clinician to send relevant clinical reminders to patients regarding medical screening examinations, regular diagnostic tests, or wellness activities (ONC 2008, 5).

According to ONC, "there is a lack of clarity about the scope of the legal medical record, particularly as it relates to secure messages sent between patients and their clinicians." This presents issues when determining the documentation requirements for secure messaging as well as any successful implementation with respect to health records (ONC 2008, 10).

> Communications sent by and to the patient may require updating the patient's specific medical records. These tools may also automatically attach all communications to and from the patient to the patient's medical record (ONC 2008, 36).

Samples of patient inquiries may be under the following circumstances:

- **General medical question**—These communications are perhaps the least amenable to structure since, by definition, the range of questions that could be communicated is completely unknown. Free text is probably most appropriate in this situation though it may still be useful to include categories of information that might be relevant for any and all questions.

- **New medical issue**—A patient may want to report on, or ask about, a new medical problem. A particular set of data such as symptoms or possibly relevant problem background may be useful to help with initial clinical consideration. These data may be similar to what might be asked during a patient interview during a face-to-face visit or what an advice nurse might ask during a telephone advice line conversation. Clearly, some free text as a part of this communication may be appropriate.

- **Question about medical tests/procedures**—Patients who receive medical test results or are considering future treatments or procedures may have specific questions or comments about them. Some of this information could be requested and conveyed within the context of patient educational information, and a structure that reflects the range of tests, procedures, and/or treatments may be most appropriate. A free text "additional comments" option may be appropriate at the end of the communication (ONC 2008, 39–40).

Samples of patient-provided data may be under the following circumstances:

- **Existing medical issue**—Patients may have information to report about a known condition for which there are new data. As an example, this type of transaction may be related to remote monitoring of a chronic condition. Some level of structure may assist in this communication, and in fact may be more relevant given it is a known condition. Some free text may be appropriate for this type of transaction.

- **Pre-visit data capture and communication**—One possible use of secure messaging is for the capture of information from the patient as a head start for obtaining the information normally gathered during the initial patient interview. As such, there is a significant set of data that could be gathered, according to a specific structure. Items such as personal medical history, family medical history, allergies, current medications, and other topics could be candidates for this structuring. Free text may be appropriate within some of these areas. General free text outside of this structure may not be appropriate or useful (ONC 2008, 40).

Samples of patient service requests may be under the following circumstances:

- **Referral request**—Patient requests of referrals for additional services may be an area in which a highly structured interaction with a provider might be appropriate. Free text may add limited value to this interaction.

- **Prescription renewal request**—A patient request to have a prescription renewed, perhaps when the number of prescribed refills has been exhausted, is a common need that could be satisfied by a highly structured communication. Specific data needs for this communication might include prescription number, prescription date, number of refills ordered and filled, pharmacy identifying information, and other data. In addition, the Centers for Medicare and Medicaid Services (CMS) e-Prescribing initiative would have a bearing on the appropriate data for consideration within this transaction. Free text may have limited value to this interaction (ONC 2008, 40).

Samples of clinician-initiated communications may be under the following circumstances:

- **Post-visit summary**—Another use for secure messaging is that of a provider-initiated communication that summarizes a recent face-to-face visit. As a part of patient visits, many providers are now including physical documents that accompany the patient at the end of a visit. These materials could also be included within a secure message. Sample data types could include patient measurements, diagnoses, treatments, prescribed medications (with explanation of rationale for prescription, side-effects, and so forth), home care instructions, and other patient education materials. Free text may also be appropriate.

- **Clinical reminders**—Providers, or their surrogates, may initiate messages for patients that remind patients of a possible need for a regular appointment or a wellness activity. Cancer screenings, annual checkups, and other reminders may best serve the needs of patients and providers, and be accomplished through the use of highly structured secure messages. Free text would probably not be utilized as many of these messages may be automatically generated by an EHR.

- **New data relevant for patient(s)**—Providers, or their surrogates, may initiate messages for patients and their surrogates to make them aware of new information that may be related to new research, new drugs, or new treatments (ONC 2008, 41).

Additionally, there may be requests from patients for appointments, billing questions, patient demographic updates, and other administrative questions. "At the conclusion of the communication exchange, the patient, the clinical support staff, and the clinician complete information related to the communication event and perform documentation of the event as required. This may be supported by automated tools that archive messages and associate them with patient medical records" (ONC 2008, 16).

Check Your Understanding 1.1

1. Which of the following general documentation practices is false?
   a. Format and content of health record should be uniform.
   b. Entries should be made at the time of service or immediately after the service.
   c. Erasures should remove documentation completely, so that erroneous entries cannot be seen.
   d. Original reports should always be maintained in the health record.

2. What type of health record consists of the database, problem list, initial plan, and progress note?
   a. Source-oriented health record
   b. Integrated health record
   c. Problem-oriented health record
   d. Basic health record

3. The problem list includes all of these listed items except for one. Which item is not part of the problem list?
   a. Confirmed diagnoses
   b. Rule-out diagnoses
   c. Completed procedures
   d. Allergies

4. The medication list includes all but the one of following items. Which item is not included in the medication list?
   a. Name of medications and dosages
   b. Date prescription was written
   c. Date prescription was discontinued
   d. Pharmacy name filling the prescription

5. According to the multisystem examination documentation guidelines, which of the following bulleted items are not included in a cardiology physical examination?
   a. Auscultation of renal arteries
   b. Palpation of chest
   c. Palpation of the heart
   d. Examination of pedal pulses

6. Which of the following describes the four parts to a SOAP note?
   a. Subjective, objective, assessment, and process
   b. Suspected, objective, analysis, and plan
   c. Subjective, objective, assessment, and plan
   d. Suspected, objective, analysis, and practice

7. According to the documentation guidelines for diagnostic imaging findings, which of the following items is not a necessary component?
   a. Date of the examination
   b. Name or type of examination
   c. Report of findings
   d. Signature of the patient if a self-referral

8. What type of report provides the ordering clinician an opinion or advice for the care of the patient?

   a. History and physical examination report
   b. Telephone contact report
   c. Consultation report
   d. Discharge summary

9. Which type of records may be documented in paper-based or electronic versions?

   a. Progress notes
   b. Flow sheets
   c. Immunization records
   d. All of the above

10. According to the ONC, which of the following is not an example of patient–provider secure messaging?

    a. Patient-provided data
    b. Clinician-initiated communications
    c. Pharmacy service requests
    d. Patient service requests

Urgent (Emergent) Care Records

According to the American Academy of Urgent Care Medicine (AAUCM), urgent care medicine is defined as the delivery of ambulatory medical care outside of a hospital emergency department on a walk-in basis without a scheduled appointment (AAUCM 2009). The expansion of operating hours is beyond the typical medical practice—in that urgent care medicine facilities are usually open later in the evenings, and open on weekends and many holidays. Because the delivery of urgent care medicine may be limited to episodes at the urgent care center, the extent of documentation is limited to the presenting problem and the treatment provided. Often this treatment does not resolve the patient's complaint completely and the patient is either referred to another provider for follow-up care or told to return to the urgent care center for a follow-up appointment. It is important to thoroughly document patient instructions as well as the presenting complaint, evaluation, and assessment. Sufficient details should be provided to justify reimbursement, protect the facility or the patient in legal proceedings, and ensure continuity of care.

The following information must be entered into the patient's health record for each urgent care visit:

- Patient identification (or the reason it could not be obtained)

- Time and means of arrival

- Name of provider and profession (for example MD, DO, NP, PT, RN, and so forth)

- Chief complaint or purpose of visit

- Pertinent history of the illness (including the length of time the patient has been ill) or injury (including the date of injury) and physical findings (including the patient's vital signs)

- Current medications and any allergies (including allergies to medications)

- Emergency care given to the patient prior to arrival

- Diagnostic and therapeutic orders

- Clinical observations, including the results of treatment

- Reports of procedures, tests, and results (including any medications administered, route site time, and patient reaction)

- Diagnostic impression

- Conclusion at the termination of evaluation/treatment, including final disposition, the patient's condition upon discharge or transfer, and any instructions given to the patient and/or the patient's representative for follow-up care

- Documentation of cases when the patient left the facility against medical advice or missed an appointment

- Authentication and verification of contents by the provider

Usually, patient, provider, and encounter data items are recorded on one form, with separate forms for orders and progress notes. For every patient visit, the physician signs or initials each form, whether electronically or manually, on which he or she made entries, and nurses sign or initial every intervention or service they provided, including the taking of vital signs.

The Urgent Care Association of America notes detailed clinical practice guidelines that reflect the documentation requirements for each diagnosis at http://www.ucaoa.org/resources_guidelines.php. These guidelines can be found for specific topics, such as asthma, back pain, headache, hernia, low back pain, otitis media, pneumonia, upper respiratory tract infection, and urinary tract infection, to name a few.

Health Record Content for Specialty Care

Although all health records maintained by a healthcare team contain the same basic information (such as chief complaint/reason for visit, history and physical, progress notes, diagnostic test results, and orders), various medical specialties have documentation requirements unique to their fields. Medical societies such as the American College of Obstetricians and Gynecologists (ACOG) and the American Society of Anesthesiologists (ASA) have adopted standards of care and documentation guidelines. Special forms can be used to facilitate data collection in these areas. The following subsections discuss documentation requirements for some of the medical specialties: surgery, obstetrics and gynecology, pediatrics, chiropractic, and physical therapy.

Surgery Records

Surgical procedures require a unique set of documentation that encompasses the preoperative, operative, and postoperative time frames. The anesthesiologist and the surgeon are both responsible for evaluating the patient's history and monitoring his or her health status during each stage of care.

The anesthesia records include areas for preoperative, intraoperative, and postoperative documentation. Along with the anesthesia record, there are valid surgical consent forms and operative reports.

Surgeon's Preoperative Evaluation

The surgeon's preoperative evaluation is a record of examinations and diagnostic tests performed to verify a patient's candidacy for surgery. This evaluation should document pertinent history, the results of a physical, and indications for surgery, and be performed no more than seven days prior to the surgery. Special attention should be given to areas that, when not corrected or properly monitored, could put the patient at surgical risk, including nutritional status, immune status, pulmonary and cardiac function, and drug allergies. The results of diagnostic tests such as blood chemistry, urinalysis, chest x-ray, and electrocardiogram should be filed in the record, along with a note indicating that the surgeon reviewed the results prior to surgery.

Informed Consent

The surgeon is responsible for explaining to the patient and/or the patient's guardian the indications for surgery, the procedure to be performed, alternative treatments, benefits, complications, and risks. This discussion should include an explanation of what will happen in the operating room and the recovery room, as well as how the patient may feel. The patient and/or legal representative must sign a consent form indicating that the procedure and its risks were explained. (A more detailed discussion of consent forms is provided later in this chapter.)

Anesthesiologist's Preoperative Assessment

The anesthesiologist and certified registered nurse anesthetists (CRNA) perform a separate preoperative examination to assess the patient's health status, determine the appropriate anesthesia type, and explain the plan of anesthesia to the patient or the patient's legal representative. The ASA's standards (ASA 2008) for the preanesthesia care require:

- Patient interview to assess:
    1. Patient and procedure identification
    2. Verification of admission status (inpatient, outpatient, "short stay," etc.)
    3. Medical history
    4. Anesthetic history
    5. Medication/allergy history
    6. NPO (nothing by mouth) status
- Appropriate physical examination, including vital signs and documentation of airway assessment
- Review of objective diagnostic data (for example, laboratory, ECG, x-ray) and medical records
- Medical consultations when applicable
- Assignment of ASA physical status, including emergent status when applicable
- Formulation of the anesthetic plan and discussion of the risks and benefits of the plan (including discharge issues when indicated) with the patient or the patient's legal representative and/or escort
- Documentation of appropriate informed consent(s)
- Appropriate premedication and prophylactic antibiotic administrations (if indicated) (ASA 2008)

Documentation must be completed in the health record indicating that the above items have been performed. Documentation should include information on any previous surgeries performed and reactions to anesthesia, any current and previous medications, any physical condition(s) that will affect the administration and management of anesthesia, and an indication that the anesthesiologist has reviewed the results of the diagnostic workup and ordered any necessary tests or consultations. The preoperative assessment should be performed immediately before the surgery.

Preoperative Orders

Both the surgeon and the anesthesiologist determine appropriate preoperative medications and instructions and record this information in the health record. Orders may relate to any of the following:

- Diet/intake
- Hydration level
- Bowel preparation
- Preanesthesia medications
- Discontinuance/continuance of prescription medications

Nurse's Preoperative Assessment

The nurse completes a preoperative assessment form, which is available in the health record before the patient enters the operating room. This form is used as a checklist to verify that all preoperative orders have been completed, that all required reports are in the health record, and that the patient is prepared for surgery. Checklist items include, but are not limited to:

- Preoperative orders
- Routine tests (date ordered, date completed, and results)
- History and physical in health record
- Signed consents
- Consultations
- Vital signs
- Allergies
- Time patient last voided
- Time of last meal/fluids
- Blood type and cross-match
- Patient identification verified
- False teeth, prostheses, hearing aids, glasses, contact lenses removed
- Hairpins, nail polish, lipstick removed
- Jewelry and valuables removed

(An example of a preoperative assessment record is provided in the Sample Forms folder on the CD-ROM accompanying this book.)

Operative Report

The operative report is a formal document that describes the events surrounding a surgical procedure or operation and identifies the principal participants in the surgery (AHIMA 2010). The operative report or other high-risk procedure report should contain the following information:

- Patient identification
- Date of surgery
- The name(s) of the licensed independent practitioner(s) who performed the procedure and his or her assistant(s)
- The name of the procedure performed
- A description of the procedure
- Findings of the procedure
- Any estimated blood loss
- Any specimen(s) removed
- The postoperative diagnosis
- Signature, credentials and date operative report was documented (Joint Commission 2009, RC.02.01.03, Item 6)

Additionally, documentation elements to include in the operative report are as follows:

- Patient's preoperative diagnoses and indications for surgery
- Patient's medical condition before, during, and after the surgery
- Duration of surgery

If the electronic or hard-copy operative report is not immediately available in the health record, then a separate documented note is necessary and should include the name(s) of the primary surgeon(s) and his or her assistant(s), procedure performed and a description of each procedure finding, estimated blood loss, specimens removed, and postoperative diagnosis (Joint Commission 2009, RC.02.01.03, Item 7).

Anesthesia Record

While the patient is under anesthesia, the anesthesiologist is responsible for documenting an assessment of the patient's health immediately before surgery and continuous monitoring of the patient during surgery.

ASA standards for intraoperative documentation are as follows:

- Immediate review prior to initiation of anesthetic procedures:
    1. Patient re-evaluation (re-verification of NPO status)
    2. Check of equipment, drugs, and gas supply

- Monitoring of the patient (for example, recording of vital signs and use of any non-routine monitors)

- Doses of drugs and agents used, times and routes of administration, and any adverse reactions

- The type and amounts of intravenous fluids used, including blood and blood products, and times of administration

- The technique(s) used and patient position(s)

- Intravenous/intravascular lines and airway devices that are inserted including technique for insertion and location

- Unusual events during the administration of anesthesia

- The status of the patient at the conclusion of anesthesia (ASA 2008)

In consideration of the legal purpose of the health record, it also is prudent to document that all of the anesthesia equipment (intubation devices, cardiac monitor, tourniquets, suction devices, defibrillator, and the like) was checked and found to be functional before surgery. Because the patient's health status may change rapidly during surgery, the anesthesiologist continuously monitors and records the patient's oxygenation, ventilation, circulation, and temperature. (An example of an anesthesia record is provided in the Sample Forms folder on the CD-ROM accompanying this book.)

Postoperative Progress Notes

Immediately after surgery and before the patient leaves the operative room, the surgeon completes the postoperative progress note detailing the findings and techniques of the operation. It should include:

- Name of primary surgeon and any assistants
- Preoperative diagnosis
- Postoperative diagnosis
- Description of procedure performed
- Specimens removed
- Estimated blood loss
- Signature of surgeon and date

This progress note serves as a communication tool prior to the operative report's availability. The activities carried out by the nursing staff during surgical procedures also should be documented.

Recovery Room Record

After the patient arrives in the postoperative recovery area, nurses observe and monitor the patient until he or she is stable and ready for discharge. The patient's status is documented immediately upon arrival in the recovery area and at predetermined time intervals thereafter.

Recovery area nurses usually use an established rating system for evaluating the patient's level of oxygenation, ventilation, and circulation. ASA postanesthesia documentation guidelines include:

- Patient evaluation on admission and discharge from the postanesthesia care unit

- A time-based record of vital signs and level of consciousness

- A time-based record of drugs administered, their dosage and route of administration

- Type and amounts of intravenous fluids administered, including blood and blood products

- Any unusual events including postanesthesia or postprocedural complications

- Postanesthesia visits (ASA 2008)

According to the Joint Commission's *Ambulatory Accreditation Requirements* (Joint Commission 2009, RC.02.01.03.09), "the clinical record contains documentation that the patient was discharged from the recovery phase of the operation or procedure either by the licensed independent practitioner responsible for his or her care or according to discharge criteria."

Postoperative Telephone Calls

After leaving the surgical facility, the patient assumes responsibility for the remainder of the recovery process. Even when follow-up instructions were thorough and the patient has indicated his or her complete understanding, questions may arise. Many practices routinely telephone patients at home to follow up on their condition a few days after surgery, although the AAAHC, the Joint Commission, and Medicare do not require such follow-up.

When a facility decides to incorporate postoperative follow-up calls into its routine procedures, a report of the telephone call should be entered in the patient's health record. Documentation should be made part of the progress notes, but delays in calling may result as a logistical issue in locating the paper-based health record. A separate form that incorporates pertinent patient data regarding the surgery may be utilized. This is not the case with an EHR. Such a form would include:

- Patient's name

- Patient's health record number

- Patient's age

- Telephone number

- Name of responsible party/guardian

- Procedure

- Date of procedure

- Anesthesia type

- Complications before discharge

- Date called

- Time called

- Patient's comments/complaints
- Practitioner's advice/teaching/referral/reassurance
- Practitioner's signature

(An example of a postoperative follow-up telephone call report form is provided in the Sample Forms folder on the CD-ROM accompanying this book.)

Pathology Report

Specimens or foreign bodies removed during surgeries must be reported to pathology. A pathology report is a type of health record or documentation that describes the results of a microscopic and macroscopic evaluation of a specimen removed or expelled during a surgical procedure. In the medical practice setting, this is typically completed by an outsourced company and not performed on-site at the medical practice. The written pathology report includes the following information:

- Patient identification
- Date of examination
- Description of the tissue examined
- Findings of the microscopic and macroscopic examination of the specimen
- Diagnosis or diagnoses
- Name, credential, and signature of the pathologist

Gynecology and Obstetrics Records

To manage obstetrics and gynecology patients effectively, it is essential that the documentation include a comprehensive history (personal or family history of breast disease, difficult pregnancies, and so on), a detailed physical, a treatment plan, and patient instructions.

Gynecology Records

The ACOG has made the following recommendations:

> An accurate medical record must be maintained for each patient in a secure, confidential, and accessible way. The patient's name should appear on each page of the record, pertinent information should be firmly attached, and a problem list should be maintained. The record should be legible, concise, cogent, and complete. It should be completed promptly and signed by the qualified healthcare practitioner. Every entry should have identifying data and should be dated. Pertinent information, including allergies, should be readily accessible. Some symbols and abbreviations can be confusing and should be avoided (ACOG 2007, 117).

Quality guidelines have been established for patients with different age groups. Since the obstetrician-gynecologist may be the only healthcare provider seeing a healthy woman, consideration should be made for a multisystem examination. However, the American Medical Association has published documentation guidelines specific for female genitourinary physical examinations that can be found in the 1997 CMS Documentation Guidelines for Evaluation and Management, pages 27–30. This document is located on the CD-ROM accompanying this book.

According to CMS (2006), Section 4102 of the Balanced Budget Act of 1997 provides for coverage of screening pelvic examinations (including a clinical breast examination) for all female beneficiaries, subject to certain frequency and other limitations. A screening pelvic examination (including a clinical breast examination) should include at least 7 of the following 11 elements:

- Inspection and palpation of breasts for masses or lumps, tenderness, symmetry, or nipple discharge

- Digital rectal examination including sphincter tone, presence of hemorrhoids, and rectal masses

- Pelvic examination (with or without specimen collection for smears and cultures) including:

  — External genitalia (for example, general appearance, hair distribution, or lesions)

  — Urethral meatus (for example, size, location, lesions, or prolapse)

  — Urethra (for example, masses, tenderness, or scarring)

  — Bladder (for example, fullness, masses, or tenderness)

  — Vagina (for example, general appearance, estrogen effect, discharge lesions, pelvic support, cystocele, or rectocele)

  — Cervix (for example, general appearance, lesions, or discharge)

  — Uterus (for example, size, contour, position, mobility, tenderness, consistency, descent, or support)

  — Adnexa/parametria (for example, masses, tenderness, organomegaly, or nodularity)

  — Anus and perineum (CMS 2006)

Additional screening documentation consists of a medical history, physical examination, laboratory testing, and medical recommendations as part of the medical decision-making component of the visit.

- Medical history

  — Reason for visit

  — Health status: medical, surgical, family

  — Dietary/nutritional assessment

  — Physical activity

  — Tobacco, alcohol, other drugs, concurrent medications

  — Abuse/neglect

  — Sexual practices

- Physical examination

  — Height, weight, blood pressure

  — Oral cavity

  — Head and neck, adenopathy, thyroid

- — Breasts, axillae
- — Abdomen
- — Pelvic and rectovaginal area
- Immunizations (based upon time intervals or patient risk)
  - — Tetanus-diphtheria booster
  - — Influenza vaccine
  - — Pneumococcal vaccine
  - — MMR vaccine
  - — Hepatitis B vaccine
  - — Hepatitis A vaccine
  - — Varicella vaccine
- Periodic laboratory testing (interval varies based on age)
  - — Pap test
  - — Mammography
  - — Cholesterol, high-density lipoprotein cholesterol
  - — Fecal occult blood test
  - — Sigmoidoscopy
- Laboratory testing for high-risk groups
  - — Hemoglobin
  - — Bacteriuria testing
  - — Fasting glucose test
  - — Sexually transmitted disease testing
  - — HIV testing
  - — Genetic testing
  - — Tuberculosis skin test
  - — Lipid profile
  - — Thyroid-stimulating hormone test
  - — Colonoscopy
  - — Bone density testing

Evaluation and counseling items include sexuality, fitness, psychosocial evaluation, cardiovascular risk factors, and health-risk behaviors specific to each category.

- Sexuality
  - — High-risk behaviors
  - — Contraceptive options

- — Sexually transmitted disease
- — Sexual functioning
- Fitness
  - — Hygiene, including dental
  - — Dietary/nutritional assessment
  - — Exercise: discussion of program
- Psychosocial evaluation
  - — Family relationships
  - — Domestic violence
  - — Job/work satisfaction
  - — Lifestyle/stress
  - — Sleep disorders
  - — Age-specific items
- Cardiovascular risk factors
  - — Family history
  - — Hypertension
  - — Dyslipidemia
  - — Obesity/diabetes mellitus
  - — Lifestyle
- Health/risk behaviors
  - — Injury prevention
  - — Breast self-examination
  - — Skin exposure to ultraviolet rays
  - — Suicide: depressive symptoms
  - — Tobacco, alcohol, other drugs

Antepartum Obstetrics Record

Beginning with the patient's first prenatal visit, health information is collected, monitored, and added throughout the pregnancy. Obstetric health data present a unique set of information, as they are collected from the mother, yet include health information from the developing fetus. Information may contain the patient's last menstrual period; current pregnancy and past obstetric outcomes; medical and social history; dietary assessment; physical findings; estimated date of delivery; laboratory tests (hemoglobin or hematocrit; urinalysis, including microscopic examination and infection screen; blood group and Rh-type determinations; antibody screen; rubella antibody titer measurement; syphilis screen; cervical cytology; hepatitis B virus screen); and risk assessment. The risk assessment may include special testing, such as genetic laboratory testing. At each follow-up visit, blood pressure, weight, uterine size, and heart rate should be assessed. The patient should be asked about fetal movement at each visit after she reports quickening. Urine should be checked to detect protein and glucose. At selected intervals, ultrasounds and fetal stress testing may be performed. Any change in pregnancy risk assessment should be recorded after each evaluation and an appropriate management plan outlined. Continuous risk assessment should be a standard part of antepartum care.

Postpartum Obstetrics Record

Documentation of the postpartum examination should include:

- Information on the delivery (date, route, anesthesia, presence/absence of an episiotomy, baby's weight, complications during labor or pospartum)
- Breast-feeding
- Contraception desired
- Physical exam (breasts, abdomen, vulva, vagina, cervix, uterus, adnexa, rectum)

The first postpartum visit(s) may be in the hospital, birthing center, or patient's home (depending upon where the delivery occurred). An additional postpartum visit for an uncomplicated delivery and recovery is completed in the medical practice six weeks after the delivery. (Examples of prenatal and postpartum forms and templates may be found in the Sample Forms folder on the CD-ROM accompanying this book.)

Pediatric Records

The periodic examination of children during their development is imperative for early diagnosis of physical and/or psychological problems. The effectiveness of medical interventions relies, in part, on complete documentation of both normal and abnormal developmental and behavioral observations. The provider should document a comprehensive history and physical and record all observations as well as the plan of treatment for each evaluation.

History and Physical

A complete pediatric history and physical is recorded at the time of the child's first visit. The history reflects past medical history, birth history, family history, immunization history, nutritional history, growth and development history, and review of systems. The physical examination consists of a report of physical findings by the provider. Data recorded at each interval are used to monitor and analyze the child's development. The provider should date and sign both the history and the physical.

The following information should be documented in a comprehensive pediatric initial history:

- Past medical history
  — Maternal health
  — Birth history
  — Nutritional history
  — Growth and development

- — Sleep patterns and behaviors

- — Illnesses

- — Immunizations

- — Allergies, drug sensitivities

- — Operations

- — Current medications

- Birth history

  - — Mother's health before and during pregnancy: diet, illnesses, medications, weight gain, and procedures

  - — Birth weight

  - — Duration of pregnancy

  - — Duration of labor

  - — Type of delivery

  - — Complications of delivery

  - — Apgar scores

  - — Color (cyanosis, jaundice)

  - — Respiratory distress

  - — Congenital anomalies

  - — Feeding problems

  - — Convulsions

  - — Crying

- Nutritional history

  - — Breast feeding: frequency, duration of each feeding, complications, weaning

  - — Formula: type, concentration, amount, frequency, complications, weaning

  - — Vitamin supplement: type, amount, frequency, duration

  - — Solid foods: date started, type, amount, self-feeding, eating habits, likes and dislikes

- Personal history: description of the patient's lifestyle, habits, academic achievement, interpersonal relationships, including information on eating habits, sleeping habits, recreation habits, relationships with parents, relationships with friends

- Family history: hereditary diseases of relatives and health of immediate relatives; social, ethnic, and religious background; family relationships. Some of these factors are listed:

  - — Diabetes

  - — Cardiovascular disease

  - — Tuberculosis

  - — Anemia

— Cancer

— Kidney disease

— Neurologic disease

— Psychiatric disorders

— Family size

— Neighborhood

— Living conditions

— Safety measures (car seats, outlet covers, door locks)

— Parents' attitudes

— Parents' work schedules

- Growth and development record: a record of the age at which developmental landmarks are achieved:

— Holding head up

— Rolling over

— Sitting alone

— Standing

— Walking

— Saying sounds or words

— Making sentences

— Tying shoes

— Dressing without help

— Controlling bladder and bowels

— Height, weight, and head circumference (recorded at various intervals and compared to national percentiles) (The Sample Forms folder on CD-ROM accompanying this book contains an example of a growth chart form.)

- Review of systems

— General: unusual weight gain or loss, fever, fatigue

— Skin: color, texture, jaundice, rashes, itching, changes in hair or nails

— Eyes: vision, glasses, redness, lacrimation, pain, blurring

— Ears: hearing, infection, discharge, earaches

— Nose: frequent colds, nosebleeds, stuffy nose

— Mouth and throat: sore throat, condition of teeth and gums, redness

— Neck: lump in neck, swollen glands, goiter, neck pain

— Cardiovascular: chest pain, syncope, tachycardia

— Respiratory: dyspnea, cough, wheezing, sputum, asthma, bronchitis, pneumonia

— Gastrointestinal: vomiting, diarrhea, constipation, abdominal pain, frequency of bowel movements, consistency of stool

— Genitourinary: frequency, polyuria, nocturia, pyuria, hematuria, urinary infections, incontience, vaginal discharge, menstrual history, abnormalities of penis or testes

— Musculoskeletal: joint pain, stiffness, weakness, postural deformities, gait, exercise tolerance

— Neurologic: headaches, fainting, dizziness, tingling, seizures

— Endocrine: disturbance of growth, excessive thirst, excessive sweating, hunger, urination

— Hematologic: anemia, easily bruised, history of transfusions

— Psychiatric: nervousness, tension, moodiness, depression

Well-Child Visits

A pediatric history and physical is documented at various intervals during the child's growth. Visits, often referred to as well-child checks, usually are scheduled at the following ages: newborn (2 to 3 weeks), 2 months, 4 months, 6 months, 9 months, 12 months, 15 months, 18 months, 2 years, 3 years, 4 years, 5 years, 6 years, 7 or 8 years, 9 or 10 years, 10 to 12 years, 12 to 15 years, 16 years, and 18 years. Data recorded at each of these intervals are used to monitor and analyze the child's development. (Examples of growth charts may be found in the Sample Forms folder on the CD-ROM accompanying this book.)

The following information should be documented during every well-child visit:

- Nutritional history

   — Breast feeding: frequency, duration of each feeding, complications, weaning

   — Formula: type, concentration, amount, frequency, complications, weaning

   — Vitamin supplement: type, amount, frequency, duration

   — Solid foods: date started, type, amount, self-feeding, eating habits, likes and dislikes

- Growth and development record

   — Holding head up

   — Rolling over

   — Sitting alone

   — Standing

   — Walking

   — Saying sounds or words

   — Making sentences

   — Tying shoes

— Dressing without help

— Controlling bladder and bowels

— Height, weight, and head circumference (recorded at various intervals and compared to national percentiles)

- Social development

— Eating

— Sleeping

— Recreation

— Elimination habits

— Parent's use of discipline and child's response

— Year schooling began and child's academic development

— Child's relationship with friends and family

— Bed-wetting

— Thumb sucking

— Temper tantrums

— Tics

— Head banging

— Smoking, alcohol/drug use, sexual activity, use of birth control pills (adolescent health record only)

- Past illness

— Type

— Age

— Severity

— Complications

- Immunization Record

The 2009 immunization schedule as recommended for patients aged 0 through 18 years are approved by the Advisory Committee on Immunization Practices (http://www.cdc.gov/vaccines/recs/acip), the American Academy of Pediatrics (http://www.aap.org), and the American Academy of Family Physicians (http://www.aafp.org) and published by the Department of Health and Human Services, Centers for Disease Control and Prevention. The specific immunization schedules are divided between patient's ages 0 to 6 years, 7 to 18 years, as well as those patients who are a month behind in immunizations (which patients may follow the catch-up schedule) can be found in figures 1.6, 1.7, and 1.8.

When administering immunizations, the following information should be documented:

— Patient name and identifier

— Date of administration

— Name of vaccine manufacturer

Figure 1.6. Immunization schedule ages 0 to 6 years

Recommended Immunization Schedule for Persons Aged 0 Through 6 Years—United States • 2009
For those who fall behind or start late, see the catch-up schedule

Vaccine ▼ Age ►	Birth	1 month	2 months	4 months	6 months	12 months	15 months	18 months	19–23 months	2–3 years	4–6 years
Hepatitis B[1]	HepB	HepB		see footnote 1		HepB					
Rotavirus[2]			RV	RV	RV[2]						
Diphtheria, Tetanus, Pertussis[3]			DTaP	DTaP	DTaP	see footnote 3	DTaP				DTaP
Haemophilus influenzae type b[4]			Hib	Hib	Hib[4]	Hib					
Pneumococcal[5]			PCV	PCV	PCV	PCV				PPSV	
Inactivated Poliovirus			IPV	IPV		IPV					IPV
Influenza[6]					Influenza (Yearly)						
Measles, Mumps, Rubella[7]						MMR		see footnote 7			MMR
Varicella[8]						Varicella		see footnote 8			Varicella
Hepatitis A[9]						HepA (2 doses)				HepA Series	
Meningococcal[10]										MCV	

Range of recommended ages

Certain high-risk groups

This schedule indicates the recommended ages for routine administration of currently licensed vaccines, as of December 1, 2008, for children aged 0 through 6 years. Any dose not administered at the recommended age should be administered at a subsequent visit, when indicated and feasible. Licensed combination vaccines may be used whenever any component of the combination is indicated and other components are not contraindicated and if approved by the Food and Drug Administration for that dose of the series. Providers should consult the relevant Advisory Committee on Immunization Practices statement for detailed recommendations, including high-risk conditions: http://www.cdc.gov/vaccines/pubs/acip-list.htm. Clinically significant adverse events that follow immunization should be reported to the Vaccine Adverse Event Reporting System (VAERS). Guidance about how to obtain and complete a VAERS form is available at http://www.vaers.hhs.gov or by telephone, 800-822-7967.

1. Hepatitis B vaccine (HepB). *(Minimum age: birth)*
At birth:
- Administer monovalent HepB to all newborns before hospital discharge.
- If mother is hepatitis B surface antigen (HBsAg)-positive, administer HepB and 0.5 mL of hepatitis B immune globulin (HBIG) within 12 hours of birth.
- If mother's HBsAg status is unknown, administer HepB within 12 hours of birth. Determine mother's HBsAg status as soon as possible and, if HBsAg-positive, administer HBIG (no later than age 1 week).
After the birth dose:
- The HepB series should be completed with either monovalent HepB or a combination vaccine containing HepB. The second dose should be administered at age 1 or 2 months. The final dose should be administered no earlier than age 24 weeks.
- Infants born to HBsAg-positive mothers should be tested for HBsAg and antibody to HBsAg (anti-HBs) after completion of at least 3 doses of the HepB series, at age 9 through 18 months (generally at the next well-child visit).
4-month dose:
- Administration of 4 doses of HepB to infants is permissible when combination vaccines containing HepB are administered after the birth dose.

2. Rotavirus vaccine (RV). *(Minimum age: 6 weeks)*
- Administer the first dose at age 6 through 14 weeks (maximum age: 14 weeks 6 days). Vaccination should not be initiated for infants aged 15 weeks or older (i.e., 15 weeks 0 days or older).
- Administer the final dose in the series by age 8 months 0 days.
- If Rotarix® is administered at ages 2 and 4 months, a dose at 6 months is not indicated.

3. Diphtheria and tetanus toxoids and acellular pertussis vaccine (DTaP). *(Minimum age: 6 weeks)*
- The fourth dose may be administered as early as age 12 months, provided at least 6 months have elapsed since the third dose.
- Administer the final dose in the series at age 4 through 6 years.

4. Haemophilus influenzae type b conjugate vaccine (Hib). *(Minimum age: 6 weeks)*
- If PRP-OMP (PedvaxHIB® or Comvax® [HepB-Hib]) is administered at ages 2 and 4 months, a dose at age 6 months is not indicated.
- TriHiBit® (DTaP/Hib) should not be used for doses at ages 2, 4, or 6 months but can be used as the final dose in children aged 12 months or older.

5. Pneumococcal vaccine. *(Minimum age: 6 weeks for pneumococcal conjugate vaccine [PCV]; 2 years for pneumococcal polysaccharide vaccine [PPSV])*
- PCV is recommended for all children aged younger than 5 years. Administer 1 dose of PCV to all healthy children aged 24 through 59 months who are not completely vaccinated for their age.

- Administer PPSV to children aged 2 years or older with certain underlying medical conditions (see *MMWR* 2000;49[No. RR-9]), including a cochlear implant.

6. Influenza vaccine. *(Minimum age: 6 months for trivalent inactivated influenza vaccine [TIV]; 2 years for live, attenuated influenza vaccine [LAIV])*
- Administer annually to children aged 6 months through 18 years.
- For healthy nonpregnant persons (i.e., those who do not have underlying medical conditions that predispose them to influenza complications) aged 2 through 49 years, either LAIV or TIV may be used.
- Children receiving TIV should receive 0.25 mL if aged 6 through 35 months or 0.5 mL if aged 3 years or older.
- Administer 2 doses (separated by at least 4 weeks) to children aged younger than 9 years who are receiving influenza vaccine for the first time or who were vaccinated for the first time during the previous influenza season but only received 1 dose.

7. Measles, mumps, and rubella vaccine (MMR). *(Minimum age: 12 months)*
- Administer the second dose at age 4 through 6 years. However, the second dose may be administered before age 4, provided at least 28 days have elapsed since the first dose.

8. Varicella vaccine. *(Minimum age: 12 months)*
- Administer the second dose at age 4 through 6 years. However, the second dose may be administered before age 4, provided at least 3 months have elapsed since the first dose.
- For children aged 12 months through 12 years the minimum interval between doses is 3 months. However, if the second dose was administered at least 28 days after the first dose, it can be accepted as valid.

9. Hepatitis A vaccine (HepA). *(Minimum age: 12 months)*
- Administer to all children aged 1 year (i.e., aged 12 through 23 months). Administer 2 doses at least 6 months apart.
- Children not fully vaccinated by age 2 years can be vaccinated at subsequent visits.
- HepA also is recommended for children older than 1 year who live in areas where vaccination programs target older children or who are at increased risk of infection. See *MMWR* 2006;55(No. RR-7).

10. Meningococcal vaccine. *(Minimum age: 2 years for meningococcal conjugate vaccine [MCV] and for meningococcal polysaccharide vaccine [MPSV])*
- Administer MCV to children aged 2 through 10 years with terminal complement component deficiency, anatomic or functional asplenia, and certain other high-risk groups. See *MMWR* 2005;54(No. RR-7).
- Persons who received MPSV 3 or more years previously and who remain at increased risk for meningococcal disease should be revaccinated with MCV.

The Recommended Immunization Schedules for Persons Aged 0 Through 18 Years are approved by the Advisory Committee on Immunization Practices (www.cdc.gov/vaccines/recs/acip), the American Academy of Pediatrics (http://www.aap.org), and the American Academy of Family Physicians (http://www.aafp.org).
DEPARTMENT OF HEALTH AND HUMAN SERVICES • CENTERS FOR DISEASE CONTROL AND PREVENTION

CS103164

Figure 1.7. Immunization schedule ages 7 to 18 years

Recommended Immunization Schedule for Persons Aged 7 Through 18 Years—United States • 2009
For those who fall behind or start late, see the schedule below and the catch-up schedule

Vaccine ▼ Age ▶	7–10 years	11–12 years	13–18 years
Tetanus, Diphtheria, Pertussis[1]	see footnote 1	Tdap	Tdap
Human Papillomavirus[2]	see footnote 2	HPV (3 doses)	HPV Series
Meningococcal[3]	MCV	MCV	MCV
Influenza[4]	Influenza (Yearly)		
Pneumococcal[5]	PPSV		
Hepatitis A[6]	HepA Series		
Hepatitis B[7]	HepB Series		
Inactivated Poliovirus[8]	IPV Series		
Measles, Mumps, Rubella[9]	MMR Series		
Varicella[10]	Varicella Series		

Range of recommended ages

Catch-up immunization

Certain high-risk groups

This schedule indicates the recommended ages for routine administration of currently licensed vaccines, as of December 1, 2008, for children aged 7 through 18 years. Any dose not administered at the recommended age should be administered at a subsequent visit, when indicated and feasible. Licensed combination vaccines may be used whenever any component of the combination is indicated and other components are not contraindicated and if approved by the Food and Drug Administration for that dose of the series. Providers should consult the relevant Advisory Committee on Immunization Practices statement for detailed recommendations, including high-risk conditions: http://www.cdc.gov/vaccines/pubs/acip-list.htm. Clinically significant adverse events that follow immunization should be reported to the Vaccine Adverse Event Reporting System (VAERS). Guidance about how to obtain and complete a VAERS form is available at http://www.vaers.hhs.gov or by telephone, 800-822-7967.

1. Tetanus and diphtheria toxoids and acellular pertussis vaccine (Tdap). *(Minimum age: 10 years for BOOSTRIX® and 11 years for ADACEL®)*
- Administer at age 11 or 12 years for those who have completed the recommended childhood DTP/DTaP vaccination series and have not received a tetanus and diphtheria toxoid (Td) booster dose.
- Persons aged 13 through 18 years who have not received Tdap should receive a dose.
- A 5-year interval from the last Td dose is encouraged when Tdap is used as a booster dose; however, a shorter interval may be used if pertussis immunity is needed.

2. Human papillomavirus vaccine (HPV). *(Minimum age: 9 years)*
- Administer the first dose to females at age 11 or 12 years.
- Administer the second dose 2 months after the first dose and the third dose 6 months after the first dose (at least 24 weeks after the first dose).
- Administer the series to females at age 13 through 18 years if not previously vaccinated.

3. Meningococcal conjugate vaccine (MCV).
- Administer at age 11 or 12 years, or at age 13 through 18 years if not previously vaccinated.
- Administer to previously unvaccinated college freshmen living in a dormitory.
- MCV is recommended for children aged 2 through 10 years with terminal complement component deficiency, anatomic or functional asplenia, and certain other groups at high risk. See *MMWR* 2005;54(No. RR-7).
- Persons who received MPSV 5 or more years previously and remain at increased risk for meningococcal disease should be revaccinated with MCV.

4. Influenza vaccine.
- Administer annually to children aged 6 months through 18 years.
- For healthy nonpregnant persons (i.e., those who do not have underlying medical conditions that predispose them to influenza complications) aged 2 through 49 years, either LAIV or TIV may be used.
- Administer 2 doses (separated by at least 4 weeks) to children aged younger than 9 years who are receiving influenza vaccine for the first time or who were vaccinated for the first time during the previous influenza season but only received 1 dose.

5. Pneumococcal polysaccharide vaccine (PPSV).
- Administer to children with certain underlying medical conditions (see *MMWR* 1997;46[No. RR-8]), including a cochlear implant. A single revaccination should be administered to children with functional or anatomic asplenia or other immunocompromising condition after 5 years.

6. Hepatitis A vaccine (HepA).
- Administer 2 doses at least 6 months apart.
- HepA is recommended for children older than 1 year who live in areas where vaccination programs target older children or who are at increased risk of infection. See *MMWR* 2006;55(No. RR-7).

7. Hepatitis B vaccine (HepB).
- Administer the 3-dose series to those not previously vaccinated.
- A 2-dose series (separated by at least 4 months) of adult formulation Recombivax HB® is licensed for children aged 11 through 15 years.

8. Inactivated poliovirus vaccine (IPV).
- For children who received an all-IPV or all-oral poliovirus (OPV) series, a fourth dose is not necessary if the third dose was administered at age 4 years or older.
- If both OPV and IPV were administered as part of a series, a total of 4 doses should be administered, regardless of the child's current age.

9. Measles, mumps, and rubella vaccine (MMR).
- If not previously vaccinated, administer 2 doses or the second dose for those who have received only 1 dose, with at least 28 days between doses.

10. Varicella vaccine.
- For persons aged 7 through 18 years without evidence of immunity (see *MMWR* 2007;56[No. RR-4]), administer 2 doses if not previously vaccinated or the second dose if they have received only 1 dose.
- For persons aged 7 through 12 years, the minimum interval between doses is 3 months. However, if the second dose was administered at least 28 days after the first dose, it can be accepted as valid.
- For persons aged 13 years and older, the minimum interval between doses is 28 days.

The Recommended Immunization Schedules for Persons Aged 0 Through 18 Years are approved by the Advisory Committee on Immunization Practices (www.cdc.gov/vaccines/recs/acip), the American Academy of Pediatrics (http://www.aap.org), and the American Academy of Family Physicians (http://www.aafp.org).

DEPARTMENT OF HEALTH AND HUMAN SERVICES • CENTERS FOR DISEASE CONTROL AND PREVENTION

Figure 1.8.   Immunization schedule catchup 4 months to 18 years

Catch-up Immunization Schedule for Persons Aged 4 Months Through 18 Years Who Start Late or Who Are More Than 1 Month Behind—United States • 2009

The table below provides catch-up schedules and minimum intervals between doses for children whose vaccinations have been delayed. A vaccine series does not need to be restarted, regardless of the time that has elapsed between doses. Use the section appropriate for the child's age.

CATCH-UP SCHEDULE FOR PERSONS AGED 4 MONTHS THROUGH 6 YEARS

Vaccine	Minimum Age for Dose 1	Minimum Interval Between Doses			
		Dose 1 to Dose 2	Dose 2 to Dose 3	Dose 3 to Dose 4	Dose 4 to Dose 5
Hepatitis B[1]	Birth	4 weeks	8 weeks (and at least 16 weeks after first dose)		
Rotavirus[2]	6 wks	4 weeks	4 weeks[2]		
Diphtheria, Tetanus, Pertussis[3]	6 wks	4 weeks	4 weeks	6 months	6 months[3]
Haemophilus influenzae type b[4]	6 wks	4 weeks if first dose administered at younger than age 12 months / 8 weeks (as final dose) if first dose administered at age 12-14 months / No further doses needed if first dose administered at age 15 months or older	4 weeks[4] if current age is younger than 12 months / 8 weeks (as final dose)[4] if current age is 12 months or older and second dose administered at younger than age 15 months / No further doses needed if previous dose administered at age 15 months or older	8 weeks (as final dose) This dose only necessary for children aged 12 months through 59 months who received 3 doses before age 12 months	
Pneumococcal[5]	6 wks	4 weeks if first dose administered at younger than age 12 months / 8 weeks (as final dose for healthy children) if first dose administered at age 12 months or older or current age 24 through 59 months / No further doses needed for healthy children if first dose administered at age 24 months or older	4 weeks if current age is younger than 12 months / 8 weeks (as final dose for healthy children) if current age is 12 months or older / No further doses needed for healthy children if previous dose administered at age 24 months or older	8 weeks (as final dose) This dose only necessary for children aged 12 months through 59 months who received 3 doses before age 12 months or for high-risk children who received 3 doses at any age	
Inactivated Poliovirus[6]	6 wks	4 weeks	4 weeks	4 weeks[6]	
Measles, Mumps, Rubella[7]	12 mos	4 weeks			
Varicella[8]	12 mos	3 months			
Hepatitis A[9]	12 mos	6 months			

CATCH-UP SCHEDULE FOR PERSONS AGED 7 THROUGH 18 YEARS

Vaccine	Minimum Age for Dose 1	Dose 1 to Dose 2	Dose 2 to Dose 3	Dose 3 to Dose 4	
Tetanus, Diphtheria/ Tetanus, Diphtheria, Pertussis[10]	7 yrs[10]	4 weeks	4 weeks if first dose administered at younger than age 12 months / 6 months if first dose administered at age 12 months or older	6 months if first dose administered at younger than age 12 months	
Human Papillomavirus[11]	9 yrs	Routine dosing intervals are recommended[11]			
Hepatitis A[9]	12 mos	6 months			
Hepatitis B[1]	Birth	4 weeks	8 weeks (and at least 16 weeks after first dose)		
Inactivated Poliovirus[6]	6 wks	4 weeks	4 weeks	4 weeks[6]	
Measles, Mumps, Rubella[7]	12 mos	4 weeks			
Varicella[8]	12 mos	3 months if the person is younger than age 13 years / 4 weeks if the person is aged 13 years or older			

1. Hepatitis B vaccine (HepB).
- Administer the 3-dose series to those not previously vaccinated.
- A 2-dose series (separated by at least 4 months) of adult formulation Recombivax HB® is licensed for children aged 11 through 15 years.

2. Rotavirus vaccine (RV).
- The maximum age for the first dose is 14 weeks 6 days. Vaccination should not be initiated for infants aged 15 weeks or older (i.e., 15 weeks 0 days or older).
- Administer the final dose in the series by age 8 months 0 days.
- If Rotarix® was administered for the first and second doses, a third dose is not indicated.

3. Diphtheria and tetanus toxoids and acellular pertussis vaccine (DTaP).
- The fifth dose is not necessary if the fourth dose was administered at age 4 years or older.

4. Haemophilus influenzae type b conjugate vaccine (Hib).
- Hib vaccine is not generally recommended for persons aged 5 years or older. No efficacy data are available on which to base a recommendation concerning use of Hib vaccine for older children and adults. However, studies suggest good immunogenicity in persons who have sickle cell disease, leukemia, or HIV infection, or who have had a splenectomy; administering 1 dose of Hib vaccine to these persons is not contraindicated.
- If the first 2 doses were PRP-OMP (PedvaxHIB® or Comvax®), and administered at age 11 months or younger, the third (and final) dose should be administered at age 12 through 15 months and at least 8 weeks after the second dose.
- If the first dose was administered at age 7 through 11 months, administer 2 doses separated by 4 weeks and a final dose at age 12 through 15 months.

5. Pneumococcal vaccine.
- Administer 1 dose of pneumococcal conjugate vaccine (PCV) to all healthy children aged 24 through 59 months who have not received at least 1 dose of PCV on or after age 12 months.
- For children aged 24 through 59 months with underlying medical conditions, administer 1 dose of PCV if 3 doses were received previously or administer 2 doses of PCV at least 8 weeks apart if fewer than 3 doses were received previously.
- Administer pneumococcal polysaccharide vaccine (PPSV) to children aged 2 years or older with certain underlying medical conditions (see MMWR 2000;49[No. RR-9]), including a cochlear implant, at least 8 weeks after the last dose of PCV.

6. Inactivated poliovirus vaccine (IPV).
- For children who received an all-IPV or all-oral poliovirus (OPV) series, a fourth dose is not necessary if the third dose was administered at age 4 years or older.
- If both OPV and IPV were administered as part of a series, a total of 4 doses should be administered, regardless of the child's current age.

7. Measles, mumps, and rubella vaccine (MMR).
- Administer the second dose at age 4 through 6 years. However, the second dose may be administered before age 4, provided at least 28 days have elapsed since the first dose.
- If not previously vaccinated, administer 2 doses with at least 28 days between doses.

8. Varicella vaccine.
- Administer the second dose at age 4 through 6 years. However, the second dose may be administered before age 4, provided at least 3 months have elapsed since the first dose.
- For persons aged 12 months through 12 years, the minimum interval between doses is 3 months. However, if the second dose was administered at least 28 days after the first dose, it can be accepted as valid.
- For persons aged 13 years and older, the minimum interval between doses is 28 days.

9. Hepatitis A vaccine (HepA).
- HepA is recommended for children older than 1 year who live in areas where vaccination programs target older children or who are at increased risk of infection. See MMWR 2006;55(No. RR-7).

10. Tetanus and diphtheria toxoids vaccine (Td) and tetanus and diphtheria toxoids and acellular pertussis vaccine (Tdap).
- Doses of DTaP are counted as part of the Td/Tdap series
- Tdap should be substituted for a single dose of Td in the catch-up series or as a booster for children aged 10 through 18 years; use Td for other doses.

11. Human papillomavirus vaccine (HPV).
- Administer the series to females at age 13 through 18 years if not previously vaccinated.
- Use recommended routine dosing intervals for series catch-up (i.e., the second and third doses should be administered at 2 and 6 months after the first dose). However, the minimum interval between the first and second doses is 4 weeks. The minimum interval between the second and third doses is 12 weeks, and the third dose should be given at least 24 weeks after the first dose.

Information about reporting reactions after immunization is available online at http://www.vaers.hhs.gov or by telephone, 800-822-7967. Suspected cases of vaccine-preventable diseases should be reported to the state or local health department. Additional information, including precautions and contraindications for immunization, is available from the National Center for Immunization and Respiratory Diseases at http://www.cdc.gov/vaccines or telephone, 800-CDC-INFO (800-232-4636).

DEPARTMENT OF HEALTH AND HUMAN SERVICES • CENTERS FOR DISEASE CONTROL AND PREVENTION

CS113897

— Vaccine lot number

— Adverse reactions

— Name/title/address of person administering the vaccine

The American Academy of Pediatrics publishes an online service entitled "Red Book Online" that provides the status of licensure and recommendations for new vaccines, and it can be found at http://aapredbook.aappublications.org/news/vaccstatus.dtl.

As with other professional services, when treatment recommendations, such as immunizations, are refused by the parent or guardian, then such refusal should be documented. Details on refusal of treatment may be found in the consent section of this chapter. (An example of a vaccine refusal form is provided in the Sample Forms folder on the CD-ROM accompanying this book.)

- Personal history

  — Eating habits

  — Sleeping habits

  — Recreation habits

  — Relationships with parents

  — Relationships with friends

- Physical examination

  — Head, ears, eyes, nose, and throat (HEENT)

  — Skin

  — Heart

  — Chest

  — Abdomen

  — Pulses (through age 6 months)

  — Hip abduction (through age 18 months)

  — External genitalia

  — Back

  — Extremities

  — Neurological

  — Hearing

  — Vision (beginning at age 15 months)

  — Oral/dental (beginning at age 15 months)

  — Blood pressure (beginning at age 3 years)

- Age-specific education, guidance, or risk testing offered

  — Lead screening

  — Hemoglobin testing

— Safety in home, recreation (bicycling, water, and such), firearms

— Car safety

— Diet

— Social development, peer contacts

— Discipline/limits

— Toilet training

— Entertainment (television/video use, stories, singing, and such)

— Readiness for school

— Sexual identity

— Physical exercise

— Alcohol/drugs/tobacco

— Driving

Other Pediatric Visits

During other pediatric visits (often referred to as sick-child visits), the history reflects the reason for the visit and child's current condition, a description of symptoms (date of onset, location, severity, duration, frequency, aggravating/alleviating factors), and medications administered. Physical findings during the examination are recorded, as well as the assessment of the provider, plans for treatment, and recommendations for follow-up. The 1995 or 1997 documentation guidelines published by the American Medical Association should be followed for accurately documenting these visits. The provider may utilize either version of the documentation guidelines—whichever is most advantageous to the provider. These documentation guidelines can be found on the CD-ROM accompanying this book.

Chiropractic Records

As noted by the CMS *Medicare Benefit Policy Manual*, chapter 15—Covered Medical and Other Health Services, Section 240.1, chiropractic services are limited to treatment by manual manipulation, which may be defined as the following:

- Spine or spinal adjustment by manual means;

- Spine or spinal manipulation;

- Manual adjustment; and

- Vertebral manipulation or adjustment (CMS 2009, Chapter 15, Section 240.1)

  Subluxation is defined as a motion segment, in which alignment, movement integrity, and/or physiological function of the spine are altered although contact between joint surfaces remains intact. A subluxation may be demonstrated by an x-ray or by physical examination" utilizing the PART system, as detailed in the following. Medicare will only pay for treatment if it is a manual manipulation of the spine to correct a subluxation that is consistent with the chief complaint (CMS 2009, Chapter 15, Section 240.1.2).

PART System

Pain and Tenderness

Identify using one or more of the following:

- Observation: You can document, by personal observation, the pain that the patient exhibits during the course of the examination. Note the location, quality, and severity of the pain.

- Percussion, Palpation, or Provocation: When examining the patient, ask them if pain is reproduced, such as, "Let me know if any of this causes discomfort."

- Visual Analog Type Scale: The patient is asked to grade the pain on a visual analog type scale from 0 to10.

- Audio Confirmation: Like the visual analog scale, the patient is asked to verbally grade their pain from 0 to10.

- Pain questionnaires: Patient questionnaires, such as the McGill pain questionnaire or an in-office patient history form, can be used for the patient to describe their pain.

Asymmetry/Misalignment

Identify on a sectional or segmental level by using one or more of the following:

- Observation: You can observe patient posture or analyze gait.

- Static and Dynamic Palpation: Describe the spinal misaligned vertebrae and symmetry.

- Diagnostic Imaging: You can use x-ray, CAT scan, and MRI to identify misalignments.

Range of Motion Abnormality

Identify an increase or decrease in segmental mobility using one or more of the following:

- Observation: You can observe an increase or decrease in the patient's range of motion.

- Motion Palpation: You can record your palpation findings, including listing(s). Be sure to record the various areas that are involved and related to the regions manipulated.

- Stress Diagnostic Imaging: You can x-ray the patient using bending views.

- Range of Motion Measuring Devices: Devices such as goniometers or inclinometers can be used to record specific measurements.

Tissue, Tone Changes

Identify using one or more of the following:

- Observation: Visible changes such as signs of spasm, inflammation, swelling, rigidity, etc.

- Palpation: Palpated changes in the tissue, such as hypertonicity, hypotonicity, spasm, inflammation, tautness, rigidity, flaccidity, etc. can be found on palpation.

- Use of instrumentation: Document the instrument used and findings.

- Tests for Length and Strength: Document leg length, scoliosis contracture, and strength of muscles that relate (ACA n.d.).

When the subluxation is based on the physical examination, two of the four criteria of the PART system are required to be documented, one of which must be **A**symmetry/misalignment or **R**ange of motion abnormality.

Initial Visit

The following documentation requirements, from the CMS *Medicare Benefit Policy Manual,* apply whether the subluxation is demonstrated by x-ray or by physical examination:

1. The history recorded in the patient record should include the following:

   • Symptoms causing patient to seek treatment;

   • Family history if relevant;

   • Past health history (general health, prior illness, injuries, or hospitalizations; medications; surgical history);

   • Mechanism of trauma, such as how did the injury or condition occur and was it gradual or sudden;

   • Quality and character of symptoms/problem, such as descriptive remarks to allow payer to fully understand the chief complaint;

   • Onset, duration, intensity, frequency, location and radiation of symptoms;

   • Aggravating or relieving factors; and

   • Prior interventions, treatments, medications, secondary complaints.

2. Description of the present illness including:

   • Mechanism of trauma;

   • Quality and character of symptoms/problem;

   • Onset, duration, intensity, frequency, location, and radiation of symptoms;

   • Aggravating or relieving factors;

   • Prior interventions, treatments, medications, secondary complaints; and

   • Symptoms causing patient to seek treatment (CMS 2009, Chapter 15, Section 240.1.2).

   These symptoms must bear a direct relationship to the level of subluxation. The symptoms should refer to the spine (spondyle or vertebral), muscle (myo), bone (osseo or osteo), rib (costo or costal) and joint (arthro) and be reported as pain (algia), inflammation (itis), or as signs such as swelling, spasticity, and so forth. Vertebral pinching of spinal nerves may cause headaches, arm, shoulder, and hand problems as well as leg and foot pains and numbness. Rib and rib/chest pains are also recognized symptoms, but in general other symptoms must relate to the spine as such. The subluxation must be causal; that is, the symptoms must be related to the level of the subluxation that has been cited. A statement on a claim that there is "pain" is insufficient. The location of pain must be described and whether the particular vertebra listed is capable of producing pain in the area determined.

3. Evaluation of musculoskeletal/nervous system through physical examination.

4. Diagnosis: The primary diagnosis must be subluxation, including the level of subluxation, either so stated or identified by a term descriptive of subluxation. Such terms may refer either to the condition of the spinal joint involved or to the direction of position assumed by the particular bone named.

5. Treatment Plan: The treatment plan should include the following:

   - Level of care (duration and frequency of visits);

   - Specific treatment goals; and

   - Objective measures to evaluate treatment effectiveness.

6. Date of the initial treatment (CMS 2009, Chapter 15, Section 240.1.2).

Subsequent Visit

The following documentation requirements, from the CMS *Medicare Benefit Policy Manual*, apply whether the subluxation is demonstrated by x-ray or by physical examination:

1. History

   - Review of chief complaint;

   - Changes since last visit;

   - System review, if relevant.

2. Physical examination

   - Exam of area of spine involved in diagnosis;

   - Assessment of change in patient condition since last visit;

   - Evaluation of treatment effectiveness.

3. Documentation of treatment given on day of visit (CMS 2009, Chapter 15, Section 240.1.2).

Necessity of Treatment

According to the CMS *Medicare Benefit Policy Manual* (CMS 2009, Chapter 15, Section 240.1), there must be a neuromuscular condition that necessitates the treatment, along with the services having a direct therapeutic impact to the patient's expected recovery or improvement of function. In this scenario, the patient must have a subluxation of the spine that is proven by x-ray or physical examination. The following categories describe most spinal joint problems:

- Acute subluxation is when the patient's condition is considered acute as with the result of a new injury. The patient's condition is expected to improve or arrest as a result of chiropractic manipulation.

- Chronic subluxation is when the patient's condition is considered chronic and is not expected to significantly improve or resolve with further treatment. There is, however, the expectation that continued therapy may result in some functional improvement. Once the clinical status is stabilized and the expectation is that there will be no further improvement, then additional manipulative treatment is considered maintenance therapy and is not covered (CMS 2009, Chapter 15, Section 240.1).

Maintenance Therapy

According to *Medicare Benefit Policy Manual* (CMS 2009, Chapter 15, Section 240.1) maintenance therapy includes services that seek to prevent disease, promote health and prolong and enhance the quality of life, or maintain or prevent deterioration of a chronic condition. When further clinical improvement cannot reasonably be expected from continuous ongoing care, and the chiropractic treatment becomes supportive rather than corrective in nature, the treatment is then considered maintenance therapy. The AT modifier (acute treatment) must not be placed on the claim when maintenance therapy has been provided. Claims without the AT modifier will be considered as maintenance therapy and denied. Chiropractors who give or receive from beneficiaries an Advanced Beneficiary Notice of Noncoverage (ABN or CMS form R-131) shall follow the instructions in Pub. 100-04, Medicare Claims Processing Manual, chapter 23, section 20.9.1.1 and include a GA (waiver of liability on file) (or in rare instances a GZ (item or service expected to be denied as not reasonable and necessary)) modifier on the claim.

Contraindications

Dynamic thrust is the therapeutic force or maneuver delivered by the physician during manipulation in the anatomic region of involvement. A relative contraindication is a condition that adds significant risk of injury to the patient from dynamic thrust, but does not rule out the use of dynamic thrust. The doctor should discuss this risk with the patient and record this in the chart. The following are relative contraindications to dynamic thrust:

- Articular hypermobility and circumstances where the stability of the joint is uncertain;
- Severe demineralization of bone;
- Benign bone tumors (spine);
- Bleeding disorders and anticoagulant therapy; and
- Radiculopathy with progressive neurological signs.

Dynamic thrust is absolutely contraindicated near the site of demonstrated subluxation and proposed manipulation in the following:

- Acute arthropathies characterized by acute inflammation and ligamentous laxity and anatomic subluxation or dislocation; including acute rheumatoid arthritis and ankylosing spondylitis;
- Acute fractures and dislocations or healed fractures and dislocations with signs of instability;
- An unstable os odontoideum;
- Malignancies that involve the vertebral column;
- Infection of bones or joints of the vertebral column;
- Signs and symptoms of myelopathy or cauda equina syndrome;
- For cervical spinal manipulations, vertebrobasilar insufficiency syndrome; and
- A significant major artery aneurysm near the proposed manipulation (CMS 2009, Chapter 15, Section 240.1).

Location of Subluxation

According to the CMS *Medicare Benefit Policy Manual* (CMS 2009, Chapter 15, Section 240.1.4), the exact level of the subluxation must be documented by the chiropractor to justify the claim for manipulation of the spine. Figure 1.9 displays the locations to be documented in the health record.

Subluxation levels may be documented as the exact bones, for example, C5, C6, and so forth or the area may be documented such as occipito-atlantal (occiput and C1 (atlas)), lumbo-sacral (L5 and sacrum), sacro-iliac (sacrum and ilium) (CMS 2009, Chapter 15, Section 240.1.4).

When documenting descriptive terms for the abnormalities, the following examples are acceptable according to the Centers for Medicare and Medicaid Services, although other terms may be documented if they clearly refer to bone or joint space or position (or motion) changes of vertebral elements:

- Off-centered

- Misalignment

- Malpositioning

- Spacing—abnormal, altered, decreased, increased

- Incomplete dislocation

- Rotation

- Listhesis—antero, postero, retro, lateral, spondylo

- Motion—limited, lost, restricted, flexion, extension, hypermobility, hypomotility, aberrant (CMS 2009, Chapter 15, Section 240.1.4)

Treatment Parameters

According to the CMS *Medicare Benefit Policy Manual,* the chiropractor should be afforded the opportunity to effect improvement or arrest or retard deterioration in such a condition

Figure 1.9. Locations of subluxation

Area of Spine	Names of Vertebrae	Number of Vertebrae	Short Form or Other Name
Neck	Occiput	7	Occ, CO
	Cervical	C1 thru C7	Cervical
	Atlas	C1	Atlas
	Axis	C2	Axis
Back	Dorsal or	12	D1 thru D12
	Thoracic	T1 thru T12	Thoracic
	Costovertebral	R1 thru R12	Costovertebral
	Costotransverse	R1 thru R12	Costotransverse
Low Back	Lumbar	5	L1 thru L5
Pelvis	Ilii, r and l		I, Si
Sacral	Sacrum, Coccyx		S, SC

Note: The Ilii, r and l (right and left) are included with the sacrum, since chiropractic manipulation may be performed on only one side.

within a reasonable and generally predictable period of time. Acute subluxation (for example, strains or sprains) problems may require as many as three months of treatment but some require very little treatment. In the first several days, treatment may be quite frequent but decreasing in frequency with time or as improvement is obtained (CMS 2009, Chapter 15, Section 240.1.5).

Chronic spinal joint condition implies, of course, the condition has existed for a longer period of time and that, in all probability, the involved joints have already "set" and fibrotic tissue has developed. This condition may require a longer treatment time, but not with higher frequency (CMS 2009, Chapter 15, Section 240.1.5).

Some chiropractors have been identified as using an "intensive care" concept of treatment. Under this approach multiple daily visits (as many as four or five in a single day) are given in the office or clinic and so-called room or ward fees are charged since the patient is confined to bed usually for the day. The room or ward fees are not covered and reimbursement under Medicare will be limited to not more than one treatment per day (CMS 2009, Chapter 15, Section 240.1.5).

Physical Therapy Records

The American Physical Therapy Association has developed specific documentations requirements (APTA 2008) which are included here in their entirety.

Physical therapy examination, evaluation, diagnosis, prognosis, and intervention shall be documented, dated, and authenticated by the physical therapist who performs the service. Intervention provided by the physical therapist or selected interventions provided by the physical therapist assistant is documented, dated, and authenticated by the physical therapist or, when permissible by law, the physical therapist assistant.

Other notations or flow sheets are considered a component of the documented record but do not meet the requirements of documentation in or of themselves.

Students in physical therapist or physical therapist assistant programs may document when the record is additionally authenticated by the physical therapist or, when permissible by law, documentation by physical therapist assistant students may be authenticated by a physical therapist assistant.

1. Types of Visits

   The following describes the main documentation elements of patient/client management: 1) initial examination/evaluation, 2) visit/encounter, 3) reexamination, and 4) discharge or discontinuation summary.

   a. Initial Examination/Evaluation

      Documentation of the initial encounter is typically called the "initial examination," "initial evaluation," or "initial examination/evaluation." Completion of the initial examination/evaluation is typically completed in one visit, but may occur over more than one visit. Documentation elements for the initial examination/evaluation include the following:

      - Examination: Includes data obtained from the history, systems review, and tests and measures.

      - Evaluation: Evaluation is a thought process that may not include formal documentation. It may include documentation of the assessment of the data collected in the examination and identification of problems pertinent to patient/client management.

- Diagnosis: Indicates level of impairment and functional limitation determined by the physical therapist. May be indicated by selecting one or more preferred practice patterns from the Guide to Physical Therapist Practice.

- Prognosis: Provides documentation of the predicted level of improvement that might be attained through intervention and the amount of time required to reach that level. Prognosis is typically not a separate documentation elements, but the components are included as part of the plan of care.

- Plan of care: Typically stated in general terms, includes goals, interventions planned, proposed frequency and duration, and discharge plans.

b. Visit/Encounter

Documentation of a visit or encounter, often called a progress note or daily note, documents sequential implementation of the plan of care established by the physical therapist, including changes in patient/client status and variations and progressions of specific interventions used. Also may include specific plans for the next visit or visits.

c. Reexamination

Documentation of reexamination includes data from repeated or new examination elements and is provided to evaluate progress and to modify or redirect intervention.

d. Discharge or Discontinuation Summary

Documentation is required following conclusion of the current episode in the physical therapy intervention sequence, to summarize progression toward goals and discharge plans.

2. General Guidelines

- Documentation is required for every visit/encounter.

- All documentation must comply with the applicable jurisdictional/regulatory requirements.

- All handwritten entries shall be made in ink and will include original signatures. Electronic entries are made with appropriate security and confidentiality provisions.

- Charting errors should be corrected by drawing a single line through the error and initialing and dating the chart or through the appropriate mechanism for electronic documentation that clearly indicates that a change was made without deletion of the original record.

- All documentation must include adequate identification of the patient/client and the physical therapist or physical therapist assistant:

  — The patient's/client's full name and identification number, if applicable, must be included on all official documents.

  — All entries must be dated and authenticated with the provider's full name and appropriate designation:

- Documentation of examination, evaluation, diagnosis, prognosis, plan of care, and discharge summary must be authenticated by the physical therapist who provided the service.

- Documentation of intervention in visit/encounter notes must be authenticated by the physical therapist or physical therapist assistant who provided the service.

- Documentation by physical therapist or physical therapist assistant graduates or other physical therapists and physical therapist assistants pending receipt of an unrestricted license shall be authenticated by a licensed physical therapist, or, when permissible by law, documentation by physical therapist assistant graduates may be authenticated by a physical therapist assistant.

- Documentation by students (SPT/SPTA) in physical therapist or physical therapist assistant programs must be additionally authenticated by the physical therapist or, when permissible by law, documentation by physical therapist assistant students may be authenticated by a physical therapist assistant.

- Documentation should include the referral mechanism by which physical therapy services are initiated. Examples include:

  — Self-referral/direct access

  — Request for consultation from another practitioner

- Documentation should include indication of no shows and cancellations.

3. Initial Examination/Evaluation

    a. Examination (history, systems review, and tests and measures)

       History

       Documentation of history may include the following:

       - General demographics
       - Social history
       - Employment/work (job/school/play)
       - Growth and development
       - Living environment
       - General health status (self-report, family report, caregiver report)
       - Social/health habits (past and current)
       - Family history
       - Medical/surgical history
       - Current condition(s)/chief complaint(s)
       - Functional status and activity level
       - Medications
       - Other clinical tests

Systems Review

Documentation of systems review may include gathering data for the following systems:

- Cardiovascular/pulmonary
  — Blood pressure
  — Edema
  — Heart rate
  — Respiratory rate
- Integumentary
  — Pliability (texture)
  — Presence of scar formation
  — Skin color
  — Skin integrity
- Musculoskeletal
  — Gross range of motion
  — Gross strength
  — Gross symmetry
  — Height
  — Weight
- Neuromuscular
  — Gross coordinated movement (for example, balance, locomotion, transfers, and transitions)
  — Motor function (motor control, motor learning)

Documentation of systems review may also address communication ability, affect, cognition, language, and learning style:

- Ability to make needs known
- Consciousness
- Expected emotional/behavioral responses
- Learning preferences (for example, education needs, learning barriers)
- Orientation (person, place, time)

Tests and Measures

Documentation of tests and measures may include findings for the following categories:

- Aerobic capacity/endurance

  Examples of examination findings include:

  — Aerobic capacity during functional activities
  — Aerobic capacity during standardized exercise test protocols

— Cardiovascular signs and symptoms in response to increased oxygen demand with exercise or activity

— Pulmonary signs and symptoms in response to increased oxygen demand with exercise or activity

- Anthropometric characteristics

Examples of examination findings include:

— Body composition

— Body dimensions

— Edema

- Arousal, attention, and cognition

Examples of examination findings include:

— Arousal and attention

— Cognition

— Communication

— Consciousness

— Motivation

— Orientation to time, person, place, and situation

— Recall

- Assistive and adaptive devices

Examples of examination findings include:

— Assistive or adaptive devices and equipment use during functional activities

— Components, alignment, fit, and ability to care for the assistive or adaptive devices and equipment

— Remediation of impairments, functional limitations, or disabilities with use of assistive or adaptive devices and equipment

— Safety during use of assistive or adaptive devices and equipment

- Circulation (arterial, venous, lymphatic)

Examples of examination findings include:

— Cardiovascular signs

— Cardiovascular symptoms

— Physiological responses to position change

- Cranial and peripheral nerve integrity

Examples of examination findings include:

— Electrophysiological integrity

— Motor distribution of the cranial nerves

— Motor distribution of the peripheral nerves

— Response to neural provocation

— Response to stimuli, including auditory, gustatory, olfactory, pharyngeal, vestibular, and visual

— Sensory distribution of the cranial nerves

— Sensory distribution of the peripheral nerves

- Environmental, home, and work (job/school/play) barriers

Examples of examination findings include:

— Current and potential barriers

— Physical space and environment

- Ergonomics and body mechanics

Examples of examination findings for ergonomics include:

— Dexterity and coordination during work

— Functional capacity and performance during work actions, tasks, or activities

— Safety in work environments

— Specific work conditions or activities

— Tools, devices, equipment, and work-stations related to work actions, tasks, or activities

Examples of examination findings for body mechanics include:

— Body mechanics during self-care, home management, work, community, or leisure actions, tasks, or activities

- Gait, locomotion, and balance

Examples of examination findings include:

— Balance during functional activities with or without the use of assistive, adaptive, orthotic, protection, supportive, or prosthetic devices or equipment

— Balance (dynamic and static) with or without the use of assistive, adaptive, orthotic, protective, supportive, or prosthetic devices or equipment

— Gait and locomotion during functional activities with or without the use of assistive, adaptive, orthotic, protective, supportive, or prosthetic devices or equipment

— Gait and locomotion with or without the use of assistive, adaptive, orthotic, protective, supportive, or prosthetic devices or equipment

— Safety during gait, locomotion, and balance

- Integumentary integrity

  Examples of examination findings include:

  Associated skin:

  — Activities, positioning, and postures that produce or relieve trauma to the skin

  — Assistive, adaptive, orthotic, protective, supportive, or prosthetic devices and equipment that may produce or relieve trauma to the skin

  — Skin characteristics

  Wound:

  — Activities, positioning, and postures that aggravate the wound or scar or that produce or relieve trauma

  — Burn

  — Signs of infection

  — Wound characteristics

  — Wound scar tissue characteristics

- Joint integrity and mobility

  Examples of examination findings include:

  — Joint integrity and mobility

  — Joint play movements

  — Specific body parts

- Motor function

  Examples of examination findings include:

  — Dexterity, coordination, and agility

  — Electrophysiological integrity

  — Hand function

  — Initiation, modification, and control of movement patterns and voluntary postures

- Muscle performance

  Examples of examination findings include:

  — Electrophysiological integrity

  — Muscle strength, power, and endurance

  — Muscle strength, power, and endurance during functional activities

  — Muscle tension

- Neuromotor development and sensory integration

  Examples of examination findings include:

  — Acquisition and evolution of motor skills

  — Oral motor function, phonation, and speech production

  — Sensorimotor integration

- Orthotic, protective, and supportive devices

  Examples of examination findings include:

  — Components, alignment, fit, and ability to care for the orthotic, protective, and supportive devices and equipment

  — Orthotic, protective, and supportive devices and equipment use during functional activities

  — Remediation of impairments, functional limitations, or disabilities with use of orthotic, protective, and supportive devices and equipment

  — Safety during use of orthotic, protective, and supportive devices and equipment

- Pain

  Examples of examination findings include:

  — Pain, soreness, and nocioception

  — Pain in specific body parts

- Posture

  Examples of examination findings include:

  — Postural alignment and position (dynamic)

  — Postural alignment and position (static)

  — Specific body parts

- Prosthetic requirements

  Examples of examination findings include:

  — Components, alignment, fit, and ability to care for prosthetic device

  — Prosthetic device use during functional activities

  — Remediation of impairments, functional limitations, or disabilities with use of the prosthetic device

  — Residual limb or adjacent segment

  — Safety during use of the prosthetic device

- Range of motion (including muscle length)

  Examples of examination findings include:

  — Functional ROM

  — Joint active and passive movement

  — Muscle length, soft tissue extensibility, and flexibility

- Reflex integrity

  Examples of examination findings include:

  — Deep reflexes

  — Electrophysiological integrity

  — Postural reflexes and reactions, including righting, equilibrium, and protective reactions

  — Primitive reflexes and reactions

  — Resistance to passive stretch

  — Superficial reflexes and reactions

- Self-care and home management (including activities of daily living and instrumental activities of daily living)

  Examples of examination findings include:

  — Ability to gain access to home environments

  — Ability to perform self-care and home management activities with or without assistive, adaptive, orthotic, protective, supportive, or prosthetic devices and equipment

  — Safety in self-care and home management activities and environments

- Sensory integrity

  Examples of examination findings include:

  — Combined/cortical sensations

  — Deep sensations

  — Electrophysiological integrity

- Ventilation and respiration

  Examples of examination findings include:

  — Pulmonary signs of respiration/gas exchange

  — Pulmonary signs of ventilatory function

  — Pulmonary symptoms

- Work (job/school/play), community, and leisure integration or reintegration (including instrumental activities of daily living)

  Examples of examination findings include:

  — Ability to assume or resume work (job/school/plan), community, and leisure activities with or without assistive, adaptive, orthotic, protective, supportive, or prosthetic devices and equipment

  — Ability to gain access to work (job/school/play), community, and leisure environments

  — Safety in work (job/school/play), community, and leisure activities and environments

b. Evaluation

Evaluation is a thought process that may not include formal documentation. However, the evaluation process may lead to documentation of impairments, functional limitations, and disabilities using formats such as:

- A problem list

- A statement of assessment of key factors (for example, cognitive factors, co-morbidities, social support) influencing the patient/client status.

c. Diagnosis

Documentation of a diagnosis determined by the physical therapist may include impairment and functional limitations. Examples include:

- Impaired Joint Mobility, Motor Function, Muscle Performance, and Range of Motion Associated With Localized Inflammation (4E)

- Impaired Motor Function and Sensory Integrity Associated With Progressive Disorders of the Central Nervous System (5E)

- Impaired Aerobic Capacity/Endurance Associated With Cardiovascular Pump Dysfunction or Failure (6D)

- Impaired Integumentary Integrity Associated With Partial-Thickness Skin Involvement and Scar Formation (7C)

d. Prognosis

Documentation of the prognosis is typically included in the plan of care.

e. Plan of Care

Documentation of the plan of care includes the following:

- Overall goals stated in measurable terms that indicate the predicted level of improvement in function

- A general statement of interventions to be used

- Proposed duration and frequency of service required to reach the goals

- Anticipated discharge plans

4. Visit or Encounter

Documentation of each visit/encounter shall include the following elements:

- Patient/client self-report (as appropriate).

- Identification of specific interventions provided, including frequency, intensity, and duration as appropriate. Examples include:

    — Knee extension, three sets, ten repetitions, 10# weight

    — Transfer training bed to chair with sliding board

    — Equipment provided

- Changes in patient/client impairment, functional limitation, and disability status as they relate to the plan of care.

- Response to interventions, including adverse reactions, if any.

- Factors that modify frequency or intensity of intervention and progression goals, including patient/client adherence to patient/client-related instructions.

- Communication/consultation with providers/patient/client/family/significant other.

- Documentation to plan for ongoing provision of services for the next visit(s), which is suggested to include, but not be limited to:

  — The interventions with objectives

  — Progression parameters

  — Precautions, if indicated

5. Reexamination

Documentation of reexamination shall include the following elements:

- Documentation of selected components of examination to update patient's/client's impairment, function, and/or disability status

- Interpretation of findings and, when indicated, revision of goals

- When indicated, revision of plan of care, as directly correlated with goals as documented

6. Discharge or Discontinuation Summary

Documentation of discharge or discontinuation shall include the following elements:

- Current physical/functional status.

- Degree of goals achieved and reasons for goals not being achieved.

- Discharge/discontinuation plan related to the patient/client's continuing care. Examples include:

  — Home program

  — Referrals for additional services

  — Recommendations for follow-up physical therapy care

  — Family and caregiver training

  — Equipment provided

Additional Specialty Records

There are many different specialties for physicians and providers. A listing of the CMS Specialty Codes may be found in appendix C. This listing will be utilized during the enrollment process and will drive the claims payment or denials of services performed by the provider. Utilizing this list, medical practices may verify that each physician or provider is enrolled correctly.

Once the enrollment specialty has been verified, there are many other resources to assist with the appropriate documentation required in medical practice. Specialty associations offer a wealth of information specific to each specialty regarding clinical protocols and documentation requirements. Some of the resources are listed in the following paragraphs.

Regardless of the specialty, all evaluation and management visits (except time-based and preventive medicine visits) must follow either the 1995 or 1997 documentation guidelines—whichever is most advantageous to the provider. Many, but not all, EHR systems follow the

1997 documentation guidelines. It is necessary to identify which version of the documentation guidelines are being utilized when using any electronic documentation system. When medical practice documentation is assisted by use of a documentation tool, such as a preprinted form for patient visits, then either the 1995 or 1997 documentation guidelines must be applied as the template to ensure documentation compliance. Detailed information on evaluation and management documentation guidelines may be found in chapter 2. The 1995 and 1997 documentation guidelines may be found on the CD-ROM accompanying this book.

Additionally, CMS publishes the *Medicare Claims Processing Manual* and the *Medicare Benefit Policy Manual,* which provide policies and procedures that may assist in identifying the necessary documentation to support the services provided. Web links to both of these documents may be found on the CD-ROM accompanying this book. The *Medicare Claims Processing Manual* provides guidance for claims processing with sections divided by the source of the claim, along with information on appeals and proper completion of the billing forms (CMS-1500 and CMS 1450 forms). The *Medicare Benefit Policy Manual* provides coverage policies by the site/provider of service, along with documentation guidelines or exclusions of coverage.

CMS also publishes a searchable database for National Coverage Determinations (NCD) and Local Coverage Determinations (LCD). NCDs are national medical necessity and reimbursement regulations, whereas LCDs are coverage rules, at a carrier or fiscal intermediary (FI) level, that provide information on what diagnoses justify the medical necessity of a test. LCDs vary from state to state, unlike the NCD which apply equally to all states. Some NCDs or LCDs provide explicit documentation that must appear in the health record in order for the medical necessity to be supported and a claim be paid.

Check Your Understanding 1.2

1. The surgeon's preoperative evaluation should include all of the following requirements, except:

   a. Be performed no more than four days prior to the surgery
   b. Pertinent history
   c. Results of a physical
   d. Indications for surgery

2. Which of the following is included within surgery records?

   a. Preoperative, intraoperative, and postoperative anesthesia record
   b. Operative report
   c. Consent form
   d. All of the above

3. Which physician(s) are responsible for determining the appropriate preoperative medications and instructions?

   a. Surgeon
   b. Anesthesiologist
   c. Primary care provider
   d. Both A and B

4. Coverage guidelines for screening pelvic examinations are documented by the Centers for Medicare and Medicaid Services. Which of the following statements is false?

   a. The examination must include 6 of the 66 elements documented in the National Coverage Determination.
   b. The National Coverage Determination documents limitations of coverage, including frequency limitations.
   c. The examination may include the cervix, uterus, vagina, and anus.
   d. The examination may include the urethra meatus, urethra, bladder, and adnexa.

5. The rotavirus vaccine (RV) is administered to children at which interval?

   a. Administer the first does in the hospital with two additional doses at 1–2 months and 6–18 months.
   b. Administer the first dose at age 6–14 weeks (maximum age: 14 weeks 6 days). Vaccination should not be initiated for infants aged 15 weeks or older (namely, 15 weeks 0 days or older). Administer the final dose in the series by age 8 months 0 days.
   c. Administer annually to children aged 6 months to 18 years.
   d. Administer to all children aged 1 year (namely, aged 12–23 months). Administer two doses at least six months apart.

6. For chiropractic services, a subluxation may be demonstrated by which of the following?

   a. An x-ray
   b. A history of subluxation
   c. A physical examination
   d. Both a and b
   e. Both a and c

7. In reference to a physical therapy health record, which of the following statements is false?

   a. Completion of the initial examination/evaluation is typically completed in one visit, but may occur over more than one visit.
   b. Documentation of the reexamination includes the documentation of selected components of examination to update patient's/client's impairment, function, and/or disability status; interpretation of findings and, when indicated, revision of goals; and when indicated, revision of plan of care, as directly correlated with goals as documented.
   c. Documentation elements for the initial examination/evaluation include the examination, evaluation, diagnosis, prognosis, and discharge.
   d. Documentation of the plan of care includes the overall goals stated in measurable terms that indicate the predicted level of improvement in function, a general statement of interventions to be used, proposed duration and frequency of service required to reach the goals, and anticipated discharge plans.

(continued on next page)

Check Your Understanding 1.2 *(continued)*

8. In which of the following documents may information on appeals and proper completion of the billing forms be found?
   a. *Medicare Benefit Policy Manual*
   b. 1995 or 1997 Documentation Guidelines for evaluation and management coding
   c. *Medicare Claims Processing Manual*
   d. Specialty Code Listing

9. In regard to National and Local Coverage Determinations, which of the following statements is false?
   a. Local and National Coverage Determinations are the same policies, but have different titles.
   b. National Coverage Determinations are federal guidelines that apply to all states.
   c. Some National and Local Coverage Determinations provide explicit documentation that must appear in the health record in order for the medical necessity to be supported and a claim be paid.
   d. Local Coverage Determinations are state-specific guidelines and published for each state.

10. Which specialty listed below is not required to follow 1995 or 1997 documentation guidelines for evaluation and management visits?
    a. Obstetrics and gynecology
    b. Pediatrics
    c. Ophthalmology
    d. All of the above specialties must follow either 1995 or 1997 documentation guidelines for evaluation and management visits

Consent Forms

The practice of obtaining consent before medical and surgical procedures are performed is based on the legal definition of battery, which is the unlawful touching of a person without implied or expressed consent. *Implied* consent is inferred when a patient voluntarily submits to treatment, the rationale being that it is reasonable to assume that the patient understands the nature of the treatment or would not submit. *Expressed* consent is that which is spoken or written. Although courts have recognized both forms, spoken consent is more difficult to prove.

Decisions regarding which situations require a written consent (as opposed to the physician documenting informed consent in the progress notes) are set by facility policy. Generally, procedures that involve interference with body tissues, significant risks, or possible dispute concerning the patient's agreement require written consent. State law also may mandate written consent forms (for example, consent for HIV testing). Some common written consents include:

- Authorization to treat a minor child (kept on file for times when the parent does not accompany the child to a visit or when the parent is out of town and the child is being cared for by another person) (An example of a patient authorization for Personal Representative is included in the Sample Forms folder on the CD-ROM accompanying this book.)

- Colonoscopy

- Experimental drugs or medications used for reasons not approved by the FDA
- Flexible sigmoidoscopy
- HIV testing
- Minor surgery or biopsy
- Sigmoidoscopy
- Sterilization
- Upper gastrointestinal endoscopy
- Use of contrast material during a radiologic procedure
- Use of experimental drugs
- Vaccination (often incorporated into the vaccine administration record)

For a written consent to be legally valid, the following conditions must be met:

- The patient must be legally competent (consent should be obtained from a legal guardian or another legal representative of mentally incapacitated patients or minors as determined by state law)
- Consent must be obtained voluntarily
- Consent must be informed, which means that the patient has received the information necessary to make a reasonable decision and understands the following:
  — Plan of treatment
  — Explanation of treatment in nontechnical language
  — Need for treatment
  — Alternative treatments
  — Risks associated with the procedure
  — Probability of success
  — Prognosis if treatment were not provided

General consent forms should be used with caution because they do not necessarily mean that the patient understands the treatment. Special consent forms, used for nonroutine treatments, inform the patient of the nature and purpose of the treatment in addition to any risks involved. Special consent forms should be obtained under the following circumstances:

- Major or minor surgery involving an entry into the body, through either an incision or a natural body opening
- All procedures involving use of anesthesia, regardless of whether an entry into the body is involved
- Nonsurgical procedures, including the administration of medicines, that involve more than a slight risk of harm to the patient or that may cause a change in the patient's body structure (such procedures include, but are not limited to, chemotherapy for cancer, hormone treatments, and diagnostic procedures such as myelograms, arteriograms, and pyelograms)

- All forms of radiological therapy

- Electroconvulsive therapy

- All experimental procedures

- All other procedures that require a specific explanation to the patient as determined by the medical staff

Any doubts about the necessity of obtaining a special consent from the patient for a procedure should be resolved in favor of obtaining the consent. The Sample Forms folder on the CD-ROM accompanying this book contains the following examples of consent forms:

- Consent to treat

- Consent for anesthesia

- Consent for an operation

- Consent for an HIV test

- Consent for ultrasound

According to the ACOG Resource Manual, if a patient refuses to sign a recommended test, treatment, or procedure, this refusal should also be documented (ACOG 2007). Documentation should include the following:

- That the clinician recommended a particular test, treatment, or procedure to the patient

- That the clinician explained the need for the test, treatment, or procedure, and the benefits and risks involved

- That the clinician explained the consequences of the refusing the recommendation

- That the patient refused the test, treatment, or procedure and the patient's reason for refusal

- Practitioners also should comply with specific state and federal informed consent laws and regulations that apply to specific treatments or procedures (ACOG 2007, 125).

Conclusion

Accreditation standards, state and federal laws, and facility policies all contribute to the content and format of a medical practice health record. Although these influences are important and must be complied with, it is important to keep in mind the primary purpose of the health record: to facilitate effective patient healthcare. Whether in electronic or paper-based format, health records need to be organized so that information is easily retrievable, complete, and leads to wise treatment decisions on the part of the healthcare provider.

References

American Academy of Urgent Care Medicine. 2009. http://aaucm.org/default.aspx.

American Chiropractic Association. n.d. Commentary on Centers for Medicare and Medicaid Services (CMS)/ PART clinical documentation guidelines. http://www.acatoday.org/pdf/part_process.pdf.

American College of Obstetricians and Gynecologists. 2007. *Guidelines to Women's Health: A Resource Manual.* Washington, DC: ACOG.

American Health Information Management Association. 2010. *Pocket Glossary for Health Information Management and Technology,* Chicago: AHIMA.

American Medical Association. 1999. *New Framework Documentation Guidelines.* Chicago: AMA.

American Physical Therapy Association. 2008 (December). *Guidelines: Physical Therapy Documentation of Patient/Client Management BOD G03-05-16-41.* Alexandria, VA: APTA.

American Society of Anesthesiologists. 2008. *Statement on Documentation of Anesthesia Care.* Park Ridge, IL: ASA.

Centers for Medicare and Medicaid Services. 2006. National coverage determination for screening pap smears and pelvic examination for early detection of cervical or vaginal cancer (210.2). http://www.cms.hhs.gov/mcd/viewncd.asp?ncd_id=210.2&ncd_version=3&basket=ncd%3A210%2E2%3A3%3AScreening+Pap+Smears+and+Pelvic+Examinations+for+Early+Detection+of+Cervical+or+Vaginal+Cancer.

Center for Medicare and Medicaid Services. 2009. *Medicare Benefit Policy Manual.* http://www.cms.hhs.gov/Manuals/IOM/itemdetail.asp?filterType=none&filterByDID=-99&sortByDID=1&sortOrder=ascending&itemID=CMS012673&intNumPerPage=10.

Institute of Medicine. 2007. *Preventing Medication Errors.* Washington, DC: The National Academies Press. http://books.nap.edu/openbook.php?record_id=11623&page=R1).

Joint Commission. 2009. *Comprehensive Accreditation Manual for Ambulatory Care.* Oakbrook Terrace, IL: Joint Commission.

LaTour, K.M., and S. Eichenwald Maki, eds. 2010. *Health Information Management: Concepts, Principles, and Practices,* 3rd ed. Chicago: AHIMA.

National Committee for Quality Assurance. 2009. *Standards for Managed Care Organizations.* Washington, DC: NCQA.

Odom-Welsey, B., D. Brown, and C.L. Meyers. 2009. *Documentation for Medical Records.* Chicago: AHIMA.

Office of the National Coordinator for Health Information Technology. 2008 (March 21). Patient–Provider secure messaging.

Chapter 2

Advanced Practice Nurses and Physician Assistants

Carolyn Buppert, JD, NP

Learning Objectives

- Identify the underlying purpose of documentation for billing purposes
- Gain a general understanding of the general principles of medical record documentation of medical and surgical services
- Explore a situation where "incident-to" billing would be appropriate
- Understand the appropriate minimum documentation by providers for a shared/split visit
- Explore the relationship between sufficient documentation and reimbursement for services

Key Terms

Advanced practice nurse
Certified nurse-midwife
  (CNM)
Certified registered nurse
  anesthetist (CRNA)
Chief complaint
Clinical nurse specialist
Evaluation and management
  (E/M) services

Family history
History
History of present illness
  (HPI)
Incident to
National Provider Identifier
  (NPI) number

Nurse practitioner
Past history
Physician assistant
Review of systems (ROS)
Shared/split visit
Social history

Documentation Requirements of Advanced Practice Nurses and Physician Assistants

Physician assistants and certain types of nurses may function similarly to physicians in medical practices. They may perform evaluation and management, consultations, and a variety of therapies and diagnostic procedures. The requirements of documentation for these providers are, for the most part, the same as for physicians. Namely, there are four objectives of documentation:

1. To show that the service was medically necessary

2. To justify billing the service at the level billed

3. To demonstrate that the standard of care was met, if needed, in order to defend against an action for malpractice

4. To assist providers who follow in performing subsequent care

For example, if performing and billing evaluation and management services of a new patient in the office setting, a provider would be required under Medicare's rules to document that the patient had symptoms requiring evaluation. If a level 4 established office visit (99214) was billed, the provider would need to document that he or she performed a detailed history, detailed physical examination, and medical decision making of moderate complexity, as well as a chief complaint and any counseling regarding a diagnosis or treatment. To document that the practitioner met the standard of care, the provider might need to document that he or she advised the patient to call the provider that evening if the complaint of severe headache got worse as the day went on. In addition, the provider might need to document that he or she prescribed a specific controlled substance, so that a following provider would know not to prescribe the same or similar medication a short time later.

In several states, there is a fifth objective of documentation. Some states require that a physician review a percentage of progress note generated by an advanced practice nurse or physician assistant. To determine state law on this issue, visit the Board of Nursing Web site (specifically the section on laws and regulations) or the Board of Medicine Web site (specifically the section addressing physician assistants). For contact information for boards of nursing, visit https://www.ncsbn.org/515.htm. For links to state medical boards, visit http://www.ama-assn.org/ama/pub/education-careers/becoming-physician/medical-licensure/state-medical-boards.shtml.

This chapter focuses on the requirements for documenting for billing purposes. For more information on documenting to defend a lawsuit, see *Avoiding Malpractice* by Carol Buppert.

General Principles of Health Record Documentation for Physicians, Advanced Practice Nurses, and Physician Assistants

The general principles of health record documentation of medical and surgical services are:

1. Medical records should be complete and legible.

2. Documentation of each patient encounter should include:

    a. Reason for encounter ("chief complaint") and history relevant to that complaint ("history of present illness");

    b. Physical examination findings and prior diagnostic test results;

    c. Assessment, clinical impression, and diagnosis;

    d. Plan for care; and

    e. Date and legible identity of observer.

3. Rationale for ordering diagnostic tests or ancillary services. If not documented, the rationale for ordering diagnostic and other ancillary services should be easily inferred.

4. Past and present diagnoses should be accessible for treating and/or consulting physician.

5. Appropriate health risk factors should be identified.

6. Patient's progress, response to changes in treatment, and revision of diagnosis should be documented (CMS 1997).

The Social Security Act states that all Medicare Part B services, including mental health services, must be "reasonable and necessary for the diagnosis or treatment of an illness or injury or to improve the functioning of a member" (SSA, Section 1862(a)(1)(A)). For every service billed, providers must indicate the specific sign, symptom, or patient complaint necessitating the service.

Signature Requirements

According to the *Medicare Program Integrity Manual*, "Medicare requires a legible identifier for services provided/ordered. The method used shall be hand written or an electronic signature (stamp signatures are not acceptable) to sign an order or other medical record documentation for medical review purposes. All State licensure and State practice regulations continue to apply. Where State law is more restrictive than Medicare, the contractor needs to apply the State law standard" (CMS 2009).

Figure 2.1 shows an example of signature requirements for Palmetto, Ohio's Part B carrier, which were published for implementation on April 28, 2008.

Evaluation and Management Professional Services

The Centers for Medicare and Medicaid Services (CMS) provides extensive detail about what the documentation should contain. CMS's *Documentation Guidelines for Evaluation and Management Services* is the standard for all payers, and is to be used with Medicare patients without exception. These guidelines specify the history, examination, and medical decision making that a provider must document in order to justify a bill for evaluation and management of professional services completed in medical practices. For new and established office or other outpatient visits, there are four levels of history: problem focused, expanded problem focused, detailed, and comprehensive. There are also four levels of physical examinations for these types of patient visits: problem focused, expanded problem focused, detailed, and comprehensive. The medical decision making is limited to four levels for office and other outpatient visits: straightforward, low, moderate, and high. These guidelines are at http://www.cms.hhs.gov/MLNEdwebGuide/25_EMDOC.asp. There are two versions—1995 and 1997. A provider may use either version of the documentation guidelines. Both the 1995 and 1997 documentation guidelines can be found on the CD-ROM that accompanies this book.

The documentation guidelines call for a provider to record:

- Patient history, including chief complaint, history of present illness, past medical history, past social history, family history, and review of systems

- Physical examination

- Medical decision making

Figure 2.1.   Signature requirements for Palmetto, Ohio's Part B carrier

Acceptable methods of signing records/test orders and findings include:

• Handwritten signatures or initials

• Electronic signatures:

  – Digitized signature—an electronic image of an individual's handwritten signature reproduced in its identical form using a pen tablet

  – Electronic signatures usually contain date and timestamps and include printed statements, e.g., 'electronically signed by,' or 'verified/reviewed by,' followed by the practitioner's name and preferably a professional designation. Note: The responsibility and authorship related to the signature should be clearly defined in the record

  – Digital signature—an electronic method of a written signature that is typically generated by special encrypted software that allows for sole usage

Note: Be aware that electronic and digital signatures are not the same as 'auto-authentication' or 'auto-signature' systems, some of which do not mandate or permit the provider to review an entry before signing. Indications that a document has been, 'Signed but not read' are not acceptable as part of the medical record.

Acceptable Signature Examples

• Chart 'Accepted By' with provider's name

• 'Electronically signed by' with provider's name

• 'Verified by' with provider's name

• 'Reviewed by' with provider's name

• 'Released by' with provider's name

• 'Signed by' with provider's name

• 'Signed before import by' with provider's name

• 'Signed: John Smith, M.D.' with provider's name

• Digitalized signature: Handwritten and scanned into the computer

• 'This is an electronically verified report by John Smith, M.D.'

• 'Authenticated by John Smith, M.D.'

• 'Authorized by: John Smith, M.D.'

• 'Digital Signature: John Smith, M.D.'

• 'Confirmed by' with provider's name

• 'Closed by' with provider's name

• 'Finalized by' with provider's name

• 'Electronically approved by' with provider's name

Unacceptable Signatures

• Signature 'stamps' alone in medical records are no longer recognized as valid authentication for Medicare signature purposes and may result in payment denials by Medicare

• Reports or any records that are dictated and/or transcribed, but do not include valid signatures 'finalizing and approving' the documents are not acceptable for reimbursement purposes. Corresponding claims for these services will be denied.

Unacceptable Signature Examples

• 'Signing physician' when provider's name is typed
  Example: Signing physician: _____
                                      John Smith, M.D.

• 'Confirmed by' when a provider's name is typed
  Example: Confirmed by: _____
                                  John Smith, M.D.

• 'Signed by' followed by provider's name typed and the signing line above, but done as part of the transcription.

• 'This document has been electronically signed in the surgery department' with no provider name.

• 'Dictated by' when provider's name is typed
  Example: Dictated by: _____
                                John Smith, M.D.

• Signature stamp

• 'Signature On File'

An assistant at surgery is not required to also sign the operative report in addition to the responsible surgeon when reference is made in the note that identifies the assistant, provided that the report contains an acceptable signature by the responsible surgeon.

Co-Surgeons must follow the signature requirements and provide an acceptable signature.

Signatures of scribes are not required. The scribe's name needs to be listed in the medical record and identified as a scribe. The signature requirements for the billing provider still apply.

Source: Palmetto GBA, LLC 2009.

- Counseling

- Coordination of care

Documentation Guidelines

The following material, through the section heading "Commercial Payers," is a summary of an excerpt from the CMS documentation guidelines, 1995 and 1997 versions (unless noted).

History-taking, in General

The chief complaint, review of systems, and past, social, and family history may be listed as separate elements of the history, or they may be included in the description of the history of the present illness.

A review of systems and/or a past, family, and/or social history obtained during an earlier encounter does not need to be re-recorded if there is evidence that the physician reviewed and updated the previous information. This may occur when a physician updates his or her own record or in an institutional setting or group practice where many physicians use a common record. The review and update may be documented by:

- describing any new review of system data and/or past, family, and/or social history information, or noting there has been no change in the information; and

- noting the date and location of the earlier review of systems and/or past, family, and/or social history.

The review of systems and past, family, and/or social history may be recorded by ancillary staff or on a form completed by the patient. To document that the physician reviewed the information, there must be a notation supplementing or confirming the information recorded by others.

If the physician is unable to obtain a history from the patient or other source, the record should describe the patient's condition or other circumstance that precludes obtaining a history.

Chief Complaint

The health record should clearly reflect the chief complaint.

History of Present Illness (HPI)

To qualify for a brief HPI (for example, 99201, 99202, 99212 or 99213), the health record should describe one to three elements of the present illness.

To qualify for an extended HPI (for example, 99203, 99204, 99205, 99214 or 99215), the health record should describe four or more elements of the present illness or associated co-morbidities or provide the status of three or more chronic diseases.

Review of Systems (ROS)

For a problem pertinent review of systems (for example, 99202 or 99213), the patient's positive responses and pertinent negatives for the system related to the problem should be documented.

For an extended review of systems (99203 or 99214), the patient's positive responses and pertinent negatives for systems should be documented.

For a complete review of systems (for example, 99204, 99205 or 99215), at least 10 organ systems should be reviewed. Organ systems include:

- Constitutional symptoms
- Eyes
- Ears, nose, mouth, and throat
- Cardiovascular
- Respiratory
- Gastrointestinal
- Genitourinary
- Musculoskeletal
- Integumentary
- Neurological
- Psychiatric
- Endocrine
- Hematologic/lymphatic
- Allergic/immunologic

Those systems with positive or pertinent negative responses must be individually documented. For the remaining systems, a notation indicating all other systems are negative is permissible as long as the provider can prove that the patient was asked the questions regarding these systems. In the absence of such a notation, at least 10 systems must be individually documented.

Past, Family, and/or Social History (PFSH)

For a pertinent PFSH (for example, 99203 or 99214), at least one specific item from any of the three history areas must be documented. The three history areas are: past, family, and social.

For a complete PFSH, at least one specific item from two of the three history areas must be documented for an established patient office visit (99215) and at least one specific item from each of the three history areas must be documented for a new patient office visit (99204 or 99205).

Examination

Specific abnormal and relevant negative findings of the examination of the affected or symptomatic body area(s) or organ system(s) should be documented. A notation of "abnormal" without elaboration is insufficient.

Abnormal or unexpected findings of the examination of the unaffected or asymptomatic body area(s) or organ system(s) should be described. Figure 2.2 lists the body areas and organ systems.

A brief statement or notation indicating "negative" or "normal" is sufficient to document normal findings related to unaffected areas or asymptomatic organ systems. Many providers

Figure 2.2. Physical examination body areas and organ systems

Body Area	Organ System
Head, including face	Constitutional
Chest, breasts, axillae	Eyes
Abdomen	Ears, nose, mouth, and throat
Genitalia, groin, buttocks	Cardiovascular
Back, spine	Respiratory
Each extremity	Gastrointestinal
	Genitourinary
	Musculoskeletal
	Skin
	Neurologic
	Psychiatric
	Hematologic/lymphatic/immunologic

may opt to utilize a check-off box format in the paper-based health record or menu selection clicks in the electronic health record.

For a multisystem examination, the health record should include findings from 8 or more of the 12 organ systems. The 1995 documentation guidelines state that a general multisystem exam is a comprehensive examination.

Medical Decision Making

Diagnosis and Management Options, in General

For each encounter, an assessment, clinical impression, or diagnosis should be documented. It may be explicitly stated or implied in documented decisions regarding management plans and/or further evaluation.

For a presenting problem with an established diagnosis, the health record should reflect whether the problem is a) improved, well controlled, resolving, or resolved; or, b) inadequately controlled, worsening, or failing to change as expected.

For a presenting problem without an established diagnosis, the assessment or clinical impression may be stated in the form of a differential diagnosis or as a "possible," "probable," or "rule out" diagnosis. However, diagnoses documented differentials, such as "possible," "probable," "rule out," to name a few, are not codable and thus require the symptoms to be documented in order for accurate coding to be reported on the claim form.

Unexpected examination findings of an unaffected area should be documented.

The initiation or changes in treatment should be documented. Treatment includes a wide range of management options including patient instructions, nursing instructions, therapies, and medications.

If referrals are made, consultations requested, or advice sought, the health record should indicate to whom or where the referral or consultation is made or from whom the advice is requested, along with the reason for the consultation or referral.

Data Reviewed

If a diagnostic service (test or procedure) is ordered, planned, scheduled, or performed at the time of the encounter, the type of service—such as lab or x-ray—should be documented.

The review of lab, radiology and/or other diagnostic tests should be documented. An entry in a progress note such as "WBC elevated" or "chest x-ray unremarkable" is acceptable. Alternatively, the review may be documented by initialing and dating the report containing the test results.

A decision to obtain old records or decision to obtain additional history from the family, caretaker, or other source to supplement that obtained from the patient should be documented.

Relevant findings from the review of old records, and/or the receipt of additional history from the family, caretaker, or other source should be documented. If there is no relevant information beyond that already obtained, that fact should be documented. A notation of "old records reviewed" or "additional history obtained from family" without elaboration is insufficient.

The results of discussion of laboratory, radiology, or other diagnostic tests with the physician who performed or interpreted the study should be documented.

The direct visualization and independent interpretation of an image, tracing, or specimen previously or subsequently interpreted by another physician should be documented.

Risk of Significant Complications, Morbidity, and/or Mortality

Comorbidities, underlying diseases, or other factors that increase the complexity of medical decision making by increasing the risk of complications, morbidity, and/or mortality should be documented.

Risk is evaluated based on the impression of the problem as it exists after the current evaluation.

If a surgical or invasive diagnostic procedure is ordered, planned, or scheduled at the time of the evaluation and management encounter, the type of procedure (for example, laparoscopy) should be documented.

If a surgical or invasive diagnostic procedure is performed at the time of the evaluation and management encounter, the specific procedure should be documented.

The referral for or decision to perform a surgical or invasive diagnostic procedure on an urgent basis should be documented or implied.

Appendix D documents a sample table of risk for medical decision making.

Counseling and Coordination of Care

If the physician elects to report the level of service based on counseling and/or coordination of care, the total length of time of the encounter (face-to-face or floor time, as appropriate) should be documented and the record should describe the counseling and/or activities to coordinate care (CMS 1995, 1997).

In the case where counseling and/or coordination of care dominates (more than 50% of) the provider/patient and/or family encounter (face-to-face time in the medical practice or other outpatient setting, floor/unit time in the hospital or nursing facility), time is considered the key or controlling factor to qualify for a particular level of evaluation and management service. The documentation requirements for timed-based evaluation and management services are as follows:

- Total length of time of the encounter (face-to-face or floor time, as appropriate)

- Proof that more than 50% of the total time was spent counseling and/or coordinating care

- Detailed description of the counseling and/or activities to coordinate care

Figure 2.3. **Time-based evaluation and management typical times**

Office or Outpatient Visit	Face-to-face Time (minutes)
99201	10
99202	20
99203	30
99204	45
99205	60
99211	5
99212	10
99213	15
99214	25
99215	40

Figure 2.3 lists the total minutes as documented in the American Medical Association's Current Procedural Terminology.

Commercial Payers

Although many commercial payers follow CMS documentation guidelines, they may publish additional and sometimes more specific guidelines that they require. Here are selected "Medical Record Documentation Standards" from CareFirst Blue Cross Blue Shield:

- Medical record is clearly organized.

- Records are organized in chronological order.

- Medical record does not contain information for other patients. Exception: Family members in one record must be clearly separated.

- Patient name or an identification number is found on each page of record.

- Handwritten entries are legible to a reader other than the author.

- Content of records is presented in a standard format that allows a reader, other than the author, to review without the use of separate legend/key.

- Entries and updates to a record are dated.

- Documentation of medical encounters must be in the record within 72 hours or three business days of occurrence.

- Entries are initialed or signed by the author.

- Author identification may be a handwritten signature, unique electronic identifier, or initials. (Applies to practitioners and members of their office staff who contribute to the record.)

- When initials are used, there is a designation of signature and status maintained in the office.

- Includes information necessary to identify patient and insurer and to submit claims.

- Information may be maintained in a computerized database as long as it is retrievable and can be printed as needed to transfer the record to another practitioner or for monitoring purposes.

- Name of the PCP for the patient is indicated in the record (in a group practice, the designated PCP may be documented in the office records).

- Initial history and physical examinations for new patients are recorded within 12 months of a patient first seeking care or within three visits, whichever occurs first. If applicable, there is written evidence that the practitioner advised the patient to return for a physical examination. The records of a complete history and physical, included in the medical chart, and done within the past 12 months by another physician, will satisfy this standard. In pediatric practices well-child visits satisfy this standard.

- History and physical documentation contains pertinent information such as age, height, vital signs, past medical and behavioral health history, preventive health maintenance and risk screening, physical examination, medical impression, and the ordering of appropriate diagnostic tests, procedures, and medications. Self-administered patient questionnaires are acceptable to obtain baseline past medical history and personal information. There is written documentation to explain the lack of information contained in the medical record regarding the history and physical (for example, poor historians, patient's inability or unwillingness to provide information).

- Patient record contains immediate family history or documentation that it is non-contributory.

- Pediatric records should include gestational and birth history documentation and should be age and diagnosis appropriate.

- Medication allergies or history of adverse reactions to medications are displayed in a prominent and consistent location or noted as "none" or "NKA." (Examples of where allergies may be prominently displayed include on a cover sheet inside the chart, at the top of every visit page, or on a medication record in the chart.)

- When applicable and known, there is documentation of the date the allergy was first discovered.

- Primary care physician must have documentation in the record regarding smoking habits, sexual behavior, and history of alcohol use and substance abuse for patients 12 years of age and older who have been seen three or more times.

- A problem list that summarizes important patient medical information, such as a patient's major diagnoses, past medical and/or surgical history, and recurrent complaints.

- Continuity of care between multiple practitioners in the same practice is demonstrated by documentation and review of pertinent medical information.

- A patient's chief complaint or purpose for a visit, as stated by the patient, is recorded. The documentation supports that the patient's perceived needs/expectations were addressed.

- Telephone encounters (phone contact) relevant to medical issues are documented in the medical record and reflect practitioner review.

- Clinical assessment and/or physical findings are documented and correspond to the patient's chief complaint, purpose for seeking care, and/or ongoing care for chronic illnesses.

- Working diagnoses or medical impressions that logically follow from the clinical assessment and physical examination are recorded.

- Proposed treatment plans, therapies, or other regimens are documented and logically follow previously documented diagnoses and medical impressions.

- Rationale for treatment decisions appear medically appropriate and substantiated by documentation in the record.

- Laboratory tests are performed at appropriate intervals.

- The medical record shows clear justification for diagnostic and therapeutic procedures.

- Continuity of care from one visit to the next is demonstrated when follow-up of unresolved problems from previous visits is documented in subsequent visit notes.

- Return to office (RTO) in a specified amount of time is recorded at time of visit, or as follow-up consultation, laboratory, or other diagnostic reports.

- Follow-up is documented for patients who require periodic visits for a chronic illness and for patients who require reassessment following an episodic illness.

- Patient involvement in the coordination of care is demonstrated through patient education, follow-up, and return visits.

- Information regarding current medications is readily apparent from review of the record.

- Changes to medication regimen are noted as they occur. When medications appear to remain unchanged, the record includes documentation of at least annual review by the practitioner.

- When the patient is being seen by multiple practitioners, such as specialists or behavioral health practitioners, there is documentation of consideration of medication interaction.

- Education may correspond directly to the reason for the visit—to specific diagnosis-related issues such as dietary instruction to reduce cholesterol.

- Examples of patient noncompliance are documented.

- Each patient record includes documentation that preventive services were ordered and performed, or that the practitioner discussed preventive services with the patient and the patient chose to defer or refuse them. Practitioners may document that a patient sought preventive services from another practitioner—for example, OB/GYN.

- The patient record includes documentation of immunizations administered from birth to present for members. When prior records are unavailable, practitioners may document that a child's parent or guardian affirmed that immunizations were administered by another practitioner and the approximate age or date the immunizations were given.

- If a consultation, the clinical assessment supports the decision for a referral for a consultation.

- Referrals are provided in a timely manner according to the severity of the patient's condition.

- Results of all lab and other diagnostic tests are documented in the medical record.

- Records demonstrate that the practitioner reviews laboratory and diagnostic reports and makes treatment decisions based on report findings. Reports within the review period are initialed and dated by the practitioner, or another system of ensuring practitioner review is in place.

- Patients are notified of abnormal laboratory and diagnostic results and advised of recommendations regarding follow-up or changes in the treatment. The record documents patient notification of abnormal results. A practitioner may document that the patient is to call regarding results; however, the practitioner is responsible for ensuring that the patient is advised of any abnormal results.

- Consultation reports reflect practitioner review.

- Primary care physician records include consultation reports/summaries (within 60 to 90 days) that correspond to specialist referrals, or documentation that physician attempted to obtain reports that were not received.

- Subsequent visit notes reflect results of the consultation as may be pertinent to ongoing patient care.

- Specialist records include a consultation report/summary addressed to the referral source.

- When a patient receives services at or through another provider, such as a hospital, emergency care, home care agency, skilled nursing facility, or behavioral health specialist, there is evidence of coordination of care through consultation reports, discharge summaries, status reports, or home health reports. The discharge summary includes the reason for admission, the treatment provided and the instructions given to the patient (CareFirst Blue Cross Blue Shield 2008).

Documentation Requirements Specific to Nurse Practitioners and Physician Assistants

Nurse practitioners and midwives are the two categories of advanced practice nurses most likely to be employed by medical practices and practicing in the office setting, so this chapter will discuss documentation relevant to those two categories of nurses. The documentation requirements are identical for nurse practitioners and nurse midwives. Generally, the documentation requirements for nurse practitioners and nurse midwives are the same as for physicians.

The documentation requirements for physician assistants are the same as for nurse practitioners, nurse midwives, and physicians. Some states require that physician assistants' charts be cosigned by a physician, while other states have no requirement for chart cosignature by physicians in a law or rule (AAPA 2009). Appendix E reveals the state-by-state regulations for cosignature requirements for physician assistants.

Incident-to Billing and Shared/Split Visits

In certain circumstances, Medicare allows visits performed by advanced practice nurses or physician assistants to be billed under a physician's National Provider Identifier (NPI) number. The rules addressing these circumstances are called the "incident to" rules and the "shared/split visits" rules. Both sets of rules include requirements regarding documentation. If the rules are followed, a practice can receive 100% of the physician fee schedule rather than 85%. In general, procedures performed by nurse practitioners and physician assistants are reimbursed by Medicare at 85% of the physician fee schedule rate. (Commercial payers and Medicaid may have similar reimbursement policies.) Both the incident-to and shared/split visit rules call for documentation of physician involvement, in addition to the documentation of services the nurse practitioner or physician assistant has performed.

The rules are complicated and frequently misunderstood. Here are the basic requirements of the rules.

Incident-to Billing

When a physician and nurse practitioner or physician assistant both are working in an office or clinic, Medicare may allow the physician to bill services performed by a nurse practitioner under the physician's NPI number. When billing "incident-to," adherence to the rules is imperative as a practice that bills inappropriately may be required to repay 15% of each claim, along with fines and interest. In addition, the government may mandate compliance activities.

The rules on incident-to billing are found in the *Medicare Benefit Policy Manual*, Chapter 15—Covered Medical and Other Health Services, Section 50.3 for drugs and biologicals, Section 60.1 to 60.3 for office and clinic professional services, Section 230.5 for physical therapy, occupational therapy, and speech-language pathology services, and Section 300.4.1 for diabetes self-management training services.

The requirements for billing a nurse practitioner's services incident to a physician's services as stated in the *Medicare Benefit Policy Manual* are:

   a. The services must be an integral, although incidental, part of the physician's professional service.

   b. The services must be commonly rendered without charge or included in the physician's bill.

   c. The services must be of a type commonly furnished in physician's offices or clinics.

   d. The services must be furnished under the physician's direct personal supervision. Direct supervision does not require the physician's presence in the same examination room, but the physician must be present in the same office suite and immediately available.

   e. Incident-to billing is not an option when services are performed in a hospital or nursing facility, unless a physician has an office in the nursing facility.

   f. When services are performed in the patient's home, incident-to billing is an option only when both the physician and nurse practitioner are present in the patient's home at the time services were performed.

   g. The services must be furnished by an individual who is an employee, leased employee, or independent contractor of the physician of the practice that employs or contracts with both physician and nurse practitioner.

   h. The physician must perform "the initial service and subsequent services of a frequency which reflect his or her active participation in the management of the course of treatment" (CMS 2003, Chapter 15, Section 60.1 B).

   i. The physician or other provider under whose name and NPI number the bill is submitted must be the individual present in the office suite when the service is provided.

   j. The medically necessary service must be one that would be covered if furnished by the physician.

Example

A physician who employs a nurse practitioner evaluates a patient and diagnoses hypertension. The physician initiates treatment. The nurse practitioner conducts follow-up visits with the patient, monitoring and treating the hypertension over weeks, months, or years. The physician sees the patient every third visit, under a policy adopted by the medical practice. The nurse practitioner's services (the follow-up visits) may be billed under the physician's NPI number, and the practice will receive Medicare's Physicians Fee Schedule rate (Medicare payment plus patient copay amount) for the services performed by the nurse practitioner.

However, if the hypertensive patient arrives for a visit with the nurse practitioner, and announces a new complaint—sinusitis, for example—incident-to billing is inappropriate. Among auditors and providers, there may be differing interpretations of the phrase "the physician must perform an initial service," found in the incident-to rules. The CMS has not defined "initial service." Providers may interpret this rule to mean that the first visit to the practice must be conducted by the physician. However, auditors interpret "perform an initial service" as referring to an episode of illness, namely if there is a new problem, the nurse practitioner must make a choice—bill under his or her own NPI number or send the patient to the physician for an initial service for the new complaint.

Because CMS has not elaborated on the phrase "subsequent services of a frequency which reflect his/her active participation in and management of the course of treatment," it is not possible to provide clear direction about the frequency of physician involvement that CMS expects. For example, active participation may mean chart review, care oversight through discussions with a nurse practitioner, or periodic face-to-face visits, depending upon the reader's interpretation. It is unlikely, given this vague language, that prosecutors could make a case that a physician did not see a patient often enough to engage in incident-to billing if a physician had documented any involvement in the care of a patient. If active participation means periodic visits, CMS has not provided guidance as to the frequency of physician visits that would indicate "active participation."

However, auditors or prosecutors could prove that incident-to rules were not followed if a practice billed a CPT code for a new patient visit under a physician's NPI number and supported the bill with a progress note written by a nurse practitioner. Furthermore, prosecutors could prove that the incident-to rules were not followed if a practice billed a visit under a physician's NPI number, supported the bill with a progress note written by a nurse practitioner, and could not establish that the physician was in the suite at the time of the visit.

Documentation to Support Incident-to Billing

If a Medicare contractor conducts an audit with incident-to billing in mind, the investigator will look for evidence that the rules were followed. First, an auditor will examine bills for new patient visits, and the accompanying documentation, to determine whether any visits conducted by an advanced practice nurse or physician assistant were billed under a physician's NPI number. Second, the auditor will review documentation for established patient visits, to see whether a physician provided an initial service and whether a physician has remained involved in the care of the patient. Third, the auditor will peruse the appointment books to determine whether a physician was on-site at the medical practice on days and times when a nurse practitioner or physician assistant's service were billed incident-to a physician's service. Fourth, the auditor will review consultation services to ensure that all consultations were billed under the provider performing the service. Fifth, the auditor will review the place of service codes for professional services submitted in hospitals, skilled nursing facilities, nursing facilities, domiciliary care facility, and home care visits, because these places of service are not eligible for incident-to professional services.

Here are instructions from a Medicare contractor regarding documentation to support incident-to billing:

> To ensure proper reimbursement according to the fee schedule, Medicare requires that documentation submitted to support billing 'incident-to' services must clearly link the services of the non-physician practitioner to the services of the supervising physician. For 'incident-to' services that are billed and undergoing medical review, documentation sent in response to the carrier's request should clearly show the link. Evidence of the link may include:
>
> - Co-signature or legible identity and credentials (i.e., MD, DO, NP, PA, etc.) of both the practitioner who provided the service and the supervising physician on documentation entries.
>
> - Some indication of the supervising physician's involvement with the patient's care. This indication could be satisfied by:
>
> Notation of supervising physician's involvement (the degree of which must be consistent with clinical circumstances of the care) within the text of the associated medical record entry.
>
> or,
>
> Documentation from other dates of service (e.g., initial visit, etc.) other than those requested, establishing the link between the two providers.
>
> Failure to provide such information may result in denial of the claim for lack of documentation from the billing provider (Trailblazer Health Enterprises, LLC 2009).

Payers Other Than Medicare

The incident-to rules are Medicare's rules, and other payers may or may not follow those rules. Medicaid requires that all services be billed under the name and number of the rendering provider. Commercial payers often direct practices to bill an employed nurse practitioner's services under an employer physician's name and/or provider number. Practice managers will need to check each commercial insurer to determine the company's policy on this matter.

Shared/Split Visits

There is no opportunity to bill professional services performed in an inpatient hospital under the incident-to rules, as the incident-to rules do not apply to the inpatient hospital setting. However, in 2003 Medicare made a significant change in rules that allows for "shared/split" billing for evaluation and management visits conducted in hospitals by a non-physician practitioner, limited to a nurse practitioner, clinical nurse specialist, certified nurse midwife, or physician assistant, and a physician employed by the same practice both for a patient on the same calendar day.

That language says:

> If a nurse practitioner performs physician services and a physician provides any face-to-face portion of the evaluation and management encounter on an inpatient service, in an emergency room, or outpatient department, such as observation, the service may be billed under either the physician's or the nurse practitioner's provider number. However, if there was no face-to-face encounter between the patient and the physician (even if the physician reviewed the medical record) then the service must be billed under the nurse practitioner's provider number (CMS 2002, Chapter 12, Section 30.6.1).

Shared/split services do include discharge day management professional services; however, exceptions to the rules of shared/split services deal with consultations and critical care services. Although consultation and critical care services are included as evaluation and management services, they are exempt from the shared/split services rules and cannot be billed as shared/split services.

The manual provides the following guidance:

Office/Clinic Setting—In the office/clinic setting when the physician performs the E/M service, the service must be reported using the physician's UPIN/PIN. When an E/M service is a shared/split encounter between a physician and a non-physician practitioner (NP, PA, CNS or CNM) the service is considered to have been performed 'incident-to' if the requirements for 'incident-to' are met and the patient is an established patient. If 'incident-to' requirements are not met for the shared/split E/M service, the service must be billed under the non-physician practitioner's UPIN/PIN, and payment will be made at the appropriate physician fee schedule payment.

Hospital Inpatient/Outpatient/Emergency Department Setting—When a hospital inpatient/hospital outpatient or emergency department E/M is shared between a physician and a non-physician practitioner from the same group practice and the physician provides any face-to-face portion of the E/M encounter with the patient, the service may be billed under either the physician's or the non-physician practitioner's UPIN/PIN number. However, if there was no face-to-face encounter between the patient and the physician (e.g., even if the physician participated in the service by only reviewing the patient's medical record) then the service may only be billed under the non-physician practitioner's UPIN/PIN. Payment will be made at the appropriate physician fee schedule rate based on the UPIN/PIN entered on the claim (CMS 2002, Chapter 12, Section 30.6.1).

Examples of Shared Visits

1. If the non-physician practitioner sees a hospital inpatient in the morning and the physician follows with a later face-to-face visit with the patient on the same day, the physician or the non-physician practitioner may report the service.

2. In an office setting the non-physician practitioner performs a portion of an E/M encounter and the physician completes the E/M service. If the 'incident-to' requirements are met, the physician reports the service. If the 'incident-to' requirements are not met, the service must be reported using the non-physician practitioner's UPIN/PIN (CMS 2002).

To document a shared/split visit, the nurse practitioner, clinical nurse specialist, nurse midwife, or physician assistant should document what he or she has performed in the way of history, physical examination, and medical decision making. The physician under whose name the visit will be billed should document what history, physical examination, or medical decision making he or she performed, and, at minimum, that the physician had a face-to-face visit with the patient.

Key issues to consider when billing for a shared/split E/M service are:

- The service must be within the scope of practice for the non-physician practitioner.

- For physician assistant services, physician collaboration and general supervision requirements must also be met.

- The service must be "reasonable and necessary" as defined by Title XVIII of the Social Security Act, Section 1862(a)(1)(A).

- The code selected should be based upon the content of the service and the summed value of services provided by both providers.

- The health record must clearly identify both the non-physician practitioner and the physician who shared/split the service.

- The physician personally documents his or her encounter with the patient at the time of the service, not a scribing service.

- The non-physician practitioner documents his or her encounter with the patient at the time of the service.

- Physician documentation should be linked to the non-physician practitioner documentation of the shared/split service, and state one (or more) element(s) of the encounter.

The shared/split visit rules apply to Medicare only, unless other payers specifically adopt Medicare's rules. There is no law governing commercial payers on this matter.

Documentation Requirements of Medicare's Conditions for Participation

Nurse practitioners do not have the legal authority to bear sole responsibility for hospitalized patients covered by Medicare, even where state law would permit it. A physician must be involved in the process of care for hospitalized patients covered by Medicare because, under Federal law governing conditions of participation by hospitals, a hospital's governing body "must ensure that . . . every Medicare patient is under the care of a doctor of medicine or osteopathy . . . , a doctor of dental surgery . . . , a doctor of podiatric medicine . . . , a doctor of optometry . . . , a chiropractor . . . , or a clinical psychologist. . . ." (42 CFR 482.12). Under federal law, a doctor of medicine may delegate tasks to other qualified health personnel. Licensed practitioners other than physicians may admit to hospitals if permitted by state law, and if the patient is under the care of a doctor of medicine or osteopathy (42 CFR 482.12).

Therefore, if a medical practice has nurse practitioners assigned to deliver care to hospitalized patients, the medical record must include documentation that a physician is the attending provider.

The Watchdogs: Who Are They and What Are They Looking For?

The Office of Inspector General is the investigation arm at the Department of Health and Human Services. The Federal Bureau of Investigation (FBI) also conducts investigation of health fraud.

The Office of Inspector General Work Plans is a good place to go to get an idea of what these watchdogs are looking for each year.

As documented in the OIG's 2009 Work Plan under the section entitled "Physicians' Medicare Services Performed by Non-physicians," it states "We will review services physicians bill to Medicare but do not perform personally. Such services, called 'incident to,' are typically performed by non-physician staff members in physicians' offices. The Social Security Act, Section 18610(s)(2)(A), provides for Medicare coverage of services and supplies performed 'incident to' the professional services of a physician. However, these services may be vulnerable to overutilization or put beneficiaries at risk of receiving services that do not meet professionally recognized standards of care. We will examine the qualifications of non-physician staff that perform 'incident to' services and assess whether these qualifications are consistent with professionally recognized standards of care" (OIG 2009).

As documented in the OIG's 2008 Work Plan under the section entitled "Medicare 'Incident to' Services," it states "We will review Medicare claims for services furnished 'incident to' the professional services of selected physicians. Medicare Part B generally pays for services 'incident to' a physician's professional service; such services are typically performed by a non-physician staff member in the physician's office. Federal regulations at 42 CFR § 410.26(b) specify criteria for 'incident to' services. We will examine the Medicare services that selected physicians bill 'incident to' their professional services and the qualifications and appropriateness of the staff who perform them. This study will review medical necessity, documentation, and quality of care for 'incident to' services" (OIG 2008).

As documented in the OIG's 2007 Work Plan under the section entitled "Evaluation of 'Incident to' Services," it states "The purpose of this study is to evaluate the appropriateness of Medicare services performed 'incident to' the professional services of physicians. We will identify services performed 'incident to' physicians' professional services and will determine the extent to which the services met Medicare standards for medical necessity, documentation, and quality of care" (OIG 2007).

So, the government clearly is serious about reviewing the documentation in medical practices to determine whether the incident-to rules are being followed.

In their investigations, FBI agents have asked physicians and nurse practitioners questions like the ones listed here:

- "Did you (or your employer) have policies regarding incident-to billing?"
- "Did your employer ever tell you about the incident-to rules, and how the practice needed to comply with them?"

Investigators will look at appointment books to see whether a physician was on-site and seeing patients on a day when a nurse practitioner's services were billed under the physician's NPI number.

Investigators will review progress notes to see whether a visit billed as a new patient visit conducted by a physician was documented by a physician.

Investigators will review consultation reports, since this type of evaluation and management service is not eligible for a shared/split service.

Investigators will be reviewing the correct place of service codes, since inaccurate reimbursements may be provided to providers who report facility and non-facility charges inappropriately.

Coding Errors

Investigators also will examine health records to determine whether the documentation for each visit justifies the visit as medically necessary and whether the documentation conforms to Medicare's "Documentation Guidelines for Evaluation and Management" requirements for the procedure code billed. If documentation does not support the level of claim billed, the provider or facility is deemed to have erred, and any payments made must be returned.

Auditors have identified these errors:

- Coding nearly every encounter as equal in complexity
- No documentation of reasons for lab tests or ancillary services
- Inadequate documentation to back up coding
- Coding for a service that was never performed
- Duplication of coding a single service that was performed
- Unbundling services when a single code is available
- Incorrect date(s) of service submitted on claim form
- Incorrect place of service based upon service billed

There are a multitude of reasons why a payer may not reimburse for a service submitted on a claim form. Coding errors are one category of such denials. For more information on reimbursement issues, see chapter 6.

Conclusion

While standards for documentation are generally the same for advanced practice nurses and physician assistants as for physicians, there are some differences. If a practice intends to bill under the incident-to rules or the rules on shared visits, the documentation must show that the physician was involved to the extent that the rules require physician involvement. For example, auditors do look for evidence that a physician from the same group had a face-to-face visit with a patient on the same day as a physician assistant visit, if an encounter with a physician assistant is billed under a physician's provider number. Assuming the additional documentation required when billing incident-to or under the shared visit rules is completed, the physician assistant or nurse practitioner should focus on ensuring the documentation for the patient visit justifies the medical necessity of the encounter as well as the supports the level of code billed.

Check Your Understanding

1. A nurse practitioner is defined as _____.
   a. a licensed practical nurse
   b. a nurse who actually practices, as compared with a research nurse or administrator
   c. a registered nurse with advanced academic and clinical experience, which enables him or her to diagnose and manage most common and many chronic illnesses
   d. a nurse who is studying to be a doctor

2. Physician assistants _____.
   a. do not have the same documentation requirements as nurse practitioners
   b. are found in only a few states
   c. are prohibited from documenting in the health record
   d. practice medicine with physician supervision

(continued on next page)

Check Your Understanding *(continued)*

3. Advanced practice nurses _____.

   a. is an umbrella term used to describe nurse executives and administrators
   b. refers to nurse practitioners, clinical nurse specialists, nurse midwives, and nurse anesthetists
   c. cannot document in the same health record that physicians use
   d. have the same documentation requirements as all other nurses

4. "Incident-to" billing _____.

   a. is a Medicare term
   b. applies to every third-party payer
   c. refers to state laws regarding certain incidents
   d. applies to billing for Good Samaritan acts

5. One of the major purposes of health record documentation is to _____.

   a. prove the qualifications of the provider
   b. provide family members with a diary of all that has been done for their loved one
   c. provide evidence of medical necessity for the treatment and/or tests
   d. avoid deportation of illegal aliens

6. The rules on incident-to billing may be applied _____.

   a. in a patient's home, if a nurse is present
   b. in a medical practice
   c. in a hospital
   d. in a patient's room in a nursing facility

7. Blue Cross has the same documentation requirements as _____.

   a. Aetna
   b. United Health Care
   c. Medicare
   d. None of the above

8. The patient's chief complaint _____.

   a. should appear in the documentation of every office visit
   b. isn't appropriate for the health record, but should be addressed by a health advocate
   c. if documented, is likely to lead to legal problems for the practice
   d. is recorded in medical terms, not the patient's words

9. When documenting physical examination _____.

   a. specific abnormal and relevant negative findings of the examination of the affected or symptomatic body area(s) or organ system(s) should be documented
   b. a notation of "abnormal" without elaboration is insufficient
   c. a brief statement or notation indicating "negative" or "normal" is sufficient to document normal findings related to unaffected areas or asymptomatic organ systems
   d. All of the above

10. If consultations are ordered, then the consultations are requested or advice is sought. Which of the following statements is true?

    a. The record should indicate to whom or where the consultation is made, from whom the advice is requested, and the reason for the advice or opinion.
    b. The referring provider will not receive third-party payment for the visit.
    c. The patient made a mistake in visiting the physician assistant or nurse practitioner.
    d. Do not note a request for advice in the medical record if the patient is covered by Medicare.

References

42 CFR 410.26(b): Services and supplies incident to a physician's professional services: Conditions. 2008 (Oct. 1).

42 CFR 482.12: Condition of participation: Governing body. 2008 (Oct. 1).

American Academy of Physician Assistants. 2009. Summary of co-signature requirements. http://www.aapa.org/advocacy-and-practice-resources/state-government-and-licensing/supervision/898.

CareFirst Blue Cross Blue Shield. 2008. Medical record documentation standards. http://www.carefirst.com/providers/attachments/BOK5129.pdf.

Centers for Medicare and Medicaid Services. 1995. Documentation guidelines for evaluation and management services. http://www.cms.hhs.gov/MLNEdwebGuide/25_EMDOC.asp.

Centers for Medicare and Medicaid Services. 1997. Documentation guidelines for evaluation and management services. http://www.cms.hhs.gov/MLNEdwebGuide/25_EMDOC.asp.

Centers for Medicare and Medicaid Services. 2002 (Oct. 26). Transmittal 1776, incorporated into the *Medicare Claims Processing Manual*.

Centers for Medicare and Medicaid Services. 2003. *Medicare Benefit Policy Manual*.

Centers for Medicare and Medicaid Services. 2009. *Medicare Program Integrity Manual*. http://www.cms.hhs.gov/manuals/.

Office of Inspector General. 2007. OIG's 2007 work plan. http://oig.hhs.gov/publications/workplan_archive.asp#2007.

Office of Inspector General. 2008. OIG's 2008 work plan. http://oig.hhs.gov/publications/workplan_archive.asp#2008.

Office of Inspector General. 2009. OIG's 2009 work plan. http://oig.hhs.gov/publications/workplan_archive.asp#2009.

Palmetto GBA, LLC. 2009. Medicare Part B medical records: Signature requirements, acceptable and unacceptable practices. http://www.palmettogba.com/palmetto/Providers.nsf/DocsCat/Ohio%20Part%20B%20Carrier~Browse%20by%20Specialty~Chiropractic~8525746A00550AA3852575A100724A89.

Social Security Act, Section 1862(a)(1)(A): Exclusions from coverage and Medicare as secondary payer. http://www.ssa.gov/OP_Home/ssact/title18/1862.htm.

Trailblazer Health Enterprises, LLC. 2009. 'Incident to' services manual. http://www.trailblazerhealth.com/Publications/Training%20Manual/incident_to.pdf?DomainID=1.

Resources

Buppert, C. 2006. *Avoiding Malpractice: 10 Rules, 5 Systems, 20 Cases*. Bethesda, MD: Law Office of Carolyn Buppert. http://www.buppert.com.

Buppert, C. 2008. *The Nurse Practitioner's Business Practice and Legal Guide*. Sudbury, MA: Jones & Bartlett. http://www.jbpub.com.

Office of Inspector General. 2010. OIG's 2010 work plan. http://oig.hhs.gov/publications/docs/workplan/2010/Work_Plan_FY_2010.pdf.

Chapter 3

Other Clinical Staff

Carolyn Buppert, JD, NP

Learning Objectives

- Identify the classes of clinicians who must meet Medicare's documentation requirements
- Understand Medicare's requirements for documentation of physical therapy, occupational therapy, and speech therapy
- Understand Medicare's requirements for documentation of psychotherapy performed by licensed clinical social workers
- Recognizing the necessity of consulting state law when determining the authorized functions of a medical assistant
- Understand the exception to the general rule that a registered nurse's service is not reimbursed by Medicare Part B

Key Terms

Diabetes educator	Nonphysician practitioner	Physical therapy (PT)
Licensed practical nurse	Occupational therapy	Speech-language therapy
Medical assistant		

Documentation by Other Medical Staff

Like physicians, advanced practice nurses, and physician assistants, other clinical staff document to prove that the standard of care was met, to inform clinicians who follow, and to support bills for services. In general, any individual who provides clinical services to a patient should document what was done. Hospitals and other facilities may have policies that determine the qualifications an individual must have to perform any clinical service and may designate the classes of clinicians with authority to document in a patient's health record. In recent years, it has been the third-party payers (Medicare and others) who set the rules for documentation. It is not so much a matter of who can document as what must be documented in order for the hospital, physician, or therapist to be paid.

This chapter addresses clinical staff other than physicians, physician assistants, and advanced practice nurses; namely, physical therapists, occupational therapists, speech therapists, certified diabetes educators, certified social workers, registered nurses, licensed practical nurses, and medical assistants. The chapter focuses on Medicare's rules, but examples of commercial payers' policies also are included.

Reimbursement by Medicare and other third-party payers is available for physical therapists, occupational therapists, speech therapists, certified diabetes educators, and certified social workers but not for registered nurses, licensed practical nurses, and medical assistants. Therefore, the payers, and specifically Medicare, set the requirements for documentation by physical therapists, occupational therapists, speech therapists, certified diabetes educators, and certified social workers. Aside from payer requirements, professional organizations sometimes develop standards for practice, including documentation. The consequence of failing to meet payer requirements is failure to be paid. A consequence of failing to meet a standard set by the profession may be loss of a lawsuit for malpractice, loss of accreditation of the facility or practice, or poor performance on an inspection or audit conducted by an organization, state, or federal agency.

Medicare Requirements Regarding Physical Therapy, Occupational Therapy, and Speech-Language Therapy

The Centers for Medicare and Medicaid Services (CMS) has established certain requirements for documentation by the clinicians who are authorized to bill Medicare. Medicare contractors may conduct audits of medical records to determine whether the criteria have been met for the procedure code billed. If a clinician has not met the criteria for billing the specific procedure code that was billed, the Medicare contractor may decline payment or may reduce payment to the amount associated with the procedure code for which criteria were met.

Medical necessity is the foundation requirement for submitting a bill to Medicare. Documentation is necessary to show the payer that a service was provided, was medically necessary, and conforms to specific requirements associated with the procedure code billed. The general requirements for therapy (physical therapy, occupational therapy, and speech therapy) are:

- Services were reasonable, necessary, specific, and effective

- Services were ordered by a physician or non-physician practitioner

- Patient required the skills of a therapist

- Treatment was dictated by a written treatment plan, which included specific and measurable goals

- Documentation of a reasonable estimate of when the patient is going to attain the goals (CMS 2008a, Chapter 15, Section 220.1.2; 42 CFR 410.61)

Therapy records should provide evidence that the patient is under the care of a physician or non-physician practitioner (NPP), through documentation of the physician/NPP's certification of the plan of care and through other evidence of physician/NPP involvement, such as orders/referrals, conference or team meeting notes, and correspondence.

Note: The following information, including the section titled "Minimum Requirements," is adapted from the Medicare Benefit Policy Manual, *Chapter 15, Section 220.3.*

Therapists' notes must show that the patient needed therapy and required a therapist's skill; that is, more than an assistant or caretaker could provide. This may be accomplished by documenting the skilled treatment provided, changes made to the treatment due to the therapist's assessment of patient's needs, or changes due to progress the clinician judged sufficient to modify the treatment toward the next more complex or difficult task.

For example, a patient may have an unstable fracture such that a skilled therapist is needed to perform an activity that might otherwise be done independently by the patient at home. Or, if a patient is learning swallowing techniques, a therapist may need to perform cervical auscultation and identify changes in voice and breathing that might signal aspiration.

Therapists' notes must show that the services are of appropriate types, frequency, intensity, and duration for the individual needs of the patient. If the patient requires more services than typical, the therapist's notes need to show why.

Documentation should provide evidence that the patient is making progress toward specific, listed goals. If the patient is not making progress, the notes needs to state reasons for lack of progress and justification for continued treatment. Factors that demonstrate a patient's need for therapy include the patient's diagnoses, complicating factors, age, severity, time since onset/acuity, self-efficacy/motivation, cognitive ability, prognosis, and/or medical, psychological, and social stability.

Specifically, Medicare requires the following type of documentation of therapy services:

- Evaluation and plan of care, including an initial evaluation and any reevaluations relevant to the episode

- Certification (physician or non-physician practitioner approval of the plan) and recertification

- Progress reports (including discharge notes)

- Treatment notes for each treatment day

- If the provider wishes to assure the Medicare contractor understands the reasoning for services that are more extensive than typical for the condition treated, a separate justification statement

Minimum Requirements

Here are Medicare's minimum requirements for each type of documentation.

Evaluation

An evaluation includes a diagnosis and description of specific problems to be evaluated and/ or treated. If relevant, include both a medical diagnosis and an impairment-based treatment diagnosis. (In many states, only physicians or specified non-physician practitioners may make medical diagnoses. Therapists may or may not be authorized, under state law, to make medical diagnoses. However, therapists always can document a medical diagnosis provided by the referring clinician and describe the patient's condition that requires the therapist's attentions.) For example, a physician may provide the diagnosis of cerebrovascular accident; however, the treatment diagnosis or condition description for a physical therapist may be gait abnormality. For an occupational therapist, the condition description may be hemiparesis. For a speech-language pathologist, the condition description may be dysphagia. Include, for PT and OT, the body part evaluated. Include all conditions and complexities that may impact the treatment.

Results of measurement instruments are recommended but not required. Instruments include National Outcomes Measurement System (NOMS) by the American Speech-Language Hearing Association, Patient Inquiry by Focus on Therapeutic Outcomes (FOTO), Activity

Measure—Post Acute Care (AM-PAC), and OPTIMAL by Cedaron through the American Physical Therapy Association. If not including a result of one of these measurement instruments, include documentation to indicate objective, measurable patient physical function, including:

- Functional assessment individual item and summary scores (and comparison to prior assessment scores) from commercially available therapy outcomes instruments other than those listed above; or

- Functional assessment scores (and comparisons to prior scores) from tests and measurements validated in the professional literature that are appropriate for the condition being measured; or

- Other measurable progress towards identified goals for function in the home environment at the conclusion of this therapy episode of care.

Reevaluation

Reevaluation is indicated when the professional assessment of the clinician indicates a significant improvement, or decline, or change in the patient's condition or functional status that was not anticipated in the plan of care. The documentation must support the need for further tests and measurements after the initial evaluation. Document the minutes spent on reevaluation.

Plan of care

The plan of care is the course of treatment determined by the clinician to reach targeted outcomes by the patient. It should include at minimum, the diagnoses, long-term treatment goals, and type, amount, duration, and frequency of therapy services. The evaluation may be attached and is considered incorporated into the plan.

Progress report

A progress report must be completed at least once every 10 treatment days or at least once each 30 calendar days, whichever is less. The progress report provides an accurate detailing of a patient's care throughout the course of treatment. A progress report must include:

- Date of the beginning and end of the reporting period

- Date the report was written

- Signature, professional identification, and date on which dictated, if dictated

- Report of patient's subjective statements, if relevant

- Objective measurements or description of changes in status relative to each goal being addressed in treatment, if they occur

- Assessment of improvement, extent of progress or lack thereof for each goal

- Plans for continuing treatment, reference to additional evaluation results, and/or treatment plan revisions

- Changes to long- or short-term goals, discharge or an updated plan of care that is sent to the physician/NPP for certification of the next interval of treatment

Treatment Note

The purpose of the treatment note is to record all treatments and skilled interventions and to record the time of the services in order to justify the billing codes on the claim. Document every therapy service. There is no required format. It is not necessary to document the medical necessity or appropriateness of the service in the treatment note. Nonskilled interventions need not be recorded. For each treatment, document these required elements:

- Date of treatment

- Identification of each specific intervention/modality provided and billed, for both timed and untimed codes

- Total timed code treatment minutes and total treatment time in minutes

- Signature and professional identification of the qualified professional who furnished or supervised the services and a list of each person who contributed to that treatment

If a treatment is added or changed under the direction of a clinician during the treatment days between the progress reports, the change must be recorded and justified on the medical record, either in the treatment note or the progress report.

Why So Many Rules?

It may be useful to know why Medicare has these rules. The rules stem from investigations that showed that the government was not getting what it paid for. The U.S. Office of Inspector General (OIG) conducted an investigation of therapy services in 1999 and found that 14% of services billed were not medically necessary. The investigators also found that many patients were not appropriate candidates for therapy, that treatment goals were met but therapy continued, that therapy goals were not achieved and reevaluation was not conducted, and that skilled therapy was provided when routine maintenance would have sufficed. The OIG found that Medicare was paying millions of dollars ($20 million in a six-month period) for care that was not documented or inadequately documented (OIG 1999).

Professional Association Standards

Although Medicare documentation requirements often serve as a model and must be followed in order to receive reimbursement, professional associations, healthcare provider organizations, and commercial payers have established their own policies and templates to guide practitioners.

Dependent upon your practice or organization, you may or may not need to reference and follow other association and organizational guidelines. This section will discuss two other main associations.

Physical Therapy

The American Physical Therapy Association has extensive guidelines on documentation of physical therapy, which can be found at http://www.apta.org.

Occupational Therapy

Occupational therapist associations also have guidelines for documentation.

An American Occupational Therapy Association (AOTA) official document, *Guidelines for Documentation of Occupational Therapy* (available at http://www.apta.org), "provides an outline which, if followed, ensures a comprehensive and professional format for documentation of occupational therapy services" (AOTA 2008).

The following excerpt from the AOTA fact sheet on Medicare documentation requirements for evaluations covers some of the key factors of documentation for occupational therapy.

The key to documenting objective, measurable beneficiary physical function is to spell out how the patient information gathered shows the patient's function limitations and relates to the patient's functional goals (occupational performance). This documentation should contain the following elements:

1. List all standardized/nonstandardized assessments administered during evaluation and the results;

2. Document how the assessments selected measure performance deficits and functional problems identified in the evaluation;

3. Document results of assessments and how they relate/what they mean in terms of performance deficits;

4. Document client performance observed (skilled observation) by therapist; and

5. Summarize and interpret the results of assessments and observations as they relate to the person's occupational performance (ADL, IADL, social participation) and as they form a foundation for the plan of care and goals.

These components should support the presumption that the occupational therapy services are reasonable and necessary. This means that the services are considered under accepted standards of medical practice to be safe and effective treatment for the client's condition and that there is an expectation that the client's condition will improve materially in a reasonable (and generally predictable) period of time based on the assessment of the client's restoration potential and unique medical condition (42 CFR 409.44; AOTA 2008).

Commercial Payer Standards

Payers other than Medicare may have their own policies on documentation. Many of these other reimbursement entities include commercial insurance companies. For example, here is Aetna's policy on occupational therapy, which essentially follows Medicare policy:

Occupational therapy services are considered medically necessary only if there is a reasonable expectation that occupational therapy will achieve measurable improvement in the member's condition in a reasonable and predictable period of time.

Documentation Requirements:

The following care plan is required to document the medical necessity of occupational therapy:

- Occupational therapy must be provided in accordance with an ongoing, written plan of care. The purpose of the written plan of care is to assist in determining medical necessity.

- The plan of care must include sufficient information to determine the medical necessity of treatment.

- The plan of care must be specific to the diagnosis, presenting symptoms, and findings of the occupational therapy evaluation.

- The plan of care must be signed by the member's attending physician and occupational therapist.

- The plan of care should include:

— The date of onset or exacerbation of the disorder/diagnosis;

— Specific statements of long-term and short-term goals;

— Quantitative objectives;

— A reasonable estimate of when the goals will be reached;

— The specific treatment techniques and/or exercises to be used in treatment; and

— The frequency and duration of treatment.

- The plan of care should be ongoing (that is, updated as the member's condition changes) and treatment should demonstrate reasonable expectation of improvement (as defined below):

— The member should be reevaluated regularly, and there should be documentation of progress made toward the goals of occupational therapy.

— The treatment goals and subsequent documentation of treatment results should specifically demonstrate that occupational therapy services are contributing to such improvement (Aetna 2009).

Speech-Language Pathologists

The American Speech-Language-Hearing Association (ASHA) lists the following components of clinical recordkeeping:

- Identifying information

- Client history

- Assessment of current client status

- Treatment plan

- Documentation of treatment

- Discharge summary

- Record of consultation (with other professionals; with client/caregivers) (Sutherland Cornet 2006)

Social Workers

Medicare covers therapeutic visits with clinical social workers when Medicare has credentialed the social worker as a provider. Medicare Part B will pay a portion of the social worker's charge for outpatient mental health services, including individual and group therapy. Other payers also may reimburse clinical social workers.

The general principles of medical record documentation for mental health services are the same as for documentation of other medical and surgical services. Documentation must provide evidence of medical necessity. The Social Security Act states that all Medicare Part B services, including mental health services, must be "reasonable and necessary for the diagnosis or treatment of an illness or injury or to improve the functioning of a malformed body member" (SSA, Section 1862(a)(1)(A)). For every service billed, providers must indicate the specific sign, symptom, or patient complaint necessitating the service. The following list presents additional documentation requirements from Medicare:

- Medical records should be complete and legible.

- Documentation of each patient encounter should include:

— Reason for encounter and relevant history;

— Physical examination findings and prior diagnostic test results;

— Assessment, clinical impression, and diagnosis;

— Plan for care; and

— Date and legible identity of observer

- If not documented, the rationale for ordering diagnostic and other ancillary services should be easily inferred.

- Past and present diagnoses should be accessible for treating and/or consulting physician.

- Appropriate health risk factors should be identified.

- Patient's progress, response to changes in treatment, and revision of diagnosis should be documented

- CPT and ICD-9-CM codes reported on the health insurance claim should be supported by documentation in the medical record (CMS 2008b).

Individual psychotherapy can be billed according to time spent—20 to 30 minutes, 45 to 50 minutes, or 75 to 80 minutes. Practitioners are required to document in the medical record the time spent with the patient. If no time is documented, services should be billed at the lowest possible time period.

Clinical social workers may also provide an evaluation and management service along with psychotherapy. If so, the clinician must document the evaluation and management (E/M) services and psychotherapy in the medical record. If only psychotherapy is documented, the practitioner should bill the CPT codes only for psychotherapy. Clinical social workers should follow Medicare's Documentation Guidelines for Evaluation and Management.

Documentation Deficiencies in Mental Health Services

An OIG report found that the majority of miscoded individual psychotherapy claims lacked documentation to justify the time billed. Miscoding for psychotherapy services also occurred when documentation in the health record indicated that the actual services were not psychotherapy but something else, such as evaluation and management, medication management, psychological evaluation, and group psychotherapy (CMS 2008b).

Coding errors can occur from any of the following three different scenarios: 1) up-coding, 2) down-coding, or 3) miscoding. Up-coded services are billed at a level higher than the actual level of the service performed and documented. For example, a 20- to 30-minute individual psychotherapy service billed as a 45- to 50-minute service is an up-coded service. Conversely, a down-coded service is billed at a lower level than the actual level of the service performed and documented.

Miscoding for E/M services can occur when the E/M services are billed at a higher level than the health record documentation supports. E/M services levels vary based on:

- The extent of the patient history obtained

- The extent of the examination performed

- The complexity of the medical decision making

Additional causes of E/M coding errors reported in an OIG report include:

- Billing an E/M service for an initial visit when the services were rendered during a subsequent visit. (Reimbursement rates for subsequent E/M visits are typically less than those for initial visits.)

- Billing an E/M service when the services should have been billed as psychiatric diagnostic interview, examination, consultation, or psychotherapy, which are reimbursed at a lower rate.

- Billing an E/M service where the place of service—for example inpatient—does not match the place of service indicated in the health record—for example, outpatient (CMS 2008b).

Registered Nurses and Licensed Practical Nurses

Generally, Medicare and other third-party payers do not directly reimburse the services of registered nurses. (Payments for nurses' services are included in comprehensive payments to hospitals for episodes of care, but nursing services are not reimbursed separately.) However, if Medicare's incident-to rules are followed, some services of registered nurses may be billed under the national provider identifier number of a physician, advanced practice nurse, or physician assistant. For a description of the incident-to rules, see chapter 2. For example, if a physician sees a patient and, on examination, the patient's blood pressure is elevated, the physician may ask the patient to return in 10 days for a blood pressure check that is documented in the health record. A registered nurse may take the patient's blood pressure and convey that information to the physician. The physician may bill CPT 99211. The documentation required of the registered nurse is the reporting of the blood pressure and a notation that it is in follow-up to the physician's initial service for elevated blood pressure. Be careful about adding a CPT 99211 when an evaluation is not medically necessary. For example, when performing an immunization, if a nurse evaluates and manages a separate and significant complaint or problem prior to the injection, a CPT 99211 may be billed along with the procedure code for the immunization. But not all immunizations require evaluation and management prior to the immunization and CPT 99211 should not be routinely added to the bill for injections, immunizations, or venipuncture (AMA 2005, 1).

For all of these examples, the nurse would document what was done, date, and sign the note.

The focus for nurses is to document what was done, by whom, when, and how. Nursing documentation is used to prove that services were rendered in a careful manner. Nursing documentation also is integral in showing that a medical practice deserves accreditation and in defending an allegation of malpractice. Perhaps more importantly, nurses rely on the documentation of their coworkers in order to coordinate the flow of care. The health record is the best evidence that care has been provided.

The American Nurses Association has a published document, available only to members, that recaps the general principles regarding documentation found in chapter 1 of this book and directs nurses to follow organizational policies and procedures related to documentation.

Certified Diabetic Educators

Diabetes self-management training (DSMT) is the ongoing process of facilitating the knowledge, skill, and ability necessary for diabetes self-care. DSMT is a service that Medicare and other payers reimburse, if provided by a certified diabetic educator.

Orders for DSMT

DSMT must be documented as medically necessary in order to obtain reimbursement from Medicare. In an order from the physician or qualified non-physician practitioner, the following documentation for an individual or group DSMT training session is required in the patient's health record to support medical necessity.

- Treating physician or non-physician practitioner (NPP) order with the number of hours for initial and/or follow-up training

- Plan of care showing the medical need for training

- Supporting medical records of the time spent and topic and/or areas of coverage in the training session.

Specific Medicare regulations are in the IOM Publication 100-02, Chapter 15, Section 300, NCD 40.1.42 and 42 CFR 410.140-140.146. The direct web link for National Coverage Determination can be found in the Web Links document on the CD-ROM accompanying this book.

Documentation Content

The content to be covered and documented should include:

- Pathophysiology of diabetes

- Nutrition

- Exercise and activity

- Diabetes medications (including skills related to the self-administration of injectable drugs)

- Self-monitoring and use of the results

- Prevention, detection, and treatment of acute complications

- Prevention, detection, and treatment of chronic complications

- Foot, skin, and dental care

- Behavior change strategies, goal setting, risk factor reduction, and problem solving

- Preconception care, pregnancy, and gestational diabetes

- Relationships among nutrition, exercise, medication, and blood glucose levels

- Stress and psychosocial adjustment

- Family involvement and social support

- Benefits, risks, and management options for improving glucose control

- Use of healthcare systems and community resources (42 CFR 410.144(a)(5))

The entity providing diabetes education is required under federal law to document certain outcome measures. Specifically, the entity must collect and record "in an organized systematic manner the following patient assessment information at least on a quarterly basis for a beneficiary who receives training" (42 CFR 410.146(A)(1-2)):

Medical information that includes the following:

- Duration of the diabetic condition

- Use of insulin or oral agents

- Height and weight by date

- Results and date of last lipid test

- Results and date of last HbA1c

- Information on self-monitoring (frequency and results)

- Blood pressure with the corresponding dates

- Date of the last eye exam

- Other information that includes educational goals, assessment of educational needs, training goals, a plan for a follow-up assessment of achievement of training goals between 6 months and 1 year after the beneficiary completes the training, and documentation of the training goals assessment (42 CFR 410.146(A)(1-2))

Medical Assistants

In some states there is a clear definition and scope of practice for medical assistants, but in other states there is no law on the matter. As shown in figure 3.1, the following states have specific language pertaining to medical assisting scope of practice.

Where there is no law, the threshold question is: Can a medical assistant legally perform any specific services? If it is not clear that a medical assistant has the authority to perform a service, the assistant should not be performing the service and therefore should not be documenting that the service was performed. Table 3.1 outlines some of the tasks medical assistants can and cannot perform.

Of course, a list on a Web site is not law, but the list provided in table 3.1 accurately describes the law in several states. For example, in California, "medical assistant" is defined, and there is a scope of practice for a medical assistant. In California, "Medical assistant means a person who may be unlicensed, who performs basic administrative, clerical, and technical supportive services in compliance with this section and Section 2070 for a licensed physician and surgeon or a licensed podiatrist, or group thereof, for a medical or podiatry corporation, or for a healthcare services plan, who is at least 18 years of age, and who has had at least the minimum amount of hours of appropriate training pursuant to standards established by the Division of Licensing. The medical assistant shall be issued a certificate by the training institution or instructor indicating satisfactory completion of the required training. A copy of the certificate shall be retained as a record by each employer of the medical assistant" (California Business & Professions Code, Sections 2069, 2070, 2071).

In California, a medical assistant may perform the following services:

1. Administer medication orally, sublingually, topically, vaginally, or rectally, or by providing a single dose to a patient for immediate self-administration. Administer medication by inhalation if the medications are patient-specific and have been or will be routinely and repetitively administered to that patient. In every instance, prior to

Figure 3.1. Key state scope of practice laws

Arizona

- Arizona Administrative Code: R4-16-4 Medical Assistants
  http://www.azmd.gov/Regulatory/MA/
- Content Requirements for CAAHEP Accredited Medical Assisting Programs
  http://aama-ntl.org/resources/library/CAAHEP_Content_Competencies.doc

California

- Medical Board of California: Medical Assistants
  http://www.mbc.ca.gov/allied/medical_assistants.html
- Medical Board of California: Medical Assistants—Frequently Asked Questions
  http://www.mbc.ca.gov/allied/medical_assistants.html

Florida

- 2008 Florida Statutes: 458.3485 Medical Assistant
  http://www.flsenate.gov/Statutes/index.cfm?App_mode=Display_Statute&Search_String=&URL=Ch0458/
  SEC3485.HTM&Title=-%3e2008-%3eCh0458-%3eSection%203485#0458.3485

Illinois

- "Illinois Nurse Law Safeguards Physician Delegation to Medical Assistants"
  http://www.aama-ntl.org/CMAToday/archives/publicaffairs/details.aspx?ArticleID=567

Maryland

- Code of Maryland Regulations: 10.32.12
  http://aama-ntl.org/resources/library/MD_10_32_12.pdf

New Jersey

- New Jersey Board of Medical Examiners: 13:35-6.4
  http://aama-ntl.org/resources/library/NJ_13_35_6_4.pdf

Ohio

- Ohio Administrative Code: 4731-23 Delegation of Medical Tasks
  http://codes.ohio.gov/oac/4731-23

South Dakota

- South Dakota Board of Nursing: Medical Assistants
  http://doh.sd.gov/Boards/Nursing/medasst.aspx

Virginia

- "Virginia Law Permits Delegation to Unlicensed Professionals"
  http://www.vmgma.org/newsletter/09winter/scopeofpractice.htm

As defined scope of practice laws develop, refer to the American Association of Medical Assistants (AAMA) at http://aama-ntl.org/employers/laws.aspx. There is also a form that may be submitted to the AAMA legal counsel if a particular state is not listed above and clarification is required for medical assistants' scope of practice.

Source: AAMA 2009.

administration of medication by the medical assistant, a licensed physician or podiatrist, or another person authorized by law to do so shall verify the correct medication and dosage. Nothing in the section shall be construed as authorizing the administration of any anesthetic agent by a medical assistant.

2. Perform electrocardiogram, electroencephalogram, or plethysmography tests, except full-body plethysmography. Nothing in this section shall permit a medical assistant to perform tests involving the penetration of human tissues except for skin tests . . . or to interpret test findings or results.

Table 3.1. Tasks medical assistants can and cannot perform

Medical assistants can:	Medical assistants cannot:
• Perform clinical and administrative tasks to keep the workflow going, if supervised by a physician or other healthcare practitioner	• Independently perform telephone triage (medical assistants are not legally authorized to interpret data or diagnose symptoms!)
• Determine the acuity of a visit and the visit length for appointment scheduling purposes using an office protocol provided by the supervising physician	• Independently diagnose or treat patients
• Measure and record vital signs	• Independently prescribe medications
• Record patient demographics and basic information about the presenting and previous conditions that is limited to the review of systems and past medical/family/social history	• Independently give out medication samples
• Use medical terminology and accepted charting abbreviations	• Independently refill prescription requests
• Escort patients to the exam room and prepare them for an exam	• Independently do triage
• Use scientific methods to solve problems and choose a mathematical method or formula to solve problems	• Inject medications into a vein (most states) unless permitted by state law
• Convey clinical information on behalf of the physician	• Start, flush, or discontinue IVs (most states) unless permitted by state law
• Arrange examining room instruments and equipment	• Provide medical treatment, analyze or interpret test results
• Change wound dressings and obtain wound cultures	• Advise patients about their condition or treatment regimen
• Remove sutures or staples from superficial incisions or lacerations	• Make assessments or perform any kind of medical care decision making
• Operate diagnostic equipment but cannot interpret tests	• Administer any anesthetic agent (except topical numbing agents such as EMLA cream)
• Provide patient information and instructions	• Perform tests that involve the penetration of human tissues except for skin tests and drawing blood as provided by law
• Provide a single dose of oral medication as ordered by the physician to a patient for immediate self-administration under observation	• Interpret the results of blood or skin tests
• Administer medications topically, sublingually, vaginally, rectally, and by injection	• Operate laser equipment
• Perform CPR and render first aid in an emergency	
• Prepare patients for examination, including draping, shaving, and disinfecting treatment sites	
• Perform aseptic procedures such as wound care	
• Collect blood specimens via capillary and venipuncture technique	
• Obtain specimens by noninvasive techniques, such as wound cultures	
• Perform simple laboratory and screening tests customarily performed STAT in a medical office, such as urinalysis	
• Administer different types of cryotherapy to reduce pain or swelling	
• Do filing and bookkeeping	
• Process insurance claims	
• Transcribe medical dictation for medical records	
• Call in prescription orders or refills to the pharmacy, but only as ordered and approved by physician, nurse practitioner, or physician assistant	

Source: Advanced Medical Assistant Custom Web Design 2009.

3. Apply and remove bandages and dressings; apply orthopedic appliances such as knee immobilizers, envelope slings, orthotics, and similar devices; remove casts, splints, and other external devices; obtain impressions for orthotics, padding, and custom-molded shoes; select and adjust crutches to patient; and instruct patient in proper use of crutches.

4. Remove sutures or staples from superficial incisions or lacerations.

5. Perform ear lavage to remove impacted cerumen.

6. Collect by noninvasive techniques, and reserve specimens for testing, including urine, sputum, semen, and stool.

7. Assist patients in ambulation and transfers.

8. Prepare patients for and assist the physician, podiatrist, physician assistant, or registered nurse in examinations or procedures including positioning, draping, shaving, and disinfecting treatment sites; prepare a patient for gait analysis testing.

9. As authorized by a physician or podiatrist, provide patient information and instructions.

10. Collect and record patient data including height, weight, temperature, pulse, respiration rate, and blood pressure, and basic information about the presenting and previous conditions.

11. Perform simple laboratory and screening tests customarily performed in a medical office.

12. Cut the nails of otherwise healthy patients (California Business & Professions Code, Section 1366).

After a 2002 act of the California Legislature, medical assistants in California may also:

1. Administer medication by intradermal, subcutaneous, or intramuscular injection if they are so authorized and supervised by a physician. In certain clinics, a nurse practitioner may authorize a medical assistant to administer intradermal, subcutaneous, or intramuscular injections (California Business & Professions Code, Section 2069).

2. Administer injections of scheduled drugs if the dosage is verified and the injection is intramuscular, intradermal, or subcutaneous and if the supervising physician or podiatrist is on the premises (California Business & Professions Code, Section 2069).

3. Perform venipuncture or skin puncture for the purposes of withdrawing blood, upon specific authorization of a physician, physician assistant, nurse practitioner, or nurse midwife (California Business & Professions Code, Section 2070).

Medical assistants in California are specifically prohibited from independently performing telephone triage.

Most states' laws on medical assistants are not as detailed as California's. Those who are working with a medical assistant should check their respective state statutes and regulations to determine the scope of practice. In some states, medical assistants are overseen by the Board of Nursing and the law can be accessed through the board's Web site. In others, it is the Board of Medicine that oversees medical assistants. In some states, there is no agency overseeing medical assistants at all. In that case, practices should write a policy stating what the medical assistant may do (and may not do), and stating that the physician in charge delegates the stated duties to the medical assistant.

Once the appropriate clinical function of a medical assistant has been determined and if it has been determined that the medical assistant will perform clinical functions, the medical assistant must document what he or she did, to whom, and date and sign the health record. In some states, such as California, a physician must write an order for a procedure to be performed by a medical assistant.

Conclusion

Payers, particularly Medicare, issue new rules daily. As the rules are complicated and becoming more complicated every day, it is important that clinicians and those billing for clinicians check the payers' Web sites monthly, at minimum, and subscribe to listservs and newsletters that announce changes and updates. Medicare has a variety of monthly "Open Door Forums," accessible by telephone, during which time CMS staff detail policy changes and take questions from participants. For information on these forums, visit http://www.cms.hhs.gov/opendoorforums/.

Check Your Understanding

1. The foundation requirement for submitting a bill to Medicare is

   a. safety
   b. medical necessity
   c. recognition within the profession
   d. standard of care

2. Documentation by a physical therapist, occupational therapist, or speech therapist must state why the therapy is _____.

   a. medically necessary
   b. accepted within the profession
   c. effective
   d. free of risk

3. An occupational therapist is one who _____.

   a. provides services for patients with speech disorders
   b. needs to be licensed by the federal government
   c. uses purposeful activity or intervention to improve or restore the highest possible level of independence of an individual with an injury, illness, cognitive impairment, developmental disability, or other disorder or condition
   d. counsels individuals about their jobs

4. In order to receive reimbursement for diabetes self-management training, a diabetes educator must _____.

   a. be certified as a diabetes educator
   b. have a master's degree
   c. be a former school teacher
   d. have a clear criminal record

(continued on next page)

Check Your Understanding *(continued)*

5. In all states, a medical assistant is authorized to _____.

   a. draw blood
   b. take patient vital signs
   c. give telephone advice
   d. None of the above

6. Documentation by registered nurses is necessary _____.

   a. in order to get reimbursement under Medicare Part B
   b. to mount a defense in case of a malpractice lawsuit
   c. to alert nurses on the following shift of what has been done and what has not been done
   d. B and C

7. Miscoding for evaluation and management (E&M) services provided by clinical social workers can occur when _____.

   a. the E&M services are billed at a higher level than the health record documentation supports
   b. the social worker is performing testing for attention deficit
   c. the social worker is using the ABC codes
   d. the social worker is not certified

8. Medicare does not pay for the services of _____,

   a. physical therapists
   b. occupational therapists
   c. clinical social workers
   d. medical assistants

9. Which of the following is not a purpose of health record documentation?

   a. To justify a bill
   b. To tell other professionals involved in the patient's care what you have done
   c. To provide evidence in case of a lawsuit
   d. To get a tax credit

10. Which of the following is a part of a speech pathologist's documentation?

   a. Client history
   b. Driving record
   c. Childhood immunizations
   d. Last job held

References

42 CFR 409.44(e): Skilled services requirements. 2009 (Oct. 1). http://www.access.gpo.gov/nara/cfr/waisidx_04/42cfr410_04.html.

42 CFR 410.144(a)(5): Training content. 2008 (Oct 1.). http://www.access.gpo.gov/nara/cfr/waisidx_04/42cfr410_04.html.

42 CFR 410.61: Plan of treatment requirements for outpatient rehabilitation services. 2008 (Oct. 1). http://www.access.gpo.gov/nara/cfr/waisidx_04/42cfr410_04.html.

42 CFR 410.140-140.146. http://www.access.gpo.gov/nara/cfr/waisidx_04/42cfr410_04.html.

42 CFR 410.146(a)(1-2): Diabetes outcome measurements. 2008 (Oct. 1). http://www.medicalassistant.net/can_and_cannot_do.htm.

Aetna. 2009. Clinical policy bulletin: Occupational therapy services. http://www.aetna.com/cpb/medical/data/200_299/0250.html.

American Association of Medical Assistants. 2009. Key state scope of practice laws. http://aama-ntl.org/employers/laws.aspx.

American Medical Association. 2005 (April). *CPT Assistant*.

American Occupational Therapy Association. 2008. AOTA fact sheet on Transmittal 63: New Medicare documentation requirements for evaluations. http://cnhs.fiu.edu/ot/pdf/Medicar.doc.

California Business & Professions Code, Sections 2069, 2070, 2071. *California Code of Regulations.* http://www.rn.ca.gov/regulations/title16.shtml.

California Business & Professions Code, Title 16, Section 1366. *California Code of Regulations.* http://www.rn.ca.gov/regulations/title16.shtml.

Centers for Medicare and Medicaid Services. n.d. Publication 100-02, Medicare Benefit Policy, Section 220.12.

Centers for Medicare and Medicaid Services. 2008a. *Medicare Benefit Policy Manual.*

Centers for Medicare and Medicaid Services. 2008b. Medicare Payments for Part B Mental Health Services: MLN: SE0816. http://www.arkmedicare.com/provider/viewarticle.aspx?pf=yes&articleid=6628.

Office of Inspector General. 1999. Draft report: Physical, occupational and speech therapy for Medicare nursing home patients OEI-09-99-00560.

Social Security Act, Section 1862(a)(1)(A): Exclusions from coverage and Medicare as secondary payer. http://www.ssa.gov/OP_Home/ssact/title18/1862.htm.

Sutherland Cornet, B. 2006. Clinical documentation in speech-language pathology. *The ASHA Leader* 11(10): 8–9, 24–25, citing Paul & Hasselkus, 2004. http://www.asha.org/Publications/leader/2006/060905/f060905b.htm.

Resources

American Occupational Therapy Association. 2007. *Guidelines for Documentation of Occupational Therapy.* http://www.apta.org.

American Physical Therapy Association. 2009. *Guidelines: Physical Therapy Documentation of Patient/Client Management.* http://www.apta.org/AM/Template.cfm?Section=Policies_and_Bylaws&TEMPLATE=/CM/ContentDisplay.cfm&CONTENTID=31688.

Centers for Medicare and Medicaid Services. 1995. Documentation guidelines for evaluation and management services. http://www.cms.hhs.gov/MLNEdwebGuide/25_EMDOC.asp.

Centers for Medicare and Medicaid Services. 1997. Documentation guidelines for evaluation and management services. http://www.cms.hhs.gov/MLNEdwebGuide/25_EMDOC.asp.

Chapter 4

Health Information Management

Susan Grennan, RHIA

Learning Objectives

- Compare and contrast the different methods of record identification systems

- Explore the differences between serial and unit numbering as well as advantages and disadvantages

- Understand what is meant by unit numbering system

- Demonstrate an understanding of terminal digit filing and list advantages and disadvantages of the filing system

- Learn the benefits to color coding records for different filing methodologies

- Explore the differences between a manual and an automated record tracking system

- Understand the steps to be taken in the analysis of a new form or revisions of an existing form

- Understand the guidelines to be followed when designing a form

Key Terms

Alphabetic filing system
Master patient index (MPI)

Outguide
Serial filing system

Serial numbering system
Terminal digit filing system

Introduction

Health information management (HIM) professionals can provide valuable assistance in the development of a health record system that provides both efficiency and effectiveness in the maintenance and control of the health record. As medical practices migrate towards the electronic record, HIM professionals will continue to develop and manage the hybrid record (part paper and part electronic) during this transitional time (Hall 2008). When up-to-date patient care data are readily available, care can be provided more effectively and efficiently. The Joint Commission Standards RC 01.01.01 and RC 02.01.01 (Ambulatory and Hospital Accreditation Requirements) necessitate that all relevant patient information is to be available when needed for patient care, treatment, and services. These standards even note that tracking the location of all components of the health record is to be possible whether done manually or through an automated mechanism (Joint Commission 2009). Health information management (HIM) professionals can provide valuable assistance in the development of integrated systems that improve the continuity of patient care. HIM professionals are qualified to design systems for the maintenance and timely retrieval of healthcare data.

This chapter discusses different record filing systems available for maintaining health record documentation. It also discusses how patient information can best be managed in terms of organization and retrieval. Finally, the chapter describes the development and control of forms filed in the patient's health record.

Record Control

Regardless of where the health records are stored, someone must be responsible for all of them. This responsibility should be assigned to a health information manager. Filing systems will need to be established for paper records as well as records stored electronically, whether the records are scanned or stored in an electronic health record (EHR).

HIM professionals should develop or be involved in the development of procedures that specify who may have access to a file area or information contained in an EHR. Further, adequate controls should be in place to ensure that records are available when needed by providers for patient appointments, phone calls, or situations involving the treatment of the patient. Policies and procedures should include who is authorized to check out a record, how long a record may be kept out of the file, and what to do if a record is given to another individual within the medical practice. They should also make it clear that the individual requesting the record is responsible for returning it in good condition and within a specified time frame. When the HIM department's workload or volume of records warrants the expense, installation of a computerized tracking system can create increased efficiency. An automated system should be capable of checking a health record in and out, displaying its location, managing multiple record volumes on a patient, and identifying outstanding charts checked out for a specified period of time. In addition, policies and procedures should clarify how the health record is to be organized, and where all components of the legal health record are located, in the case of the hybrid record, so that critical patient information can be retrieved easily.

Record Identification and Filing Systems

The goal of every record identification and filing system is to make it possible to retrieve health records promptly and efficiently. The collection of patient identification data and the assignment of a medical record number or verification of an existing number is the first step in identifying a record needed for a patient visit. Filing systems are based on the type of identification assigned to individual records. Identification may be either alphabetic or numeric.

Alphabetic Identification and Filing

Solo practitioners or medical practices with a small volume of patients or little or no computerization may elect to identify records by the patient's name and file the records alphabetically. Such a system is easy to learn and does not require keeping a file index. However, alphabetic systems are prone to filing errors due to misspelling of names, names that sound alike but are spelled differently, name changes, and duplication of names. Spelling accuracy of the patient's full name needs to be stressed with staff. A system should be developed to cross-reference patient name changes in order to identify previous locations of a patient folder. Some rules to follow when filing alphabetically include:

- Place the patient's last name, first name followed by the middle name or initial on the folder

- If you have identical last and first names, use the middle name for sequencing

- File names with an apostrophe (O'Connor) as if the apostrophe does not exist

- If the patient's first name is listed as initials (J T O'Connor), file the name with J first before a name such as John

- Do not abbreviate names, such as Pat for Patricia

- Do not include titles when determining filing order, such as Dr., Mr., or Sister (Abdelhak et al. 2001)

Assignment of Health Record Numbers

Health record numbers can be assigned either manually or electronically. In either case, the system should accommodate the growth of the medical practice. Most medical practices assign a six-digit number, which usually meets the demand for new numbers for several years. Starting a new numbering series for each year with a letter or number prefix is not advisable because any error in the prefix makes record retrieval extremely difficult. After all six digits have been used (99-99-99), the next logical number to be assigned would be 100-00-00.

When the medical practice assigns its numbers manually, the HIM or patient registration/access department usually maintains a control book. The location of the control book depends on the medical practice; however, the control book should be maintained where the most accurate and trouble-free operation exists. When the medical practice's number assignment system has been automated, the computer can maintain control over the issuance of numbers by issuing the next number to the next new patient registration. In addition, the computer can search the master patient index to determine whether the patient already has an assigned medical record number.

The department responsible for patient registration must emphasize accuracy. The registration/access staff must ask the patient for the correct spelling of his or her legal name. Also, it is a best practice to ask the patient whether he or she has been a patient at the medical practice before or has ever registered under another name. By registering the patient accurately and determining whether the patient has been registered previously, record duplication and the need for costly master patient index (MPI) cleanups can be avoided. This also promotes continuity of patient care.

Numeric Identification and Filing

Most medical practices with a large volume of patients prefer some type of numeric record identification and filing system. A numeric record system requires the use of an MPI to cross-reference the patient's name with the unique medical record number. There are two main systems of numbering health records.

Serial Numbering and Filing

Serial numbering systems assign a health record number for each visit to the medical practice. The patient is treated as a new patient with a new number each time they visit a medical practice. Serial numbering is not used extensively and is only useful in a medical practice in which return patient visits are low or a frequently changing population with serial numbering systems. These numbers are assigned and filed sequentially. Most of the filing in this type of system is concentrated in one area of the file system, which can cause congestion and a space issue, because all current folders are filed sequentially at the end of the filing space.

Unit Numbering and Filing

Unit numbering is a popular system for assigning numbers to health records because patient health information is filed in one place under one number and is easy to retrieve. With unit numbering, the patient is assigned a unique number that is recorded on the file folder and on all subsequent reports filed for that patient. (New numbers are assigned serially.) Although the unit numbering system is efficient and cost-effective, it is important to remember to leave space throughout the files to allow individual patient records to expand with each new visit.

In a unit numbering system, it is imperative that those individuals who assign health record numbers complete a thorough search of the system (manual or computer) to determine whether the patient has been seen at the medical practice before assigning the patient a new health record number. If it is discovered that a patient has been assigned a duplicate record, the contents of all records must be moved to one record, which in most case is the first number assigned.

Advantages of using a unit number for filing include:

- The number is unique to the patient
- The number does not change regardless of how often a person has visits to the medical practice
- Patient information is filed in a single folder in one place

Disadvantages of using a unit number for filing include:

- Records may become thick, thus requiring additional folders/volumes be created
- Space needs to be properly allocated to allow for the expansion of records

Terminal Digit Filing

In terminal digit filing, the record number is broken down into three distinct parts. The number is read from left to right for identification purposes and right to left (terminal digit) for filing purposes. Usually, each part contains two digits; for example, the two primary digits are located on the right-hand side of the number, the two secondary digits are located in the middle, and the two tertiary digits are the first digits on the left-hand side of the number. The staff begins the filing task by considering the primary digits and taking the records with the same primary digits to the corresponding primary section of the file room, where he or she groups the records according to the secondary digits. In the second step, the staff then finds the correct secondary digit section and files the records in numerical order according to the tertiary digits. In this way, the staff can concentrate on two digits at a time and so is less likely to transpose the numbers. Figure 4.1 displays an example of terminal digit filing utilizing six digits.

In figure 4.2, an example of the correct sequencing in a terminal digit filing system may be viewed.

Figure 4.3 provides an example of the correct sequencing in a terminal digit system utilizing seven digits.

Figure 4.1. Terminal digit filing

46	52	02
Tertiary digits	Secondary digits	Primary (terminal) digits
Step 3	Step 2	Step 1

Figure 4.2. Proper sequencing in terminal digit filing system

46-52-02
47-52-02
48-52-02
49-52-02
90-05-26
99-05-26
00-06-26
01-06-26
98-99-30
99-99-30
00-00-31
01-00-31

Figure 4.3. Proper sequencing in a seven-digit terminal digit filing system

123-45-67
123-45-68
123-45-69

When more digits are used, such as nine digits, the number can be broken down several ways. However, the last group of four digits usually is broken down into two sections. The remaining five digits are used for sequential filing, as follows: 123-45-6790 becomes 12345-67-89.

Although users may need more time to learn terminal digit filing, the system is used widely throughout larger medical practices because it is considered more efficient and less prone to error than straight numeric or alphabetic filing. Moreover, using color-coded folders that correspond to the number or numeric record tabs place on the folder in conjunction with a terminal digit numbering systems makes it easier to visually detect filing errors.

Social Security Numbers

The use of a social security number as a unique identifying number is discouraged for many reasons. The following lists the disadvantages of utilizing social security numbers as unique identifying numbers:

- Patient may not have a social security number

- There may be an increased risk of a privacy breach

- There may be an increased opportunity for identity theft or medical identity theft

- Patient may not wish to provide the medical practice with the security number

- Nine digits is a long number for filing purposes

Family Numbering

A variation of the unit numbering system is the family numbering system. In this system, a unit number is assigned to a family and a prefix is assigned for each member of the family. Each prefix also designates the patient's place in the family, for example:

01   Head of household

02   Spouse

03   First child

04   Second child

Information on each family member is maintained in a separate folder but filed under the number used to designate the family unit. This system can be extremely effective in a primary care practice, where the family is often seen as a unit, for example, when the children from one family are brought in together for immunizations. In addition, this system makes it easy to purge inactive records for an entire family. The major disadvantage of the family numbering system occurs when record numbers must be reassigned due to a shift in family composition, such as marriage and divorce. In such circumstances, a new household number must be assigned, resulting in an entirely new record. Other disadvantages include the difficulty of integrating the numbering of a family file system into a system-wide MPI based on a health record for each patient. Further, because they hold and organize data for entire families, family files take up more space and cost more to maintain than individual files. Finally, when the medical practice uses an alphabetic filing system, family files can be more difficult to locate when the individual family members have different last names.

Multiple Volumes

Some health records may become so thick that additional folders are needed to house the complete record. One method of creating multiple volumes of a record is to write or place a sticker on each volume to indicate that multiple volumes exist. For example, the first folder could be labeled as Volume 1 of 2, the second is labeled Volume 2 of 2, and so on. However, all of the folders for one patient would need to be relabeled each time an additional volume was added. For facilities that utilize a computerized record tracking system, the system can track each record volume for a patient. Volumes can be named and potentially be filed in separate file rooms in those cases when a medical practice has multiple locations where patients are treated.

Color Coding

A color-coding system of file folders can help to prevent misfiles and can help in the efficiency and speed in which records are filed and retrieved. Records can be sorted easier and faster. There are several different methods of color coding folders or adding colored bars or numbers to the folder to aid in the decrease of potential misfiles. (See figure 4.4.)

Year labels can also be affixed to a folder on the first visit of each year the patient is seen for a visit. When records become inactive for a period determined by the medical practice, based on the amount of filing space available and the frequency of encounters with the typical patient, records can be easily purged by viewing the year label affixed to the record folder.

Figure 4.4.   Illustration of color coding for terminal digit filing

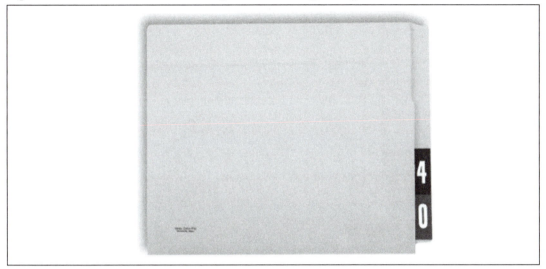

Record Tracking

Knowing the location of a health record out of the file can be one of the biggest challenges of a record management system. The medical practice needs to develop a system to track records that are retrieved from the file area whether the system is manual or automated.

Manual Record Tracking Systems

In manual tracking systems, outguides are placed in the file when a record is pulled from the file. Outguides can either be cardboard or plastic with pockets. When cardboard outguides are used, the individual removing the record from the file will write the patient's name, medical record number, date removed, and location/individual on the outguide to indicate who the record is signed out to, along with the volume number if multiple volumes exist. Outguides with plastic pockets can be used in a similar way, however there is usually a requisition slip with the patient's name, medical record number, volume number, date requested, and location recorded on it that can be placed in a plastic pocket and a pocket to file loose reports for the patient while the record is out of the file. If a record is transferred to another location, the outguide must be updated. When the record is returned to refile, remove the outguide and interfile any loose sheets that were placed in the plastic pocket.

Disadvantages to manual record tracking systems include:

- Amount of time spent updating outguides when a record changes location
- Time lags in updating outguides can result in difficulty locating a record due to inaccurate information on the outguide
- Frustration on the part of the staff to locate a record out of the file

Automated Record Tracking

When utilizing an automated record tracking system, current and past locations of all records and record volumes (when multiple records exist for a patient) are tracked. Automated systems usually include an outguide slip or label that is printed out of the system that can be used in conjunction with the cardboard or plastic outguides. These outguides can serve as a place-holder in the file system for easier refiling of the record or to store loose reports. The outguide found in the file is not necessarily the current location of the record, but merely a placeholder for the file. The automated record tracking system should be utilized to determine current location of a record, to change/update the location of a record, and to place a pending request for a record that is out of the file. The following lists the advantages of automated record tracking systems:

- Online inquiry or record location by anyone with privileges to view record location

- Tracking of multiple record volumes for a patient

- Updating the change of record location can be completed quickly and efficiently

- When records are returned, staff can be alerted to any outstanding requests for the record

- Records can be requested online by the individual

- Records can be checked in or out utilizing barcode technology, which makes the process more accurate and often faster than keying in the information

- Management reports can be produced from automated systems to determine records checked out that are overdue, or reports of pending requests that have yet to be fulfilled

- Some record tracking systems work in conjunction with appointments and scheduling systems to automate the record retrieval process for patients with scheduled appointments

Expansion of the File

The choice of record identification and filing system affects planning for file expansion. For any identification and filing system, additional storage room must be left to allow for expansion of individual health records and/or additional records for new patients, depending on how long the medical practice wants to maintain records in on-site storage. (See table 4.1 for a formula for determining the amount of filing space needed.)

In alphabetic filing systems, the letters of the alphabet appear in any given volume of records with a predictable average frequency. These frequencies can be used to predict the percentage of file space that should be allowed for the records. (See table 4.2.)

To plan space for a straight numeric identification and filing system, one can think of the file room as a circle. As inactive records are removed from the lower-numbered areas, these areas can be consolidated forward, thus creating additional room for the end of the number series to grow into. This method is far easier than moving the entire contents of the file area back to the starting point whenever the end of the number series reaches the end of the filing space.

Terminal digit identification and filing requires space to accommodate the growth of records that are distributed equally throughout the system. To determine the size of each primary section in a new file area, the lengths of the shelves or drawers are measured to find the available inches of filing space. This number then is divided by 100. The result is the number of inches of filing space available for each primary digit combination (00–99). Although this approach may leave considerable space between primary sections, it saves the time required to shift the records later as the file grows.

Table 4.1.   Formula for calculating the number of filing units required

Step 1:	Number of records to be stored per year divided by the average number of records per inch equals the number of filing inches needed per year (A) # Records stored per year / # Records per inch = # Inches needed per year (A)
Step 2:	Number of filing inches needed per year (A) multiplied by the total number of years the records are to be maintained on-site equals total filing inches required (B) # Inches needed per year (A) × Total number of years on-site = Total filing inches (B)
Step 3:	Actual number of filing inches per shelf (34", 36", 42", 48") multiplied by 0.75 equals the total number of usable inches per shelf (C) # Filing inches per shelf × 0.75 = Total number of usable inches per shelf (C)
Step 4:	Total filing inches required (B) divided by total number of usable inches per shelf (C) equals the number of shelves required (D) Total number of filing inches (B) / Total number of usable inches per shelf (C) = # of shelves required (D)
Step 5:	Number of shelves required (D) divided by the number of shelves per unit (5, 7, 8) equals the number of filing shelf units required (If the answer is a fraction, round up to next whole number) # Shelves required (D) / # Shelves per unit = # Filing shelf units

Table 4.2   Predictable percentages that the alphabet requires for filing systems

A—3%	G—5.05%	M—9.5%	S—10.2%
B—9.38%	H—7.38%	N—1.85%	T—3.37%
C—7.18%	I—0.38%	O—1.52%	U—0.24%
D—4.84%	J—2.59%	P—4.93%	V—1.24%
E—1.87%	K—4.24%	Q—0.17%	W—6.31%
F—3.72%	L—4.85%	R—5.05%	X, Y, Z—1.14%

Forms/Information Capture Control

A well-designed health record facilitates communication among providers as well as performance improvement activities, clinical research, legal defense activities, and reimbursement verification. The recording and retrieval of information for all these purposes is the goal of a forms design and control program for a paper-based system. Such a program must consider the design of forms, use of forms, sequence of information, arrangement of sections, and order of pages.

General design principles to be considered when developing a form or a computer screen design are:

- Needs of users

- Purpose of the form or view

- Selection and sequencing of items

  — A list of required data should be compiled to insure the collection of essential data and the elimination of unnecessary or redundant data

  — The flow of data should be logical and also take into consideration the manner in which data are collected

- Standard terminology, abbreviations, and format
  - The use of standard terminology and data definitions is recommended; however when a standard definition is not available, the form or view should supply the definition
  - Words, numbers, and abbreviations should be standardized
  - Data should be placed in the same sequence on similar forms or views with similar layouts facilitates rapid entry and retrieval
- Instructions
  - Instructions can briefly identify who is to complete the data items
  - Identification and distribution of forms should be specified
- Simplification
  - Keep forms or views simple
  - Only create a form or view when there is an established need to collect the data that aren't being handled with an existing form or view
  - Simplification saves in time, effort, and material (Abdelhak et al. 2001)

In a paper-based environment, forms control includes forms inventory, forms identification, forms analysis (ongoing review and revision of existing forms), and forms purchasing. In a computer-based system, data elements inventory takes the place of forms inventory and programming logic takes the place of forms identification. The management of forms or computer views should be a collaborative process that involves several members of the healthcare team such as:

- Health information management
- Information systems
- Healthcare providers
- Others as needed

Paper-based System

The forms history file should be reviewed and updated periodically. Folders on discontinued or obsolete forms should be removed from the active file and placed in a separate, discontinued history file for the amount of time required by the medical practice's records retention schedule.

Forms Identification

Forms control requires that all forms be titled and identified appropriately. Usually, forms identification is a number issued sequentially, prefixed or suffixed by a code for the originating department, edition date, and revision date, when performed. An example of a nursing department form would be: 0001a-10/1/99 ND.

When a form is backprinted (printed on both sides) or comprises several pages, the primary form number (the sequential number) should have as its last character a lowercase alphabetic character, such as an "*a*" to represent the first page and a "*b*" to represent the reverse side of the form or the next page, and so forth.

A forms control register is essential for the proper control of form numbers issued, as well as for other identifying information. It can be maintained either manually or electronically. The register should include the following information:

- Form number
- Title
- Form size
- Edition date
- Revision date
- Name of originating department

Ongoing Review and Revision

Ongoing review and revision of forms, or forms analysis, is a critical step in forms control. It should begin with a regular review of each form, not just when the supply runs out or a change is requested. A forms analysis may be prompted in response to any of the following:

- Reimbursement issues, such as charge slip with outdated CPT, HCPCS, and ICD-9-CM codes
- Operational problems, such as backlogs, bottlenecks, unusual time lags, repetition, or numerous errors
- Areas suggested by top management for potential savings and improvement
- Suggestions for revisions made by the providers or staff

Steps in the form analysis process are as follows:

- The first step in the forms analysis process is to issue a questionnaire to all users. The questionnaire may be completed by the form users or by the forms analyst as an interview guide.
- The second step is to do a fact comparison. Facts about a form are summarized and presented to each user for review. A comparison might show, for example, that some staff still need data that other staff no longer use.
- To assess the value of both newly proposed and existing forms, the following types of questions should be asked:
    1. Who needs the data?
    2. Who collects the data?
    3. Who files the form in the health record?
    4. What purpose does the form serve?
    5. What forms or computer systems already collect these data elements/fields?
    6. What form will this form replace?

7. What will the form cost?

8. Where is the form initiated?

9. Where is the form sent?

10. Where is the form filed in the health record?

11. Where will the data on the form come from?

12. Why is this form needed?

13. Why are the data important?

14. When are the data collected?

15. Can this form be faxed, copied, transmitted electronically, microfilmed, or scanned?

The use of barcoding can prove to be a significant time-saver and the combination of standardized barcoding schemes and automated scanning software reduces errors in indexing document data when used in conjunction with scanning documents into an electronic record system.

According to Dunn, "Patient data can be embedded in barcodes that are printed directly on patient forms from electronic records systems, or other computerized form systems. This saves providers time when applying labels or writing in demographic data, as well as avoids the potential for mislabeling documents" (Dunn 2006).

When it is determined that the form is necessary, a forms flow chart can be used to analyze the distribution of the form and/or its copies. In addition to its overall merit and distribution, the form's content should be analyzed. Does each item serve the stated purpose? What would be the consequence if individual data elements/fields were omitted? Can the data be shortened or eliminated?

Forms analysis also includes a review of the specifications and elements of design related to paper color and weight, ink color, font style and size, hole punching, and so on. Every medical practice should develop its own checklist of standard form design considerations, which spells out its policy on titles, number of copies, head-to-toe or front-to-back format, and so forth.

The following guidelines can be applied to forms design:

- The medical practice name and logo should appear in a consistent location on every form.

- A descriptive title should appear in a consistent location on every form.

- All forms should contain space (for example, upper right or lower left) for patient and provider identification.

- All forms should contain space for barcoding in the event a form would need to be scanned.

- Holes in forms for attachment in the health record should be standardized and should not obliterate data.

- Spacing requirements for margins should be specified.

- Vertical and horizontal lines should be aligned as much as possible to make the form appear less busy.

- Check boxes or lines can be time-savers for providers and also conserve space on the form. They should be consistently to the immediate left or right of the caption and aligned vertically when possible.

- The use of color, shading, font, and point size should be prescribed.

- Form size should be standardized or the use of mounting sheets should be specified.

- Preprinted instructions for completing the form should include purpose, use, and steps in completion.

- Instructions for printing two-sided reports should be provided (for example, "second side printing starts at the top of the page"). All forms within the health record should be printed so that they can be easily attached in the record folder.

- Each person who enters data should arrange the data on the form into groups, data should be sequenced within each group in the order they were collected, and data should be aligned from left to right and from top to bottom.

- Spacing should be planned according to the number of lines per inch for typewritten entries, handwritten entries, or computer printouts.

- Space should be designated for signature(s) and date on each form that requires authentication.

- Multiple pages of the form should be assigned individual page numbers (for example, "page 2 of 6 pages").

- Each form should be identified with a number and printing/revision date.

Forms Inventory

A forms inventory lists all the forms that exist in the system. The inventory should be kept up-to-date at all times. A forms history file provides a complete picture of each form in the medical practice, from development to current status. The forms inventory should be arranged according to the numbering system used to identify forms.

A forms history file can be set up by establishing a folder for each form and filing the folders by form number. Each folder should contain the following materials:

- A copy of the current version of the form and any previous versions

- Drafts showing significant stages of development and pertinent correspondence

- Final approval for the printing or reproduction and issuance of the form

- A record of all actions taken on the form

Electronic Views/Screen Format Design

Automated forms or computer screen views allows the user to electronically enter data into online, digital forms and electronically extract various data for collection purposes. Typically, online form documents are stored in a form format—as the user sees it on the screen. Computer screen views/formats should be designed to meet the needs of the user. The users not only include providers and patients, but also administrative, financial staff, and other external users who use the collected data for a variety of reasons such as planning and research.

According to Abdelhak et al., a well-designed screen views/forms for data entry should include the following:

- Organize fields for data entry in a logical order

- Brief instructions on screens or fields

- Make the screens attractive through the use of color, lines, borders, and so forth

- Use default values in a field to eliminate the need for repeated data entry (e.g., date fields could default to today's date)

- All screens should be user friendly with good menus and system prompts

- Highlighting of required fields can help bring attention to a field for the individual entering data (Abdelhak et al. 2001).

In addition, H. Rhodes considers the following important:

- All views need to have key identification data in same locations for all views (e.g., n, etc.)

- There needs to be an audit trail of views to ensure that all data elements are completed before electronically signing or completing a form

- Test the system with data to determine whether there are any database structure or system design errors that could result in poor data quality

- Screen form must include a paper output

- Sequence of the computer fields should follow the flow of work for the task being performed

- Whenever possible, information should be entered only once and then shared by all appropriate users in the medical practice

- Determine the correct size of the document. Too much information will make the screen difficult to read; too little information on the screen may require the user to scroll through numerous screens for the required information (Rhodes 1997)

Additional information on electronic health records (EHR) models may be found in chapter 5.

Conclusion

Efficient health information management refers not only to the accuracy of the record's content, but also to the ease with which health records are organized and can be retrieved. The medical practice health information department should choose a filing system that meets both the needs of its staff and the requirements of its physical space. After a filing system has been selected, it must be reviewed continuously to ensure that it will meet the medical practice's needs over time. A well-designed forms management program is a process that enables the recording and retrieval of information the many activities within the medical practice. The value of good health record management cannot be overestimated. When health information is clearly organized and easily accessible, the medical practice is better able to realize its goal of reducing the cost of providing high-quality care for its patients.

Check Your Understanding

1. Name two different record identification systems.

   a. Numerical and serial
   b. Alphabetical and numerical
   c. Serial and unit
   d. Unit and terminal digit

2. This type of record identification system is most practical in a small healthcare practice.

   a. Alphabetical
   b. Numerical
   c. Terminal digit
   d. All of the above

3. Advantages of a unit number for filing are _____.

   a. the number is unique to the patient
   b. the number does not change regardless of how often a person has visits to the medical practice
   c. patient information is filed in a single folder in one place
   d. All of the above

4. Which example of terminal digit filing order is correct?

   a. 23-30-29
      24-30-29
      25-30-29
   b. 23-30-20
      23-30-21
      23-30-22
   c. 23-31-31
      24-31-31
      24-32-31
   d. All of the above

5. What is the major advantage of terminal digit filing as opposed to straight numeric or alphabetic filing?

   a. The system is easy to learn and doesn't require a file index.
   b. There may be an increased risk of a privacy breach.
   c. The system is considered more efficient and less prone to error.
   d. All of the above.

6. Color coding a folder can aid in a record system for all of the reasons listed below except _____.

   a. records are sorted easier and faster
   b. misfiles are prevented
   c. purging records
   d. decrease in the potential misfiles

(continued on next page)

Check Your Understanding (continued)

7. When placing a manual outguide in the file, what information should be placed on the outguide?

   a. Date
   b. Medical record number and volume number if one exists
   c. Location/individual the record is checked out to
   d. Patient's name
   e. All of the above

8. Forms control is not necessary for which of the following reasons?

   a. To prevent creation of useless forms
   b. To facilitate the collection of data
   c. To protect existing forms from unauthorized revision
   d. When only one provider will be the user of the form

9. All forms should contain the following information except _____.

   a. form number
   b. title of the form
   c. revision date
   d. name of originator of the form

10. Electronic views of forms do not require which of the following?

    a. Paper output
    b. Menus with choices for data entry
    c. Highlighting of required fields to help bring attention to those doing data entry
    d. Establishment of rules and validation checks

References

Abdelhak, M., S. Grostick, M.A. Hanken, and E. Jacobs. 2001. *Health Information: Management of a Strategic Resource*. Philadelphia: W.B. Saunders Co.

Dunn, R. 2006. Quick scan of bar coding. *Journal of AHIMA* 77(1):50–54. http://library.ahima.org/xpedio/groups/secure/documents/ahima/bok1_029034.hcsp.

Hall, T.M. 2008. Minimizing hybrid records: Tips for reducing paper documentation as new systems come online. *Journal of AHIMA* 79(11):42–45. http://library.ahima.org/xpedio/groups/secure/documents/ahima/bok1_040779.hcsp?dDocName=bok1_040779.

Joint Commission. 2009. Ambulatory and Hospital Accreditation Requirements, RC 01.01.01 and RC 02.01.01. http://www.thejointcommission.org.

Rhodes H. 1997. Practice brief: Developing information capture tools. *Journal of AHIMA* 68(3).

Resources

Hyde, C.S. 2008. Planning forms automation. *Journal of AHIMA* 79(11):34–37. http://library.ahima.org/xpedio/groups/public/documents/ahima/bok1_040780.hcsp?dDocName=bok1_040780.

Kloss, L. 2008. A new era in records management. *Journal of AHIMA* 79(11):25.

Liette, E., C. Meyers, and K. Olenik. 2008. Is document imaging the right choice for your organization? *Journal of AHIMA* 79(11):58–60.

Westhafer, K. 2005. The forms management process: Keeping pace with EHR development. *Journal of AHIMA* 76(8):66–67.

Chapter 5

Electronic Health Record

Margret Amatayakul, MBA, RHIA, CHPS, CPHIT, CPEHR, CPHIE, FHIMSS
President, Margret\A Consulting, LLC

Learning Objectives

- Develop a clear definition of EHR and its benefits over paper-based charts

- Describe the functionality one should expect to have in an EHR

- Compare EHRs in medical practices with EHRs in hospitals and describe level of adoption in these respective care delivery organizations (CDOs)

- Discuss EHR interoperability and the impact on integrated delivery networks

- Understand that there is some EHR terminology confusion in the industry

- Prepare medical practices to adopt EHR in light of the many government and other efforts to promote their use

- Discuss the EHR marketplace and how an EHR may be acquired

- Describe the process recommended for preparing an organization for EHR, the steps in vendor selection, the nature of implementation, and how to optimize use

- Provide information on other health information technology (HIT), including e-prescribing, e-registries, health information exchange, personal health records, and telehealth

- Develop a method to keep up on the rapidly changing landscape of HIT

Key Terms

Ancillary systems
Application service provider (ASP)
Barcode medication administration record (BC-MAR)
Best of breed
Best of fit
Chart conversion
Clinical decision support (CDS)
Clinical systems

Computerized provider order entry (CPOE)
Continual quality improvement (CQI)
Continuity of care document (CCD)
Due diligence
Electronic document management system (EDMS)
Electronic health record (EHR)

Electronic registry
e-Prescribing (eRx)
Health information exchange (HIE)
Health information organization (HIO)
Hospital information system (HIS)
Integrated delivery network (IDN)
Interoperability
Legacy systems

Picture archiving and communication system (PACS)	Pre-load	Software as a service (SaaS)
Practice management system (PMS)	Results management	System build
	Results review	Telehealth/telemedicine
	S.M.A.R.T. goals	Workflow and process redesign

The principles of good documentation are important when physicians move to electronic health records (EHRs). However, it must be recognized that an EHR is more than just electronic documentation. In fact, a good way to think about the move to an EHR is that the chart is not being automated, but the *information* needed to take care of patients in an effective and efficient way is being automated.

Definition of EHR

The federal government, in the stimulus legislation known as the American Recovery and Reinvestment Act (ARRA) of 2009 and its associated Health Information Technology for Electronic and Clinical Health (HITECH) Act provisions, defines an EHR as:

> . . . an electronic record of health-related information on an individual that includes patient demographics and clinical health information, such as medical history and problem lists, and has the capacity to:
>
> - provide clinical decision support,
>
> - support physician order entry,
>
> - capture and query information relevant to healthcare quality, and
>
> - exchange electronic health information with and integrate such information from other sources (ARRA 2009)

This definition is in keeping with that described in the original Institute of Medicine reports:

> Merely automating the form, content, and procedures of current patient records will perpetuate their deficiencies and will be insufficient to meet emerging user needs (Dick and Steen 1991; Dick et al. 1997).

> The EHR "encompasses a broader view of the patient record than is current today, moving from the notion of a location or device for keeping track of patient care events to a resource with much enhanced utility in patient care, management of the healthcare system, and extension of knowledge" (Dick and Steen 1991; Dick et al. 1997).

These concepts continue to define EHR functionality (Tang 2003) and use of computational technology in health care (Stead and Lin 2009).

EHR vs. Paper-based Health Records

The benefits of an EHR may best be considered when comparing an EHR to paper-based health records. While paper-based health records are familiar and have some other advantages,

Table 5.1. EHR vs. paper-based health records

Paper-based Health Record	Electronic Health Record
Cheap	Expensive
Familiar	New to many
Focus on information that only clinicians choose to document	Focus on guided data collection to support information and knowledge generation
Unstructured, narrative annotation—static	Structured, discrete data points—dynamic
Paper health record may incorporate patient-generated documents, such as health history questionnaires, but these are not well integrated into the record	EHR enables patients or caregivers to enter data directly into the record, identifiable as patient-entered data that can be verified by clinician to reduce the clinician's data entry burden
Separate films, monitoring strips, photographs	Digital images incorporated into EHR
No "downtime," except when health record or content is missing, lost, or being used elsewhere	Downtime should be able to be avoided through redundant computing capability
One user at a time	Simultaneous access by many
Often illegible, sometimes cryptic; narrative notes provide something of a story about the patient	Always legible, sometimes too many data points that are not brought together to relate a story unless the EHR has been programmed to do so
Requires manual abstraction to retrieve and report on data	Able to automatically retrieve data and generate reports if constructed to do so
Requires "manual" communication for carrying out tasks—may provide for socialization	Automated tasking and communication—conscious effort may be needed to address socialization
Flippable—it is not necessary to go page by page to find the yellow form; but it can be difficult to find a specific data point	Searchable—specific data points can be readily identified either through sophisticated preprogramming or a literal search for a data point
No access controls or audit logs. Loss or theft may be confined to one or small number of patients' health records, or many in a paper destruction process	Access controls and audit logs as well as many other security services can make EHR very secure, but volume of loss can be significantly greater if it occurs. Perception often is that EHR is not as secure, though can be made more secure
There is no specific support for clinical decision making other than the fact that information may be available in the health record for a person to think about. Paper-based health records do not address the human failing of selective memory, especially in light of the time- and resource-pressured environment in which care is practiced today	Clinical decision support provides reminders, alerts, context-sensitive data collection, drug selection support, differential diagnosis aids, and access to context-sensitive knowledge sources. However, unless the system is sufficiently sophisticated as to learn individual clinician preferences and enable flexible leveling of such support, there can be alert fatigue

they are lacking in a number of ways. This is not to suggest that EHRs are perfect or that there are not barriers to their use. In addition, there is a fair amount of variability in how EHRs work—when they meet the baseline criteria for product certification. Understanding the differences between paper-based health records and EHR capabilities, such as those illustrated in table 5.1, should enable medical practices to enter the information age.

EHR Functionality

The IOM reports previously cited describe the following functionality that EHRs should possess in order to achieve the benefits brought about by the enhanced utility enabled by automation:

- Improve quality of healthcare through data availability and links to knowledge sources

- Enhance patient safety with context-sensitive reminders and alerts, clinical decision support, automated surveillance, chronic disease management, and drug/device recall capability

- Support health maintenance, preventive care, and wellness through patient reminders, health summaries, tailored instructions, educational materials, and home monitoring/ tracking

- Increase productivity through data capture and reporting formats tailored to the user, streamlined workflow support, and patient-specific care plans, guidelines, and protocols

- Reduce hassle factors/improve satisfaction for providers, consumers, and caregivers by managing appointment scheduling, registration, referrals, medication refills, and work queues

- Support revenue enhancement through accurate and timely eligibility and benefit information, cost-efficacy analysis, clinical trial recruitment, rules-driven coding assistance, external accountability reporting/outcomes measures, and contract management

- Support predictive modeling and develop evidence-based healthcare guidance

- Maintain patient confidentiality and exchange data securely among all key stakeholders

EHR in Hospitals vs. Medical Practices

The definitions and benefits described in the preceding have two key elements. First, an EHR is not a replication of paper-based health records but provides significant additional functions (such as enhanced utility); and second, it is desirable for information systems within and across organizations to exchange data (which is called *interoperability*). Both of these elements are challenging to achieve and have also led to some confusion in terminology used to describe clinical automation.

Hospitals may have literally hundreds of information system applications. Those typically found in a hospital are identified in figure 5.1.

While different hospitals may go about acquiring their information system applications in somewhat different sequences, in general, most hospitals follow the sequence in which the applications are listed in figure 5.1. The biggest potential difference relates to the sequencing of clinical application implementation. Some hospitals start with point-of-care documentation, while others start with CPOE. Often what the hospital's primary vendor has available is a determining factor. Another factor includes whether the HIS and ancillary systems are sufficiently up-to-date to support all or only some of the clinical system applications. Yet another factor is how likely the hospital thinks it is that physicians will adopt the EHR components designed for physician use—for example CPOE, results management, and point-of-care documentation. Clinical components are especially challenging to adopt because so many physicians (and nurses) do not use computers on a routine basis. (In fact, many nurses and physicians still to this day have never used a computer!) Finally, just as clinical applications are the last to be acquired, they have also been the last to be developed by vendors. As a result, the clinical applications are generally still the most immature of all the information system applications available to hospitals.

Whatever the sequence of clinical system applications, it is these applications that result in the achievement of an EHR. The Certification Commission on Health Information Technology (CCHIT), which began certifying inpatient EHR products in 2007, required products to have foundational HIS and ancillary systems and at least CPOE and EMAR in order to be certified. In the first two years of the certification process, only about half of the potential vendors (namely, 11 out of 24) were able to meet the certification criteria for inpatient EHR.

Figure 5.1. Hospital EHR functions

- Hospital information systems (HIS) that capture **patient demographics** and insurance information, provide patient registration and admission-discharge-transfer (R-ADT) services, master person index (MPI), capture charges for patient financial services (PFS), and support health information management (HIM) such as chart tracking, deficiency analysis, release of information, encoders, and groupers, to name a few.
- Ancillary systems that primarily aid the operation of the department that uses them, such as a laboratory information system (LIS), radiology information system (RIS), pharmacy information system (Rx), surgery information system (SIS), food and nutrition system (FNS), and many others.
- Results review systems are those that enable viewing of **laboratory reports**, **radiology reports** and other **diagnostic studies reports** (in contrast to results management, to be described next). Results review also includes the incorporation of **consulting physician reports** into the EHR.
- Specialty care systems may include those for use in intensive care units, emergency department, obstetrics, and cardiology, to name a few.
- Electronic document management systems (EDMS), as described above, are used to scan paper documents and electronically feed documents in digital form, such as those from digital dictation systems, transcription systems, e-mail, efax, and so forth.
- Picture archiving and communication system (PACS) is a special type of system that captures **radiology images** and other **diagnostic studies images** and stores them in digital form for review. Such digital images may then be enlarged, rotated, sliced, and enhanced in numerous ways.
- Smart peripherals are medical devices that collect information to support their use, such as smart infusion pumps, robotics for medication dispensing, and monitors.
- Clinical systems are generally those that are used at the point of care, directly by physicians, nurses, therapists, and others. These include:
  - Electronic medication administration record (EMAR) systems, often with barcode support for positive patient identification and then called BC-MAR
  - Computerized provider order entry (CPOE) systems that enable orders for **consultations**; **laboratory**, **radiology**, and other diagnostic studies; **medications**; **nursing services**; nutrition and food services; therapies; to name a few
  - Point-of-care documentation, such as for recording **nursing assessments**, history and physical exams, **physician notes**, **discharge summaries**, **medication lists**, **problem lists**, and **advance directives**
  - Results management systems that enable laboratory results and other diagnostic studies results to not only be viewed, but processed into tables, trend lines, and comparisons—such as comparing a patient's lab results and vital signs against medication administration.
- Clinical decision support (CDS), in various forms, may be incorporated into each of the clinical systems described. Clinical decision support provides context-sensitive **clinical guidelines** for point-of-care documentation; **reminders** (such as health maintenance, preventive services, and chronic care); **drug alerts for allergies**, **drug alerts for contraindications with other drugs**, **alerts where drugs are contraindicated in light of laboratory results**; for examp, a specific drug should not be taken if the patient has poor liver function, and **dosing support** is incorporated into both BC-MAR and CPOE; and integration of more sophisticated data and knowledge-based information resources aids in differential diagnosis, outcomes analysis, population health, predictive modeling for generation of best practices, and data for clinical trials and research protocols. As CDS becomes more sophisticated, a CDS system may be used to manage the data integration and interactions that are provided.
- Security services should afford confidentiality, data integrity, and availability—in other words, the CIA of security.

The level of adoption of EHR in hospitals is even more dismal. Although many hospitals utilize EDMS to create a paperless environment postdischarge, some hospitals do not even have all the foundational applications, and many are just starting to deploy CPOE, EMAR, and other clinical applications. In 2008, researchers from Boston surveyed 3,037 hospitals and found that just 1.7% had fully implemented across all units of their hospitals a "comprehensive" EHR that had all 24 key functions as selected by a panel of IT experts. (These 24 functions are identified in figure 5.1 as bolded functions.) Only 7.9% had a "basic" EHR with 9 of the 24 functions, and 12% had an even more basic EHR with 7 of the 24 functions (DesRoches et al. 2008).

Medical practices have applications that are similar to those in hospitals, though generally the applications are more integrated for a medical practice than for a hospital. The information system applications most commonly found in medical practices that lead to an EHR are described in figure 5.2.

EHRs in medical practices tend to be more integrated than in hospitals; where in hospitals the EHR is comprised of many different components—often operating quite independently of one another. Interestingly, while medical practices may have adopted automation more recently than hospitals, their adoption has accelerated more rapidly than in hospitals. The Boston researchers cited for conducting a study of hospital EHR adoption also conducted a survey in late 2007 and early 2008 of 2,758 physicians on 16 key factors they used to define an EHR (bolded in figure 5.2). They found that 4% of physicians reported having an extensive, fully functional EHR system, and 13% reported having a basic system (which excluded the order management functions except for eRx and excluded all the CDS functions) (Jha et al. 2009).

Figure 5.2.   Medical practices EHR functions

- A Practice management system (PMS) is used for capturing **patient demographics** and insurance information, scheduling patients, possibly managing patient flow throughout the office to reduce wait time, and capturing charges and billing. The PMS in many medical practices may be a "legacy system" based on older technology.

- An E-prescribing (eRx) system may be a stand-alone system used by physicians to be guided in medication selection based on drug-drug or drug-allergy interactions and on formulary information (that is, what drugs are covered by the patient's insurance benefits). Such a system significantly reduces errors in prescribing drugs that are contraindicated and typically recommends lower-cost generic equivalents to brand name drugs. The e-prescribing system then is used to transmit a prescription transaction to a retail pharmacy, where it goes directly into the pharmacy information system at Walgreens, Osco, CVS, Target, or WalMart, to name a few, eliminating prescription transcription—and the potential for error often caused by illegible or incomplete prescriptions and reducing the constant need for a pharmacist to call back the clinician. An e-prescribing system also aids in managing approval of prescription renewals, as the system can generate an automated request to the medical practice from the pharmacy. (If the clinician uses an eRx system that is integrated with the EHR, the renewal processing is further aided by eliminating the need to pull health records to review recent lab results and other information needed to determine whether a prescription should be renewed or the patient called back for an appointment.)

- Electronic registries are generally stand-alone systems that capture information about a specific disease, such as diabetes. Paper-based health records may be abstracted onto bubble sheets that get sent to the organization maintaining the registry for scanning into the registry database; or the paper charts may be abstracted using a template on the registry organization's Web site. In some cases, the registry is used only for quality measure reporting; in other cases, the registry generates a paper form for the next visit that contains documentation and service reminders, such as that a diabetic patient requires a hemoglobin A1c test, foot exam, or retinal exam.

- Ancillary systems may be present in some medical practices. Depending on their size and nature of practice, they may have a LIS and/or RIS. Some practices have a PACS. If the medical practice does not have its own ancillary systems, it may use a portal to access such information from a hospital and/or receive lab results or PACS from another external facility via an interface—either to its PMS or EHR. A document imaging system or simple scanning system is generally considered an ancillary system for a physician office because it serves only to supplement the EHR by scanning externally received documents.

- EHR—When a physician office acquires an EHR, it generally incorporates much of the clinical system functionality described for a hospital (as applicable). This would include **problem lists**, **medication lists**, **clinical notes**, **medical history and follow-up**, and both the ability to **write** and electronically **transmit orders for prescriptions** (eRx), **laboratory tests**, radiology tests, and orders for other tasks (such as notifying a nurse when a patient is ready for an injection). The EHR also enables **viewing laboratory results** and **imaging results** as well as **retrieving imaging results** (such as from a PACS). Examples of CDS functionality include **warnings of drug interactions or contraindications**, **out-of-range test levels being highlighted**, and **reminders regarding guideline-based interventions or screening**; for example, chronic disease care or health maintenance reminders.

- Security services should afford confidentiality, data integrity, and availability (that is, the CIA of security).

Interoperability

The second important element relating to EHR is the ability to exchange data. This is perhaps even more challenging to achieve than enhanced utility. There are generally considered to be three primary aspects of interoperability that must be present to fully enable exchange of meaningful data. These relate to the technical aspects of data exchange—hardware, software, and networking standards; semantics—using standard vocabulary; and process—standard workflows, user roles, and so forth.

Technical Interoperability

Technical interoperability relating to hardware and networking used in healthcare generally is achieved through using technology that meets generic standards across all industries. Technical standards for software, however, are specific to healthcare. Figure 5.3 lists the standards development organizations (SDOs) that develop standards for healthcare information systems. (Some organizations are referred to by their acronyms only.)

Because so many CDOs have "legacy" systems, acquired as many as 10, 20, or even more years ago, the systems do not incorporate the latest technology that might enable better interoperability. For example, some of the newer, Web-based technology is not backward compatible with older technology. This means that a CDO wishing to adopt new technology must replace all of its old systems—an investment many CDOs are unwilling to make because it is a major undertaking or unable to do because of the cost.

However, it is not simply the adoption of new technology for EHR components that would enable better interoperability. The foundational systems that many CDOs have are highly proprietary, meaning the vendor does not conform strictly to technical standards that easily enable exchange of data. These vendors have believed that if they make their systems proprietary, the CDO will be forced to buy all applications from the same vendor. This has come to be

Figure 5.3.   SDOs developing technical standards for healthcare

- American National Standards Institute (ANSI) Accredited Standards Committee (ASC) X12—Develops standards for the exchange of financial and administrative transactions (mandated by HIPAA) for enrollment and premium payment, eligibility inquiry and response, prior authorization, claims, claim status, remittance (explanation of benefits), and claims attachments.

- ASTM International—Primarily an SDO that develops standards for industrial manufacturing, such as for grades of motor oil or size of railroad ties. Its Committee E31 on Healthcare Informatics develops a small number of standards for healthcare, largely relating to the content of data that should be exchanged among referring physicians, for transcription of healthcare documents, and so forth.

- Digital Imaging and Communications in Medicine (DICOM)—Develops standards for the exchange of clinical images in PACS.

- Health Level Seven (HL7)—This is the predominant SDO in healthcare, developing standard protocols for most types of information system applications within CDOs. HL7 has developed a version of its standards that supports Web services architecture, but it is not backward compatible with its earlier "message format" standards.

- Institute of Electrical and Electronics Engineers, Inc. (IEEE) (pronounced Eye-triple-E)—An industrial engineering SDO that develops standards for such things as wireless networks; for example, 802.11. Although its generic standards for hardware and networking are used in healthcare, its early standards for the exchange of data between medical devices and information systems are not as widely used as those developed by HL7 for this purpose.

- National Council for Prescription Drug Programs (NCPDP)—Develops standards for retail pharmacy claims and eligibility verification, as well as for the exchange of prescriptions and other prescription-related information exchanges between medical practices and retail pharmacies.

described as a "best-of-fit" acquisition strategy and has actually worked well in the vendors' favor.

In a best-of-fit situation, the applications exchange data among themselves reasonably well, but do not exchange data as well with other vendors' systems. Despite the disparity between information system applications, some CDOs have not wanted to buy from a single vendor, preferring a "best of breed" approach. In this situation, the practice management system (PMS) or hospital information system (HIS) may be from vendor A, a laboratory information system (LIS) from vendor B, a radiology information system (RIS) from vendor C, and so forth. Extensive interface programs then must be written to get each application to exchange data with other applications. This is very expensive not only because it requires negotiation between two competing vendors to write the initial interface, but because anytime one vendor updates its application, the interface from it to all other applications must be reviewed and potentially rewritten. Because of the workload, the interfaces are written to exchange only the absolute minimum amount of data necessary and feasible to exchange.

Finally, it should be observed that just because two applications are purchased from one vendor does not mean that the vendor developed both applications. The vendor may well have acquired the two products from different vendors, through a merger or acquisition. As a result, the two products may be able to exchange data reasonably well because they have an interface maintained by the one vendor, but they will never exchange data as well as if they were both developed using a common software strategy. Some medical practices have found out about this issue after buying an EHR from the hospital's vendor, only to find that it is at best an acquired product, and sometimes only a product from a vendor with which the hospital vendor has a partnership agreement.

Semantic Interoperability

Semantic interoperability ensures that when data are exchanged they carry the same meaning in any usage. However, just as with healthcare software, many vendors have developed EHRs using proprietary vocabularies—again wanting to keep their clients, but also because the vocabularies have only recently become standardized. In addition, some of the standard vocabularies are not always as user friendly as desired. For instance, the term "mole" is a lay term and not a standard term included in the standard vocabulary SNOMED. As a result, a provider wanting to add the term mole to a patient's problem list in an EHR that has adopted SNOMED exclusively as its standard vocabulary would have to select a more comprehensive term, such as a specific type of skin lesion. (A number of products are starting to use SNOMED as a standard vocabulary, but doing so at the "back end" and mapping this to a proprietary vocabulary that is used at the "front end," or the user-facing part of the EHR.) Vocabularies recommended for use in EHRs include those described in figure 5.4. (Note: There is no government mandate as yet to require adoption of these vocabularies in EHRs as required standards. Instead, they have been recommended for use by the National Committee on Vital and Health Statistics [NCVHS] and are starting to be adopted and tested in federal agencies using health data, such as the Department of Veterans Affairs [VA].)

Process Interoperability

Process interoperability may be the most difficult to standardize. It is particularly challenging to automatically exchange data between medical practices and hospitals because their workflows and processes are different. For instance, a medication order written for an inpatient is sent to the hospital's clinical pharmacy, whereas a retail pharmacy requires a specific set of

Figure 5.4. Recommended standard vocabularies for EHR

- SNOMED is an international, multi-axial vocabulary that provides a comprehensive set of medical concepts. Originally created by the College of American Pathologists, it is now maintained by the International Healthcare Terminology Standards Development Organization based in Denmark. The United States, through the National Library of Medicine, has acquired a perpetual license to incorporate SNOMED into EHRs used in the United States. SNOMED has mapping capability to many of the classification systems, such as ICD-9-CM, ICD-10-CM, CPT, and CDT, and to some of proprietary terminology systems, such as MEDCIN.

- Logical Observations Identifiers and Names and Codes (LOINC) provides a standard vocabulary to encode lab results and other observational data, such as vital signs. It is maintained by the Regenstrief Institute under grants and contracts from the federal government, funding from the Regenstrief Foundation, and other sources.

- RxNorm is a naming system for clinical drugs that links its names to many of the drug vocabularies used in pharmacy management and drug knowledge databases, such as First Databank, Micromedex, MediSpan, Gold Standard Alchemy, and Multum. It has been developed as a joint effort between the National Library of Medicine and the Food and Drug Administration.

- Universal Medical Device Nomenclature System (UMDNS) provides an international naming and computer coding system for medical devices. It has been developed by ECRI Institute, a nonprofit organization dedicated to supporting applied scientific research in the discovery of best medical procedures, devices, drugs, and processes. It is designated as a Collaborating Center of the World Health Organization (WHO) and an Evidence-Based Practice Center by the U.S. Agency for Healthcare Research and Quality (AHRQ).

data to constitute a prescription. Similarly, hospitals require medication administration support to ensure the medication "five rights," namely, right patient, right drug, right dose, right route, and right time, because they administer many medications to their inpatients. Except for a few medical specialties, most medical practices only occasionally administer medications to their ambulatory patients. Unlike in hospitals, medical practices do not need to be reminded to administer medications at specific times and therefore can document the administration as part of a progress note, ambulatory surgery note, or specialty flow sheet. Because of workflow and process differences, SDOs have developed separate technical standards for these two environments. It has only been recently that some of the SDOs are collaborating to understand where there are differences and similarities, and when it is necessary to exchange data across these environments. The result has been a process where standards from different organizations or for different purposes are being "harmonized" for use in both environments.

Integration for Health Information Exchange

Although an alternative to achieving interoperability is for both medical practices and hospitals to adopt an EHR from the same vendor that has addressed both types of organizations' requirements, this is not always a feasible or desirable solution. There are not many vendors in the marketplace that have been able to fully integrate information system applications for the two environments. In fact, there is only one vendor that was certified as meeting the CCHIT enterprise criteria in its first year being offered (2008).

In addition to the workflow and process differences between inpatient and ambulatory care, there are other issues that may best be described as political. While many integrated delivery networks (IDNs) include hospitals and medical practices within a single ownership structure, there are many independent providers as well. Many independent providers do not want to be tied to any one hospital or its information system. Some medical practices that are owned by an IDN have also been known to pull out of the ownership arrangement.

Even if the independent medical practices do want to utilize the IDN system, there can be technical challenges. The approach taken by most vendors who are attempting to develop an enterprise solution is to utilize a single Active Directory that essentially merges all records for a given patient into one database. (Active Directory is a central component of the Microsoft Windows platform that provides the means to manage the identities and relationships that make up network environments.)

From a patient care perspective, this should be an ideal scenario—where all information is available across the continuum of care. However, keeping proprietary information relating to a given medical practice separate is only achieved logically by access controls. This has been something many independent practices have a difficult time accepting. They may not want to be a part of the quality monitoring within the IDN; or, they may fear that the hospital is monitoring the number of patients the practice admits to that hospital in comparison to other hospitals in the community. In some cases, the result has been the creation of "shadow records," or supplementary records within medical practices for certain information that then may not be included in the patient's primary EHR.

The integration of the medical practice's patient records into the enterprise system relies on matching a practice's existing records with records in the Active Directory. This can be very difficult, especially where a practice's records are often not very complete or accurate with respect to patient demographics, or where different standards have been used to create patient demographic data. As a result, the desired benefit of "one record-one patient" is often not fully realized, at least not initially. Compounding this scenario is the fact that the IDN may have multiple systems it interfaces with, so there may be a match for the primary vendor system but not for some of the interfaced systems, such as a commercial lab. Such an environment could pose a patient safety issue if providers attempt to rely exclusively on the presence or absence of information within the "enterprise system," which may not be completely merged.

Finally, once the information is successfully merged, if the medical practice wants to pull out of the IDN, separating that practice's generated information from all other information for the practice's patients becomes a matter of both definition of what constitutes each practice's legal health record and technical feasibility where audit logs must be used to determine who entered what data.

In some cases, the solution for exchange of information has not been an integrated environment, but a health information organization (HIO) that supports health information exchange (HIE). An HIO can serve as a negotiating party to either point-to-point exchange of data among participants in the HIO, or as a data exchange service where each participants' data are retained in a centrally hosted location but maintained in separate physical databases. The latter is much like the application service provider (ASP) model where a vendor hosts the EHR software and stores data for a CDO at its remote data center. Although there is no provision of access across CDOs using an ASP; in an HIE environment, specific permissions are required to identify where patient data are located and to retrieve that data, either from the individual hosts or the individual databases centrally hosted.

Terminology Confusion

As previously mentioned, the industry has suffered somewhat by use of multiple terms, sometimes with slightly different meanings, to describe automation of paper-based health records and even to describe health information exchange.

The EHR as currently being promoted by the federal government and in its most comprehensive sense is not just an automated form of a paper-based health record; for example, a collection of scanned or electronically generated paper documents. An EHR has much enhanced utility. Discrete data are required for clinical decision support, alerts to potential drug-drug contraindications, preventative care reminders, registry functionality, and other patient safety and quality of care aids. However, because the EHR in a hospital is comprised of many components, it can take several years before all of them are fully implemented. Therefore, an electronic document management system (EDMS) can afford improved access to information that was originally captured on a form or other digital media, such as digital dictation, e-mail, or e-fax. Such systems are bridge strategies that provide complementary capability to create a paperless state until such time as all components of the EHR are implemented. EDMS are limited in their functionality and primarily serve to support postcare delivery processes. Where a hospital has adopted an EDMS to achieve a paperless state, the system is sometimes called an electronic medical record (EMR). Often the intent is to distinguish the "paperless record system" from a system with more enhanced utility that would be used at the point of care, which some hospitals then call an EHR. Many hospitals are at the stage in their information systems acquisition where they have some elements of both this "EMR" and "EHR."

Alternatively, many medical practices call their information system EMRs, even though they typically are not based on an EDMS. Their systems do support enhanced utility beyond documentation. Some use of the term EMR in the medical practice is probably based on habit—this was the term most commonly used by vendors initially for ambulatory products. However, some observers suggest—perhaps being somewhat derogatory—that providers use the term because they continue to cling to the medical model of healthcare rather than a wellness model or patient-centric model. Whatever the reason, the use of the term EMR to suggest subtle distinctions based on location of care or type of system is confusing.

Tasked by the federal Office of the National Coordinator for Health Information Technology (ONC) to distinguish between EMR and EHR, the National Alliance for Health Information Technology (NAHIT) has also created definitions that do not match either of the distinctions described previously. NAHIT defines an EMR as "an electronic record of health-related information on an individual that can be created, gathered, managed, and consulted by authorized providers and staff *within one healthcare organization*;" it defines an EHR as "an electronic record of health-related information on an individual *that conforms to nationally recognized interoperability standards* and that can be created, managed, and consulted by authorized providers and staff *across more than one healthcare organization*" (NAHIT 2008) (italics added to emphasize differences). Because interoperability is an issue both within an organization (where multiple systems from multiple vendors exist) as well as externally among organizations, the distinction made by NAHIT seems somewhat artificial. In addition, neither NAHIT definition seems to describe the enhanced utility that the IOM originally called for, or which the federal government is mandating through the HITECH Act of 2009.

Federal Incentives for Use of EHR

The federal government has been promoting adoption of EHR in a variety of ways for a number of years. In 2009, an eRx incentive was initiated, where eligible professionals can receive 2% increase in Medicare Part B charges in 2009 and 2010, 1% in 2011 and 2012, and 0.5% in 2013. Eligible professionals who do not adopt eRx by 2012 will earn only 99% of the physician fee schedule for covered Medicare Part B services, with this moving to 98.5% by 2013, and 98% by 2014 (CMS 2009). Some health plans, such as some of the BlueCross BlueShield plans and others, have already started providing medical practices with free eRx systems and incentives for use of eRx as part of their contracting.

Under the stimulus legislation introduced in 2009, both significant monetary incentives as well as leadership are being funded for EHR adoption. Medicare and Medicaid incentives are being provided for both hospitals and eligible professionals who make meaningful use of EHR, starting in 2011. Eligible professionals may earn as much as $44,000 over a five-year period if they start using an EHR by 2011 or 2012. If an eligible professional is not using EHR by 2014, an adjustment in the level of reimbursement will be made, not exceeding a 5% lower payment by 2017 and thereafter. Meaningful use for eligible professionals requires use of a certified EHR, including eRx, exchange of health information to improve quality of healthcare, and submission of health information on clinical quality measures or other selected measures (ARRA 2009).

In addition to retrospective incentives to providers, federal funding is also being provided to states that may be used for various forms of technical assistance, grants, and no- or low-cost loans. There are also specific programs to fund up-front costs of EHRs for federally qualified health centers and certain other programs for providers not eligible for other support. Funding is also being made available immediately to shore up infrastructure—investing in standards development, training in informatics, infrastructure and tools for telemedicine, improvements in uses of health information technology by public health departments, and other uses.

EHR Marketplace and Acquisition

For a given medical practice, the incentives mean understanding the EHR marketplace and acquiring an EHR system.

The first step in understanding the EHR marketplace is to obtain a solid understanding of what an EHR is. Because many providers do not use computers to any great extent, they often are surprised by the variety of functionality available in an EHR. In other words, many physicians still view an EHR as an automated form of the paper-based health record rather than a tool that provides enhanced utility. A good way to learn more about EHRs is to view demos online, attend trade shows where vendors exhibit their products, talk with colleagues who have EHRs, participate in online social networking tools, and read the literature on EHR characteristics and use. It is also important to plot a strategy for how the EHR will be selected, implemented, and optimized for use (see next section).

While it is important for providers and others in the office to learn as much as possible about what an EHR can do, it is also important to ensure that the EHR is recognized for what it is—a highly useful and sophisticated tool, but a tool nonetheless. It is not a substitute for professional judgment. In fact, many vendors write into their licensure contracts the requirement for customers to acknowledge that EHRs are not medical devices, but require personal vigilance to use. Figure 5.5 provides an example of language that some vendors use in their contracts to this effect.

The second step in preparing for an EHR acquisition is to assess the practice's readiness and to take steps to make improvements as applicable. The phrase "garbage in-garbage out" was coined for a reason: Organizations—in any sector of society—that do not have appropriate leadership, vision and goals, financing, IT support, and efficient workflows and processes today will very likely find that a computer system will only exacerbate these problems. Unfortunately, many medical practices think that an EHR is a silver bullet that will solve their people, policy, and process issues. Table 5.2 provides a list of types of readiness assessments that should be performed in advance of EHR selection. "Getting your house in order" will help determine the nature of EHR product to acquire and make implementation go much more smoothly. In fact, virtually every medical practice that has undertaken an EHR project reports that if the practice had the opportunity to do the project again they would focus much more attention on readiness, planning, workflow and process redesign, and change management.

In addition to addressing the findings of various assessments, thorough planning should also be performed in advance of EHR selection and implementation. Table 5.3 describes a number of planning steps and their purpose.

Figure 5.5. EHR requires professional judgment to use

Example of "hold harmless" language that may be included in an EHR contract:

Medical Diagnosis and Treatment. Customer acknowledges and agrees that all medical treatment and diagnostic decisions are the responsibility of the Customer's professional healthcare providers. Customer further acknowledges and agrees that:

a) The software does not make medical decisions and is not a substitute for competent, properly trained, and knowledgeable staff who bring **professional judgment** and analysis to the information presented by the software.

b) Customer is responsible for **verifying the accuracy** of all patient information and determining the data necessary for Customer's users to make medical decisions, as well as for complying with all laws, regulations, and licensing requirements applicable to Customer's delivery of healthcare services.

c) Customer is responsible for establishing and maintaining reasonable **quality control** procedures to ensure the accuracy of input to the software.

Copyright © 2009, Margret\A Consulting, LLC. Used with permission.

Table 5.2. EHR readiness assessment strategies

Assessment	Purpose and Potential Actions
Understand the culture of the medical practice, its ability to change, attitudes that exist about its leadership, and concerns about automation	A medical practice where there is less openness, less willingness to change, lax adherence to policies, and concerns about automation will not be conducive to the level of change brought about by EHR. The focus in such medical practices tends to be on using an EHR for documentation rather than for clinical quality and productivity improvement. It may be necessary to consider using facilitated assistance in changing the culture of the medical practice.
Analyze the operations of the medical practice using workflow and process mapping techniques, often accompanied by continual quality improvement (CQI) strategies such as Lean, Six Sigma, Balanced Scorecard	A medical practice that uses a CQI strategy to improve and maintain the practice's workflows and processes will gain immediate benefit and be better prepared to adopt automation. When staff members see for themselves how inefficient or ineffective current processes are, desire is created for automated aids. Many practices start a formal CQI process in advance of acquiring an EHR.
Assess the level of computer skills present in all members of the medical practice	Computer skills can be learned in advance of acquiring an EHR through a variety of online tools, local software, and classes. Skills should be reinforced by requiring use of e-mail for internal communications and adoption of automation aids, such as electronic signature of transcribed documents, online viewing of lab results, maintaining a personal schedule on a PDA, accessing the patient schedule from the PMS online, using a stand-alone eRx or at least a stand-alone drug knowledge database, to name a few.
Conduct a review of finances, including current productivity, staffing ratios, debt, and financing options. Prepare a cost/benefit analysis and perhaps pro forma financial statements to learn of the impact an EHR will have on the medical practice's finances. Initiate conversations with the bank, the hospital, members of the community, state and federal granting agencies, and potential other sources to assess funding opportunities	It is essential to understand what an EHR costs—up front and ongoing, what financial resources are available to pay for an EHR, what type of EHR may be feasible to acquire, and what form of financing should be used; for example, straight licensure or ASP. This is not the time to be shy—describing intentions to acquire an EHR to others can not only aid in understanding financing options that may be available but can also support improved relationships with the hospital, community, employers, health plans, and others who may be in a position to provide some form of funding or other support. Many of the workflow and process improvement opportunities identified in an operations analysis can aid in improving internal performance that strengthens a medical practice's financial picture.
Assess information technology (IT) support and infrastructure. If necessary, use an external IT auditor to evaluate your current computer systems and staffing. Also consider the fact that by January 1, 2012 the federal government is requiring use of a new version of the claim, so the PMS or billing system will need significant upgrading. In addition, by October 1, 2013, the federal government is requiring use of ICD-10-CM, with much expanded code structure and specificity that will also impact the PMS or billing system.	Although it will be necessary to acquire additional information technology for an EHR, understanding what you have today and what you may be able to acquire in advance can ease the burden of acquiring everything at once. Some medical practices experiment with different types of input devices prior to EHR acquisition. Some practices set up a wireless network during this time. Most medical practices find they need some external support during an EHR selection and implementation, and often find they need staff to acquire new data analytical skills to optimize use of EHR.

Copyright © 2009, Margret\A Consulting, LLC. Used with permission.

Table 5.3. EHR planning strategies

Planning Steps	Purpose and Potential Actions
Identify project leadership:	
• EHR steering committee	An EHR steering committee should include representatives of every type of staff member in the medical practice, including physicians and other providers, nursing staff, ancillary support staff, and managers of administrative support services. If the medical practice has IT staff, there should be a representative, but caution must be applied in not turning the EHR project into an IT project. The EHR steering committee should have a focus on clinical quality improvement.
• Clinician champion(s)	At least one clinician should assume leadership for the EHR project. Other clinicians must be engaged in the steering committee and other activities. It not advisable for the clinician champion to be a "techno-doc," but rather a mainstream clinician who is a peer to all others. However, it can be helpful to include a naysayer on the steering committee to ensure concerns are always heard and addressed. A large practice may employ a chief medical informatics officer or medical director of information systems, at least part time.
• Project manager	An individual with strong organizational skills should be put in charge of the day-to-day project activities. In a small medical practice, this may be part of a staff member's time; but once a practice is at least nine or more clinicians, the project manager is almost always needed full time. This rarely is a temporary position, as the individual usually turns into a data analyst.
Describe project governance	Especially in medium and large medical practices, it is necessary to describe who has authority and responsibility for making certain types of decisions. This includes everything from who has authority to sign the contract to who may decide to turn off a clinical decision support rule.
Plan for ongoing communication, including celebration of successes and course correction as needed	Use a communication plan to identify from the very start of the project through successful utilization who will be conveying what messages about the project to whom, when, and how. Communication is vitally important. Missteps here can result in valuable staff leaving the medical practice for fear they will lose their jobs, clinicians who unknowingly introduce bias into the selection process, vendors who may raise prices or find ways to sabotage your project because they do not want to lose the business, nurses who become disenchanted with the EHR before it is ever implemented because they were not informed or given an opportunity to contribute to the selection process, and board or owner disappointment in EHR results because they are not regularly informed of milestone achievement and other successes.
Develop a vision statement and S.M.A.R.T. goals	As part of the medical practice's education about EHR, there should be an overall vision of what the system will do for the practice and specific, measurable, achievable, right, and time-based goals that can be used to monitor and celebrate accomplishments or correct course as needed.
Adopt formal change management strategies, including engaging all clinicians and staff members	While change is inevitable in all aspects of life, change through an EHR is sudden and transforming. Adapting to change takes time, so it is essential to start early in the project and adopt various change management strategies and tactics to introduce change, help people prepare themselves for the change, and assist people in coping with the change. The importance of change management should not be underestimated.

EHR Selection, Implementation, and Optimization

While readiness assessment and planning should be done in advance of EHR selection, many of the elements in assessment and planning do not end with the initiation of a formal selection process—but rather serve to enhance it. Certainly, many of the change management and CQI processes will be ongoing.

Selection

Selection has become a relatively formal process, considering the size and type of investment being made. Many medical practices have rarely, if ever, made such an investment, and some are reluctant to put a lot of time or effort into selection. However, following a formal process can keep a practice from second-guessing itself later. It is important to take some time to understand the steps that comprise selection and then determine a schedule for following the steps. This can be helpful to avoid getting into analysis paralysis after months of aimless looking around. Figure 5.6 lists steps in selection commonly performed for EHR acquisition.

In addition to selecting the EHR application, medical practices will also need to select hardware. If the practice is going to acquire a client/server EHR, it will need to add one or more servers and storage devices. Most EHR vendors will provide advice about what types of these hardware devices to acquire. An important caveat here is to request information about

Figure 5.6. EHR selection steps

1. Use a code of conduct to ensure that the vendor selection process is performed without bias and in a manner that preserves necessary confidentiality. The best selection process is one where the medical practice is an informed consumer and able to make a choice based on objective criteria.

2. Conduct a requirements analysis. While it is necessary to select a certified EHR product, there are many of such in the market, and they do differ in a variety of often subtle but potentially powerful ways—including both from a functional and technical perspective as well as from a vendor characteristic perspective. It is important for the medical practice to understand its own requirements and establish specific, differentiating criteria for selection. For instance, if the practice includes an urgent care center, it may be desirable to have a special dashboard feature that monitors where each of several patients are in the care process. Different specialties have different needs. Dermatologists may want to incorporate many "before" and "after" photographs, including the ability to draw on these or to use them to create "future" state images for patients. Pediatricians may need special calibration techniques for drug dosing. Obstetricians may want to keep a series of visits open as a single encounter. A medical practice that has several locations where patients are seen at more than one of these locations may need to ensure there is a single master person index to take extra care in not opening more than one chart for a patient. There are many such requirements that are unique to any given medical practice that should be identified and used to screen products.

3. Canvass the marketplace to identify vendors to whom to send a request for proposal. CCHIT has certified over 75 vendors out of a potential 250 vendors offering ambulatory EHRs. In the future, there may be another certifying body or bodies. It is impossible to thoroughly evaluate more than a half a dozen. Therefore, the medical practice needs to pare down the number of vendors to consider. To do so, medical practices frequently evaluate the EHR offering from its incumbent PMS—if the PMS offers an EHR, the EHR offering from its hospital, and then two to four vendors who are most commonly used in their locale, by their specialty, and for their size of practice. Some other aspects to prequalify vendors may include their reputation for implementation service and ongoing support, their success in equivalent size and type of practices, and their viability—for example, how long have they been in business and selling EHRs, are they rumored to be a takeover target, and are they growing too fast or too slow. This information is readily available by talking to colleagues in medical practices with EHRs.

4. Prepare and send a request for proposal (RFP) to a small number of candidate vendors. There are a number of RFP models on the Web. At a minimum, the RFP should identify to whom the response should be sent, describe the nature of the medical practice in full so that a pricing proposal can be accurately made, request evidence that the vendor is certified, ask the vendor to describe how it meets the practice's unique functional and technical requirements, seek information on numbers and types of clients the vendor serves in addition to requesting specific references, and request a copy of a typical implementation plan, service level agreement, and contract. The RFP should request that the pricing proposal be supplied separately. The vendors may need four to six weeks to complete the response.

5. Once all responses are received, the steering committee should develop a plan to review them in depth, usually using a scoring system to evaluate and rank the vendors. One member of the medical practice staff should review the pricing proposals and set up a spreadsheet to compare them. However, most experts recommend not sharing the pricing information with the selection committee at this time. Every contract is negotiable. Vendors vary significantly in their potential ability to meet return on investment goals. Practices have rejected products that appear to be too expensive, only to realize later that the product might have had a faster payback period, or priced its product a la carte and not all product components were needed. Ideally, the review of responses to the RFP should help the medical practice narrow the field to only two or three vendors to which further due diligence will be applied.

6. Due diligence performed on a few vendors generally includes a series of formal product demonstrations in the medical practice, site visits to other practices using the product, and reference checks—calling additional offices, speaking or even visiting with corporate personnel, and checking partnership references as may be applicable.

7. Once all due diligence is performed, ideally there will emerge a vendor of choice. If there appears to be more than one feasible vendor, it may then come down to which vendor will offer the best contract terms, price, and payment schedule.

8. Approval from the medical practice's owners is usually required prior to negotiating a contract. When obtained, the vendor should be asked to review the response to the RFP, update it as applicable, and finalize its offer by providing a best and final contract. This contract should be reviewed by an expert in IT contracts and the practice's legal counsel. An issues letter should be developed outlining any issues. These may be in what components or modules are included, when and how upgrades will be supplied (especially important relative to the new versions of the financial transactions and ICD-10-CM), how much training is provided, discounts, service level agreements, payment schedule (less down payment and more paid after go-live), to name a few. The issues letter begins the negotiation process, which concludes when all issues have been addressed to the satisfaction of both parties and the contract signed.

what hardware would ensure that the EHR software runs "optimally." Many EHR vendors are reluctant to describe optimal hardware configuration because they fear the price will scare the practice. However, without optimal hardware, the EHR may work too slowly, run out of capacity quickly, or present connectivity issues. Often practices who acquire minimally necessary hardware find they have to replace the hardware fairly soon after implementing their EHR.

If the practice will use a third-party data center to host the servers only, or use an ASP or newer SaaS acquisition strategy, it will not be necessary to acquire servers and storage devices. However, network connectivity and client-side computing devices will be needed. Many medical practices spend considerable time evaluating and debating the merits of mobile computing using a wireless network versus stationary computing and a wired network. Some of the pros and cons of these are described in table 5.4.

It should be observed that rarely does a medical practice rely solely on a wireless network. It is important to have redundancy in all aspects of computing. Any form of host (data center, ASP, or SaaS) should provide server redundancy, including automated failover to virtually eliminate downtime, backup, and disaster recovery. In fact, that is one of the key advantages to such an acquisition strategy—saving the medical practice considerable money in not having to create such redundancy. But if the medical practice has only one form of connectivity and that goes down, obviously the best redundancy at the host site will not afford access to the EHR. Network redundancy would include at a minimum two forms of connection to the host, such as a dedicated trunk line and cable, DSL, or even "plain old telephone service" (POTS) connection. Within the practice, redundancy can be achieved with both wired and wireless networking. Wireless networking is more expensive, however, so some practices prefer to use only the wired network. In addition to cost, the wireless network has been slower than a wired network. The standard, 802.11 used to support wireless is still working on version 802.11n to increase speed and reduce interference.

Table 5.4. Comparison of computing devices

Characteristics	Stationary Devices	Mobile Devices
Type of device	Desktop PC (Note: any of the mobile devices can be used in a stationary mode when connected to a wired network)	• Tablet (slate, convertible) • Notebook/laptop • Personal digital assistant (PDA) • Wireless computers on wheels (WOWs)
Suitability	• Many options for monitors, keyboards, and navigational devices • Always available from network and power perspective	• Affords mobility • Requires wireless network; potential issues of speed and interference • Requires long battery life, extra/swappable batteries, power cords, or power stations • Small screens may be difficult to read • Weight and heat may be issues for some users
Security	Requires log on and off with every use to avoid patient access when not in room	• Enables staying logged on as user moves • Subject to loss and/or destruction
Space requirements	• Thick clients require associated box • Footprint size may be overcome by wall mounting, using a keyboard tray	Minimal space requirements, but some place to put device during patient examination is necessary
Cost	• Generally less expensive device • Wired network generally less expensive	• Generally more expensive device • Wireless network generally more expensive

Implementation

Implementation begins shortly after a contract is signed. As with selection, there are a number of tasks to be accomplished in implementation, however, unlike selection, not all the tasks are performed in a sequential manner. For instance, the medical practice may immediately send a staff member who will be a superuser for training at the vendor's corporate headquarters. Training for all other "end users" will be performed after the hardware and software are fully installed and customized to meet the medical practice's specific needs. Likewise, there are a number of points in the implementation where testing needs to occur.

Implementation should begin with the practice's project manager sitting down with the vendor's project manager and reviewing, in depth, the implementation plan. If any significant changes have been made to the terms of the contract, these should also be reviewed with the vendor's project manager, as it is unlikely this individual has been involved in the contract negotiation. Next, an issues management log should be created by the practice's project manager. Although many vendors use an online issues management system for the medical practice to report problems and check off their resolution, it is always a good idea to maintain an internal system for issues that do not relate to the vendor. This may also include a change control process, where changes made during the "system build" phase of implementation are annotated.

After the initial preparatory work, implementations may vary depending on the vendor. Suffice it to say, the following are implementation steps that must be performed:

- Hardware and software installation. Even if the medical practice chooses to use an ASP or SaaS form of EHR acquisition, the practice must set up a network and install input devices, printers, scanners, and so forth. In some cases, these may require new furnishings, shelves to be built, or wall mounts to be installed. If the practice does not use remote hosting, then a data center needs to be created. If networking needs to be updated or a wireless network installed, this would be performed at this time as well.

- Workflow and process redesign is sometimes called the "discovery" phase of the implementation because it enables the medical practice to identify additional opportunities for improvement with its EHR. During this phase, the practice may choose among various options for workflows and processes if the EHR is customizable. It is also the opportunity to document whatever changes are made in policies and procedures.

- System build, which is configuring the system to meet the medical practice's specific requirements. This varies considerably among vendors. Some will simply add the name of the practice to the system, load providers and staff information, and prepopulate a few other tables. At the opposite end of the spectrum, some products are highly customizable, where practices can insert their own practice guidelines as templates and create their own clinical decision support. Most EHR products are somewhere in between these extremes.

- If there are interfaces to be written, they would be written at this time as well. Often practices replace a legacy PMS at the time they acquire an EHR because so many EHRs now come with highly integrated PMS and the incremental cost of adding the PMS is often less than the interface between an existing PMS and the EHR. If a new PMS is acquired, a decision needs to be made as to whether the existing data will be converted or if the old system will be retained until most of the accounts receivable have been run down. Interfaces would also be required to receive lab data and potentially other ancillary systems.

- Testing should be conducted as the hardware is installed, the system build occurs, for each interface, and to ensure all parts of the system work together.

- Most medical practices do some form of health record conversion or data preload. This may entail scanning some active patient health records, scanning key parts of active patient health records, and/or staff entering key data, such as the problem list, medication list, allergy information, immunizations, and some lab values. In general, the more discrete data values that can be entered the better off the new users will be on go-live. Many practices are finding that unless they need the file room space for other purposes, scanning paper-based health records is not as desirable as preloading data. Most providers do not like to find and view images. The more data that can be preloaded, the less data entry will be required on go-live and the more clinical decision support will be immediately functional.

- A roll out strategy is usually selected unless the medical practice is very small and all providers can go live at once.

- Training of end users should occur as close to completion of all of the above elements and just before go-live. In addition, there is often a "go-live rehearsal," in which staff and providers role play to become accustomed to the system. This is often performed on a Saturday prior to a Monday go-live.

- The day of go-live, and often for a week or so after go-live, the medical practice usually tries to reduce the number of patients seen or extend the work day so everyone has more time to enter data and complete their health records as they see patients. It is very important to get users into the habit of doing this, or the value of clinical decision support at the point of care will be negated. Appropriate patient scheduling is critical during the first week.

- Acceptance testing is not a test to determine that the system is working, as described previously, but is a process usually occurring 30, 60, or 90 days after go-live to evaluate that everything is working properly, that users are actually using the system, and that there are no outstanding vendor issues. At that time, the final payment is usually made and the maintenance agreement kicks in.

Optimization

Optimization is then the ongoing process of using all the EHR features and functions to their fullest extent and to realize achievement of the medical practice's goals. Optimization should focus on monitoring goals to ensure patient safety improvement; quality assurance, improvement, and reporting; productivity enhancements, user satisfaction, patient satisfaction, and financial return on investment.

Optimization depends on a well-executed implementation, but also on ongoing system maintenance. The EHR vendor will regularly supply patches and upgrades. Subscriptions to drug knowledge databases, clinical practice guidelines, and other knowledge sources will be updated daily, weekly, or at other applicable intervals. In addition, as users learn to use the system, they will want to see certain changes made, such as data elements added to or deleted from templates, clinical decision support alerts added or turned off, new reports created, and even new uses made of the data being collected.

Other HIT

Optimization of the EHR also may entail adding new modules or other forms of health information technology. Some medical practices wait until the EHR is stable and being used fully by all providers to add technology such as a personal health record (PHR), telemedicine, continuity of care record (CCR), medical device connections to the EHR, or even participation in an HIO. There are many potential new opportunities and new technology being introduced on a regular basis. Vendors may add new utilities or a medical practice may decide to add utilities that were not part of the base product, such as an automated patient history-taking kiosk, differential diagnosis support, clinical data warehousing with predictive modeling, to name a few.

In some cases, medical practices develop a migration path that starts before they acquire an EHR. A migration path may begin with clinical messaging among care delivery organizations, using a provider portal to the hospital and other practices and/or using a patient portal for scheduling, provision of results, and for e-visits. Because of the eRx incentives, some practices have adopted a stand-alone eRx before an EHR. Table 5.5 distinguishes between stand-alone and integrated eRx systems. Practices that see a lot of patients with chronic disease may start using a disease-specific registry. Table 5.6 distinguishes between a registry and EHR. Practices that have a small lab may decide to adopt a laboratory information system (LIS); or, they may have an older LIS and find they need to replace it to support its use with the EHR. Depending on the specialty of the medical practice, it may also consider acquiring a radiology information system (RIS) and picture archiving and communication system (PACS).

Some of the technology being added is definitely bordering on being very high-tech; but other technology may actually make sense to consider adopting earlier than later. For instance, some medical practices are adopting an automated patient history-taking kiosk even before the EHR. This gets their patients accustomed to using automation and provides useful information

Table 5.5. Stand-alone vs. integrated eRx

Stand-alone eRx	eRx Integrated with EHR
Lower cost of software (free software available)	Higher cost of software
Computing device costs could be the same, although buying for stand-alone may spread payment for eventual EHR use over time	Computing device costs could be the same. Additional servers likely to be needed unless a hosted model is used
Less complex to install and use	More costly and complex to install and use
Good segue to EHR	More to learn than just eRx
Requires interface to practice management system for patient demographics and, ideally, appointment schedule when processing renewals	No separate interface to practice management system required
No certification as yet for eRx except SureScripts connectivity certification	CCHIT-certified since 2008 ensures meets definition of qualified eRx for incentives
Issue of where "official" medication list resides	No issue of potentially multiple medication lists; or patient safety issue of no paper medication list available to clinicians who do not use system
Conversion of data from eRx to EHR is unproven	No issue of data conversion
Does not have access to data to perform drug-lab checking	Enables access to full information about patient, including demographics, appointment schedule, medical and medication history, lab results, and other information for all eRx uses
Does not lessen burden of chart pulls for renewal processing	

Table 5.6. Registry vs. EHR

Attribute	Registry	EHR
Definition	An electronic tool that captures and tracks data for a patient population with a particular disease or health state	An electronic record of health-related information on an individual that conforms to nationally recognized interoperability standards and that can be created, managed, and consulted by authorized clinicians and staff across more than one healthcare organization (NAHIT 2008)
Costs	• Some public domain registries; some sponsored by local medical societies, quality improvement organizations, clinic consortia, independent practice associations (IPA), health plans, federal government, or pharmaceutical companies • Less than EHR; varies depending on whether bought or built (building requires knowledge of database development) • Interfaces (from practice management, lab, billing system—if desired and if feasible) • Staff time to enter data, or manage patient matching if source of data is from external feed	• More expensive than registry; cost varies widely depending on level of sophistication, customization requirements, and interfaces • Registry functionality may not fully exist in EHR so staff time to abstract data or create reports to provide registry functionality still may be required
Barriers	• Limited data set requires adherence to standard data elements and their definitions • Contributing to multiple registries with similar but not precisely the same data requirements or definitions may be confusing and time consuming; this issue may increase with the incentive	• Cost is most frequently cited barrier • Other barriers include interoperability issues, privacy and security concerns, questions about legality, and concerns for product obsolescence (although all of these issues are largely addressed today)
People challenges	• Chart abstraction may not be timely, and can be error prone • Chronic disease reminders on separate papers can get lost with the assumption that there are no current reminders • Change management and workflow issues need to be addressed	• Resistance to use of computers at the point of care by some providers and other staff • Time consuming to implement and maintain, especially where there is a high degree of customization capability • Process and workflow changes often under estimated and not well planned
System challenges	• Limited R&D to expand capabilities • Weak implementation support • Often not scalable • Cannot document entire clinical note; no other health record functionality • Registries are not often HL7 compliant for interoperability with other systems • Ad hoc reporting may require knowledge of database design even if registry is a commercial product	• Handles one patient, one problem at a time • Weak population management functions; although these are improving with increasing incentives • Some products have little or no care/case management functionality • Ad hoc reporting may require light programming skills
Benefits	• Easier to use (than EHR) for stratifying, targeting, and tracking all patients in a given population (e.g., all diabetics in the practice) • Organizes data within a condition around guidelines and adherence • Designed for tracking patients outside of point of care, including generating call lists and/or mailing labels • Population-based data available for variety of purposes, including quality improvement, credentialing, incentive reporting, contracting	• Used for all patients, all data results in timely, anytime, anywhere access • Complete and legible visit documentation • Clinical decision support through alerts, reminders, templates, and other aids • Strong research and development and support (from major vendors) • Communication with other providers, continuity of care, on call coverage, referrals, patients • Support for patient safety—avoiding medication errors, communicating test results, immunization recording

Table 5.6. Registry vs. EHR *(continued)*

Attribute	Registry	EHR
Incentives	• "Qualified registries" may be used for contributing data for some incentive programs • Other and local incentives may be available for certain types of providers • No certification program at this time	• Physician Quality Reporting Initiative (PQRI) does not require EHR but EHR greatly facilitates reporting • HITECH Act of 2009 requires certified EHR for retroactive incentives covering some or all of cost of acquisition • Certification Commission for Health Information Technology (CCHIT) exists
Summary	Database that tracks population of (chronic care) patients	Sophisticated software that supports clinical decision making at point of care

for the patient assessment. If added as part of the initial EHR, it can greatly reduce the data entry burden for nurses and providers alike. Such functionality can also be a part of a PHR function or contribute to a later acquisition of a PHR (see chapter 9). Similarly, many providers are frustrated with the lack of needed information when referrals are made. The CCR is standard data content developed by the ASTM International SDO for the purpose of exchanging data in a referral situation. It has been merged with the HL7 clinical document architecture (CDA) to become the continuity of care document (CCD). It is the ideal way to exchange data with other providers, and it is also being used as the basis for many PHRs. It may be a utility to be included in the EHR earlier than later.

Finally, some medical practices have moved to adopt one or more forms of telehealth/telemedicine. The term "telemedicine" generally connotes use of remote connectivity to link a provider to a patient for the purpose of patient care monitoring, an actual patient care encounter, or a consultation. Telehealth is generally broader, and may also include training, simulation, conferencing, language translation services, and many other uses. Telehealth/telemedicine may use somewhat simple technology where there is only audio or audio/visual connectivity through a phone line; or may use highly sophisticated technology such as robotics to perform remote surgery or retrieval of wounded from a battlefield. Home monitoring is another element of telehealth/telemedicine. Home monitoring may include devices that only the individual uses, such as a pedometer or thermometer. Information from these devices may never get reported to a provider, only verbally communicated. Home monitoring also includes use of personalized diagnostics, such as home pregnancy tests or tests for HIV that may be sent to a designated lab. In general, when home monitoring is used as part of a telehealth/telemedicine encounter or consultation it includes transmission of biometric data from sensors applied to a patient in a remote setting back to a base station. Some examples would be cardiac monitoring, fetal monitoring, and vital sign reporting. There are many advantages of telehealth/telemedicine, including reduced transportation costs, ability to treat a patient more rapidly, avoiding emergency department visits, and reducing length of stay in a hospital or even avoiding an admission. Perhaps the biggest impediments to use of telehealth/telemedicine include cost of devices and connectivity, lack of FDA approval of devices that then must remain within the research domain, and provider licensure and reimbursement issues. Most states have yet to address the ability for providers or nurses to practice telehealth/telemedicine in states other than those in which they are explicitly licensed. In addition, reimbursement for telehealth/telemedicine encounters and consultations is almost nonexistent. Medicare will recognize telemonitoring as an allowable cost only for certain services; Medicaid provides payment only under the fee-for-service plans in about half the states and technology is not included; and a few private insurers have only begun to look at coverage. When telemedicine reporting and monitoring is utilized within a medical practice, the documentation of telemedicine encounters and communications must be documented in the health record.

Keeping Up-To-Date

Finally, whether to optimize use of the EHR, take advantage of incentives, ensure your system is meeting all new regulatory requirements, or starting to participate in new forms of health information exchange, it is necessary to keep up-to-date. Obviously, perusing every possible new piece of information can be time consuming. However, identifying a few key e-newsletters, list serves, or other resources that summarize new information and provide links to additional information is essential. The EHR vendor should help keep medical practices informed and often has a user group that meets virtually or in person to provide tips for enhancing use and gives medical practices a forum in which to make recommendations for product enhancements.

Conclusion

Although EHRs remains a "voluntary mandate" from the federal government, there are increasingly strong incentives to move from paper charts to computer-based systems. There are many benefits that relate to provider productivity, office efficiency, reducing lost chart and pharmacy call back hassles, and—most importantly—patient safety and continual quality improvement opportunities. EHRs are definitely more than automated forms of the paper-based health records—they are sophisticated systems that should support clinical decision-making and exchange of information across the continuum of care. EHRs, however, are not perfect, and not without controversy. They are tools that require users to apply professional judgment. Just as with other tools, some EHRs are better than others, or at least some EHRs are more suited to certain practices than others. Determining a practice's readiness and planning for EHR, and then applying a formal process of vendor selection will help a practice ensure it has made the right investment. Most medical practices find that while acquiring an EHR is a major project undertaking, including implementation, testing, training, and going live, maintaining and optimizing use of the EHR is an ongoing program that supports continual quality improvement. In fact, implementing an EHR is not an IT project nor a documentation project, but the hardware, software, people, policies, and processes that transform healthcare.

Check Your Understanding

1. What is the primary difference between an EHR in a hospital and physician office?
   a. Hospital EHR has components
   b. Hospital EHR is more integrated
   c. Physician office does not use EHR to enter orders
   d. Physician office EHR has no clinical decision support

2. The level of adoption of EHR in physician offices is _____.

    a. accelerating more rapidly than in hospitals
    b. estimated to be close to 50 percent
    c. less than 2 percent
    d. primarily in small, family practice facilities

3. In which environment is e-prescribing used?

    a. Both in hospitals and physician offices to select drugs
    b. For Medicare patients only
    c. Hospital for medication ordering
    d. Physician office to transmit prescriptions to retail pharmacies

4. Which of the following is the standards development organization that defines protocols for exchange of clinical images?

    a. ASTM International
    b. Digital Imaging and Communications in Medicine (DICOM)
    c. Health Level Seven (HL7)
    d. Universal Medical Device Nomenclature System (UMDNS)

5. A naming system for clinical drugs that aids drug knowledge is _____.

    a. International Classification of Diseases
    b. National Council for Prescription Drug Programs
    c. National Drug Codes
    d. RxNorm

6. When a standard terminology is used to exchange information among providers, the interoperability is referred to as _____.

    a. functional
    b. process
    c. semantic
    d. technical

7. The number of vendors offering an enterprise solution to achieve EHR interoperability is _____.

    a. almost all inpatient vendors
    b. confined to hospital information system vendors
    c. half of all ambulatory vendors
    d. very small

8. The federal government incentive for use of EHR _____.

    a. covers the full cost of a product
    b. gives providers payment for reporting and exchanging data
    c. provides capital at low or no cost
    d. reimburses at a higher RVU rate for users

(continued on next page)

Check Your Understanding *(continued)*

9. A technique that helps assess readiness for EHR is _____.

   a. change management
   b. EHR steering committee
   c. visioning and goal development
   d. workflow and process mapping

10. The process of thoroughly investigating a product and vendor is _____.

   a. due diligence
   b. issuance of request for proposal
   c. operations analysis
   d. readiness assessment

References

American Recovery and Reinvestment Act (ARRA) of 2009. Public Law 111-5.

Centers for Medicare and Medicaid Services. 2009. E-prescribing incentive program: Overview. http://www.cms. hhs.gov/ERXincentive/.

DesRoches, C.M., et al. 2008. Electronic health records in ambulatory care—A national survey of physicians. *New England Journal of Medicine* 359:50–60. http://content.nejm.org/cgi/content/full/NEJMsa0802005.

Dick, R.S., and E.B. Steen, eds. 1991. Committee on Improving the Patient Record, Institute of Medicine. *The Computer-based Patient Record: An Essential Technology for Health Care*. Washington, DC: National Academies Press.

Dick, R.S., E.B. Steen, and D.E. Detmer, eds. 1997. Committee on Improving the Patient Record, Institute of Medicine, Revised Edition. *The Computer-based Patient Record: An Essential Technology for Health Care*. Washington, DC: National Academies Press.

Jha, A.K., et al. 2009. Use of electronic health records in U.S. hospitals. *New England Journal of Medicine*. 360(16): 1628-1638. http://content.nejm.org/cgi/content/full/NEJMsa0900592.

National Alliance for Health Information Technology. 2008. Report to the Office of the National Coordinator for Health Information Technology on defining key health information technology terms. http://healthit.hhs.gov/ portal/server.pt/gateway/PTARGS_0_10741_848133_0_0_18/10_2_hit_terms.pdf.

Stead, W.W. and H.S. Lin, eds. 2009. Committee on Engaging the Computer Science Research Community in Health Care Informatics, Institute of Medicine. *Computational Technology for Effective Health Care: Immediate Steps and Strategic Directions*. Washington, DC: National Academies Press.

Tang, P.C., Chair. 2003 (July 31). Letter report: Committee on Data Standards for Patient Safety, Institute of Medicine. Key capabilities of an electronic health record system.

Chapter 6

Reimbursement Considerations

Cheryl Gregg Fahrenholz, RHIA, CCS-P

Learning Objectives

- Explore the steps along with the details of each step of the revenue cycle

- Identify coding resources

- Illustrate the performance improvement process

- Gain an understanding of the Physician Quality Reporting Initiative (PQRI)

- Develop practical examples of coding scenarios

- Understand the standards of ethical coding

- Present the Advanced Beneficiary of Noncoverage form information

- Explore the basis for revenue audit contractors (RACs)

- Explore the basic components of an internal coding audit processes

Key Terms

Abuse
Accounts receivable (A/R)
Accounts receivable days or aging
AHIMA Standard of Ethical Coding
Ancillary services
Bad debt
Benchmarking
Best practice
Bundling
Carrier
Centers for Medicare and Medicaid Services (CMS)
Charge capture
Charge description master
Charge entry

Charge reconciliation
Charge slip
Coding Clinic for ICD-9-CM
Coding compliance plan
Collection
Collection agency
Compliance
Compliance plan
Compliance program guidance
Contractual adjustment
Copayment
CPT Assistant
Credentialing
Credit balance
Current Procedural Terminology (CPT)

Current Procedural Terminology Category I Code
Current Procedural Terminology Category II Code
Current Procedural Terminology Category III Code
Days in accounts receivable
Deductible
Denial
Denial management
Dunning message
Explanation of Benefits
False Claims Act
Fee schedule

Financial assistance

Fraud

Health Care Common
Procedural Coding System
(HCPCS)

Health Insurance Portability
and Accountability Act of
1996 (HIPAA)

International Classification
of Diseases, ninth
revision, Clinical
Modification (ICD-9-CM)

Key performance indicators

Local coverage
determination (LCD)

Lost charge

Managed care

Medically Unlikely Edits
(MUEs)

Modifier

National Correct Coding
Initiative (NCCI)

National Coverage
Determination (NCD)

No-show

Office of Inspector General
(OIG)

Office of Inspector General
Work Plan

Payer

Payer mix

Precollection

Preregistration

Registration

Remittance advice (RA)

Reserves

Revenue cycle

Revenue cycle management

Small balance

Unapplied cash

Write-off

Introduction

The revenue cycle is the process of how patient financial and health information moves into, through, and out of the medical practice, culminating with the practice receiving reimbursement for the services provided. A streamlined and efficient revenue cycle can result in a successful medical practice. Conversely, a revenue cycle that lacks efficiency, proper skills set of staff, and effective denial management can negatively impact the medical practice's bottom line.

The coding of diagnoses, signs and symptoms, services or procedures, and supplies involves the process of assigning numbers to narrative diagnostic and procedural statements. The narratives and statements become coded data that can be easily collected, stored, and manipulated for both internal and external purposes. Internally, coded data are used for a variety of purposes, including, but not limited to, marketing, budgeting, and quality improvement projects. Externally, they are used to help forecast healthcare needs, to monitor quality of care, and to reimburse healthcare providers. Clearly, the successful medical practice implements and supports efforts to ensure the integrity of these critically important data sets.

This chapter describes the major steps in the revenue cycle along with the format, structure, and conventions of the three major healthcare coding systems: International Classification of Diseases, ninth revision, Clinical Modification (ICD-9-CM); Current Procedural Terminology (CPT); and Health Care Financing Administration Common Procedure Coding System (HCPCS). In addition, it discusses the Physician Quality Reporting Initiative, advanced beneficiary notice of noncoverage, and internal reimbursement policies.

Steps in the Revenue Cycle Process

There are many fundamental elements that must be in place at a medical practice. Proper organizational structure to support the revenue cycle management, along with physician support, is a best practice foundation. Clear communication about the revenue cycle between administration and providers must include more than simply supplying monthly reports or a dashboard report to the providers. Each provider should understand how to read and interpret the monthly reports regarding the revenue cycle, as well as take action, if necessary.

Each step of the revenue cycle requires documented policies and procedures that are followed by staff and enforced by practice leadership.

Revenue Cycle Team

The revenue cycle requires a team of professionals for success. The individuals responsible for managed care contracting and business development are instrumental in establishing a solid foundation for the revenue cycle. In collaboration with the physician and information systems staff, the administrative and clinical staff completes the revenue cycle team. Key players in the revenue cycle team are:

- Vice president of Revenue Cycle Management
- Chief financial officer
- Vice president of Managed Care Contracting
- Physician/provider leadership
- Director of Business Development
- Practice administrator
- Regional leadership (for large group networks)
- Director of Patient Access/Registration
- Director of Purchasing (including pharmaceuticals)
- Director of Professional Service Billing (Business Office)
- Director of Revenue Cycle Management

In smaller practices that may not have vice president and director positions, key leaders would be represented from each of the following areas:

- Physician/provider leadership
- Revenue cycle management
- Managed care contracting (may be a contracted healthcare attorney)
- Office manager
- Patient Access/Registration
- Professional billing or outsourced billing company
- Finance/Accounting (may be contracted accounting firm)
- Clinical (may be registered nurse, licensed practical nurse, or medical assistant)
- Collections (may be an outsourced collection company)

Monitoring the revenue cycle requires highly skilled and knowledgeable professionals. The skill set requires not only a detailed-oriented professional, but also the ability to produce, dissect, and monitor a variety of reports and reporting methods. Communications skills are exceedingly important, because these professionals will be interacting with all physicians, administration, and staff.

The goals of the revenue cycle team vary slightly depending upon the specialty of the practice; however, common to all specialties would be the following goals:

- Identify opportunities in the revenue cycle flow to increase efficiency.

- Improve the accounts receivable.

- Reduce denials and streamline the appeals process.

- Identify lost charges.

- Provide continued communications on revenue cycle management issues.

- Ensure baseline knowledge of the revenue cycle with all providers and staff.

- Identify a baseline of key performance indicators for the revenue cycle.

- Establish appropriate benchmarks and goals for the revenue cycle.

- Provide useful reporting to providers and administration.

- Identify payment issues with payers.

- Complete a reimbursement analysis for all new services prior to implementation of the services or all new equipment prior to the purchase of equipment.

- Identify or facilitate the identification of best practice models for components of the revenue cycle.

Key Performance Indicators

Key performance indicators are areas identified for needed improvement through benchmarking and continuous quality improvement. In order to begin this process, the practice's baseline statistics on key areas must be documented. Improvement may only be measured if the starting place is determined. Potential areas to establish baselines and comparative benchmarking statistics are:

- Number of days in accounts receivable

- Accounts receivable aging (aging buckets of 0-30, 31-60, 61-90, 91-120, and 121+ days)

- Lag time for initial claims processing

- Total dollars of claims not initially processed

- Number of primary payer claims processed electronically

- Total charges for a day, month, and year

- Percentage of insurance coverage verifications completed

- Number of missing charge slips

- Number or percentage of clean claims (no errors in initial submission)

- Number of claims denied with associated dollar amounts

- Number of denied claims with associated reason codes

- Write off dollars for specific reason codes

- Total dollars unapplied

- Total number of claims as credit balances with associated dollar amounts

- Lag time for posting payments (including cash)

- Number of claims turned over to collections with the associated dollar amounts

- Number of claims deemed as bad debt with the associated dollar amounts

- Percentage of copays collected at the time of service

- Percentage of accurate registrations

- Payer mix distribution

The universal key indicator is the number of days in accounts receivable.

Revenue Cycle Flow

Credentialing and Contracting

Proper credentialing is the first step in the revenue cycle. If the credentialing process is not completed correctly, proper reimbursement for services performed is not received and denials are affected. The credentialing process is a tedious task and requires a detailed-oriented, multitasking professional who can monitor and document extensive follow-up. Although the credentialing process may sometimes take three to nine months for a particular payer, many payers complete their credentialing process within six months.

In some practices the credentialing process is completed manually, while in other, mostly larger practices, the credentialing process is automated utilizing credentialing software. Although the initial loading of key data into the software may be time-consuming, the recredentialing and maintenance process is streamlined and runs more efficiently than manual systems. Automated credentialing systems also produce useful reports and reminders.

One oversight in the credentialing process is that some providers think once they are credentialed, they can start billing for their services and will receive the appropriate reimbursement. On the contrary, there is an additional step with the majority of the payers, and a patient's financial responsibilities, such as copayments, may be increased if this step is not completed correctly. The contracting step must be completed. This will ensure that in-network reimbursements are received from commercial payers. With some payers, it is only after both the credentialing and contracting steps are completed that the effective dates for the providers are issued. Even if credentialing is completed, if the effective date is not entered into the payer's computer system, the reimbursements will not be correct.

Fee Schedule

Each medical practice will establish fees for the professional services that are performed. This listing of CPT and HCPCS codes along with the corresponding charge will comprise the fee schedule. The process of reviewing payer reimbursement for a given charge should be performed continuously as payments are received. If at any time the payment received from a payer equals the charge amount, the practice is leaving money on the table. This translates that the payer would have reimbursed more for the line item billed, but the practice's charge was too low. If a payer's reimbursement amount is higher than billed charges, the payer may

Figure 6.1.   Frequently asked questions regarding fee schedule changes

---

Commonly asked questions from physicians and providers

- Why are we changing our fees?
- Will the patient have to pay more or will the insurance companies cover the fee?
- How often will these increases occur?
- How is this going to affect my productivity target and compensation?
- Why aren't we adjusting our fees to the high end of the market?
- How did we arrive at this fee schedule?

Commonly asked questions from practice leadership

- Why are we changing our fees?
- Will staff get a raise?
- How did we arrive at this fee schedule?
- How is this going to affect the physician's productivity target and compensation?
- Why aren't we adjusting our fees to the high end of the market?
- Didn't we just raise our fees?
- What if self-pay patients can't afford these fees?
- Why didn't you give us some additional notice?

Commonly asked questions from staff

- Why are we changing our fees?
- Will the patient have to pay more or will the insurance companies cover the fee?
- How often will these increases occur?
- When will I receive a raise?

---

reimburse the practice the billed charge. The payer will not automatically reimburse the practice the higher payment or the current reimbursement rate for a given CPT/HCPCS code.

Once charges are set and a fee schedule is developed, the maintenance of the fee schedule must not be forgotten. The maintenance process occurs continuously throughout the fiscal year; however, major adjustments in fees occur annually with the release of the Centers for Medicare and Medicaid's Physician Fee Schedule. Close attention to pharmaceuticals should be paid, because the costs for these products may change drastically from one shipment to another—especially if a generic drug is taken off the market and only the brand name pharmaceutical is available for purchase. For detailed information on fee schedule calculations, see chapter 10.

When fees are adjusted, then proper communication must be made to the physicians, providers, practice staff, and patients. It is a best practice to develop an FAQ (frequently asked questions) sheet as part of the communication plan. Commonly asked questions may be found in figure 6.1.

First Contact by the Patient

Oftentimes the first contact with a patient is over the telephone or through a Web site question from the potential patient. Whether the interaction is with a clinical or administrative staff member, accurate information must be collected, such as demographic information. Denial rates significantly increase when the incorrect demographic information is entered into the EHR, practice management, or billing systems.

Preregistration or Registration

Accuracy of data entry is of vital importance to ensure proper reimbursement. Many practices utilize technology to reduce human error in data entry. One example is the ability to swipe the patient's insurance card, which automatically populates the required data fields in the EHR. Whether advanced technology is utilized or registration data is keyed manually by staff, a copy of the patient's insurance card and photo identification should be made at the patient's first visit. For each visit thereafter, the patient's insurance card and photo identification should be reviewed for accuracy. The current information should always be updated in the EHR, practice management, and billing systems.

Some practices utilize online registration forms that may be completed on the practice's Web site, or the registration form may be printed from the Web site, completed manually by the patient, and brought to the first patient visit. When technology is utilized, there is still the human error opportunity by the patient, so this demographic information should be verified by the practice staff.

Depending upon the location and population of the practice's patients, it may be required that registration forms be available in multiple languages. In multicultural locations, such as New York City, registration forms and other patient forms are provided in a multitude of languages.

Insurance Verification and Preauthorization

As with any service performed at a medical practice, insurance verification should be completed prior to the service being performed. Many payers have online eligibility that may be utilized for the most time-efficient responses. At times, a phone call to the payer may be required, especially in cases where surgical procedures are planned. Supporting documentation, such as test results or visit notes, may be required by the payer prior to preauthorization.

Some vendors offer software programs that allow the practice to manage the eligibility in a sophisticated manner. These programs may allow report-sorting functionalities that expedite report review, such as sorting by payer. Figure 6.2 illustrates an example of an eligibility screen from RealMed's Revenue Cycle Management software.

In a paper-based environment, a best practice reference would be a payer grid or spreadsheet that details by CPT or HCPCS code the requirements by payers, such as which CPT codes require a referral or preauthorization. This reference will save practice staff valuable time, as well as reduce errors and denials. For services requiring preauthorizations, this task is often completed by clinical staff, since they may have the best knowledge base for the actual service ordered.

However, in a computerized environment, programs may offer the enhanced ability to automatically verify eligibility with payers prior to performed services, as well as monitoring claims eligibility throughout the submission and payment process. Additional benefits of automated eligibility are the reduction in manual phone calls to the payer, increased report functionalities, and reduced denials.

Patient Scheduling

Although the majority of medical practices utilize an automated patient scheduling system, this system is only as good as the staff making the appointments. Accurately determining the appropriate appointment times is critical to efficient patient scheduling. An overflow of

Figure 6.2. RealMed Eligibility Management

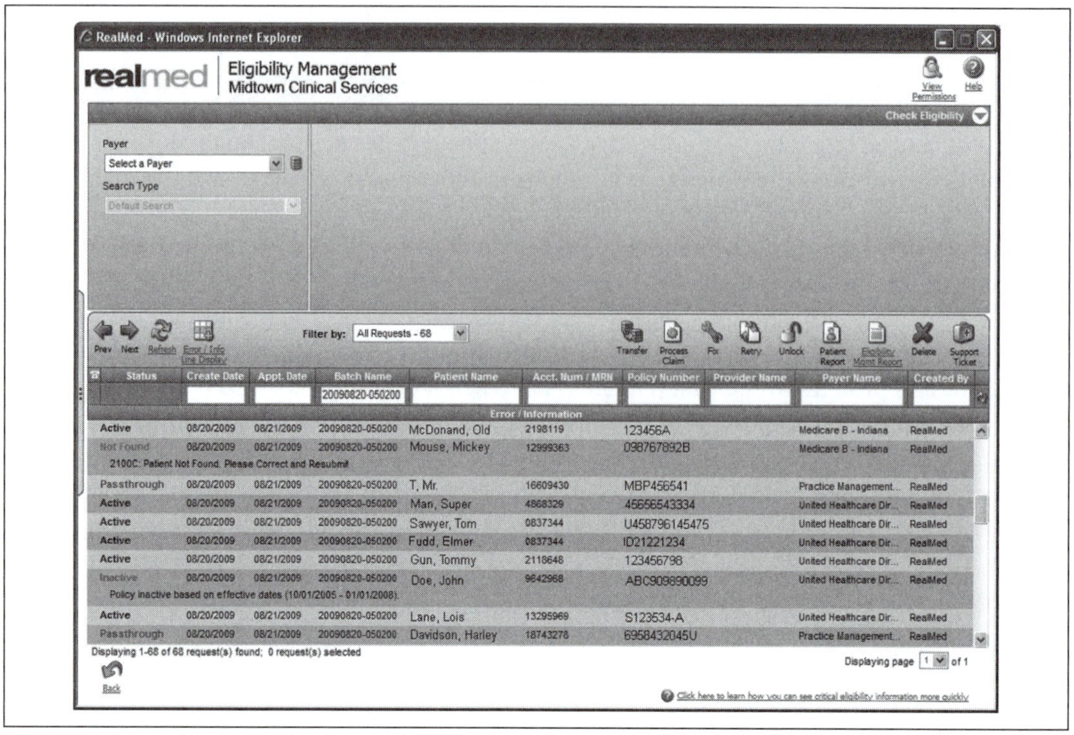

© RealMed Corporation. Reprinted with permission.

patients in the reception area or an empty reception area is the first indication of poor patient scheduling. The documentation required for accurate scheduling may include:

- Patient full name
- Patient identifier, such as birth date or unique identifying number
- Reason for appointment, such as preventive visit or procedure
- Length of appointment
- Provider to be seen
- Practice location to be seen (for large multilocation practices)
- Additional demographic information, such as primary insurance

By utilizing the patient schedule as the source document, monitoring patient flow throughout the entire patient care process is also vital to an efficiently running medical practice. An example of Greenway's EHR clinical desktop that identifies the location of patients within the office may be found in figure 6.3.

Furthermore, account balances should be available and accessed by the scheduling staff. Patient balances should be communicated to patients at the time of scheduling an appointment or procedure. If the payment is not collected during the phone call, such as with a credit card

The author wishes to acknowledge RealMed for providing screens from its award-winning Revenue Cycle Management software (v. 9.1).

Figure 6.3. Greenway clinical desktop

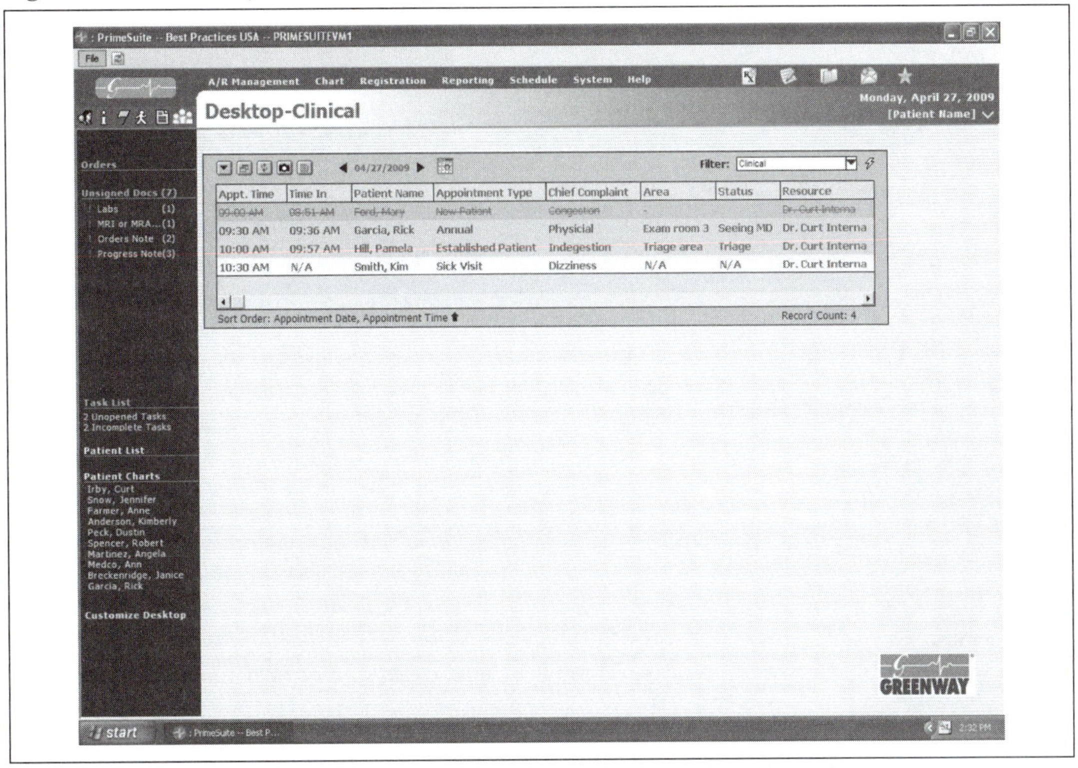

The author wishes to acknowledge Greenway for providing screens from its electronic health record system.

payment, the patient should be prepared to pay balances or make payment arrangements at the time of service.

No-show statistics should be documented and monitored, and resolutions should be determined. To reduce no-show percentages, automated phone or e-mail reminders may be utilized. Reminder communication is especially important for visits associated with higher costs, such as procedures and lengthy appointment times.

Charge Capture and Entry

The charge capture process includes entering codes for all services, procedures, and supplies provided during patient care, along with the corresponding ICD-9-CM diagnosis codes. Although this sounds easy to accomplish, it is oftentimes only as complete as the information supplied by the physician, provider, or clinical staff. In the EHR, the charge entry function may occur automatically from the point of care to the claims data. However, the documentation must be present in the EHR in order for the charge data to transfer. In the paper-based environment, a charge slip is utilized to capture the services performed during a single patient visit. If service items are not accurately marked, the charges will not be billed and, consequently, those services will not be reimbursed. A sample of Greenway's EHR charge slip summary may be found in figure 6.4.

Although it is a best practice to complete all charge entry functions on-site at the practice location, some medical practices utilize an outsourced billing company to complete the charge entry process. This option presents many documentation, coding, and communication issues and should be avoided when possible.

Figure 6.4. Greenway charge slip summary

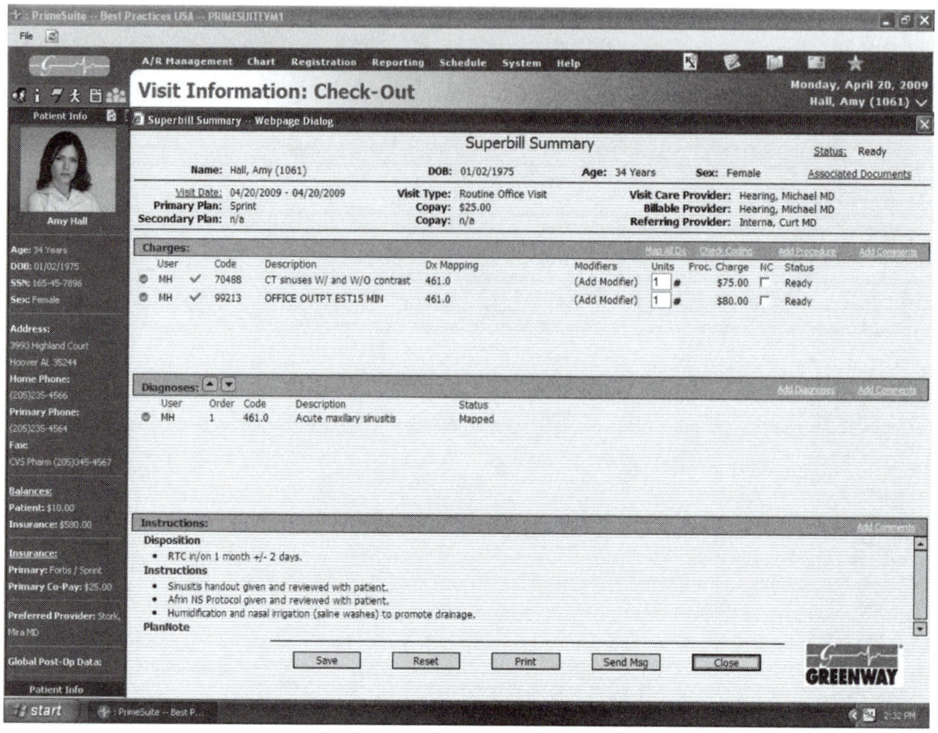

The author wishes to acknowledge Greenway for providing screens from its electronic health record system.

A copy of the charge slip, whether printed from the EHR or from a paper-based charge slip, is provided to the patient as a receipt of services. The charge capture process flow in a medical practice may be seen in figure 6.5.

Coding

Coding of services performed should be completed by a certified coder. A highly skilled professional with experience unique to the specialty of services provided at the medical practice will offer accurately coded claims. The accuracy of coded claims increases the correctness of reimbursements.

The charge slip, charge description master, managed care modules, and other paper-based or electronic sources where ICD-9-CM, CPT, and HCPCS codes reside must be coded to the highest level of specificity using only the current year's code sets. Allowing any one of these sources to become outdated will increase the practice's denial rate. More information on accurate coding can be found later in this chapter.

Health Record

The health record plays a key role in the revenue cycle, since it provides the documentation to support the services provided as well as the claims submission data. Details on health record content and format may be found in chapter 1.

Figure 6.5. Charge capture process flow

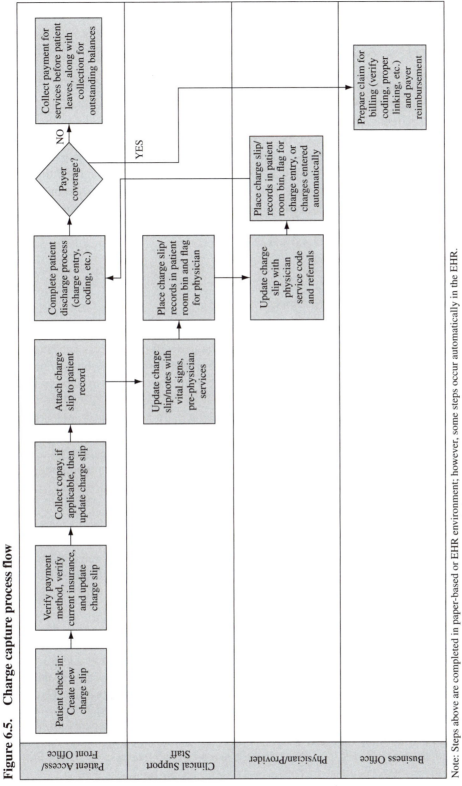

Charge Reconciliation and Lost Charges

Reconciling charges is the act of reviewing charges entered for claims submission by the charge entry process. Although the provider of service initially marked the charge slip or supplied entries into the EHR, charge reconciliation ensures that all services, procedures, and supplies (including pharmaceuticals) are available to pass to the claim form.

Lost charges are those services, procedures, or supplies that were provided or administered during a patient visit yet never marked on the charge slip or entered into the EHR. These services, procedures, or supplies are never billed to the payer or patient and thus result in free services. Lost charges are oftentimes difficult to identify unless an audit is performed. For example, if a particular dosage of medication is administered to the patient and the CPT and/or HCPCS codes are captured as charges, it is difficult to identify if the correct units were noted at charge entry. The documentation in the health record must be reviewed and compared with the billed charges to determine the accuracy of the charges. Many practices do not accurately capture the units of service (especially with pharmaceuticals), which results in an expense to the practice that is not reimbursed.

Statement Processing and Cycle

Each medical practice should establish time cycles for the initial submission of claims to the payers. The shorter the cycle time, the sooner the practice will have the opportunity to be reimbursed for the services performed. A quick turnaround time for claims submission also reduces the chance for a concurrent care denial. If the cycle time is long (also known as lag time), accounts receivable will be impacted.

Statement processing to patients should initially be daily, yet further statement processing cycles should meet the requirement for each practice. For example, a practice may submit the initial patient statement utilizing the daily cycle, yet revert to a 29-day cycle thereafter. This would result in a timely initial patient statement and monthly patient statements if full payment was not received in the first month.

Electronic Claims Processing

Many practices utilize software to screen claims for accuracy prior to claims submission. This is oftentimes performed through a clearinghouse or internal claims scrubber. Once accurate data is included on the claim form, the claim is submitted to the payer for payment consideration. This process is performed electronically.

According to Casto and Layman:

> The Health Insurance Portability and Accountability Act of 1996 (HIPAA) added a new part to the Social Security Act entitled Administrative Simplification. The purpose of this section is to improve the efficiency and effectiveness of the healthcare delivery system. Through this section, Medicare has established standards and requirements for the electronic exchange of certain health information (HHS 2003b, 8381). The Final Rule on Standards for Electronic Transactions and Code Sets, also known as the Transaction Rule, identified eight electronic transactions and six codes sets. [See tables 6.1 and 6.2.] This rule ensures that all providers, third-party payers, claims clearinghouses, and so forth use the same sets of codes to communicate coded health information, therefore ensuring standardization for systems and applications across the healthcare continuum. Not only does this support standardization, but it also supports administrative simplification. Providers can now maintain a select number of code sets at their current version, rather than maintaining different versions (current and old) of many code sets based on payer specification as required in the past. (Casto and Layman 2008, 210–211)

Table 6.1. HIPAA electronic transactions

Healthcare claims or equivalent encounter information
Eligibility for a health plan
Referral certification and authorization
Healthcare claim status
Enrollment and disenrollment in a health plan
Healthcare payment and remittance advice
Health plan premium payments
Coordination of benefits

Source: HHS 2003b.

Table 6.2. HIPAA code sets

International Classification of Diseases, ninth revision, Clinical Modification, Volumes 1 and 2
International Classification of Diseases, ninth revision, Clinical Modification, Volume 3
National Drug Codes
Code on Dental Procedures and Nomenclature
Health Care Financing Administration Common Procedure Coding System
Current Procedural Terminology, fourth edition

Source: HHS 2003a.

Primary and Secondary Claims Submission

There is a correct sequence for claims submission. The primary payer receives the claim submission first, then the secondary payer, and then the tertiary payer (if applicable). This process typically occurs electronically and automatically through the use of information systems. Monitoring claim volumes allows the practice to identify new trends or potential problems. As with all reporting, the product may yield a statistical report or a graphic report. When identifying trends and issues, graphic reports permit more immediate identification. Figure 6.6 illustrates a graphic report for claims volume from RealMed's Revenue Cycle Management software.

Remittance Processing and Payment Posting

Once the payer has processed the claim, a remittance advice (RA) is electronically sent to the provider. In some practices where billing is outsourced, the RA may be sent directly to the billing company. Payments and RA are transmitted directly to the provider's bank. This electronic transfer ensures the timeliest receipt of funds from payers.

Although technology is available for electronic remittance advice (ERA) processing, some medical practices continue to process RAs manually. Figure 6.7 displays an example of the remittance file download screen from RealMed's Revenue Cycle Management software.

The manual processing of RA not only delays the accuracy of the accounts receivable, but also permits the opportunity for human error in posting payments to the correct patients and account for the same patient. When working in a manual RA mode, the lag time is extremely sensitive to the availability of qualified staff. If staffing is low or there is an attendance issue at the practice, the lag time for payment posting will increase. If payments are posted manually (including cash payment postings), this task should be completed within 24 hours of receipt of cash or RA. Manual payment posting, along with many other factors mentioned in this chapter, directly affect the practice's bottom line.

Figure 6.6.   RealMed Practice Profile of claims volume

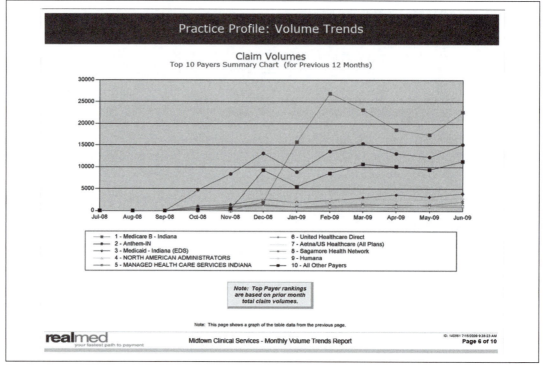

© RealMed Corporation. Reprinted with permission.

Figure 6.7.   RealMed Remittance File Download

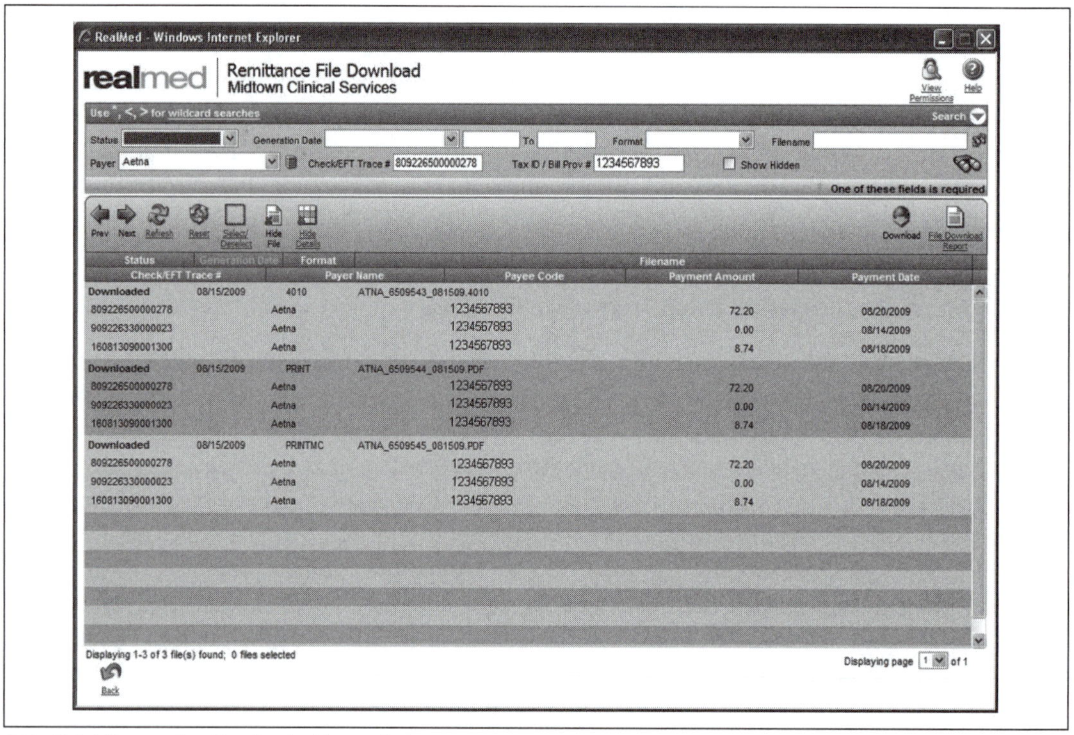

© RealMed Corporation. Reprinted with permission.

The author wishes to acknowledge RealMed for providing screens from its award-winning Revenue Cycle Management software (v. 9.1).

Contractual Adjustments

A contractual adjustment is the difference between what is charged by the healthcare provider and what is paid by the managed care company or other payer. Contractual adjustments are a direct reflection of the provider's negotiations with the payer. The reimbursements received from the payer are based upon the calculations documented in the contract.

Many practices use managed care modules within the EHR, practice management, or billing systems to accurately monitor correct payments by payers for the services provided and billed. It is a poor practice to rely upon staff to manually monitor that correct payments were received. For example, the practice should be reimbursed $50 for a certain CPT code based upon the contract; however, the payer reimbursed only $40. In this scenario, it is unlikely that the practice staff would recognize the incorrect payment by a single payer. The difference of $10 could easily be lost if not identified immediately and appropriate action taken.

It is important to have detailed reason codes for each adjustment. These adjustment codes must be compliant with the HIPAA data sets. At the Washington Publishing Company Web site (http://www.wpc-edi.com/codes), lists may be found for the following code set standards:

- Claim Adjustment Reason Codes
- Remittance Advice Remark Codes
- Claim Status Codes
- Claim Status Category Codes
- Health Care Provider Taxonomy Code Set
- Provider Characteristics Codes
- Health Care Services Decision Reason Codes
- Insurance Business Process Application Error Codes

Discount and Financial Assistance

Financial counseling and charity care standards should be available at every medical practice. As with all steps in the revenue cycle, documented policies and procedures must be established and enforced for charity care and financial counseling. It is extremely important that any policies and procedures or charity care be followed as documented. Any unfair inducements to entice patients are disallowed by CMS, such as offering free initial visits or discounted transportation to visits.

Self-pay discounts may be offered; however, these discounts must be documented in the practices financial policy and made available to all patients. Examples of guidelines may include:

- Make certain that the hardship and discount policies are followed as documented.

- Monitor the number of patients receiving the discount. If a large percentage of patients receive the discount, this discounted fee may be considered the practice's "usual and customary fee" from the payer's perspective.

- Utilize federal poverty levels in the documented policy. Each state has specific poverty levels based upon individual and household income. These levels change each year and should be revised at the practice level on an annual basis. The poverty guidelines for 2008 may be found in table 6.3 for the 48 contiguous states, DC, Alaska, and Hawaii. Additional information may be found at http://aspe.hhs.gov/poverty/09poverty.shtml.

Table 6.3. 2009 HHS poverty guidelines

Persons in Family or Household	48 Contiguous States and DC	Alaska	Hawaii
1	$10,830	$13,530	$ 12,460
2	14,570	18,210	16,760
3	18,310	22,890	21,060
4	22,050	27,570	25,360
5	35,790	32,250	29,660
6	29,530	36,930	33,960
7	33,270	41,610	38,260
8	37,010	46,290	42,560
For each additional person, add	3,740	4,680	4,300

Source: HHS 2009, 4199–4201.

- Never bill a service as "insurance only" or "take what insurance pays."
- Always collect copays and deductibles. Never write them off for any reason, including small balance write-offs.
- Offer self-pay discounts to those who pay in full at the time of service.
- Consider sliding scales for indigent patients.

Unapplied Cash

When payment is received and the specific patient and/or account cannot be identified, the funds are posted to a separate account called an unapplied account. Some practices title this account as unidentified funds. Whatever the title of the account, these dollars must be resolved immediately. It is very easy to let these dollars sit until they become unmanageable, which in turn affects the accuracy of the accounts receivable and aging, as well as individual patient accounts. At a maximum, unapplied dollars should be resolved within 30 days of receipt.

Collections and Payer Follow-up

It is imperative to the medical practice's bottom line that accounts are followed up and collection policies are documented and enforced. The U.S. Department of Commerce reports that accounts over 90 days old depreciate at one-half (0.5) percent per day. In other words, accounts lose 15 percent of their value every month after the first three months. The sooner accounts are collected, the better the success of collections.

In many states, there are prompt pay regulations that may be used by practices to ensure timely payment of services for clean claims submitted. These regulations may even have a penalty of interest, such as 18 percent, for payments not reimbursed by payers. If payers are not following these regulations, practices may contact the state's Department of Insurance for assistance. For specific information regarding state laws on prompt pay, go to http://www.naic.org/state_web_map.htm and select the appropriate state.

Self-Pay Collections

As with all collections, the Federal Trade Commission's Fair Debt Collection Practice Act must be followed. This document was revised in 2009 and can be found on the CD-ROM accompanying this book. However, self-pay collections should occur at the time of service. Any outstanding balances should also be collected or payment plans determined and enforced.

Many practices designate key staff to monitor and follow up with self-pay accounts. As documented in the practice's financial policies, payment plans may be offered to self-pay patients and patients with outstanding balances. The payment policy should document specific dollar amounts expected and time intervals for payment. For example, if an account balance is $500, the practice must document in the financial policy what dollar amount is expected each month and how many months the balance may remain while payments are being made, such as $100 per month for five months or $250 for two months.

Effective dunning messages should be added to each statement that reflect the action that will be taken if payment is not received. Although always polite in language, dunning messages typically increase in their severity as the number of statements increases. As with all policies, it is extremely important that the action documented in the dunning statement is followed through. If a dunning statement documents that the patient will be turned over to a collection agency if payment is not received, this action must be completed or all of the practice's credibility will be lost.

It is extremely important to begin self-pay collections immediately after the date of service. The longer the balance remains outstanding, the less opportunity to collect for a multitude of reasons—for instance, change of address, disconnected telephone, and so forth. All federal and state laws regarding unclaimed funds must be followed.

Denial Management

Note: This section was adapted from the article "Bringing down denials: Successfully managing denials in medical practices" by Cheryl Gregg Fahrenholz, which was published in the August 2009 issue of the Journal of AHIMA.

A denial by definition is the circumstance when a bill has been accepted by a payer, but payment has been denied for a specific reason (for example, sending the bill to the wrong primary or secondary payer, patient not having current coverage, inaccurate coding, lack of medical necessity, and so on).

Every medical practice's goal should be a clean claim on the first submission. Appealing a denied claim requires money as well as time. The average cost to process a first appeal ranges from $20 to $25 per claim. The cost rises if a claim requires additional appeals. Profits diminish quickly when claims are not clean on first submission. There are even situations when an appeal would cost the practice more money than it could recoup. For example, a $25 appeal on an $11 denial loses the practice $14.

Denial management falls into three broad steps: logging and responding to denials, understanding root causes, and creating an action plan for preventing future denials. The ultimate goal of every denial management program should be prevention.

Accurate collection of demographic data, including current insurance information, is the first step in preventing claims denials. Verifying a patient's insurance coverage prior to any professional service is a best practice, but using technology to capture accurate insurance information is a "must" in a strong prevention program (for example, swiping, scanning, or copying the patient's current insurance card). Staff should verify coverage at each patient visit.

Receiving the Denial

A common roadblock in denial management happens with the response to this question: What to do when a denied claim is received? One typical reaction is to set the denial aside and work on another step of the billing process—something more familiar, namely processing that day's claims. Unresolved denials quickly accumulate to a proportion that appears unmanageable. As time passes, the likelihood of addressing them diminishes, as does the opportunity to appeal them.

Practices benefit when they establish a simple process for receiving denials. If the practice completes its billing internally, monitoring denials is easier. If billing is completed by an out-sourced company, the practice must rely upon someone else to respond and resolve the denial on the practice's behalf. Some practices may not even know their denial rates by physician or provider.

A denial is easy to identify because 0 dollars are reimbursed. Claims denied as duplicate claims should be investigated. The first step is to verify the number of times that the service was performed. Some services are actually performed more than once a day. For example, a patient may receive laboratory services in the office during a scheduled morning appointment—such as glucose testing—and return in the afternoon for the test to be repeated. Without the appropriate modifier attached to the claim, the payer may perceive the second laboratory service as duplicative and produce a denial.

More difficult to identify are correct reimbursements based upon currently contracted reimbursement rates with a particular payer. Payers are not always correct with the reimbursement (dollar amount) they issue. Without the use of software such as managed care modules to the practice management or billing systems, this is difficult for the practice staff to identify.

Understanding the Denial

Essential to accurately processing a denial is understanding why the claim was denied. Inaccurate appeals cost the practice. Common issues in denied claims include registration errors, medical necessity, bundled services, and coding errors. The key to understanding why a claim was denied resides in the denial reason codes. It is critical that the practice obtain a thorough understanding of each denial reason code in order to accurately process appeals. Acknowledging what the payer needs to approve the claim—such as operative reports, consultation orders, or history report—will also assist with the payment of a denied claim.

Preventing Denials

As stated previously, collecting and entering accurate patient demographics and payer information is critical in the prevention of denials. Properly trained staff with current resources, as well as determining the top denials in a medical practice and developing a denial management action plan, will reduce the opportunity for new denials and resolve existing denials.

Follow these steps as one way to analyze denials:

1. Identify the top 10 payers through a payer mix report from the practice management or billing system.

2. Identify the top procedure codes that are denied, along with the corresponding denial reason codes.

3. Compare these lists.

4. Review payer Web sites, newsletters, and administrative manuals.

5. Review the National Coverage Determinations (NCDs) and Local Coverage Determinations (LCDs) for coverage guidelines. Some of these guidelines will list acceptable frequencies of service along with a listing of diagnosis codes that support the medical necessity.

Additionally, payer policy and procedures for appeals may be located in manuals, newsletters, and online. The practice has one chance at the first step to appeal each denied claim. Understanding the correct appeal process for each payer is essential to overturning a denied claim.

The appeal may include, but is not limited to, clinical documentation of the service performed, the physician's clinical necessity for providing the service, and additional supporting documentation, such as Medicare coverage guidelines, AMA's CPT coding book references, scientific research, specialty medical society supporting statements or published research, and more. Copying patients on this correspondence lets them know the practice is working on their behalf.

Denial Action Plan

Understanding and properly appealing denied claims is only part of the denial process. Practices must have a formal method for monitoring denials—often called denial management. At the heart of denial management is a denial action plan. The plan includes a denial database that contains the identification and explanation of all denial reason codes; electronic file receipts; deadline dates; and profiles based on payer, reason, diagnosis, procedure, or service (CPT or HCPCS code), and physician or provider.

Key to identifying areas of focus is tracking and trending denial data. Computerized tracking programs or spreadsheets assist with denial management. Samples of two hard-copy tracking tools may be found in figures 6.8 and 6.9.

The practice may choose to monitor specific areas or departments, or it may break down the analysis by other variables such as office location, provider, specialty, payer, or specific procedure. The data will reveal patterns or trends in denials. For example, the practice may be experiencing consistent denials for one physician.

Figure 6.8.   Denial database summary report

				Denial Database Summary				
				Month _____				
Payer	Total Open Accounts	New Accounts	Total Dollars Pending	Percentage of Dollars at Risk	Closed Accounts Won	Dollars Recovered	Closed Accounts Lost	Dollars Lost
1								
2								
3								
4								
5								
6								
Total								

© Preferred Healthcare Solutions, LLC. 937-848-6080. Reprinted with permission.

Figure 6.9. Denial tracking form

Denial Tracking Form

Payor _____

Physician _____

	Patient Name	Account Number	Date of Service	CPT Code	ICD-9-CM Code	Date Denial Issued	Denial Code	Charges on Claim	Denied Dollar Amount	Date Requested	Action Taken	Recovered Amount
1												
2												
3												
4												
5												
6												
7												
8												
9												
10												
11												
12												
13												
14												
15												
16												
17												
18												
19												
20												
21												
22												
23												
24												
25												

Identifying the denial issues, investigating the potential solutions, communicating the findings with the provider and appropriate staff, and monitoring the results are all steps in finding a resolution. Resulting good news should be noted and shared, too, such as declines in specific denials or dollars recovered.

Trending denials also helps the practice determine the top denials by payer. This information may be coordinated with the denial resolution for each type of denial. The team then documents, publishes, and distributes the details of denial trending and resolution by payer, including sample appeal letters, to practice staff. This information will speed the appeal process for the staff working on the denials. Included in the denial action plan are benchmarks for the practice.

Benchmarks may be set by the answers to the following questions:

- What percentage of claims is rejected? This should be less than 5 percent of all electronic claims submitted.

- What percentage of claims is denied by payer? This rate should be a single digit.

- What is the dollar amount of the denied claims? This varies greatly based upon specialty.

- What are the top denial reasons, and are there consistencies by physician, provider, or payer? Once analyzed, the practice may discover that many of the denials are a result of one issue or are produced by one provider.

- What is the appeal rate by payer? This should be dissected by CPT and HCPCS code to fully understand the denials and find a resolution.

- What is the overturn rate on appeal? A higher percentage in this category simply reflects that the payer may not have a comprehensive system in place to pay claims appropriately the first time the claims are submitted.

As with any initiative, good intentions may only go as far as the staff can provide assistance. Many practices use consultants to analyze their revenue cycles, including steps in the denial management process such as charge capture, reporting, appeal processes, and action plan development. Whether practices tackle their denials internally or with outside help, the best solution is to resolve them. Practices that take the time necessary to understand the denial process and make the necessary clinical or administrative changes to resolve denials see a benefit to their bottom line.

Small-Balance Accounts

Every medical practice has small balances. Written policies and procedures on this subject must be documented and enforced. As mentioned earlier in this chapter, copays and deductibles may be a small amount but may never be written off of the account. Some practices have determined that a small balance is $5, $10, $15, or $20. For accounts determined to have small balances, a practice may decide that statements may not be sent and dollars may be written off, except for copays and deductibles. One example would be if a practice has the majority of their patients' copays equaling $10, then perhaps the small balance would be established at $9.99. This would avoid mistakenly writing off a non-paid copay of $10.

Credit Balances

Just as with unapplied cash, credit balances affect the accuracy of accounts receivable statistics. Credit balances are positive dollar amounts posted to an account. One instance when this may happen is when a staff member posts cash receipts to the correct patient, but not to the correct date of service for that patient. Credit balances also may be a result of a patient paying for services performed that were not expected to be covered by the payer; however, the payer did reimburse the practice for the services. In this instance, there would be a credit balance (positive dollar amount) on the account and this money would belong to the patient. All federal and state laws regarding unclaimed funds must be followed.

Credit balance processing is the responsibility of all business office staff. Unfortunately, in some medical practices, the priority is to "get the claims out the door" for the current day, then complete other responsibilities such as working older accounts. The fact of the matter is that many staff members want to bring money into the practice rather than give it away. This false assumption places the practice under a great compliance risk.

If this credit balance belongs to the patient and the practice has attempted to return the money, yet receives the mailing as returned to sender, address unknown, or no one at this address by that name, then proper steps should be taken to comply with state laws regarding unclaimed funds. These state laws have time frames that require compliance.

If the credit balance belongs to a payer, then many payers will identify the credit and recoup the dollars during future claims, and these recovered amounts will be withheld in remittance advice to the providers. If the practice identifies the credit balance, then proper communications must occur to the payer and the funds must be returned.

Credit balances should be resolved within 30 days of receipt to avoid interest penalties. CMS states that credit balances fall under reasonable care in the billing process and acceptance of payments. Keeping improper payments or excess payments could lead to false claims charges and whistleblower suits. A sample demand letter that the practice may receive can be viewed in figure 6.10.

Precollection and Collection

Precollection (also known as soft collections) is the act of collecting on outstanding accounts prior to turning accounts over to a collection agency. This task may be completed in-house by practice staff or may be outsourced to a collection agency for a fee. Depending upon the delinquency of the outstanding accounts, some practices find success in performing precollections in-house. This allows the practice to retain the entire amount of funds received. Precollections performed by an outsourced agency typically have lower fees than other collection protocols.

Precollection steps tend to be kinder and may involve a series of phone calls or letters. Oftentimes a payment plan can be agreed upon by the patient and must be documented in the billing section of the practice's software. If payment plan arrangements are not followed by the patient, consideration must be made for immediate release to a collection company.

The Centers for Medicare and Medicaid Services states that the collection process ". . . must involve the issuance of a bill on or shortly after discharge or death of the beneficiary to the party responsible for the patient's personal financial obligations. It also includes other actions such as subsequent billings, collection letters and telephone calls or personal contacts with this party which constitute a genuine, rather than a token, collection effort. The provider's collection effort may include using or threatening to use court action to obtain payment . . . The provider's collection effort should be documented in the patient's file by copies of the bill(s), follow-up letters, reports of telephone and personal contact, etc. . . . If after reasonable and customary attempts to collect a bill, the debt remains unpaid more than 120 days from the date the first bill is mailed to the beneficiary, the debt may be deemed uncollectible" (CMS 2008d, Chapter 3, Section 310).

Once a patient is turned over to a collection agency, the practice should have policies and procedures in place to determine if the patient will be discharged from the practice. This decision must be documented and consideration for reentry into the practice may be made after the balance is paid in full. This decision is sometimes difficult when one family member is turned over to collection, yet the remaining family members are being treated.

Figure 6.10. Sample demand letter

Date
Certified Mail
Name/Address
Re: Provider Number
Claims Accounts Receivable

Dear _____:

On _____, a claim adjustment was entered in our system under provider _____ for $_____. Since then, adjustments were made to the claim and a balance in the amount of $_____ has been outstanding for 60 days. As this amount has not been recouped through claims submission, the purpose of our letter is to request that this amount be repaid to our office. For your reference, a copy of the Claims Accounts Receivable Transaction Summary is enclosed. (Insert the name of the detailed summary report enclosed. This report should include sufficient information needed by the provider to identify the overpayment).

Submit your check payable to _____, to the following address:
                Street
                City, State Zip code

In order to ensure that your check is credited to this overpayment, please enclose a copy of this letter with your payment.

Until payment in full is received or an acceptable extended repayment request is received all payments due to you are being withheld. (This includes claims, settlement amounts, or interim payments.) If you have reason to believe that withhold should cease you must notify our office before _____ and provide documentation as to why this withholding action should not continue. We will review your documentation, but will not delay recoupment during the review process. This is not an appeal of the overpayment determination.

In addition, in accordance with 42 C.F.R. §405.378, simple interest at the rate of ____% will be charged on the unpaid balance of the overpayment, beginning on the 31st day. Interest is calculated in 30-day periods and is assessed for each full 30-day period that payment is not made on time. Thus, if payment is received 31 days from the date of this letter, one 30-day period of interest will be charged. Each payment will be applied first to accrued interest and the remaining amount to principal.

Additional interest of $___ will be assessed against the principal balance on ____ and will continue to assess at the rate of ___% a year for each 30-day period the principal amount remains unpaid. In addition, please note that Medicare rules require that payment be either received in our office by ___ or United States Postal Service postmarked by that date in order for the payment to be considered timely. A metered mail postmark received in our office after ___ will cause an additional month's interest to be assessed on the debt.

We request that you refund this amount in full. If you are unable to make refund of the entire amount at this time, please advise our office immediately so that we may determine if you are eligible for a repayment schedule (see enclosure for details). Any repayment schedule (where one is approved) would run from the date of this letter. If we do not hear from you, your interim payments will continue to be withheld and applied towards the outstanding overpayment balance. Any amount withheld will not be refunded.

If you feel you have reason to appeal this adjustment, please refer to the original remittance advice dated _____ for additional instruction.

If you have filed a bankruptcy petition or are involved in a bankruptcy proceeding, Medicare financial obligations will be resolved in accordance with the applicable bankruptcy process. Accordingly, we request that you immediately notify us about this bankruptcy so that we may coordinate with both the Centers for Medicare & Medicaid Services and the Department of Justice so as to assure that we handle your situation properly. If possible, when notifying us about the bankruptcy, please include the name the bankruptcy was filed under and the district where the bankruptcy is filed.

If you have a question regarding why these adjustments were made, please contact our _____ at _____. If we can assist you further in the resolution of this matter, we will be glad to do so. We look forward to hearing from you shortly.

Sincerely,

(name and title)

Source: CMS 2008c, Chapter 3, Section 40.2.

Bad Debt, Write-offs, and Reserves

Bad debt is considered the receivables of an organization that are uncollectible for services that have already been performed. According to CMS, the accounting period for bad debt as outlined in Section 314 of the Bad Debt, Charity, and Courtesy Allowances portion is uncollectible deductibles and coinsurance amounts that are recognized as allowable bad debts in the reporting period in which the debts are determined to be worthless (CMS 2008d). Allowable bad debts must be related to specific amounts that have been determined to be uncollectible. Since bad debts are uncollectible accounts receivable and not receivable, the provider should have the usual accounts receivable records-ledger cards and source documents to support its claim for a bad debt for each account included. Examples of the types of information to be retained may include, but are not limited to, the beneficiary's name and health insurance number, admission/discharge dates for Part A bills and dates of services for Part B bills, date of bills, date of write-off, and a breakdown of the uncollectible amount by deductible and coinsurance amounts. This proposed list is illustrative and not obligatory.

As stated in Sections 320.1 and 320.2 of the Bad Debt, Charity, and Courtesy Allowances portion of CMS online manual, there are two methods of determining bad debt expense. The first method is a direct charge-off. "Under the direct charge-off method, accounts receivable are analyzed and a determination made as to specific accounts which are deemed uncollectible. The amounts deemed to be uncollectible are charged to an expense account for uncollectible accounts. The amounts charged to the expense account for bad debts should be adequately identified as to those which represent deductible and coinsurance amounts applicable to beneficiaries and those which are applicable to other than beneficiaries or which are for other than covered services. Those bad debts which are applicable to beneficiaries for uncollectible deductible and coinsurance amounts are included in the calculation of reimbursable bad debts" (CMS 2008d, Chapter 3, Section 320).

Reserves are dollars set aside to cover unexpected expenses, such as bad debt. Under the second method (reserve method), "bad debt expenses computed by use of the reserve method are not allowable bad debts under the program. However, the specific uncollectible deductibles and coinsurance amounts applicable to beneficiaries and charged against the reserve are includable in the calculation of reimbursable bad debts. Under the reserve method, providers estimate the amount of bad debts that will be incurred during a period, and establish a reserve account for that amount. The amount estimated as bad debts does not represent any particular debts, but is based on the aggregate of receivables or services" (CMS 2008d).

Write-off is the action taken to eliminate the balance of a bill after the bill has been submitted, partial payment has been made or payment has been denied, and all avenues of collecting the payment have been exhausted. All billing systems, whether through a practice management system or EHR, have reason codes that describe the circumstance of a particular scenario, such as a denial or write-off reason. Reason codes must be detailed in their description and provide a specific explanation. The more specific the reason code description, the more effective the reason code will be in reporting and analyzing the accounts receivable. Reason codes such as past filing limits or no preauthorization obtained provide a wealth of information in order to resolve denials and reduce write-offs.

Account Balance Zero

An obvious last step in the revenue cycle is when the patient balance equals $0. As stated in this chapter, there are a multitude of documented steps that must take place to reach this goal;

however, a well-organized, streamlined, and efficient revenue cycle management process will achieve the $0 account balance goal sooner than those practices that do not have the necessary protocols, policies, and procedures in place for revenue cycle management.

Staff Training and Development

As with all the computerized application and policies and procedures discussed, they are only as good as the staffs who are trained to use and apply them. Documented training programs should be established for new hires as well as established physicians, providers, and staff. Training should be done continually through each year as new developments, regulations, versions of software, and so forth are utilized at the medical practice.

All training plans should be incorporated into the medical practice's compliance plan. This includes attendance signature sheets, program content, and evaluation forms.

Check Your Understanding 6.1

1. The first step in the revenue cycle is which of the following?
   a. When the patient appears in the medical practice for an appointment
   b. Proper credentialing and contracting
   c. Patient scheduling
   d. Submission of claim to payer

2. Which of the following is not considered a goal of the revenue cycle team?
   a. To reduce denials and streamline the appeals process
   b. To identify payment issues with payers
   c. To improve the accounts receivable
   d. To increase days in accounts receivable

3. The collection of copayments is primarily the responsibility of which position of the medical practice?
   a. Physician
   b. Collection agency staff
   c. Patient access/front office staff
   d. Practice administrator

4. Which of the following is a true statement?
   a. As long as a provider is contracted with a payer, credentialing is not necessary.
   b. It is not necessary to complete the credentialing or contracting steps with a payer to receive in-network provider reimbursement.
   c. Both credentialing and contracting must be properly completed in order for accurate reimbursement to be received by a payer.
   d. Once a provider is credentialed, then claims may be submitted to the payer and proper reimbursement will be received.

(continued on next page)

Check Your Understanding 6.1 *(continued)*

5. According to the best practices of the preregistration or registration process, which of the following is/are important to obtain from the patient?

   a. Correct patient name as displayed on the patient's insurance card and photo identification
   b. Correct insurance coverage information
   c. Patient identifier, such as birth date or unique indentifying number
   d. All of the above

6. According to the Washington Publishing Company, which of the following is NOT a HIPAA-compliant data set?

   a. Insurance Services Taxonomy Code Sets
   b. Claim Status Codes
   c. Claim Adjustment Reason Codes
   d. Health Care Provider Taxonomy Code Set

7. Unapplied cash is what?

   a. The receivables of an organization that are uncollectible for services that have already been performed
   b. The difference between what is charged by the healthcare provider and what is paid by the managed care company or other payer
   c. Payments received without specific patient and/or account numbers associated
   d. Dollars set aside to cover unexpected expenses

8. When analyzing denials, which of the following resources would be beneficial?

   a. National and Local Coverage Determinations
   b. Payer guidelines and administrative manuals
   c. Listing of the top procedures denied
   d. All of the above

9. Which of the following is typically not a component of a denial tracking tool?

   a. ICD-9-CM and CPT codes
   b. Patient's date of birth
   c. Date of denial, denial reason code, and dollars denied
   d. Action taken to resolve the denial

10. Credit balances should be resolved within how many days?

    a. Not to exceed 30 days
    b. Not to exceed 45 days
    c. Not to exceed 60 days
    d. Not to exceed 75 days

Resources for Coding Professionals

The person assigned responsibility for coding must have knowledge of the pertinent coding systems, as well as medical terminology, anatomy, and physiology. In addition, he or she must keep abreast of coding changes, make appropriate updates, and be proficient with coding software.

To help physicians and staff to assign diagnostic and procedural codes correctly, the following publications and documents should be available and close at hand:

- A current ICD-9-CM diagnosis code book (updated annually effective October 1)

- A current CPT code book, copyrighted and published by the American Medical Association (AMA) (updated annually effective January 1)

- A current HCPCS code book (updated annually effective January 1)

- Online access to the National Correct Coding Initiative (http://www.cms.hhs.gov/NationalCorrectCodInitEd/)

- Online access to National Coverage Determinations (NCDs) and Local Coverage Determinations (LCDs) (http://www.cms.hhs.gov/mcd/search.asp?)

- Online access to Medicare manuals, transmittals, bulletins, or newsletters provided by the Centers for Medicare and Medicaid Services or the Medicare carrier

- *Medicaid Provider Billing Manual,* provided by Medicaid

- Online access to Medicaid provider newsletters or bulletins

- Access to payer administrative manuals, billing manuals, newsletters, and bulletins

- Documentation of all telephone contacts with Medicare, Medicaid, and all payers regarding coding/billing issues

- Subscriptions to coding publications that provide current coding requirements—for example, *CPT Assistant* and *Coding Clinic*

- Subscriptions to specialty-specific coding publications based upon the specialty of the medical practice

The official source for ICD-9-CM coding is available on CD-ROM from the U.S Department of Health and Human Services. The National Center for Health Statistics (http://www.cdc.gov/nchs/icd.htm) also supplies current information on ICD-9-CM. Because ICD-9-CM codes are in the public domain, many versions of ICD-9-CM code books are on the market, and several publishers distribute code books that include the annual updates. Whereas each of these code books may offer special features, the ICD-9-CM codes themselves are the same in every code book. Many publishers also offer electronic single- and multiple-user versions of ICD-9-CM. Several of the ICD-9-CM code books, as well as other coding materials related to ICD-9-CM and CPT/HCPCS, can be purchased from the American Health Information Management Association (AHIMA) and other sources.

Coding Clinic, published by the American Hospital Association (AHA), is the official source of ICD-9-CM coding advice (http://www.ahacentraloffice.org). Coding staff personnel should refer to *Coding Clinic* continuously for the most current information on ICD-9-CM coding and also try to improve their knowledge of disease processes by keeping on hand various resource books such as a recent medical dictionary and an anatomy and physiology textbook. *CPT Assistant*, published by the American Medical Association (AMA), is the official source of CPT coding advice (http://www.ama-assn.org). Coders must always utilize this reference when directed by the CPT code book. In addition, coding staff should never hesitate to query providers about unfamiliar conditions, services, or procedures and should attend any educational programs conducted for coders by the medical staff, as well as participate in online educational opportunities for coders.

The coding function must never be anything less than efficient. It is up to health information management leadership staff to ask the right questions and answer them with data. Is the number of records to be coded per day appropriate? The answer lies in the volume and scope of the medical practice's clinical services, patient demographics, and billing procedures. Does the practice have enough coders? Changes in the composition of the physicians will affect coding staff requirements as well. How many claims are rejected and for what reasons? By analyzing these numbers, the health information management leadership staff can identify coding weaknesses and document the need for any changes in staff size, qualifications, and education.

AHIMA Standards of Ethical Coding

In this era of payment based on diagnostic and procedural coding, the professional ethics of health information coding professionals continue to be challenged. A conscientious goal for coding and maintaining a high-quality database is accurate clinical and statistical data. The following standards of ethical coding, developed by AHIMA's Coding Policy and Strategy Committee and approved by AHIMA's House of Delegates in September 2008, are offered to guide coding professionals in this process.

The Standards of Ethical Coding are based on the AHIMA Code of Ethics (see appendix F). Both sets of principles reflect expectations of professional conduct for coding professionals involved in diagnostic and/or procedural coding or other health record data abstraction.

A code of ethics sets forth professional values and ethical principles and offers ethical guidelines to which professionals aspire and by which their actions can be judged. Health information management (HIM) professionals are expected to demonstrate professional values by their actions to patients, employers, members of the healthcare team, the public, and the many stakeholders they serve. A code of ethics is important in helping to guide the decision-making process and can be referenced by individuals, agencies, organizations, and bodies (such as licensing and regulatory boards, insurance providers, courts of law, government agencies, and other professional groups).

The AHIMA Code of Ethics is relevant to all AHIMA members and credentialed HIM professionals and students, regardless of their professional functions, the settings in which they work, or the populations they serve. Coding is one of the core HIM functions, and due to the complex regulatory requirements affecting the health information coding process, coding professionals are frequently faced with ethical challenges. The AHIMA Standards of Ethical Coding are intended to assist coding professionals and managers in decision-making processes and actions, outline expectations for making ethical decisions in the workplace, and demonstrate coding professionals' commitment to integrity during the coding process, regardless of the purpose for which the codes are being reported. They are relevant to all coding professionals and those who manage the coding function, regardless of the healthcare setting in which they work or whether they are AHIMA members or nonmembers.

The Standards of Ethical Coding were revised in 2008 to reflect the current healthcare environment and modern coding practices. The previous revision was published in 1999.

Coding professionals should:

1. Apply accurate, complete, and consistent coding practices for the production of high-quality healthcare data.

2. Report all healthcare data elements (for example, diagnosis and procedure codes, present on admission indicator, discharge status) required for external reporting

purposes (for example, reimbursement and other administrative uses, population health, quality and patient safety measurement, and research) completely and accurately, in accordance with regulatory and documentation standards and requirements and applicable official coding conventions, rules, and guidelines.

3. Assign and report only the codes and data that are clearly and consistently supported by health record documentation in accordance with applicable code set and abstraction conventions, rules, and guidelines.

4. Query provider (physician or other qualified healthcare practitioner) for clarification and additional documentation prior to code assignment when there is conflicting, incomplete, or ambiguous information in the health record regarding a significant reportable condition or procedure or other reportable data element dependent on health record documentation (for example, present on admission indicator).

5. Refuse to change reported codes or the narratives of codes so that meanings are misrepresented.

6. Refuse to participate in or support coding or documentation practices intended to inappropriately increase payment, qualify for insurance policy coverage, or skew data by means that do not comply with federal and state statutes, regulations, and official rules and guidelines.

7. Facilitate interdisciplinary collaboration in situations supporting proper coding practices.

8. Advance coding knowledge and practice through continuing education.

9. Refuse to participate in or conceal unethical coding or abstraction practices or procedures.

10. Protect the confidentiality of the health record at all times and refuse to access protected health information not required for coding-related activities (examples of coding-related activities include completion of code assignment, other health record data abstraction, coding audits, and educational purposes).

11. Demonstrate behavior that reflects integrity, shows a commitment to ethical and legal coding practices, and fosters trust in professional activities (AHIMA House of Delegates 2008).

ICD-9-CM Coding

ICD-9-CM code books are divided into three volumes: Volume 1, Diseases: Tabular List; Volume 2, Diseases: Alphabetic Index; and Volume 3: Procedure Index and Procedure Tabular. Medical practices use both Volumes 1 and 2 for diagnosis coding. The third volume of ICD-9-CM contains procedural codes that are used only for inpatient hospital services.

Volume 1: Diseases: Tabular List

Volume 1 is organized into 17 chapters arranged by etiology (cause of disease) and anatomical site. Each chapter consists of category codes, which are three-digit numeric codes that represent a single disease entity or a group of similar or closely related conditions. Most three-digit category codes are divided further into four-digit subcategory codes—the three-digit category number plus a decimal digit. The subcategory codes provide specificity or more information on cause, site, or manifestation. Some fourth-digit subcategories add a fifth digit to provide even greater specificity. Fifth digits can appear at the beginning of a chapter, a section, or a three-digit category or in a fourth-digit subcategory.

Volume 1 also contains two supplementary classifications: Classification of Factors Influencing Health Status and Contact with Health Services (V Codes), and Classification of External Causes of Injury and Poisoning (E Codes).

Volume 2: Diseases: Alphabetic Index

Volume 2 contains three separate indexes:

- The Alphabetic Index to Disease and Injuries, which includes the Supplementary V Code Classification. Two tables, also alphabetic, appear within this index: a complete list of all conditions due to or associated with a main term (for example, hypertension [persistently high arterial blood pressure]) and a complete list of anatomical sites associated with a main term (for example, neoplasm [an abnormal growth]).

- The Table of Drugs and Chemicals, used to code poisonings by drugs and adverse drug reactions.

- The Alphabetic Index to External Causes of Injuries and Poisoning, used to locate the optional E codes.

The Alphabetic Index is organized by main terms printed in bold type for ease of reference. The main terms represent the following:

- Diseases (for example, influenza, bronchitis)

- Conditions (for example, fatigue, fracture, injury)

- Nouns (for example, disease, disturbance, syndrome)

- Adjectives (for example, double, large, kink/kinking)

Anatomical sites are not used for main terms. Thus, bronchial asthma is found in the entry for "Asthma, asthmatic" rather than the anatomical site "bronchial."

Coding Conventions

Coders should review the preface to Volume 1 of ICD-9-CM to familiarize themselves with abbreviations, punctuation, symbols, and other conventions used in this context.

Following are the basic steps to be followed to arrive at accurate codes:

1. Identify all main terms included in the diagnostic statement.

2. Locate each main term in the Alphabetic Index.

3. Examine any modifiers appearing in parentheses next to the main term.

4. Refer to any subterms indented under the main term. The subterms form individual line entries and describe essential differences by site, etiology, or clinical type.

5. Choose a tentative code and confirm the code in the Tabular List.

6. Read and be guided by any instructional terms in the Tabular List.

7. Use fifth-digit subclassification codes, where provided.

8. Follow cross-reference instructions if the needed code is not located under the first main entity consulted.

9. Review color coding and reimbursement prompts.

10. Confirm and assign the code.

11. Continue coding diagnostic statements until all of the component elements are fully identified.

(For a more detailed discussion of the basics of ICD-9-CM coding, as well as exercises to help learn the system, coders should consult *Basic ICD-9-CM Coding,* by Lou Ann Schraffenberger.)

Basic Coding Guidelines for Outpatient Services

The ICD-9-CM Official Guidelines for Coding and Reporting were revised with an effective date of October 1, 2009, and can be found in their entirety at http://www.cdc.gov/nchs/data/icd9/icdguide09.pdf.

The following paragraphs, through the heading "Routine Outpatient Prenatal Visits" are excerpts from the ICD-9-CM Official Guidelines for Coding and Reporting.

These coding guidelines for outpatient diagnoses have been approved for use by hospitals/providers in coding and reporting hospital-based outpatient services and provider-based office visits.

The terms "encounter" and "visit" are often used interchangeably in describing outpatient service contacts and, therefore, appear together in these guidelines without distinguishing one from the other.

Though the conventions and general guidelines apply to all settings, coding guidelines for outpatient and provider reporting of diagnoses will vary in a number of instances from those for inpatient diagnoses, recognizing that:

- The Uniform Hospital Discharge Data Set (UHDDS) definition of principal diagnosis applies only to inpatients in acute, short-term, long-term care, and psychiatric hospitals.

- Coding guidelines for inconclusive diagnoses (probable, suspected, rule out, and so forth) were developed for inpatient reporting and do not apply to outpatients.

Selection of First-listed Condition

In the outpatient setting, the term "first-listed diagnosis" is used in lieu of principal diagnosis.

In determining the first-listed diagnosis the coding conventions of ICD-9-CM, as well as the general and disease-specific guidelines, take precedence over the outpatient guidelines.

Diagnoses often are not established at the time of the initial encounter/visit. It may take two or more visits before the diagnosis is confirmed.

The most critical rule involves beginning the search for the correct code assignment through the Alphabetic Index. Never begin searching initially in the Tabular List as this will lead to coding errors.

- **Outpatient Surgery:** When a patient presents for outpatient surgery, code the reason for the surgery as the first-listed diagnosis (reason for the encounter), even if the surgery is not performed due to a contraindication.

- **Observation Stay:** When a patient is admitted for observation for a medical condition, assign a code for the medical condition as the first-listed diagnosis. When a patient presents for outpatient surgery and develops complications requiring admission to observation, code the reason for the surgery as the first-reported diagnosis (reason for the encounter), followed by codes for the complications as secondary diagnoses.

Codes from 001.0 through V89

The appropriate code or codes from 001.0 through V89 must be used to identify diagnoses, symptoms, conditions, problems, complaints, or other reason(s) for the encounter/visit.

Accurate Reporting of ICD-9-CM Diagnosis Codes

For accurate reporting of ICD-9-CM diagnosis codes, the documentation should describe the patient's condition, using terminology that includes specific diagnoses as well as symptoms, problems, or reasons for the encounter. There are ICD-9-CM codes to describe all of these.

Selection of Codes 001.0 through 999.9

The selection of codes 001.0 through 999.9 will frequently be used to describe the reason for the encounter. These codes are from the section of ICD-9-CM for the classification of diseases and injuries (for example, infectious and parasitic diseases; neoplasms; symptoms, signs, and ill-defined conditions; and so forth).

Codes That Describe Symptoms and Signs

Codes that describe symptoms and signs, as opposed to diagnoses, are acceptable for reporting purposes when a diagnosis has not been established (confirmed) by the provider. Chapter 16 of ICD-9-CM, Symptoms, Signs, and Ill-defined conditions (codes 780.0–799.9) contain many, but not all, codes for symptoms.

Encounters for Circumstances Other Than a Disease or Injury

ICD-9-CM provides codes to deal with encounters for circumstances other than a disease or injury. The Supplementary Classification of factors Influencing Health Status and Contact with Health Services (V01.0–V89) is provided to deal with occasions when circumstances other than a disease or injury are recorded as diagnosis or problems. *See Section I.C. 18 for information on V-codes.*

Level of Detail in Coding

ICD-9-CM Codes with Three, Four, or Five Digits

ICD-9-CM is composed of codes with either three, four, or five digits. Codes with three digits are included in ICD-9-CM as the heading of a category of codes that may be further subdivided by the use of fourth and/or fifth digits, which provide greater specificity.

Use of Full Number of Digits Required for a Code

A three-digit code is to be used only if it is not further subdivided. Where fourth-digit subcategories and/or fifth-digit subclassifications are provided, they must be assigned. A code is invalid if it has not been coded to the full number of digits required for that code.

See also discussion under Section I.b.3., General Coding Guidelines, Level of Detail in Coding.

ICD-9-CM Code for the Diagnosis, Condition, Problem, or Other Reason for Encounter/Visit

List first the ICD-9-CM code for the diagnosis, condition, problem, or other reason for encounter/visit shown in the medical record to be chiefly responsible for the services provided. List additional codes that describe any coexisting conditions. In some cases the first-listed diagnosis may be a symptom when a diagnosis has not been established (confirmed) by the physician.

Uncertain Diagnosis

Do not code diagnoses documented as "probable," "suspected," "questionable," "rule out," or "working diagnosis" or other similar terms indicating uncertainty. Rather, code the condition(s) to the highest degree of certainty for that encounter/visit, such as symptoms, signs, abnormal test results, or other reason for the visit.

Please note: This differs from the coding practices used by short-term, acute care, long-term care, and psychiatric hospitals.

Chronic Diseases

Chronic diseases treated on an ongoing basis may be coded and reported as many times as the patient receives treatment and care for the condition(s).

Code All Documented Conditions That Coexist

Code all documented conditions that coexist at the time of the encounter/visit, and require or affect patient care treatment or management. Do not code conditions that were previously treated and no longer exist. However, history codes (V10–V19) may be used as secondary codes if the historical condition or family history has an impact on current care or influences treatment.

Patients Receiving Diagnostic Services Only

For patients receiving diagnostic services only during an encounter/visit, sequence first the diagnosis, condition, problem, or other reason for encounter/visit shown in the medical record to be chiefly responsible for the outpatient services provided during the encounter/visit. Codes for other diagnoses (for example, chronic conditions) may be sequenced as additional diagnoses.

For encounters for routine laboratory/radiology testing in the absence of any signs, symptoms, or associated diagnosis, assign V72.5 and a code from subcategory V72.6. If routine testing is performed during the same encounter as a test to evaluate a sign, symptom, or diagnosis, it is appropriate to assign both the V code and the code describing the reason for the nonroutine test.

For outpatient encounters for diagnostic tests that have been interpreted by a physician, and the final report is available at the time of coding, code any confirmed or definitive diagnosis(es) documented in the interpretation. Do not code related signs and symptoms as additional diagnoses.

Please note: This differs from the coding practice in the hospital inpatient setting regarding abnormal findings on test results.

Patients Receiving Therapeutic Services Only

For patients receiving therapeutic services only during an encounter/visit, sequence first the diagnosis, condition, problem, or other reason for encounter/visit shown in the medical record to be chiefly responsible for the outpatient services provided during the encounter/visit. Codes for other diagnoses (for example, chronic conditions) may be sequenced as additional diagnoses.

The only exception to this rule is that when the primary reason for the admission/encounter is chemotherapy, radiation therapy, or rehabilitation, the appropriate V code for the service is listed first, and the diagnosis or problem for which the service is being performed listed second.

Patients Receiving Preoperative Evaluations Only

For patients receiving preoperative evaluations only, sequence first a code from category V72.8, Other specified examinations, to describe the preop consultations. Assign a code for the condition to describe the reason for the surgery as an additional diagnosis. Code also any findings related to the preop evaluation.

Ambulatory Surgery

For ambulatory surgery, code the diagnosis for which the surgery was performed. If the postoperative diagnosis is known to be different from the preoperative diagnosis at the time the diagnosis is confirmed, select the postoperative diagnosis for coding, because it is the most definitive.

Routine Outpatient Prenatal Visits

For routine outpatient prenatal visits when no complications are present, codes V22.0, Supervision of normal first pregnancy, or V22.1, Supervision of other normal pregnancy, should be used as the principal diagnosis. These codes should not be used in conjunction with chapter 11 codes, Complications of Pregnancy, Childbirth, and the Puerperium.

Some additional guidelines, which are not included in the official guidelines, should be followed as well.

- Conditions or reasons for encounter/visit classifiable to the supplementary classifications, V01–V89, are used, where appropriate, to designate the diagnostic code.

  Example: A routine follow-up care visit for change of surgical dressings is coded V58.31, Encounter for change or removal of surgical wound dressing, when there is no mention of any wound infection or other complications.

- To provide an easy reference to a patient's history, some providers add any previous surgery or conditions that no longer exist to the list of conditions currently being treated. However, this added material should never be coded. Keepers of documents are advised to exercise care in distinguishing among:

  — Conditions presently existing

  — Conditions no longer existing

  — Residuals (late effects) of conditions no longer existing

  — Certain postoperative status conditions that require consideration in the management of patient care and warrant coding

Example: The provider documents hypertensive cardiovascular disease, coronary atherosclerosis, status postpneumonia (six months ago), and status postappendectomy (fifteen years ago). In this case, the code assignments should reflect only the current conditions: hypertensive cardiovascular disease (402.90) and coronary atherosclerosis (414.00).

- In those cases where the provider does not document (identify) a definite condition or problem at the conclusion of a patient care encounter/visit, the coder should query the provider for clarity of the final diagnosis and documentation in the health record must support this diagnosis for this date of service.

CPT Coding

Current Procedural Terminology (CPT) codes are used to identify procedures and services performed in medical practices, hospital-based outpatient areas, and selected other ambulatory care facilities. CPT is the first level of the HCPCS coding system.

Format and Structure

CPT is a listing of codes for procedures and services performed by healthcare providers. Each procedure/service is identified with a five-digit code. Inclusion or exclusion of a procedure code does not imply any payer coverage or reimbursement policy.

The body of CPT is divided into eight sections:

- Evaluation and Management

- Anesthesia

- Surgery

- Radiology

- Pathology and Laboratory

- Medicine

- Category II Codes

- Category III Codes

The first six sections contain subsections with anatomic, procedural, condition, or descriptor subheadings. The procedures and services are presented along with their identifying codes in numeric order with the one exception of the Evaluation and Management (E/M) section (99201–99499), which appears at the beginning of the book. The listing of a service/procedure in a specific section of the code book does not restrict its use to a specific specialty group; any qualified provider may use a code for services/procedures rendered from any section of CPT. When performing a service/procedure in which there are extenuating circumstances, the provider must note the circumstances. For this purpose, modifiers—two-digit alpha or numeric characters—may be added to the base code.

The seventh section, Category II Codes, is a set of supplementary tracking codes utilized for performance measures. The assignment of these codes assists with the data collection of the quality of care performed. Although the assignment of these codes is optional, incentive payments may be associated with their use. More information on quality incentives is addressed later in this chapter.

The eighth section, Category III Codes, is a set of temporary codes assigned for emerging technology, services, and procedures. If a Category III code is available, this code must be reported rather than the unlisted Category I code (CPT codes from first six sections of the code book).

The AMA has developed CPT procedural terminology so that terms can stand alone as descriptions of medical procedures. Instead of being printed in their entirety, however, some of the procedures refer back to a common portion of the preceding entry. This is evident when one or more indentations follow an entry. The indented code description is substituted for the portion following the semicolon (;) in the main code.

The AMA offers guidelines at the beginning of each of the eight sections of the code book to assist in the appropriate interpretation and reporting of the services in that section.

Evaluation and Management Coding

Evaluation and management (E/M) services include office or other outpatient visits, consultations, inpatient services, preventive medicine, critical care, emergency department, neonatal, nursing facility, home visits, and other types of services provided by physicians and nonphysician providers (for example, nurse practitioners, certified nurse midwives, clinical nurse specialists, and physician assistants). They encompass the wide variations in skill, effort, time, responsibility, and medical knowledge required to prevent or diagnose and treat illness or injury and to promote optimal health. All physicians, regardless of specialty, may use any E/M service. For details on the documentation requirements for E/M services, see chapter 2.

Modifiers

Modifiers are available in both the CPT and the HCPCS coding systems. A modifier is a two-digit code that may be numeric, alphabetic, or alphanumeric. Use of a modifier by the reporting provider indicates that some specific circumstance has altered a service or procedure that has been performed, but the definition of the service or procedure has not been changed. Some examples of instances when modifiers may be used to further explain a service or procedure are:

- Only a professional or technical portion of a service or procedure has been performed.

- More than one provider performed a service or procedure in more than one bodily location.

- A service or procedure has been increased or reduced.

- Only part of a service was performed.

- A staged procedure or service was performed by the same provider during the postoperative period.

- A bilateral procedure was performed.

- A service or procedure was provided more than once.

- A significant, separately identifiable E/M service was performed by the same provider on the same day of the procedure or other service.

- An unusual event occurred.

- A waiver of liability statement was obtained from the patient and is on file.

- A nurse practitioner rendering the service is in collaboration with a physician.

The two-digit modifier is added at the end of the base code. For example, 20610-50 would be the appropriate code to use for a patient who had a bilateral knee injection performed.

Ambulatory surgery centers and hospital outpatient departments are expected to report certain modifiers, when applicable. These modifiers are explained in appendix A of the CPT code book.

HCPCS Coding

The Health Care Financing Administration Common Procedure Coding System (HCPCS) is an alphanumeric classification system that identifies healthcare procedures, equipment, and supplies for claim submission purposes. The two levels are as follows: I, Current Procedural Terminology codes, developed by the AMA; and II, codes for equipment, supplies, and services not covered by Current Procedural Terminology codes as well as modifiers that can be used with all levels of codes, developed by CMS.

Level I: Current Procedural Terminology

The Final Rule on Standards for Electronic Transactions and Code Sets, also known as the Transaction Rule, identified both CPT and HCPCS code sets as the approved classification system to utilize for HIPAA. The system lists descriptive terms and identifying codes that serve a wide variety of important functions in the field of medical nomenclature. Level I codes are numeric with five digits.

Because CPT is currently in its fourth edition, it often now is referred to simply as CPT-4.

Level II: National Codes

The National Codes were developed by CMS to classify physician and nonphysician services that are not included in CPT, such as ambulance services, dental services, pharmaceuticals, injections, and durable medical goods (for example, prosthetics and orthotics). National Codes are alphanumeric and begin with the letters *A* through *V* and are followed by four numeric digits.

CMS provides quarterly updates for HCPCS codes, yet the vast majority of its National Codes are updated annually with the effective dates each January 1.

(The basics of CPT/HCPCS coding, as well as exercises to help learn the system, are presented in *Basic Current Procedural Terminology and HCPCS Coding,* by Gail Smith.)

Coding Errors

Coding errors can result in delayed or incorrect payment. Generally, coding errors are caused by any of several factors:

- Coding from incomplete reports or partial health records

- Coding the procedure title from a report without reviewing the procedure description

- Failing to read the entire operative and pathology report

- Coding only one of the procedures performed

- Coding a suspected condition as a confirmed diagnosis

- Coding only from the ICD-9-CM or CPT index, without referring to the Tabular List

- Coding with outdated coding books or encoders that are not updated

- Utilizing an outdated charge slip or charge description master

- Not coding to the highest level of specificity

- Not correctly sequencing the diagnoses or procedure codes

- Misinterpreting the coding guidelines, National Correct Coding Initiative (NCCI), Medically Unlikely Edits (MUEs), payer guidelines, and so forth

- Coding from poor or illegible documentation

Errors that occur in ICD-9-CM coding are different from those that occur in CPT coding.

Common ICD-9-CM Coding Errors

Errors that commonly occur in ICD-9-CM coding include:

- Failing to apply fourth or fifth digits

- Using unspecified codes even though the record contains more specific information

- Using the manifestation code first instead of the etiology code

- Using disease codes instead of more appropriate V codes

Common CPT Coding Errors

Errors that commonly occur in CPT coding include:

- Failing to assign diagnosis(es) codes that support the procedure performed

- Failing to use additional ICD-9-CM or CPT codes as indicated by the diagnosis or procedure

- Double-coding procedures that can be reported with one code (unbundling)

- Not coding the correct units of service

- Not differentiating between screening and diagnostic code assignments

With the added scrutiny of CPT codes by the Office of Inspector General (OIG) and payers to substantiate fraud and abuse of the healthcare (namely, Medicare) system, it is very important to minimize errors that can result from incomplete documentation or inappropriate use of codes. The key to minimizing coding errors is careful review and attention to improving documentation.

The following subsections offer examples of coding errors that commonly occur when reporting conditions/procedures within specific categories and subcategories of CPT.

Evaluation and Management

Errors that commonly occur in E/M coding include:

- Using only one or two codes in a section repeatedly or clustering codes (that is, all office visits coded to one or two levels)

- Failing to address documentation requirements for history, exam, and medical decision making for codes that must meet or exceed them (in cases of new patients, consultations, and so on)

- Using time as the determinant, even though counseling and coordination of care did not dominate the encounter

- Misinterpreting new and established patient definitions

- Coding a "sick" evaluation and management service when only "well" services were performed

Removal of Skin Lesions (Integumentary System)

Errors that commonly occur when coding the removal of skin lesions include:

- Coding the wrong technique (excision versus destruction versus paring)

- Coding the incorrect site

- Choosing the incorrect skin thickness (epidermis, dermis, subcutaneous tissues, or superficial fascia)

- Choosing malignant or benign lesion codes incorrectly

- Coding size of specimen instead of size of lesion

- Using only one code when multiple lesions were removed

- Disregarding the terms "single," "each," and "each additional"

- Failing to code nerve, tendon, or laceration repairs

Repair of Wounds (Integumentary System)

Errors that commonly occur when reporting the repair of wounds include:

- Grouping or adding together wound repair sites incorrectly

- Missing layered closures (simple to complex)

- Assigning an unlisted (XXX99) CPT code in place of a more appropriate code

Endoscopic Procedures (Digestive System)

Errors that commonly occur when reporting endoscopic procedures include:

- Failing to code the proper site(s)

- Coding the biopsy instead of polyp removal (if both are done from two different sites, both procedures are coded)

- Missing esophageal dilation guide wires

- Reporting the wrong technique, endoscopy missed
- Coding both diagnostic and surgical endoscopies at same site

Cataract Extraction (Eye and Ocular Adnexa)

Errors that commonly occur when reporting cataract extractions include:

- Interchanging the terms "intracapsular" and "extracapsular"
- Assigning multiple codes for procedures that could have been reported with one code (unbundling)
- Not coding pharmaceuticals administered

Hernia Repair (Digestive System)

Errors that commonly occur when reporting hernia repair include:

- Using excision codes when a laparoscope was used
- Using the terms "reducible" and "incarcerated" interchangeably
- Failing to use additional codes for mesh/prosthesis for incisional hernia repair

Auditory System

Errors that commonly occur when reporting procedures/services performed for the auditory system include:

- Confusing myringotomy and tympanotomy and tubes
- Failing to understand the concepts of separate procedure and multiple procedures

---

Check Your Understanding 6.2

1. Which of the following is not a tenet of the Standards of Ethical Coding?
   a. Refuse to change reported codes or the narratives of codes so that meanings are misrepresented.
   b. Advance coding knowledge and practice through continuing education.
   c. Demonstrate behavior that reflects integrity, shows a commitment to ethical and legal coding practices, and fosters trust in professional activities.
   d. Protect the confidentiality of the health record when possible and refuse to access protected health information not required for coding-related activities.

2. There are basic steps to follow to accurately assign ICD-9-CM diagnosis codes. Which of the following is one of these steps?
   a. Code all evaluations and management services based upon the documentation in the health record.
   b. Code units of service based upon the code descriptions documented in the code book and the service documented in the health record.
   c. Use fifth-digit subclassification codes, when provided.
   d. Always assign codes from the alphabetic index.

3. According to the ICD-9-CM Official Coding Guidelines, which of the following is true?

   a. Codes that describe symptoms and signs, as opposed to diagnoses, are acceptable for reporting purposes when a diagnosis has not been established (confirmed) by the provider.

   b. List first the ICD-9-CM code for the diagnosis, condition, problem, or other reason for encounter/visit shown in the medical record to be chiefly responsible for the services provided.

   c. Do not code diagnoses documented as "probable," "suspected," "questionable," "rule out," or "working diagnosis" or other similar terms indicating uncertainty.

   d. All of the above statements are true.

4. For patients receiving preoperative evaluations only, which diagnosis is sequenced first?

   a. Sequence first a code for the condition that describes the reason for the surgery.

   b. Sequence first a code for the medical condition that is the reason the consultant is seeing the patient.

   c. Sequence first a code from category V72.8X, Other specified examinations, to describe the preoperative consultation.

   d. Sequence first the E code for the external reason for the patient's surgery.

5. Which of the following statements is true?

   a. Assign diagnosis codes to the highest level of specificity.

   b. All payers require the assignment of E codes.

   c. The sequence of diagnoses is not important.

   d. V codes may never be the first listed diagnosis.

6. Which of the following is not a section in the CPT code book?

   a. Evaluation and Management

   b. Radiology

   c. Neoplasms

   d. Category II Codes

7. Modifiers are appended to CPT codes for which reason?

   a. A service or procedure has been increased or reduced.

   b. Only part of a service was performed.

   c. A bilateral procedure was performed.

   d. All of the above.

8. Which of the following is not a coding CPT error?

   a. Using the full range of evaluation and management service codes for a new office visit

   b. Coding all skin lesions as if they were excised

   c. Coding all wound repairs as simple closures

   d. Coding all pharmaceuticals with a unit of one

(continued on next page)

Check Your Understanding 6.2 *(continued)*

9. Which of the following statements is true?

    a. It is a best practice to assign malignant codes to all lesions.

    b. Modifiers should be appended to all CPT codes reported from the evaluation and management section.

    c. The documentation in the health record must support the codes assigned.

    d. There are no official coding sources for ICD-9-CM, CPT, and HCPCS.

10. HCPCS Level II national codes contain all but which of the following?

    a. Pharmaceuticals

    b. Medical conditions

    c. Injections and durable medical goods

    d. Ambulance services

Physician Quality Reporting Initiative (PQRI)

As with any performance improvement process, there are specific steps to be taken. Figure 6.11 illustrates steps to be taken when participating in a performance improvement process.

Figure 6.11. Performance improvement process

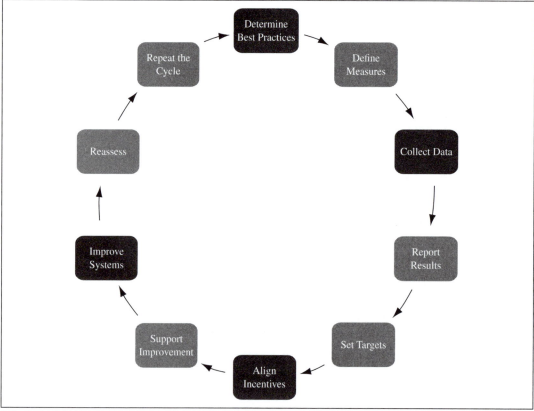

© Preferred Healthcare Solutions, LLC. Reprinted with permission.

The Physician Quality Reporting Initiative is a performance improvement process. With the PQRI, quality of care is the focus. The evidence-based measures were developed by professionals and offer a financial incentive for reporting quality measurement that results in improvements in care. Providers may report PQRI measures during the claims submission process. Unique codes are reported based upon the patient's health condition and care provided.

"The 2006 Tax Relief and Health Care Act (TRHCA) (P.L. 109-432) required the establishment of a physician quality reporting system, including an incentive payment for eligible professionals (EPs) who satisfactorily report data on quality measures for covered services furnished to Medicare beneficiaries during the second half of 2007 (the 2007 reporting period). CMS named this program the Physician Quality Reporting Initiative (PQRI)" (CMS 2009a).

As a result of the initial reporting period of 2007, additional regulations were developed resulting in the program's permanency. The "Medicare Improvements for Patients and Providers Act of 2008 (MIPPA) (Pub. L. 110-275) made the PQRI program permanent, but only authorized incentive payments through 2010. EPs who meet the criteria for satisfactory submission of quality measures data for services furnished during the reporting period, January 1, 2009–December 31, 2009, will earn an incentive payment of 2.0 percent of their total allowed charges for Physician Fee Schedule (PFS) covered professional services furnished during that same period (the 2009 calendar year)" (CMS 2009a).

As defined in the Social Security Act, Section 1861(r), eligible professionals in the PQRI are:

- Doctor of medicine
- Doctor of osteopathy
- Doctor of podiatric medicine
- Doctor of optometry
- Doctor of oral surgery
- Doctor of dental medicine
- Chiropractor

Also, eligible professionals are defined in an additional section of the Social Security Act, Section 1842(b)(18)(C), as:

- Physician assistant
- Nurse practitioner
- Clinical nurse specialist
- Certified registered nurse anesthetist
- Certified nurse-midwife
- Clinical social worker
- Clinical psychologist
- Registered dietitian
- Nutrition professional

Table 6.4. 2009 PQRI sample patient criteria table (rheumatoid arthritis)

Patient Sample Criteria Table		
Measures Group	**CPT Patient Encounter Codes**	**ICD-9-CM Diagnosis Codes**
Rheumatoid Arthritis 18 years and older	99201, 99202, 99203, 99204, 99205, 99212, 99213, 99214, 99215, 99241, 99242, 99243, 99244, 99245, 99341, 99342, 99343, 99344, 99345, 99347, 99348, 99349, 99350, 99455, 99456	714.0, 714.1, 714.2, 714.81

Source: CMS 2008a, 3

- Therapists
    - Physical therapist
    - Occupational therapist
    - Qualified speech-language pathologist

Claims data are utilized for reporting of CPT Category II codes and HCPCS temporary G-codes. These codes are reported with a $0 charge and no monies may be collected from patients for PQRI measures. The quality codes, which supply the measure numerator, must be reported on the same claims as the payment codes, which supply the measure denominator. The numerator is the upper portion of a fraction or the CPT Category II codes and G codes. The denominator is the lower portion of a fraction or the ICD-9-CM, CPT, and HCPCS codes. Patient demographics such as age and gender also come into the equation for PQRI. Additionally, there are modifiers that are two-digit alphanumeric fields, such as 1P, 2P, and 3P, which are examples of "exclusion modifiers," and 8P, which is an example of "action not performed." A sample CMS-1500 claim form for rheumatoid arthritis may be found in appendix G.

There are 153 quality measures in 7 different measure groups for the 2009 PQRI. CMS's 2009 List of Quality Measures may be found on the CD-ROM accompanying this book. Eligible professionals must select at least three measures in order to participate in the PQRI program. It is an identified best practice to select three measures that relate to a particular disease, such as diabetes. For example, A1C control, LDL control, and blood pressure control may be selected for diabetes patients. A sample patient criteria table for rheumatoid arthritis may be viewed in table 6.4.

The American Academy of Family Practice offers two sample data collection tools. The coder's PQRI data collection sheet for diabetes may be reviewed in figure 6.12. The family medicine physician's data collection tool may be found on the CD-ROM accompanying this book; note that the Excel file has two worksheets, one for physicians and one for coders.

CMS offers a wealth of information online at www.cms.hhs.gov/pqri. For medical practices that are just starting to report PQRI measures, the "Getting Started with PQRI Reporting" document will be helpful and may be found in appendix H.

Advanced Beneficiary Notice of Noncoverage

As documented in *Medicare Claims Processing Manual*, chapter 30—Financial Liability Protections, Section 40.3—Advanced Beneficiary Notice Standards, "The purpose of the ABN is to inform a Medicare beneficiary, before he or she receives specified items or services

Figure 6.12. Sample PQRI data capture tool

AAFP CODER'S PQRI DATA COLLECTION SHEET - DIABETES			
PHYSICIAN	DATE	MR#	No. of years in physician's care
PATIENT NAME		DOB	Date last seen

Lay this sheet on top of the physician's data collection form so that the headings below align and the physician's initials are visible. Report the codes next to the physician's initials for each measure.

Code (See below for modifier indications)	Measure & result	Verification & test date
Hemoglobin A1C – Patients aged 18-75. Report with 250.00-250.93, 648.00-648.04. Report at least once per reporting period.		
3044F	Most recent A1C level within 12 months <7.0%	A1C: Test date:
3045F	Most recent A1C level within 12 months 7.0% to 9.0%	A1C: Test date:
3046F	Most recent A1C level within 12 months >9%	A1C: Test date:
3046F-8P	A1C not performed within 12 months	Reason not otherwise specified
Lipid management – Patients aged 18-75. Report with 250.00-250.93, 648.00-648.04. Report at least once per reporting period.		
3048F	Most recent LDL-C level within 12 months <100 mg/dL	LDL-C value: Test date:
3049F	Most recent LDL-C level within 12 months 100-129 mg/dL	LDL-C value: Test date:
3050F	Most recent LDL-C level within 12 months ≥130 mg/dL	LDL-C value: Test date:
3048F-1P	LDL-C not performed due to medical reason	Reason documented:
3048F-8P	LDL-C not performed within 12 months	Reason not otherwise specified
Blood pressure – Patients aged 18-75. Report with 250.00-250.93, 648.00-648.04. Report at least once per reporting period.		
3074F	Most recent systolic blood pressure within 12 months <130 mm Hg *Report also appropriate code for diastolic result*	BP reading: Date:
3075F	Most recent systolic blood pressure within 12 months 130-139 mm Hg *Report also appropriate code for diastolic result*	BP reading: Date:
3077F	Most recent systolic blood pressure within 12 months ≥140 mm Hg *Report also appropriate code for diastolic result*	BP reading: Date:
3078F	Most recent diastolic blood pressure within 12 months <80 mm Hg	BP reading: Date:
3079F	Most recent diastolic blood pressure within 12 months 80-89 mm Hg	BP reading: Date:
3080F	Most recent diastolic blood pressure within 12 months ≥90 mm Hg	BP reading: Date:
3074F-1P 3078F-1P	Blood pressure not measured <u>within 12 months</u> due to medical reasons	Reason documented:
2000F-8P	Blood pressure not measured within 12 months	Reason not otherwise specified
Urine screening for microalbumin or medical attention for nephropathy - 250.00-250.93, 648.00-648.04 - aged 18-75 years - report at least once per period		
3060F	Positive microalbuminuria test result documented and reviewed	Documentation verified
3061F	Negative microalbuminuria test result documented and reviewed	Documentation verified
3062F	Positive macroalbuminuria test result documented and reviewed	Documentation verified
3066F	Documentation of treatment for nephropathy (eg, patient receiving dialysis, patient being treated for ESRD, CRF, ARF, or renal insufficiency, any visit to a nephrologist)	Documentation verified
4009F	Angiotensin converting enzyme (ACE) inhibitor or angiotensin receptor blocker (ARB) therapy prescribed	Documentation verified
3060F-8P	Nephropathy screening was not performed	Reason not specified
Performance Measure Modifier Indications		
1P Performance measure exclusion modifier due to medical reasons includes: - not indicated (absence of organ/limb, already received/performed, other) - contraindicated (patient allergic history, potential adverse drug interaction, other)		
8P – Performance measure exclusion due to action not performed, reason not otherwise specified.		

© 2008 American Academy of Family Physicians

that otherwise might be paid for, that Medicare certainly or probably will not pay for them on that particular occasion. The ABN also allows the beneficiary to make an informed consumer decision whether or not to receive the items or services for which he or she may have to pay out of pocket or through other insurance. In addition, the ABN allows the beneficiary to better participate in his/her own health care treatment decisions by making informed consumer decisions. If the provider, practitioner, or supplier expects payment for the items or services to be denied by Medicare, the provider, practitioner, or supplier must advise the beneficiary before items or services are furnished that, in its opinion, the beneficiary will be personally and fully responsible for payment" (CMS 2008b, Chapter 30, Section 40.3).

"The Financial Liability Protection provisions of the Social Security Act protect beneficiaries and healthcare providers under certain circumstances from unexpected liability for charges associated with claims that Medicare does not pay . . . " (CMS 2008e).

"Section 50 of the *Medicare Claims Processing Manual* establishes the standards for use by providers, practitioners, suppliers, and laboratories in implementing the revised Advance Beneficiary Notice of Noncoverage (ABN) (Form CMS-R-131), formerly the 'Advance Beneficiary Notice.' Beginning March 1, 2009, the ABN-G and ABN-L will no longer be valid; and notifiers must begin using the revised Advance Beneficiary Notice of Noncoverage (CMS-R-131)" (CMS 2008e, Chapter 30, Section 50.1). A copy of the CMS-R-131 can be found in appendix I.

Section 50.2.1—Applicability of Limitation on Liability (LOL) states, "The Limitation On Liability (LOL) protections of §1879 of the Act apply only when a provider believes that an otherwise covered item or service may be denied either as not reasonable and necessary under §1862(a)(1) of the Act or because the item or service constitutes custodial care under §1862(a)(9) of the Act. §1879 of the Act requires a provider to notify a beneficiary in advance when he or she believes that items or services will likely be denied either as not reasonable and necessary or as constituting custodial care. If such notice is not given, providers may not shift financial liability for such items or services to beneficiaries should a claim for such items or services be denied by Medicare" (CMS 2008b, Chapter 30, Section 50.2.1).

Section 50.5, Financial Liability Protections, states that Notifiers (healthcare providers) are required to issue ABNs whenever LOL applies. This typically occurs at three points during a course of treatment: initiation, reduction, and termination, also known as "triggering events."

Initiations

An initiation is the beginning of a new patient encounter, start of a plan of care, or beginning of treatment. If a notifier believes that certain otherwise covered items or services will be non-covered (for example, not reasonable and necessary) at initiation, an ABN must be issued prior to the beneficiary receiving the noncovered care (CMS 2008b, Chapter 30, Section 50.5).

Reductions

A reduction occurs when there is a decrease in a component of care (that is, frequency, duration, and so forth). For example, a beneficiary is receiving outpatient physical therapy five days a week and wishes to continue therapy five days; however, the notifier believes that the beneficiary's therapy goals can be met with only three days of therapy weekly. This reduction in treatment would trigger the requirement for an ABN (CMS 2008b, Chapter 30, Section 50.5).

Terminations

Termination is the discontinuation of certain items or services. An example would be when a speech therapist no longer considers outpatient speech therapy described in a plan of care reasonable and necessary. An ABN would have to be issued prior to the termination of the speech therapy. If the beneficiary wishes to continue receiving noncovered speech therapy treatments upon receiving the ABN, he or she must select Option 1 or 2 on the ABN stating that he or she wants to receive the services and agrees to be financially responsible if Medicare does not pay (CMS 2008b, Chapter 30, Section 50.5).

"A healthcare provider who fails to comply with the ABN instructions risks financial liability and/or sanctions" (CMS 2008b, Chapter 30, Section 50.2.2).

General Notice Preparation Instructions

- Minimum of two copies.

- Reproductions are permitted via photocopying, digitized technology, or other appropriate method.

- Dark ink on a pale background must be used.

- Highlighted text is not permitted.

- Font from the CMS Web site should be used; however, if system electronic restrictions exist, then Arial, Arial Narrow, Times New Roman, and Courier may be utilized.

- Italics, embossing, and bold fonts are not permitted.

- Font size should be 12-point. Font size for titles should be 14- to 16-point. Font size for insertion blanks may be no smaller than 10-point.

- Minor customization is permitted:

  — Preprinting information in blanks, such as specific tests.

  — Multiple versions may be utilized to specify different services.

  — Lettering for each section should be removed.

  — Check-off boxes may be used when listing services.

Only the modifications listed above are permitted. Additional modifications will result in an invalid ABN.

Delivery Requirements

- Delivered by a suitable individual to a capable recipient (this includes the appropriate language interpretation)

- Provided using the correct ABN form

- Completed in all sections

- Completed in person, when possible

- Provided with advanced notice

- Explained in its entirety and all beneficiary's questions answered

- Signed by the beneficiary or his/her representative

Figure 6.13 illustrates the process flow of an ABN.

Figure 6.13. Advance Beneficiary Notice of Noncoverage process flow

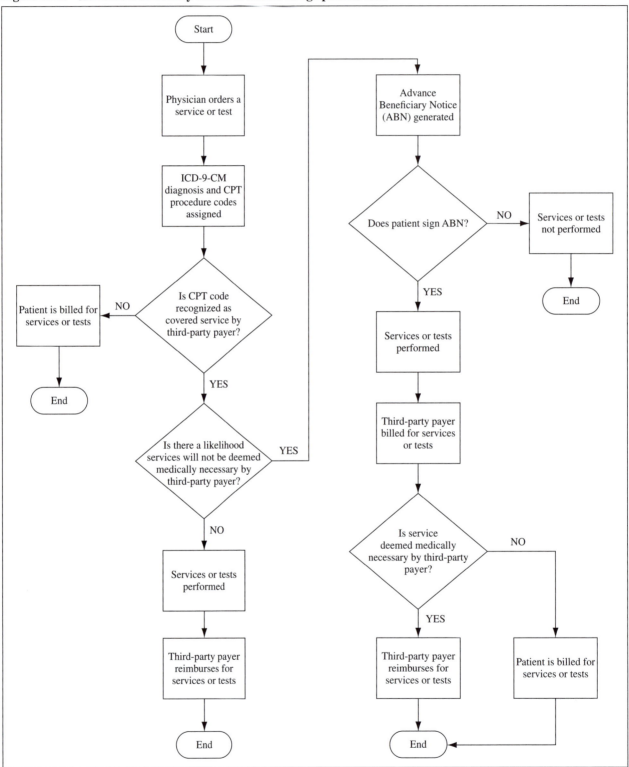

Internal Reimbursement Policies

Medicare, Medicaid, and private insurance companies have become more aggressive in auditing physician services. CMS's most recent initiative is Recovery Audit Contractors, commonly referred to as RAC. Medicare Modernization Act, Section 306 required the three-year RAC demonstration time frame. The Tax Relief and Healthcare Act of 2006, Section 302 required a permanent and nationwide RAC program no later than 2010.

The RAC began as a demonstration project (March 2005–March 2008) and is now in its permanent phase in stages. This program is aimed to detect and correct improper payments. "The RAC program's mission is to reduce Medicare improper payments through efficient detection and collection of overpayments, the identification of underpayments and the implementation of actions that will prevent future improper payments" (CMS 2006).

The phase-in approach will be effective for the permanent RAC. This phase-in schedule may be found in appendix J (and in chapter 9 as figure 9.6) or at http://www.cms.hhs.gov/RAC. Each of the four regions have subcontractor(s) to carry out the responsibilities of the RAC initiative.

Region A: DCS
Subcontractors: PRG Shultz, iHealth Technologies, and Strategic Health Solutions

Region B: CGI
Subcontractor: PRG Schultz

Region C: Connolly Consulting
Subcontractor: Viant, Inc.

Region D: HDI
Subcontractor: PRG Schultz

There are two types of reviews that may be performed: (1) automated, which does not require the review of health records, and (2) complex, which requires the submission of health record copies. Although the RAC may go back three years from when the claim was paid, the RACs may only review claims paid on or after October 1, 2007. During the transition from the RAC demonstration project into the RAC permanency, many changes were made, such as the requirement of a medical director and qualified coders.

Although there was much discussion regarding the inclusion of evaluation and management professional services during the demonstration project, CMS states, "the review of all evaluation and management (E/M) services will be allowed under the RAC program. The review of duplicate claims or E/M services that should be included in a global surgery was available for review during the RAC demonstration and will continue to be available for review. The review of the level of the visit of some E/M services was not included in the RAC demonstration. CMS will work closely with the American Medical Association and the physician community prior to any reviews being completed regarding the level of the visit and will provide notice to the physician community before the RACs are allowed to begin reviews of evaluation and management (E/M) services and the level of the visit" (CMS 2009b). Additional information, including the RAC Fact Sheet and background details of the RAC process steps, may be found at http://www.cms.hhs.gov/RAC. AHIMA has published a Recovery Audit Contractor tool kit that is available as an AHIMA member resource, along with a variety of articles.

Clearly, physicians must be more forceful in addressing their exposure to prepayment and postpayment audit activity.

At a minimum, physicians should:

- In cases of coding and billing errors, refund the overpayment and explain the error to Medicare, Medicaid, or the payer

- Develop internal policies and procedures with respect to coding, claims filing, and documentation

- Annually review office policies and procedures for coding, reimbursement processing, and patient record documentation

- Conduct internal and external health record audits

- Educate themselves and staff regarding coding, reimbursement, and documentation rules, as well as penalties and sanction possibilities

- Develop action plans, if necessary

In addition, medical practices should develop various internal policies that will ensure appropriate reimbursement and protect them from charges of fraud and abuse. The following subsections discuss some of the actions that practices may take.

Conduct a Quality Review Process

A quality review should be conducted at least annually to monitor the productivity and accuracy of coding practices. This process requires that the medical practice establish policies and procedures on the assignment of diagnostic and procedural/service codes. The significant findings of the reviews should be discussed with the relevant physician(s) and office staff.

This quality assurance process should:

- Be continuous and routine

- Include a systematic process for sampling all the records every year

- Be conducted for each physician in the group/practice (more often than annually during the first year for new physicians)

- Be conducted for each new coder (more often than annually during the first year for a new coder)

- Focus on the most frequent diagnoses/procedures

- Focus on area(s) of vulnerability, such as specialty-specific services or those services noted in OIG documents, namely the OIG's Work Plan

- Include all disciplines or services (for example, radiology and pathology)

- Review the use of CPT unlisted procedures

- Be done both prospectively (to prevent billing errors) and retrospectively (to uncover patterns of code selection over time)

- Be done on all rejected claims or claims paid on a reduced basis

- Review charge description masters, charge slips, and other coding-related forms at least annually when new codes are published

- Compare the volume of tests ordered per code to identify potential overuse and underuse of codes

Conduct a Coding Audit

Although there are various topics that are prime areas for coding audits, the OIG's Work Plan documents potential areas of concern each year. Serious consideration should be given to these topics if they are pertinent to the services provided at the medical practice. The OIG's Work Plan for 2009 may be found at http://oig.hhs.gov/publications/workplan.asp.

Other potential areas for coding audits are the following:

1. Evaluation and management services coding

2. Consultations

3. Modifier use

4. Accurate linking of diagnosis to procedure

5. Correct units of service

6. Newly provided services

7. Injections, immunizations, and their administration

8. Chemotherapy

9. Legible documentation

10. Service provided incident to

11. Professional services provided by the provider at locations other than the main medical practice location, such as satellite offices and skilled nursing facilities

Perform an Outpatient Diagnosis Coding Review

An outpatient (medical practice or clinic) diagnosis coding review should involve reviewing the sequencing of multiple diagnoses to ensure that the reason chiefly responsible for the visit is listed first. In addition, it should examine the coding of cases where a physician qualifies a diagnosis with the terms "rule out," "questionable," "suspect," and so on. Cases of the repeated coding of a single diagnosis also should be reviewed to confirm that, instead of being an old diagnosis, the condition is chronic and continues to be managed. Finally, cases coded as "history of" or "postop" in the absence of a current condition should be scrutinized carefully.

Perform a Surgery Coding Diagnosis Review

A surgery coding diagnosis review should be performed to compare preoperative, postoperative, and pathological diagnoses for consistency or reasonableness. Records coded prior to receipt of a pathology report also should be reviewed. Moreover, the review should include comparing the titles of operations to the body of the report. Finally, the surgery coding diagnosis review should compare the patient's history and examination with the operative report to identify concurrent conditions that should be coded because they may have influenced treatment.

Review the Charge Description Master (CDM)

Charge description masters have always been a challenge. Although specific areas (for example, laboratory or radiology) create special problems, the challenge of the CDM can be met by taking a systematic approach to the various elements in all its areas. For example:

- New procedure codes should be added.

- New HCPCS codes for equipment, supplies, or pharmaceuticals should be added.

- Invalid or deleted CPT codes should be removed or replaced.

- When the new CPT code book is released every year, its appendix listing should be compared with the current CDM for new, deleted, and revised codes.

- More specific codes should be found for any unlisted procedure codes (XXX99).

- Accurate code descriptions from all coding systems should be verified and parallel those descriptions documented in the official coding books.

- Charges should be verified so that they remain consistent and based on some common logic for the entire CDM.

- Carrier newsletters, bulletins, and advisories should be reviewed on a continuing basis for additions or corrections.

Moreover, it is important to note that the CDM will require updating at least three times a year (January, July, and October) to reflect changes in the CPT and ICD-9-CM coding systems. Continual updating is necessary when pharmaceutical or other highly priced susceptible items or services are included in the CDM.

Check Your Understanding 6.3

1. In the Physician Quality Reporting Initiative, which of the following is not defined as an eligible professional?

   a. Doctor of medicine
   b. Nurse practitioner
   c. Chiropractor
   d. Doctor of acupuncture

2. According to the Physician Quality Reporting Initiative, what codes are included in the reporting calculation?

   a. ICD-9-CM code
   b. CPT code
   c. HCPCS temporary G code
   d. All of the above

---

3. Which of the following statements is false?

   a. The ABN must be signed by the patient prior to the ordered service being performed.
   b. There are many different versions of a valid ABN and providers may select the one that works best for their medical practice.
   c. An ABN must be presented and explained to the patient when the provider expects payment for the services to be denied by Medicare.
   d. The purpose of the ABN is to inform the Medicare beneficiary, before he or she receives specific items or services that otherwise might be paid for, that Medicare certainly or probably will not pay for them on that particular occasion.

4. What are three triggering events that may produce the need for an ABN?

   a. Initiations, continuations, or terminations of services
   b. Reductions, continuations, or terminations of services
   c. Initiations, reductions, or terminations of services
   d. Continuations, reductions, or initiations of services

5. The RAC refers to which of the following?

   a. Revenue audit contractors
   b. Revenue audit consultants
   c. Recovery audit contractors
   d. Recovery audit consultants

6. There are two types of reviews that may be performed by the RAC. Which one requires the submission of health records?

   a. Complex review
   b. Simple review
   c. Intermediate review
   d. Composite review

7. When participating in a performance improvement process, what steps are included in this process?

   a. Determine best practices, define measures, and collect data
   b. Report results, set targets, and align incentives
   c. Support improvement, improve systems, and reassess
   d. All of the above

8. What resource would be helpful in identifying potential focus areas for a coding audit?

   a. Listing of patients receiving financial assistance
   b. OIG's Work Plan for the current year
   c. Detailed listing of those patients who no-showed for their appointments
   d. Listing of all members on the revenue cycle team

(continued on next page)

Check Your Understanding 6.3 *(continued)*

9. What is the name of the database used by medical practices to house the price list for all services provided to patients?

   a. Charge slip
   b. HIPAA database
   c. Charge description master
   d. Denial database

10. When reviewing the charge description master, which are areas to review?

    a. Invalid or deleted codes should be removed or replaced.
    b. Write off dollars for specific reason codes.
    c. Unlisted procedure codes should be replaced with more specific codes.
    d. Both A and C should be reviewed.

Conclusion

Of obvious importance in every medical practice is an efficient and streamlined revenue cycle. Many detailed steps must be monitored, analyzed, and potential action taken to ensure accurate revenue for the practice. Additionally, a team approach to the revenue cycle with strong leadership will benefit every practice. Regulatory compliance is always of utmost importance when coding and billing of professional services is involved; consequently, there are regulations and guidelines that must be followed. With the revenue audit contractors' close eye on correct payments, medical practices have entered into a time when ignoring the revenue cycle or not staying current with regulatory changes may result in sanctions. The newly revised Advanced Beneficiary Notice of Noncoverage offers more detailed attention to the medical practice's compliance. Yet the benefits of the Physician Quality Reporting Initiative and other financial incentives associated with electronic health record implementation and e-prescribing propose financial opportunities for medical practices if time frames are followed. All of these processes and programs have come together simultaneously during a tough economic time. Although some medical practices may simply think that they do not have the staff, resources, or funds to address revenue cycle issues, PQRI data collection, or EHR implementations, on the contrary, medical practices cannot afford to not address revenue cycle issues or any opportunity to increase revenue to the practice.

Diagnostic and procedural codes assigned on the basis of the information documented in the health record are used not only in-house to guide the medical practice's marketing, budgeting, and quality improvement efforts, but they also are used by outside agencies to help forecast healthcare needs and by payers to justify reimbursement. Three coding systems are used by medical practices: ICD-9-CM, CPT, and HCPCS. The accuracy of coding with these three classification systems drives the appropriate reimbursement for documented professional services.

References

AHIMA House of Delegates. 2008. Standards of ethical coding. http://www.ahima.org/infocenter/guidelines/standards.asp.

Casto, A.B., and E. Layman. 2008. *Principles of Healthcare Reimbursement,* 2nd ed. Chicago: AHIMA.

Centers for Medicare and Medicaid Services. 2006. Medicare recovery audit contractors (RACs): FY 2006 findings, corrective actions, and expansion plans. http://www.cms.hhs.gov/RAC/01_Overview.asp#TopOfPage.

Centers for Medicare and Medicaid Services. 2008a. Getting started with 2009 PQRI reporting of measures groups, version 3.0.

Centers for Medicare and Medicaid Services. 2008b. *Medicare Claims Processing Manual.*

Centers for Medicare and Medicaid Services. 2008c. *Medicare Financial Management Manual.*

Centers for Medicare and Medicaid Services. 2008d. *Provider Reimbursement Manual.*

Centers for Medicare and Medicaid Services. 2008e. Transmittal 1587, Revised form CMS-R-131, Advanced Beneficiary Notice of Noncoverage.

Centers for Medicare and Medicaid Services. 2009a. Physician quality reporting initiative: Overview. http://www.cms.hhs.gov/PQRI/01_Overview.asp#TopOfPage.

Centers for Medicare and Medicaid Services. 2009b. Revenue audit contractors: Frequently asked questions. http://questions.cms.hhs.gov/cgi-bin/cmshhs.cfg/php/enduser/std_alp.php?p_pv=4.497.

Department of Health and Human Services. 2003a (Feb. 20). Health insurance reform: Modifications to electronic data transaction standards and code sets. *Federal Register* 68(34):8381–8399.

Department of Health and Human Services. 2003b (Feb. 20). Health insurance reform: Security standards; final rule. *Federal Register* 68(34):8333–8381.

Department of Health and Human Services. 2009 (Jan. 23). Annual update of the HHS poverty guidelines. *Federal Register* 74(14):4199–4201. http://aspe.hhs.gov/poverty/09poverty.shtml.

Gregg Fahrenholz, C. 2009. Bringing down denials: Successfully managing denials in medical practices. *Journal of AHIMA* 80(8):32–38.

Schraffenberger, L.A. 2009. *Basic ICD-9-CM Coding,* 2010 ed. Chicago: AHIMA.

Smith, G.I. 2009. *Basic Current Procedural Terminology and HCPCS Coding,* 2009 ed. Chicago: AHIMA.

Social Security Act, Section 1861(r), Part E—Miscellaneous Provisions. http://www.ssa.gov/OP_Home/ssact/title18/1861.htm.

Social Security Act, Section 1842(b)(18)(C). Provisions Relating to the Administration of Part B. http://www.ssa.gov/OP_Home/ssact/title18/1842.htm.

Chapter 7

Medical Practice Accreditation Standards

Laurie A. Rinehart-Thompson, JD, RHIA, CHP

Learning Objectives

- Gain an understanding of the concept of accreditation and its benefit to medical practices

- Identify the various organizations by which medical practices can elect to become accredited

- Understand the Joint Commission chapters, standards, and elements of performance that apply to the management of health information

- Understand National Patient Safety Goals as they apply to ambulatory care and office-based surgery

- Define a sentinel event and apply a root cause analysis to it

Key Terms

Accreditation
Accreditation Association for Ambulatory Health Care
Ambulatory Care Accreditation Program
Element of performance
Improving Organization Performance

Information Management
Joint Commission
National Committee for Quality Assurance (NCQA)
National Patient Safety Goals
Nonreviewable sentinel events

Record of Care, Treatment, and Services
Reviewable sentinel events
Root cause analysis
Sentinel event
Sentinel event database
Sentinel event policy
Standard

Introduction

This chapter discusses the concept of accreditation, the advantages of being accredited, and three organizations by which a medical practice may choose to seek accreditation, including the National Committee for Quality Assurance, the Joint Commission, and the Accreditation Association for Ambulatory Health Care. The chapter emphasizes the Joint Commission, the standards and elements of performance that apply to the management of information, and the handling of sentinel events.

In addition to accreditation standards, the U.S. Senate passed a Medicare law provision in 2007 that directs the Secretary of Health and Human Services to commission an initiative to deploy uniform, evidence-based performance measures and a reporting infrastructure. The initiative provides $10 million per year for fiscal years 2009 through 2012 to:

- Set national priorities that identify reforms that will yield the biggest results

- Endorse and maintain measures that promote health, safety, and efficiency

- Promote the development of electronic health records that support performance management by making the coordination and monitoring of practices possible (NQF 2008)

The National Quality Forum's (NQF) mission is to improve the quality of American healthcare by setting national priorities and goals for performance improvement, endorsing national consensus standards for measuring and publicly reporting on performance, and promoting the attainment of national goals through education and outreach programs. This nonprofit organization was established in 1999 and is based in Washington, DC. The NQF's National Voluntary Consensus Standards for Ambulatory Care may be found in appendix K.

Advantages of Accreditation

Quality patient care is paramount to healthcare providers, patients, and payers alike. The medical practice setting is no exception. There are numerous mechanisms by which quality of care can be measured; however, one way to measure and validate quality is through the process of accreditation. *Accreditation* is a voluntary process that results in formal approval from an external accrediting body. It demonstrates that the healthcare organization has met a set of standards established by the accrediting body (Odom-Wesley and Brown 2009). Through the accreditation process, a medical practice is held to a set of national standards that is also applied to other medical practices.

Often viewed as a "gold standard" or sometimes denoted by a "gold seal of approval," accreditation enables a medical practice to hold itself out as exceeding the highest of standards. However, there are many other benefits—including concrete benefits—that derive from being accredited. For example, accreditation:

- Attracts patients, professional staff, and third-party payers

- Enhances reputation and community confidence by demonstrating a commitment to excellence

- Enables organizations to meet certain regulatory agency certification and state licensure requirements in an alternative manner

- Enables organizations to meet eligibility requirements for reimbursement from payers

- Provides a report card of the quality of an organization's performance

- Serves as an educational tool and enables continuous performance improvement (Odom-Wesley and Brown 2009)

There are a variety of organizations that accredit healthcare providers. The three accreditation organizations that are relevant to medical practices are the National Committee for Quality

Assurance (NCQA), the Joint Commission, and the Accreditation Association for Ambulatory Health Care (AAAHC).

National Committee for Quality Assurance (NCQA)

The NCQA was founded in 1990 and began accrediting managed care organizations in 1991 (Shi and Singh 2008). A private, not-for-profit organization, the NCQA identifies itself as "dedicated to improving healthcare quality" (NCQA 2009). Although recognized most prominently for its health plan accreditation, it now accredits a wide spectrum of healthcare organizations. NCQA accreditation is voluntary, but the majority of health plans in the United States participate and seek accreditation from it. Further, many large employers limit the health plans that they offer to their employees to only those that are NCQA-accredited (NCQA 2009). Finally, more than 30 states exempt NCQA-accredited organizations from state audit requirements (NCQA 2009). As with all accrediting bodies, its approval is used by providers and managed care organizations to market and advertise themselves as high-quality organizations.

Organizations accredited by NCQA must meet more than 60 standards and report on their performance in more than 40 areas that are evaluated through activities such as on-site and off-site surveys, satisfaction surveys, audits, and measurements of clinical performance (NCQA 2009). Quality practices are assessed and improved outcomes occur through measurement, analysis, and improvement based on the measurement and analysis of findings. It is through continued measurement and reporting that consumers and employers are able to make informed healthcare purchasing decisions. Accreditation by NCQA is designated by one of its "seals of approval" (NCQA 2009). Continuous standard development includes pay-for-performance and enhanced patient-centered care (NCQA 2009). NCQA evaluates programs applicable to health plans (for example, HMOs, PPOs, and consumer-directed health plans), but it also evaluates providers including medical practices (NCQA 2009). Figure 7.1 illustrates

Figure 7.1.   NCQA evaluation programs

Accreditation Programs:

- Disease Management (DM)
  http://www.ncqa.org/tabid/98/Default.aspx
- Health Plan (HP)
  http://www.ncqa.org/tabid/689/Default.aspx
- Managed Behavioral Healthcare Organization (MBHO)
  http://www.ncqa.org/tabid/94/Default.aspx
- New Health Plan (NHP)
  http://www.ncqa.org/tabid/100/Default.aspx
- Wellness & Health Promotion (WHP)
  http://www.ncqa.org/tabid/834/Default.aspx

Certification Programs:

- Credentials Verification Organization (CVO)
  http://www.ncqa.org/tabid/110/Default.aspx
- Disease Management (DM)
  http://www.ncqa.org/tabid/98/Default.aspx
- Health Information Products (HIP)
  http://www.ncqa.org/tabid/572/Default.aspx

- Physician Organization (PO)
  http://www.ncqa.org/tabid/128/Default.aspx
- Utilization Management (UM) and Credentialing (CR)
  http://www.ncqa.org/tabid/130/Default.aspx

Physician Recognition Programs:

- Back Pain Recognition Program (BPRP)
  http://www.ncqa.org/tabid/137/Default.aspx
- Diabetes Physician Recognition Program (DPRP)
  http://www.ncqa.org/tabid/139/Default.aspx
- Heart/Stroke Recognition Program (HSRP)
  http://www.ncqa.org/tabid/140/Default.aspx
- Physician Practice Connections® (PPC®)
  http://www.ncqa.org/tabid/141/Default.aspx
- Physician Practice Connection®—Patient-Centered Medical Home™ (PPC®-PCMH™)
  http://www.ncqa.org/tabid/631/Default.aspx

Source: NCQA 2009.

the types of evaluation programs offered by NCQA and their designation as accreditation, certification, or physician recognition programs.

An important quality measurement tool for health plans is the Healthcare Effectiveness and Data Information Set (HEDIS), which was created to allow purchasers (primarily employers) and consumers to compare health plan performances. Used by 90% of the health plans in the United States to collect data related to the quality of care, the performance of health plans can be compared consistently with one another through HEDIS. As a result of these comparisons, quality improvement initiatives can be instituted. It is not unusual for health plans to share their HEDIS data with employers and consumers who purchase services from a health plan. Data from HEDIS is also available to the media, which publish "report cards" that are indicators of health plan quality (NCQA 2009).

Additional information regarding details from NCQA may be found at http://www.ncqa.org.

The Joint Commission Accreditation Standards

The oldest and likely the most recognized and expansive accrediting body for healthcare providers is the Joint Commission. Preceded by a hospital inspection program created by the American College of Surgeons (ACS) in 1917, it was established as the Joint Commission on the Accreditation of Hospitals (JCAH) through a collaborative effort by the American College of Surgeons, American College of Physicians, American Hospital Association, American Medical Association, and Canadian Medical Association in 1951. Over time it has changed to meet the needs of the healthcare industry. As its original name indicates, it was initially created to set standards for the inpatient setting. As healthcare changed, however, and numerous other venues were created, it changed in both name and scope. Renamed the Joint Commission on the Accreditation of Healthcare Organizations (JCAHO) in 1987, it most recently updated its name to the Joint Commission. The service areas that the Joint Commission accredits are expansive. They are outlined in figure 7.2.

Not unlike other provider settings, the competitive and dynamic nature of ambulatory care places pressure on providers to demonstrate to payers, regulatory bodies, and managed care organizations that they provide high-quality patient care. As a result, an increasing number of ambulatory care providers, including medical practices, seek Joint Commission accreditation because its standards represent accepted practice related to quality patient care (Joint Commission 2009a). Established in 1975, the purpose of the Joint Commission Ambulatory Care Accreditation Program is "to encourage quality patient care in all types of freestanding ambulatory care facilities" (Joint Commission 2009a). Figure 7.3 lists all service types that are covered by the Ambulatory Care Accreditation Program. Evaluations of ambulatory programs seeking Joint Commission accreditation or reaccreditation are conducted by surveyors who have a minimum of five years of ambulatory leadership experience, and a minimum of a master's degree, and have completed specified educational requirements.

Figure 7.2.   Joint Commission accreditation programs

Ambulatory Care	Home Care	Long-Term Care
Behavioral Health Care	Hospitals	Office-Based Surgery
Critical Access Hospitals	Laboratory Services	

Source: Joint Commission 2009a.

Figure 7.3. Service types in the Joint Commission Ambulatory Care Accreditation Program

• Ambulatory surgery centers	• Group medical practices	• Pain management centers
• Audiology	• Imaging centers	• Plastic/cosmetic surgery
• Cancer therapy	• In vitro fertilization clinics	• Podiatric services
• Catheterization labs	• Indian Health Services	• Radiation oncology
• Chiropractic practices	• Infusion therapy services	• Recovery care/short stay
• College/university health	• Laser surgery centers	• Rehabilitative and physical therapy
• Community health centers	• Lithotripsy services	• Sleep centers
• Correctional health facilities	• Military clinics	• Telemedicine diagnostics
• Dental practices	• Mobile imaging	• Teleradiology
• Dermatology practices	• Occupational health	• Urgent care centers
• Dialysis centers	• Ophthalmology practices	• Urology services
• Ear, nose, and throat practices	• Optometry	• VA clinics
• Endoscopy centers	• Oral and maxillofacial surgery	• Women's health centers
• Family practices	• Orthopedic services	
• Gastroenterology services	• Orthotics/prosthetics	

Source: Joint Commission 2009a.

In 2001, the Joint Commission established standards and made surveys available to smaller office-based surgery practices. Referred to as the Office-Based Surgery Accreditation Program (OBS), it is aimed at surgical practices with no more than four practitioners.

Elements of Performance

The manner in which the Joint Commission's expectations have been displayed and formatted has evolved over time; however, a commitment to high-quality patient care remains. All expectations are articulated through standards, which are "statements that define the performance expectations that must be in place for an organization to provide safe and high-quality care, treatment, and service" (Joint Commission 2009a).

The Joint Commission's standards for the management of health information have historically resided in the chapter on information management. Recent changes to the structure of the Joint Commission's requirements, however, have resulted in the creation of two chapters that are relevant to those responsible for managing health information: Information Management and Record of Care, Treatment, and Services.

Each chapter contains a series of standards, which are further delineated and detailed by elements of performance, which are "specific performance expectations associated with each standard" (Joint Commission 2009a). Surveyors evaluate an organization against elements of performance to determine whether, overall, that organization is in compliance with the standard. For example, the first standard in the "Record of Care, Treatment, and Services" chapter is RC 01.01.01. It states that "The [organization] maintains complete and accurate clinical records." This standard is detailed by a series of elements of performance.

The standards and accompanying elements of performance for the Information Management chapter and the Record of Care, Treatment, and Services chapter are detailed in figures 7.4 and 7.5, respectively.

Figure 7.4. Standards and elements of performance for the Joint Commission Information Management chapter

---

Standard IM.01.01.01: The [organization] plans for managing information.

Elements of Performance

1. The organization identifies the internal and external information needed to provide safe, quality care.

2. The organization identifies how data and information enter, flow within, and leave the organization.

3. The organization uses the identified information to guide development of processes to manage information.

4. Staff and licensed independent practitioners, selected by the organization, participate in the assessment, selection, integration, and use of information management systems for the delivery of care, treatment, or services.

Standard IM.01.01.03: The [organization] plans for continuity of its information management processes.

1. The organization has a written plan for managing interruptions to its information processes (paper-based, electronic, or a mix of paper-based and electronic). (See also EM 01.01.01, EP 6)

2. The organization's plan for managing interruptions to information processes addresses the following: Scheduled and unscheduled interruptions of electronic information systems. (See also EM.01.01.01, EP 6)

3. The organization's plan for managing interruptions to information processes addressing the following: Training for staff and licensed independent practitioners on alternate procedures to follow when electronic information systems are unavailable.

4. The organization's plan for managing interruptions to information processes addresses the following: Backup of electronic information systems. (See also EM.01.01.01, EP 6)

5. The organization's plan for managing interruptions to electronic information processes is tested for effectiveness according to time frames defined by the organization.

6. The organization implements its plan for managing interruptions to information processes to maintain access to information needed for patient care, treatment, or services.

Standard IM.02.01.01: The [organization] protects the privacy of health information.

1. The organization has a written policy addressing the privacy of health information. (See also Rl.01.01.01, EP 7)

2. The organization implements its policy on the privacy of health information. (See also Rl.01.01.01, EP 7)

3. The organization uses health information only for purposes as required by law and regulation or as further limited by its policy on privacy. (See also MM.01.01.01, EP 1; Rl.01.01.01, EP 7)

4. The organization discloses health information only as authorized by the patient or as otherwise consistent with law and regulation. (See also Rl.01.01.01, EP 7)

5. The organization monitors compliance with its policy on the privacy of health information. (See also Rl.01.01.01, EP 7)

Standard IM.02.01.03: The [organization] maintains the security and integrity of health information.

1. The organization has a written policy addressing the security of health information, including access, use, and disclosure.

2. The organization has a written policy addressing the integrity of health information against loss, damage, unauthorized alteration, unintentional change, and accidental destruction.

3. The organization has a written policy addressing the intentional destruction of health information.

4. The organization defines when and by whom the removal of health information is permitted. Note: Removal refers to those actions that place health information outside the organization's control.

5. The organization protects against unauthorized access, use, and disclosure of health information.

6. The organization protects health information against loss, damage, unauthorized alteration, unintentional change, and accidental destruction.

7. The organization controls the intentional destruction of health information.

8. The organization monitors compliance with its policies on the security and integrity of health information.

Figure 7.4. Standards and elements of performance for the Joint Commission Information Management chapter *(continued)*

Standard IM.02.02.01: The [organization] effectively manages the collection of health information.

1. The organization uses uniform data sets to standardize data collection throughout the organization.

2. The organization uses standardized terminology, definitions, abbreviations, acronyms, symbols, and dose designations.

Standard IM.02.02.03: The [organization] retrieves, disseminates, and transmits health information in usable formats.

2. The organization's storage and retrieval systems make health information accessible when needed for patient care, treatment, or services. (See also IC.01.02.01, EP 1)

3. The organization disseminates data and information in useful formats within time frames that are defined by the organization and consistent with law and regulation.

Standard IM.03.01.01: Knowledge-based information resources are available, current, and authoritative.

1. The organization provides access to knowledge-based information resources during hours of operation.

Standard IM.04.01.01: The [organization] maintains accurate health information.

1. The organization has processes to check the accuracy of health information.

Source: Joint Commission 2009b.

Figure 7.5. Standards and elements of performance for the Joint Commission Record of Care, Treatment, and Services chapter

---

Standard RC.01.01.01: The [organization] maintains complete and accurate clinical records.

1. The organization defines the components of a complete clinical record.

5. The clinical record contains the information needed to support the patient's diagnosis and condition.

6. The clinical record contains the information needed to justify the patient's care, treatment, or services.

7. The clinical record contains information that documents the course and result of the patient's care, treatment, or services.

8. The clinical record contains information about the patient's care, treatment, or services that promotes continuity of care among providers.

9. The organization uses standardized formats to document the care, treatment, or services it provides to patients.

11. All entries in the clinical record are dated.

12. The organization tracks the location of all components of the clinical record.

13. The organization assembles or makes available in a summary in the clinical record all information required to provide patient care, treatment, or services. (See also MM.01.01.01, EP 1)

14. When needed to provide care, summaries of treatment and other documents provided by the organization are forwarded to other care providers.

Standard RC.01.02.01: Entries in the clinical record are authenticated.

1. Only authorized individuals make entries in the clinical record.

2. The organization defines the types of entries in the clinical record made by nonindependent practitioners that require countersigning, in accordance with law and regulation.

3. The author of each clinical record entry is identified in the clinical record.

(continued on next page)

Figure 7.5. Standards and elements of performance for the Joint Commission Record of Care, Treatment, and Services chapter *(continued)*

4. Entries in the clinical record are authenticated by the author. Information introduced into the clinical record through transcription or dictation is authenticated by the author.

   Note 1: Authentication can be verified through electronic signatures, written signatures or initials, rubber-stamp signatures, or computer key.

   Note 2: For paper-based records, signatures entered for purposes of authentication after transcription or for verbal orders are dated when required by law or regulation or organization policy. For electronic records, electronic signatures will be date-stamped.

5. The individual identified by the signature stamp or method of electronic authentication is the only individual who uses it.

Standard RC.01.03.01: Documentation in the clinical record is entered in a timely manner.

1. The organization has a written policy that requires timely entry of information into the clinical record. (See also PC.01.02.03, EP 1)

2. The organization defines the time frame for completion of the clinical record.

3. The organization implements its policy requiring timely entry of information into the patient's clinical record. (See also PC.01.02.03, EP 2)

Standard RC.01.04.01: The [organization] audits its clinical records.

1. According to a time frame it defines, the organization reviews its clinical records to confirm that the required information is present, accurate, legible, authenticated, and completed on time.

Standard RC.01.05.01: The [organization] retains its clinical records.

1. The retention times of the clinical record is determined by its use and organization policy, in accordance with law and regulation.

8. Original clinical records are not released unless the organization is responding to law and regulation.

Standard RC.02.01.01: The clinical record contains information that reflects the [patient]'s care, treatment, or services.

1. The clinical record contains the following demographic information:

   – The patient's name, address, phone number, date of birth, and the name of any legally authorized representative

   – The patient's sex, height, and weight (See also MM.01.01.01, EP 3)

   – The legal status of any patient receiving behavioral health care services

   – The patient's language and communication needs

2. The clinical record contains the following clinical information:

   – The patient's initial diagnosis, diagnostic impression(s), or condition(s)

   – Any findings of assessments and reassessments (See also PC.01.02.01, EP 1;PC.03.01.03, EPs 1 and 8)

   – Any allergies to food

   – Any allergies to medications

   – Any conclusions or impressions drawn from the patient's medical history and physical examination

   – Any diagnoses or conditions established during the patient's course of care, treatment, or services

   – Any consultation reports

   – Any progress notes

   – Any medications ordered or prescribed

   – Any medications administered, including the strength, dose, and route

   – Any access site for medication, administration devices used, and rate of administration

   – The patient's response to any medication administered

   – Any adverse drug reactions

Figure 7.5.   Standards and elements of performance for the Joint Commission Record of Care, Treatment, and Services chapter *(continued)*

  – Plans for care and any revisions to the plan for care (See also PC.01.03.01, EP 1)

  – Orders for diagnostic and therapeutic tests and procedures and their results

 4. As needed to provide care, treatment, or services, the clinical record contains the following additional information:

  – Any advance directives

  – Any informed consent, when required by organization policy (See also RI.01.03.01, EP 13)

  – Any documentation of clinical research interventions distinct from entries related to regular patient care, treatment, or services (See also RI.01.03.05, EPs 4-6)

  – Any records of communication with the patient, such as telephone calls or e-mail

  – Any referrals or communications made to internal or external care providers and community agencies

  – Any patient-generated information

 21. The clinical record of a patient who receives urgent or immediate care, treatment, or services contains the following:

  – The times and means of arrival

  – Indication that the patient left against medical advice, when applicable

  – Conclusions reached at the termination of care, treatment, or services, including the patient's final disposition, condition, and instructions given for follow-up care, treatment, or services

  – A copy of any information made available to the practitioner or medical organization providing follow-up care, treatment, or services

Standard RC.02.01.03: The [patient]'s clinical record documents operative or other high-risk procedures and the use of moderate or deep sedation or anesthesia.

 1. The organization documents in the patient's clinical record any operative or other high-risk procedure and/or the administration of moderate or deep sedation or anesthesia.

 2. A licensed independent practitioner involved in the patient's care documents the provisional diagnosis in the clinical record before an operative or other high-risk procedure is performed.

 4. For ambulatory surgical centers that elect to use the Joint Commission deemed status option: The patient's clinical record contains the results of preoperative diagnostic studies.

 5. An operative or other high-risk procedure report is written or dictated upon completion of the operative or other high-risk procedure and before the patient is transferred to the next level of care.

   Note 1: The exception to this requirement occurs when an operative or other high-risk procedure progress note is written immediately after the procedure, in which case the full report can be written or dictated within a time frame defined by the organization.

   Note 2: If the practitioner performing the operation or high-risk procedure accompanies the patient from the operating room to the next unit or area of care, the report can be written or dictated in the new unit or area of care.

 6. The operative or other high-risk procedure report includes the following information:

  – The name(s) of the licensed independent practitioner(s) who performed the procedure and his or her assistant(s)

  – The name of the procedure performed

  – A description of the procedure

  – Findings of the procedure

  – Any estimated blood loss

  – Any specimen(s) removed

  – The postoperative diagnosis

 7. When a full operative or other high-risk procedure report cannot be entered immediately into the patient's clinical record, a note is entered immediately. This note includes the name(s) of the primary surgeon(s) and his or her assistant(s), procedure performed and a description of each procedure finding, estimated blood loss, specimens removed, and postoperative diagnosis.

(continued on next page)

Figure 7.5. Standards and elements of performance for the Joint Commission Record of Care, Treatment, and Services chapter *(continued)*

8. The clinical record contains the following postoperative information:

   – The patient's vital signs and level of consciousness (See also PC.03.01.05, EP 1; PC.03.01.07, EP 1)

   – Any medications, including intravenous fluids and any administered blood, blood products, and blood components

   – Any unanticipated events or complications (including blood transfusion reactions) and the management of those events

9. The clinical record contains documentation that the patient was discharged from the recovery phase of the operation or procedure either by the licensed independent practitioner responsible for his or her care or according to discharge criteria. (See also PC.03.01.07, EP 4)

10. The clinical record contains documentation of the use of approved discharge criteria that determine the patient's readiness for discharge. (See also PC.03.01.07. EP 4)

11. The operative documentation contains the name of the licensed independent practitioner responsible for discharge.

12. For ambulatory surgical centers that elect to use the Joint Commission deemed status option: The clinical record contains the discharge diagnosis.

Standard RC.02.01.05: The clinical record contains documentation of the use of restraint.

1. The organization documents the use of restraint in the clinical record, including the following:

   – Orders for use

   – Results of patient monitoring

   – Reassessment

   – Unanticipated changes in the patient's position

   (See also PC.03.02.03, EP 1; PC.03.02.07, EPs 1 and 2)

Standard RC.02.01.07: The clinical record contains a summary list for each [patient] who receives continuing ambulatory care services.

1. A summary list is initiated for the patient by his or her third visit.

2. The patient's summary list contains the following information:

   – Any significant medical diagnoses and conditions

   – Any significant operative and invasive procedures

   – Any adverse or allergic drug reactions

   – Any current medications, over-the-counter medications, and herbal preparations

3. The patient's summary list is updated whenever there is a change in diagnoses, medications, or allergies to medications, and whenever a procedure is performed.

4. The summary list is readily available to practitioners who need access to the information of patients who receive continuing ambulatory care services in order to provide care, treatment, or services.

Standard RC.02.03.07: Qualified staff receive and record verbal orders.

1. The organization identifies, in writing, the staff who are authorized to receive and record verbal orders, in accordance with law and regulation.

2. Only authorized staff receive and record verbal orders.

3. Documentation of verbal orders includes the date and the names of individuals who gave, received, recorded, and implemented the orders.

4. Verbal orders are authenticated within the time frame specified by law and regulation.

Source: Joint Commission 2009b.

Of significance as well to the medical practice setting is the Joint Commission chapter on Waived Testing. Laboratory tests evaluate the content of substances that are removed from the human body and, subsequently, assess either a patient's condition or make a clinical decision. These tests are subject to the federal Clinical Laboratory Improvement Amendments of 1988 (CLIA). CLIA regulations categorize laboratory tests based on complexity. Waived tests are those laboratory tests determined by the FDA to be so simple that there is little risk of error or little risk of harm to a patient if the test is performed incorrectly. As a result, they are exempt from regulatory oversight or subject to less stringent requirements. Waivers may be granted to any test listed in the CLIA regulation, tests that the FDA has cleared for home use, and test systems that meet the CLIA criteria and for which the manufacturer or producer applies for a waiver and scientifically validates as having met the waiver criteria. The Centers for Medicare and Medicaid Services (CMS) does perform random on-site visits of laboratories that have received certificates of waiver (CMS 2009).

Tests specified in the CLIA regulation are:

1. Dipstick or tablet reagent urinalysis (nonautomated) for the following:

    - Bilirubin
    - Glucose
    - Hemoglobin
    - Ketone
    - Leukocytes
    - Nitrite
    - pH
    - Protein
    - Specific gravity
    - Urobilinogen

2. Fecal occult blood

3. Ovulation tests—visual color comparison tests for luteinizing hormone

4. Urine pregnancy tests—visual color comparison tests

5. Erythrocyte sedimentation rate—nonautomated

6. Hemoglobin-copper sulfate—nonautomated

7. Blood glucose by glucose monitoring devices cleared by the FDA specifically for home use

8. Spun microhematocrit

9. Hemoglobin by single analyte instruments with self-contained or component features to perform specimen/reagent interaction, providing direct measurement and readout (CMS 2009)

Nonwaived tests are those that involve moderate to high complexity and do not meet the definition of waived tests. They are subject to detailed performance requirements (FDA 2009;

Figure 7.6.   Waived Testing WT.05.01.01: The organization maintains records for waived testing

1	Quality control results, including internal and external controls for waived testing, are documented.
	Note 1: Internal quality controls may include electronic, liquid, or control zone. External quality controls may include electronic or liquid.
	Note 2: Quality control results may be located in the clinical record.
2	Test results for waived testing are documented in the patient's clinical record.
3	Quantitative test result reports in the clinical record for waived testing are accompanied by reference intervals (normal values) specific to the test method used and the population served.
	Note 1: Semiquantitative results, such as urine macroscopic and urine dipsticks, are not required to comply with this element of performance.
	Note 2: If the reference intervals (normal values) are not documented on the same page as and adjacent to the waived test result, they must be located elsewhere within the permanent clinical record. The result must have a notation directing the reader to the location of the reference intervals (normal values) in the clinical record.
4	Individual test results for waived testing are associated with quality control results and instrument records.
	Note: A formal log is not required, but a functional audit trail is maintained that allows retrieval of individual test results and their association with quality control and instrument records.
5	Quality control result records, test result records, and instrument records for waived testing are retained for at least two years.

Source: Joint Commission 2009a.

CMS 2009). Each state has a separate agency that monitors CLIA activities. A listing of state agencies may be found in appendix B.

The Joint Commission first addressed waived testing in its standards in 1992, revising the standards in 2005 due to the increasing number of waived tests and associated patient safety and quality concerns because waived tests are not, in fact, error-proof and can present serious consequences when performed improperly. The five standards in the Waived Testing (WT) chapter address topics such as the establishment of policies and procedures pertaining to waived testing; the identification and competence of staff responsible for performing and supervising waived testing; and the performance of quality checks and maintenance of records for waived testing (Joint Commission 2009a). Figure 7.6 displays the ambulatory healthcare standards for documentation of waived testing.

Check Your Understanding 7.1

Instructions: Select the phrase that best completes the following statements.

1. Accreditation is:
    a. mandatory
    b. voluntary
    c. necessary to receive payer reimbursement
    d. obtained through one national accrediting body

2. The National Committee on Quality Assurance (NCQA) is the primary accrediting body for:
    a. hospitals
    b. medical practices
    c. health plans
    d. all of the above

---

3. The Joint Commission:

    a. accredits a variety of healthcare service providers

    b. accredits only hospitals

    c. is mandatory for a medical practice to operate

    d. licenses healthcare providers

4. A Joint Commission element of performance is:

    a. broader in scope than a standard

    b. not associated with a standard

    c. a specific performance expectation

    d. all of the above

5. The Ambulatory Health Care Accreditation Program:

    a. was the first accreditation program offered by the Joint Commission

    b. applies to medical practices only

    c. will be implemented by the Joint Commission in the near future

    d. applies to all types of freestanding ambulatory care facilities

Ambulatory Care and Office-based Surgery National Patient Safety Goals

Effective in 2003, and in response to the need to address the safety of patients during treatment encounters, the Joint Commission implemented National Patient Safety Goals (NPSGs). As explained by the Joint Commission, the purpose of the NPSGs is "to promote specific improvements in patient safety . . . highlight problematic areas in healthcare and describe evidence-based and expert-based consensus to solutions to these problems" (Joint Commission 2009a). It is the responsibility of organizations that provide care, treatment, and services related to the NPSGs to implement their requirements as applicable (Joint Commission 2009a).

Certain problems resulting in compromised patient safety are common to numerous provider settings. Therefore, many of the NPSGs are uniform across care settings. Figure 7.7 outlines the ambulatory healthcare NPSGs and figure 7.8 outlines the office-based surgery NPSGs; both are accompanied by specific mechanisms required to meet those goals. As NPSGs are reviewed and updated annually, certain ones are added and others removed. However, the placeholder numbers for the deleted NPSGs remain, are identified by number, and are labeled "not applicable."

Particularly relevant to documentation in the health record are Goal 1A, the use of two patient identifiers, and Goals 2A and 2B, reading back verbal orders (2A) and creating a list of abbreviations not to use (2B). To ensure that documentation in the health record belongs to the appropriate patient, each document should be indicated by two pieces of identification, generally the patient's name and some other type of unique information (such as date of birth) that would serve as verification. The read-back of verbal orders may become less critical as practitioners move toward computerized provider order entry (CPOE) systems. Nonetheless, as many medical practices still function in paper environments, the importance of verbal orders being read back to and verified by the providers who gave them cannot be underestimated from a patient safety perspective. Just as electronic systems will reduce the need for read-backs, so too may electronic health records minimize the need to monitor unapproved (that is, unsafe) abbreviations, provided that systems are able to translate and convert unapproved abbreviations to full text. If these capabilities are not implemented, however, and to the extent that paper records continue to dominate medical practices, compliance with this NPSG will continue to be essential to patient safety.

Figure 7.7. Ambulatory healthcare National Patient Safety Goals

Goal 1—Improve the accuracy of patient identification.

A. Use of Two Patient Identifiers (revised NPSG.01.01.01)

B. Not Applicable to Ambulatory Health Care (revised NPSG.01.02.01)

C. Eliminating Transfusion Errors (revised NPSG.01.03.01)

Goal 2—Improve the effectiveness of communication among caregivers.

A. Reading Back Verbal Orders (revised NPSG.02.01.01)

B. Creating a List of Abbreviations Not to Use (revised NPSG.02.02.01)

C. Timely Reporting of Critical Tests and Critical Results (revised NPSG.02.03.01)

D. Not Applicable

E. Managing Hand–Off Communications (revised NPSG.02.05.01)

Goal 3—Improve the safety of using medications.

A. Not Applicable

B. Not Applicable

C. Managing Look Alike, Sound Alike Medications (revised NPSG.03.03.01)

D. Labeling Medications (revised NPSG.03.04.01)

E. Reducing Harm from Anticoagulation Therapy (revised NPSG.03.05.01)

Goal 4—Not Applicable

Goal 5—Not Applicable

Goal 6—Not Applicable

Goal 7—Reduce the risk of health care-associated infections.

A. Meeting Hand Hygiene Guidelines (revised NPSG.07.01.01)

B. Sentinel Events Resulting from Infection (revised NPSG.07.02.01)

C. Not Applicable to Ambulatory Health Care (revised NPSG.07.03.01)

D. Preventing Central-Line Associated Blood Stream Infections (revised NPSG.07.04.01)

E. Preventing Surgical Site Infections (revised NPSG.07.05.01)

Goal 8—Accurately and completely reconcile medications across the continuum of care.

A. Comparing Current and Newly Ordered Medications (revised NPSG.08.01.01)

B. Communicating Medications to the Next Provider (revised NPSG.08.02.01)

C. Providing a Reconciled Medication List to the Patient (revised NPSG.08.03.01)

D. Settings in Which Medications are Minimally Used (revised NPSG.08.04.01)

Goal 9—Reduce the risk of patient harm resulting from falls.

A. Not Applicable to Ambulatory Health Care (revised NPSG.09.02.01)

Goal 10—Reduce the risk of influenza and pneumococcal disease in institutionalized older adults.

A. Not Applicable to Ambulatory Health Care (revised NPSG.10.01.01)

B. Not Applicable to Ambulatory Health Care (revised NPSG.10.02.01)

C. Not Applicable to Ambulatory Health Care (revised NPSG.10.03.01)

Figure 7.7.   Ambulatory healthcare National Patient Safety Goals *(continued)*

Goal 11—Reduce the risk of surgical fires.

A. Preventing Surgical Fires (revised NPSG.11.01.01)

Goal 12—Not Applicable

Goal 13—Encourage patients' active involvement in their own care as a patient safety strategy.

A. Patient and Family Reporting of Safety Concerns (revised NPSG.13.01.01)

Goal 14—Prevent health care associated pressure ulcers (decubitus ulcers).

A. Not Applicable to Ambulatory Health Care (revised NPSG.14.01.01)

Goal 15—The organization identifies safety risks inherent in its patient population.

A. Not Applicable to Ambulatory Health Care (revised NPSG.15.01.01)

B. Not Applicable to Ambulatory Health Care (revised NPSG.15.02.01)

Goal 16—Improve recognition and response to changes in a patient's condition.

A. Not Applicable to Ambulatory Health Care (revised NPSG.16.01.01)

Universal Protocol

A. Conducting a Pre-Procedure Verification Process (revised UP.01.01.01)

B. Marking the Procedure Site (revised UP.01.02.01)

C. Performing a Time-Out (revised UP.01.03.01)

Source: Joint Commission 2009b.

Figure 7.8.   Office-based surgery National Patient Safety Goals

---

Goal 1—Improve the accuracy of patient identification.

A. Use of Two Patient Identifiers (revised NPSG.01.01.01)

B. Not Applicable to Office-Based Surgery (revised NPSG.01.02.01)

C. Eliminating Transfusion Errors (revised NPSG.01.03.01)

Goal 2—Improve the effectiveness of communication among caregivers.

A. Reading Back Verbal Orders (revised NPSG.02.01.01)

B. Creating a List of Abbreviations Not to Use (revised NPSG.02.02.01)

C. Timely Reporting of Critical Tests and Critical Results (revised NPSG.02.03.01)

D. Not Applicable

E. Managing Hand–Off Communications (revised NPSG.02.05.01)

Goal 3—Improve the safety of using medications.

A. Not Applicable

B. Not Applicable

C. Managing Look Alike, Sound Alike Medications (revised NPSG.03.03.01)

D. Labeling Medications (revised NPSG.03.04.01)

E. Not Applicable to Office-Based Surgery (revised NPSG.03.05.01)

Goal 4—Not Applicable

Goal 5—Not Applicable

(continued on next page)

Figure 7.8. Office-based surgery National Patient Safety Goals *(continued)*

Goal 6—Not Applicable

Goal 7—Reduce the risk of health care-associated infections.

A. Meeting Hand Hygiene Guidelines (revised NPSG.07.01.01)

B. Sentinel Events Resulting from Infection (revised NPSG.07.02.01)

C. Not Applicable to Office-Based Surgery (revised NPSG.07.03.01)

D. Not Applicable to Office-Based Surgery (revised NPSG.07.04.01)

E. Preventing Surgical Site Infections (revised NPSG.07.05.01)

Goal 8—Accurately and completely reconcile medications across the continuum of care.

A. Comparing Current and Newly Ordered Medications (revised NPSG.08.01.01)

B. Communicating Medications to the Next Provider (revised NPSG.08.02.01)

C. Providing a Reconciled Medication List to the Patient (revised NPSG.08.03.01)

D. Settings in Which Medications are Minimally Used (revised NPSG.08.04.01)

Goal 9—Reduce the risk of patient harm resulting from falls.

A. Not Applicable to Office-Based Surgery (revised NPSG.09.02.01)

Goal 10—Reduce the risk of influenza and pneumococcal disease in institutionalized older adults.

A. Not Applicable to Office-Based Surgery (revised NPSG.10.01.01)

B. Not Applicable to Office-Based Surgery (revised NPSG.10.02.01)

C. Not Applicable to Office-Based Surgery (revised NPSG.10.03.01)

Goal 11—Reduce the risk of surgical fires.

A. Preventing Surgical Fires (revised NPSG.11.01.01)

Goal 12—Not Applicable

Goal 13—Encourage patients' active involvement in their own care as a patient safety strategy.

A. Patient and Family Reporting of Safety Concerns (revised NPSG.13.01.01)

Goal 14—Prevent health care associated pressure ulcers (decubitus ulcers).

A. Not Applicable to Office-Based Surgery (revised NPSG.14.01.01)

Goal 15—The organization identifies safety risks inherent in its patient population.

A. Not Applicable to Office-Based Surgery (revised NPSG.15.01.01)

B. Not Applicable to Office-Based Surgery (revised NPSG.15.02.01)

Goal 16—Improve recognition and response to changes in a patient's condition.

A. Not Applicable to Office-Based Surgery (revised NPSG.16.01.01)

Universal Protocol

A. Conducting a Pre-Procedure Verification Process (revised UP.01.01.01)

B. Marking the Procedure Site (revised UP.01.02.01)

C. Performing a Time-Out (revised UP.01.03.01)

Source: Joint Commission 2009b.

Sentinel Event Policy

Prior to the implementation of NPSGs to support patient safety and high-quality healthcare, the Joint Commission developed its sentinel event policy in 1996. Through this policy, adverse occurrences that require immediate action are identified.

A sentinel event is "an unexpected occurrence involving death or serious physical or psychological injury, or the risk thereof" (Joint Commission 2009a). The Joint Commission has defined a serious injury to include the loss of limb or function. The "or the risk thereof" portion identifies process deviations that carry a significant risk of a serious adverse outcome should this type of event occur again (Joint Commission 2009a). The term "sentinel" is significant because these types of events signal the need for a healthcare provider to take immediate action through an investigation and response plan. The Joint Commission notes that sentinel events and medical errors are not synonymous because sentinel events encompass many more types of events that just medical errors. Conversely, not all medical errors meet the sentinel event definition, which specifies death or serious injury, or the risk thereof, as a consequence (Joint Commission 2009a).

The Joint Commission's sentinel event policy has four goals, which are outlined in figure 7.9. Each Joint Commission accreditation manual, including ambulatory care, contains standards in the "Improving Organization Performance" (PI) chapter that directly address the appropriate management of sentinel events (Joint Commission 2009a). Specifically, these standards are PI.1.10, PI.2.20, PI.2.30, and PI.3.10. Although the Joint Commission has provided a definition of a sentinel event, organizations that are accredited or seeking accreditation must create their own definition in an effort to establish mechanisms for identifying, reporting, and managing sentinel events. It is expected that an organization's definition will be consistent with that of the Joint Commission; however, some discretion may be exercised in determining what comprises "unexpected," "serious," and "the risk thereof" (Joint Commission 2009a).

An organization must respond to a sentinel event in a number of ways. They include a root cause analysis (described below) that is timely, thorough, and credible; an action plan that should include improvements to diminish future risks; implementation of the improvements; and monitoring of the effectiveness of the improvements (Joint Commission 2009a).

Central to an organization's sentinel event response plan is the completion of a root cause analysis. A root cause analysis is defined as "a process for identifying the basic or causal factors that underlie variation in performance, including the occurrence or possible occurrence of a sentinel event" (Joint Commission 2009a). The Joint Commission emphasizes that root cause analyses be used to identify systemic flaws or deficiencies rather than critiquing individual behaviors or performance. An important part of the root cause analysis is the identification

Figure 7.9.   Goals of the Joint Commission sentinel event policy

1. To have a positive impact in improving patient care, treatment, and services and preventing sentinel events.

2. To focus the attention of an organization that has experienced a sentinel event on understanding the causes that underlie the event, and on changing the organization's systems and processes to reduce the probability of such an event in the future.

3. To increase the general knowledge about sentinel events, their causes, and strategies for prevention.

4. To maintain the confidence of the public and accredited organizations in the accreditation process.

Source: Joint Commission 2009a.

of changes that could potentially improve or decrease the likelihood of similar types of events occurring in the future. It is possible that a root cause analysis may reveal that no opportunities for improvement exist. However, the root cause analysis must be thorough and credible in reaching such a conclusion, or any conclusion, and the final product must be a strategic action plan that organizations can use in the future to reduce future similar incidents. The plan should include responsible parties, potential pilot testing, timelines, and means for measuring its effectiveness (Joint Commission 2009a).

A sentinel event will be either reviewable or nonreviewable by the Joint Commission. Sentinel events that are subject to Joint Commission review are occurrences that meet any of the criteria listed in figure 7.10. Although not all items on the list are relevant to the medical office setting, the Joint Commission does not differentiate care settings when creating this list.

Accredited organizations are not required to report a reviewable sentinel event to the Joint Commission; however, they are advised that there are many alternative ways that the Joint Commission may learn of a sentinel event including from patients, family member, employees, the media, or a Joint Commission surveyor. The Joint Commission encourages organizational self-reporting for a number of reasons. First, it enables collaboration with and consultation by the Joint Commission. Second, it demonstrates to the public a motivation by the organization to prevent and/or minimize the likelihood of such future occurrences. Third, the event can be added to the "lessons learned" in the Joint Commission sentinel event database (described below) and diminish the likelihood of any similar future occurrences at any location (Joint Commission 2009a).

Figure 7.11 contains examples of sentinel events that are reviewable under the Joint Commission sentinel event policy. Figure 7.12 contains examples of nonreviewable sentinel events.

Once the Joint Commission becomes aware of a reviewable sentinel event that was not reported, the organization is notified that a preliminary assessment will be completed. Sentinel events occurring greater than one year before the Joint Commission learned of them will likely require a written response that is separate from a review under the sentinel event policy (Joint Commission 2009a). For a reviewable sentinel event, an organization must prepare a root cause analysis and action plan (if it has not already done so) and submit it to the Joint

Figure 7.10.   Criteria for reviewable sentinel events

An incident that resulted in an unanticipated death or major permanent loss of function, not related to the natural course of the patient's illness or underlying condition OR

The event was one of the following (even if the above definition is not met):

- Suicide of any patient receiving care, treatment, and services in a staffed around-the-clock care setting or within 72 hours of discharge

- Unanticipated death of a full-term infant

- Abduction of a patient receiving care, treatment, and services

- Discharge of an infant to the wrong family

- Rape

- Hemolytic transfusion reaction involving administration of blood or blood products having blood group incompatabilities

- Surgery on the wrong patient or wrong body parts

- Unintended retention of a foreign object in a patient after surgery or other procedure

Severe neonatal hyperbilirubinemia (bilirubin >30 milligrams/deciliter)

Prolonged fluoroscopy with cumulative dose >1500 rads to a single field or any delivery of radiotherapy to the wrong body region or >25% above the planned radiotherapy dose

Source: Joint Commission 2009a.

Figure 7.11.   Examples of reviewable sentinel events

Any patient death, paralysis, coma, or other major permanent loss of function associated with a medication error.
A patient commits suicide within 72 hours of being discharged from a hospital setting that provides staffed around-the-clock care.
Any elopement, that is unauthorized departure, of a patient from an around-the-clock care setting resulting in a temporally related death (suicide, accidental death, or homicide) or major permanent loss of function.
A hospital operates on the wrong side of the patient's body.
Any intrapartum (related to the birth process) maternal death.
Any perinatal death unrelated to a congenital condition in an infant having a birth weight greater than 2,500 grams.
A patient is abducted from the hospital where he or she receives care, treatment, or services.
Assault, homicide, or other crime resulting in patient death or major permanent loss of function.
A patient fall that results in death or major permanent loss of function as a direct result of the injuries sustained in the fall.
Hemolytic transfusion reaction involving major blood group incompatibilities.
A foreign body, such as a sponge or forceps, that was left in a patient after surgery.
Note: An adverse outcome that is directly related to the natural course of the patient's illness or underlying condition, for example, terminal illness present at the time of presentation, is not reportable except for suicide in, or following elopement from, a 24-hour care setting.

Source: Joint Commission 2009a.

Figure 7.12.   Examples of nonreviewable sentinel events

Any "near miss" (that is, a process variation that did not affect an outcome but for which a recurrence carries a significant chance of a serious adverse outcome).
Full or expected return of limb or bodily function to the same level as prior to the adverse event by discharge or within two weeks of the initial loss of said function.
Any sentinel event that has not affected a recipient of care (patient, client, resident).
Medication errors that do not result in death or major permanent loss of function.
Suicide other than in an around-the-clock care setting or following elopement from such a setting.
A death or loss of function following a discharge "against medical advice (AMA)."
Unsuccessful suicide attempts unless resulting in major permanent loss of function.
Minor degrees of hemolysis not caused by a major blood group incompatibility and with no clinical sequelae.

Source: Joint Commission 2009a.

Commission. Failure to comply in a timely manner may result in a change to the organization's accreditation status, potentially resulting ultimately in a denial of accreditation. The Joint Commission has identified characteristics necessary for an acceptable root cause analysis and action plan. These are outlined in figure 7.13. Nonreviewable sentinel events also require the completion of a root cause analysis, but documentation is not required to be submitted to the Joint Commission.

It is reasonable that an organization may be concerned about waiving the confidentiality protections of a root cause analysis and action plan if they are sent to the Joint Commission. Because of these valid concerns, the Joint Commission has provided alternative methods by which an organization can respond to a sentinel event. These methods include hand-delivering and returning the documents to Joint Commission headquarters and returning to the accreditation organization with them; accommodating an on-site visit by a surveyor; or accommodating an on-site visit by a surveyor who does not directly view the root cause analysis documents, but instead conducts interviews and reviews other relevant documents (for example, the patient's

Figure 7.13. Characteristics of an acceptable root cause analysis and action plan

---

A root cause analysis will be considered acceptable if it does the following:

- The analysis focuses primarily on systems and processes, not on individual performance
- The analysis progresses from special causes in clinical processes to common causes in organizational processes
- The analysis repeatedly digs deeper by asking "Why?"; then, when answered, "Why?" again, and so on
- The analysis identifies changes that could be made in systems and processes (either through redesign or development of new systems or processes) which would reduce the risk of such events occurring in the future
- The analysis is **thorough** and **credible**

To be thorough, the root cause analysis must include the following:

- A determination of the human and other factors most directly associated with the sentinel event and the process(es) and systems related to its occurrence
- An analysis of the underlying systems and processes through a series of "Why?" questions to determine where redesign might reduce risk
- An inquiry into all areas appropriate to the specific type of event
- An identification of risk points and their potential contributions to this type of event
- A determination of potential improvement in processes or systems that would tend to decrease the likelihood of such events in the future, or a determination, after analysis, that no such improvement opportunities exist

To be credible, the root cause analysis must do the following:

- Include participation by the leadership of the organization and by individuals most closely involved in the processes and systems under review
- Be internally consistent (that is, not contradict itself or leave obvious questions unanswered)
- Provide an explanation for all findings of "not applicable" or "no problem"
- Include consideration of any relevant literature

An action plan will be considered acceptable if it does the following:

- Identifies changes that can be implemented to reduce risk or formulates a rationale for not undertaking such changes
- Identifies, in situations where improvement actions are planned, who is responsible for implementation, when the action will be implemented (including any pilot testing), and how the effectiveness of the actions will be evaluated

---

Source: Joint Commission 2009a.

health record) that may trace a patient encounter and ascertain the adequacy of the actions taken by the organization following the sentinel event. Inadequate follow-up by the accredited organization may result in a change to the organization's accreditation status, potentially resulting ultimately in a denial of accreditation.

Sentinel Event Database

As described previously, the Joint Commission's sentinel event database was created to increase general knowledge about the occurrence of sentinel events and ways that they may be prevented. This occurs through the collection and analysis of data related to sentinel events in accredited organizations. When information is added to the database, the confidentiality of the organization, the patient, and involved providers is maintained (Joint Commission 2009a). The database includes information related not only to the sentinel event itself, but also data related to root cause analysis and risk reduction. Data extracted from the sentinel event database serves as a basis for the creation of national patient safety goals.

Accreditation Association for Ambulatory Health Care

The AAAHC (or the Accreditation Association) is a private, not-for-profit organization formed in 1979 (http://www.aaahc.org).

AAAHC is the leader in ambulatory healthcare accreditation, with more than 4,300 organizations accredited nationwide and overseas. These include ambulatory and office-based surgery centers, managed care organizations, college health centers, Indian health centers, military healthcare clinics, and large medical and dental group practices. The AAAHC peer-based survey process uses active healthcare professionals as surveyors and is collaborative rather than prescriptive.

AAAHC serves as an advocate for the provision of high-quality healthcare through the development of nationally recognized standards and through its survey and accreditation programs. Accreditation by AAAHC is recognized as a symbol of quality by third-party payers, medical organizations, liability insurance companies, state and federal agencies, and the public. In addition, AAAHC maintains deemed status to certify healthcare organizations for Medicare by the CMS (CMS 2009).

Structured uniquely to address all aspects of ambulatory care, the AAAHC standards are housed in eight chapters in the AAAHC *Accreditation Handbook for Ambulatory Health Care* and cover:

1. Patient Rights

2. Governance

3. Administration

4. Quality of Care Provided

5. Quality Management and Improvement

6. Clinical Records and Health Information

7. Infection Control and Safety

8. Facilities and Environment

These 8 chapters are accompanied by 19 adjunct chapters that are service-specific and may or may not apply to a particular organization.

The Accreditation Association Represents Sixteen Member Organizations

The Accreditation Association has a total of 16 member organizations on its Board of Directors. Member organizations include:

- Ambulatory Surgery Foundation

- American Academy of Cosmetic Surgery

- American Academy of Dental Group Practice

- American Academy of Dermatology

- American Academy of Facial Plastic and Reconstructive Surgery

- American Association of Oral and Maxillofacial Surgeons
- American College of Gastroenterology
- American College Health Association
- American College of Mohs Surgery
- American College of Obstetricians and Gynecologists
- American Gastroenterological Association
- American Society of Anesthesiologists
- American Society for Dermatologic Surgery
- American Society for Gastrointestinal Endoscopy
- Medical Group Management Association
- Society for Ambulatory Anesthesia

Conclusion

Many ambulatory care organizations, including medical practices, choose to be accredited by one of the major accreditation bodies such as the National Committee for Quality Assurance, the Joint Commission, or the Accreditation Association for Ambulatory Health Care. By being accredited, organizations demonstrate their commitment to patient safety and high-quality care. This commitment is important in developing relationships with payers, regulatory agencies, and the public. Although accreditation is a rigorous process, the benefits of being accredited often outweigh the costs and efforts involved. A detailed listing of ambulatory care documentation standards may be found in appendix L.

Check Your Understanding 7.2

Instructions: Select the phrase that best completes the following statements.

1. National patient safety goals:
   a. apply only to the hospital setting
   b. are similar for a variety of care settings
   c. have been created only for ambulatory healthcare settings
   d. were established in 1975

2. A sentinel event:
   a. involves death
   b. is an unexpected occurrence
   c. applies only to ambulatory care settings
   d. must be reported to the Joint Commission

3. Reviewable sentinel events:

   a. must be submitted to the Joint Commission
   b. will result in a change of accreditation status for an organization
   c. include death following a discharge "against medical advice (AMA)"
   d. include patient paralysis associated with a medication error

4. A root cause analysis:

   a. must identify the person who was at fault relative to a sentinel event
   b. is always reviewable by the Joint Commission
   c. is expected following a sentinel event
   d. is not necessary for a "near miss"

5. The Accreditation Association for Ambulatory Health Care:

   a. utilizes a peer-based survey process
   b. is not associated with Medicare deemed status
   c. is a for-profit organization
   d. does not address health information in its standards

References

Centers for Medicare and Medicaid Services. 2009. Questions and answers for on site visits of CLIA certificate of waiver laboratories. http://www.cms.hhs.gov/CLIA/downloads/cliaback.pdf.

Food and Drug Administration. 2009. CLIA waivers. http://www.fda.gov//MedicalDevices/DeviceRegulationand Guidance/IVDRegulatoryAssistance/ucm124202.htm.

Joint Commission. 2009a. http://www.thejointcommission.org.

Joint Commission. 2009b. *Accreditation Manual for Ambulatory Surgical Centers.* Oakbrook Terrace, IL: Joint Commission.

National Committee for Quality Assurance. 2009. http://www.ncqa.org.

National Quality Forum. 2008. Press release: Medicare law provision will make quality front and center in America's efforts to successfully reform our nation's healthcare system. http://www.qualityforum.org/News_ And_Resources/Press_Releases/2008/Medicare_Law_Provision_Will_Make_Quality_Front_and_Center_in_ America_s_Efforts_to_Successfully_Reform_Our_Nation_s_Healthcare_System.aspx.

Odom-Wesley, B., and D. Brown, eds. 2009. *Documentation for Medical Records.* Chicago: AHIMA.

Shi, L., and D. Singh. 2008. *Delivering Health Care in America: A Systems Approach,* 4th ed. Sudbury, MA: Jones and Bartlett Publishers.

Resources

Accreditation Association for Ambulatory Health Care. http://www.aaahc.org.

Chapter 8

Regulation and Policy

Susan Grennan, RHIA

Learning Objectives

- Identify what is informed consent and what are the elements of informed consent

- Describe the purpose and functions related to health record assembly and analysis in a medical practice environment

- Compare and contrast the advantages and disadvantages regarding health record delivery when records are managed centrally as opposed to decentrally

- Describe the steps a medical practice may take when patients miss appointments

- Describe the form components of a valid permission to release information

- Learn who has the authority to sign a permission to release form

- Provide examples of situations that do not require a signed release of information form

- Describe the different options the medical practice has for the handling of health records of its patients when the medical practice decides to close

- Learn what a medical practice must consider when developing a records retention schedule

Key Terms

Advance directives
Attorney ad litem
Authentication
Centralization and
  decentralization
Clinical trial
Competency
Disclosure

Emancipated minor
Health information
  management (HIM)
Implied consent
Informed consent
Legal guardian
Minimum necessary

PHI
Power of attorney for
  healthcare
Records retention period
Record tracking
Redisclosure
Statute of limitations

Introduction

Personal health information is collected, reviewed, analyzed, transmitted, and used on every patient that visits a medical practice. Health information management (HIM) professionals manage the daily use, access, and disclosure of these health records. In maintaining these records and protecting a patient's confidentiality, HIM professionals must be aware of a variety of legal issues as they apply to the health record. The HIM professional must be knowledgeable about legal rules and regulations and apply the rules to those legal issues that exist in a medical practice. This chapter will explore legal issues such as informed consent, completion of the record, chart delivery, missed appointments, release of information, record retention, and what to do with health records when a practice closes.

Informed Consent

Informed consent is the process of understanding the risks and benefits of treatment. The process involves the communication between a patient and the provider that results in the patient's authorization to undergo a specific treatment or procedure.

Components of Informed Consent

Patients must voluntarily give consent for treatment and most medical tests and procedures. For routine procedures such as a physical exam with the provider, or a lab procedure, implied consent is assumed. For more invasive tests or treatments with significant risks or alternatives, the provider should disclose and discuss the following with their patients:

- The patient should have the capacity to make a decision regarding his or her healthcare.
- The provider must disclose the following:
  - The patient's diagnosis, if known
  - Information on the proposed treatment, test, or procedure
  - The risks and benefits of the proposed treatment, test, or procedure
  - Alternatives to the proposed treatment, test, or procedure and the risks and benefits or risks of not receiving the alternative test, procedure, or treatment
- The patient comprehends the information presented to them and the patient should have an opportunity to ask questions of their provider.
- The patient should voluntarily grant consent once all information has been provided to them and all questions have been answered (Edwards 2008).

Decision-Making Capacity

Competency to make an informed consent decision is one of the most important components of informed consent. For the patient's consent to be valid, the consent must be voluntary and the patient should feel as though he or she has participated in and not been coerced into the decision to sign a consent form. The discussion regarding the proposed treatment, test, or procedure should be conducted in layman's terms and the patient should indicate an understanding of the issues discussed. When the patient is unable to consent to the treatment because the patient is legally incompetent, a minor, or in the case of an emergency, the guardian or next of kin (designated by state law) may act as decision maker for the patient and sign the consent. In the case of a minor (barring any state law that prohibits the minor from consenting to a treatment, test, or procedure), he or she may be capable of giving informed consent, such as with an emancipated minor. Most states have laws that designate certain minors as emancipated and entitled to the same rights as an adult. When language barriers, hearing impairment, or other issues exist, the provider should take steps to ensure that the patient can understand the risks, benefits, or alternatives for the treatment he or she will be consenting to. Medical practices may develop patient education materials and consent forms in common non-English languages, or they may have staff or utilize outside sources that are competent to translate or use sign language for these patient populations.

Documentation of the Consent

For many tests and procedures, such as routine blood tests, x-rays, and so forth, consent is implied and written documentation is not required. When tests, procedures, or treatments that involve significant risk are contemplated, the patient should consent to these test or procedures in writing along with a verbal explanation. The components that are both verbally discussed and listed on the consent form are as follows:

- Description of the medical condition warranting the test, procedure, or treatment

- Benefits of the proposed test, procedure, or treatment

- Description of the proposed, test, procedure, or treatment including possible complications or adverse effects

- Discussion of alternative tests, treatments, or procedures and the risks and benefits of these alternatives

- Consequences of not having the test, procedure, or treatment

The consent form should be signed and dated by the provider and the patient prior to the patient undergoing the test, procedure, or treatment.

The Right to Refuse Treatment

Even if the decision is considered to be bad, patients who are legally competent to make medical decisions have the right to refuse treatment. In a case where a patient refuses a test, procedure, or treatment, the provider should document the refusal in the patient's health record to protect the provider from legal liability. A form documenting refusal of treatment, the patient's signature, and the signature date may also be used.

An advance directive is a legal, written document that specifies patient preferences regarding future healthcare or specifies another person who is authorized to make medical decisions in the event the patient is not capable of communicating his or her preferences; the patient must be competent at the time the document is prepared and signed. Living wills and durable power of attorney are both considered advance directives (Abdelhak et al. 2007, 13). If these documents are presented to the provider, they should be maintained in the patient's health record.

Procedures, Tests, and Treatments Requiring Informed Consent

Providers should develop policies and procedures to indicate which tests, procedures, or treatments require a consent form signed by the patient. For example, surgery, anesthesia, or other invasive procedures might require informed consent. The provider may also consult with their malpractice insurer to help in the process of determining what tests, procedures, or treatments that are routinely provided at the medical practice require informed consent.

Clinical Trials and Research

Clinical research trials or studies are sometimes used to determine whether new drugs, procedures, or treatments are safer or more effective than current drugs or treatments used. Informed consent for a clinical trial involves the informed consent document and a process of ongoing explanations used to help make informed decisions while participating in a clinical trial.

The informed consent document provides a summary of the clinical trial and the patient's rights as a participant of the clinical trial. The document should be given to the research subject and written in plain language and include:

- Why the research is being done and what the researcher hopes to accomplish

- Description of the procedures, tests, or treatments that will be done and how long the patient will be required to participate

- The potential risks and benefits, and alternatives to the treatment, test, or procedure

- The informed consent document should be signed prior to enrollment into the study

According to Burrington-Brown and Wagg (2003) these additional items need to be included:

- A statement describing the extent, if any, to which confidentiality of records identifying the subject will be maintained

- For research involving more than minimal risk, an explanation as to whether any compensation and an explanation as to whether any medical treatments are available if injury occurs and, if so, what they consist of or where further information may be obtained

- Contact information for answers to pertinent questions about the research and research subjects' rights and in the event of a research-related injury to the subject

- A statement that participation is voluntary, refusal to participate will involve no penalty or loss of benefits to which the subject is otherwise entitled, and the subject may discontinue participation at any time without penalty or loss of benefits to which the subject is otherwise entitled (Burrington-Brown and Wagg 2003)

In the case of a minor, the parents or legal guardians shall act in the best interest of the child when deciding whether or not to participate in the study.

The researcher should always keep the participant well informed, both throughout and after the procedure or treatment is completed. The process should be interactive and not a one-time session.

Records Completion

Patient health records shall be reviewed for documentation accuracy and completeness. The analysis of health records ensures that the required documentation and authentication of entries in the patient's health record are present. The medical practice shall meet all documentation requirements as defined by the state or accrediting agency affiliated with the medical practice.

In the traditional retrospective data analysis and collection process, performed tasks include the following:

- Assembly of the health record in a prescribed order
- Review of the health record for required documentation and authentication
  - Authentication for all entries in the record shall be through signature, initials, or computer key
- Presence of:
  - Reason for visit
  - Patient history
  - Physical examination
  - Ancillary tests, such as laboratory and cardiology results
  - Diagnosis
  - Plan of treatment
  - Disposition
- Presence of ordered diagnostic studies, consultations, or other requested records
- Presence of proper patient identification on every page of all forms (both front and back)

For more detailed information on the content of the health record, see chapter 1.

General Documentation Guidelines

Guidelines for documenting in the medical practice health record may be found in chapter 1 under figure 1.1.

When a health record is found to be incomplete or signatures are missing, a deficiency slip may be prepared for the record that itemizes missing documents or signatures. Pages in the record can then be flagged to assist the provider in locating missing signatures. Figure 8.1 displays a sample of a deficiency form.

An audit of record deficiencies can be completed by the provider by placing the health records in a designated area within the medical practice; or, when a provider maintains a private office within the medical practice, health records can be routed to his or her private office for completion.

Chart Delivery

Delivery of patient health records becomes an issue for the health information specialist to consider when records are centralized or decentralized. Access to patient health information affects the efficiency of the medical practice and the quality of healthcare delivery. Whether paper-based health records are centralized or decentralized, some of the advantages and disadvantages are detailed in figure 8.2.

Figure 8.1.   Deficiency slip

Patient's Name: _____		Record Number _____
Date of Visit: _____	Provider: _____	

Documentation Requirements	Missing Documentation	Needs Signature	N/A
Significant diagnosis/surgeries are entered on the Summary List			
Current and past medications are listed on the Medication Reconciliation form			
Presence or absence of allergies			
Each visit contains documentation of: • Chief complaint • History of present illness • Past, family, and social history as needed • Physical exam • Diagnosis or impression • Plan of treatment • Disposition			
Immunization record is up to date			
Diagnostic test results are dated and initialed			
Preanesthesia evaluation			
Operative report			

Figure 8.2.   Advantages and disadvantages of centralized and decentralized paper-based health records

Centralized	Decentralized
Reduced duplication of effort with regard to record creation, maintenance, and storage	Retrieval and delivery time is usually decreased for records located within the clinic
Lower overall expenditure for space and equipment	Increased risk for the patient because the provider may not have access to the entire health record, unless components of the health record are electronic
Standardized policies and procedures for record storage and maintenance	Release of information is more difficult when the potential for multiple volumes in different locations exist
Improved record control and security	Need for superior tracking systems for multiple volumes
Consistent supervision of staff is easier	Potential inconsistency in recordkeeping policies and procedures can exist when records exist in numerous medical practices that maintain patient health records
Requesting and receiving a health record may take an unacceptable amount of time, depending on the location of medical practices	Supply costs for storage equipment and multiple folder volumes are increased
Centralized systems demand superior chart-tracking and secure transportation systems, especially when medical practices are located outside the building where the centralized records are located	Record control is more difficult to maintain with the possibility of multiple volumes existing in multiple locations
	Organization of the health record can be more flexible for the provider when multiple record volumes exist

Record Control

Regardless of whether health records are stored centrally in one location or decentralized in multiple locations, the HIM department manager should develop consistent policies and procedures for the maintenance of all records. Policies and procedures for paper-based health records should include:

- Who has access to the file area and how records should be checked out of the file
- When records may be removed/checked out of the file
- How long records may be kept out of the file

Regardless of the system, controls should be in place to ensure that health records are accessible when needed. When the HIM manager is managing a large number of health records or the records are located in multiple locations, an expense of an automated chart-tracking system may be warranted. Installation of a computerized tracking system can create increased efficiency. An automated system should be capable of the following:

- Checking a health record in and out
- Displaying the record's current and historical location
- Tracking of multiple volumes of a record
- Tracking of multiple file room locations for each record or volume
- Allowing authorized users to electronically request a record
- Providing alerts to the individual checking in a health record that the record has a request
- Offering management and statistical reports that identify:
  - Outstanding charts checked out
  - Inactive charts
  - Unfulfilled requests for records
  - Total records checked out by reason and location for a specified time period

Finally, there should be policies and procedures that define how the health record is organized so that patient information can be retrieved easily. (This is especially helpful when portions of records are maintained in locations outside of the HIM department.) Chapter 1 provides detail on the organization of the health record.

Delivery of the Record

When patient health records need to be delivered to medical practice locations outside the centralized file location, the HIM manager should determine how often and when records need to be delivered. The medical practice should determine who and how records can be delivered to outside practice locations. Options for delivery of records include a contracted courier service, or personnel within the organization whose job is to securely transport health records and possibly other items such as lab work, supplies, or payment records. Records that are delivered out of the building should be placed in secure containers. Pickup and delivery of records to medical practices should be determined based on what days and times the various patient appointments are scheduled. When same day appointments are scheduled, the HIM manager must determine whether it is possible to deliver health records prior to the patient's appointment. When it is not possible to deliver a patient record prior to their appointment, policies and procedures should exist that define how patient information can be delivered to the provider and what types of information the provider needs for the appointment.

Depending on whether electronic systems exist, information could be accessed electronically at the medical practice. Information available electronically might include lab and x-ray results and transcribed patient reports, to name a few. Patient information could also be faxed prior to the appointment in the absence of electronic systems. Regardless of what types of systems exist, the details of delivery of patient information to the provider should be predetermined.

For more information on electronic health records, see chapter 5.

Missed Appointments

Missed appointments, or "no-shows," means the patients have not kept their appointments and the providers suddenly find themselves with time on their hands that should be filled with patient visits. While this short break from a hectic clinical day may give the provider an opportunity to catch up on paperwork, the appointment time can never be recovered and the medical practice/provider also loses revenue.

This becomes more problematic when appointment demands are high, especially during the flu and cold season or when parents are trying to get mandated school or sport physical appointments for their children.

To help combat appointment no-shows, the medical practice should set up an appointment reminder system to call patients one or two days before their scheduled appointment. Practices can either make these appointment reminder calls themselves or they could purchase an automated reminder system that can be interfaced to the practice management system. These automated reminder systems make calls to patients with scheduled appointments with the appointment date and time. At a minimum, patients with longer appointment times should be called, such as for preventive medicine visits or procedures. A reminder system, whether manual or automated, provides an opportunity for patients to cancel or reschedule their appointment, thus, freeing a bookable appointment for someone else.

Medical practices should develop policies regarding missed appointments. When a patient misses an appointment, the provider or designee should review the patient's record to determine what actions need to be taken based on the practice's policy of missed appointments. Because of liability reasons, the provider's actions might include:

- Contact the patient by phone

- Send the patient a certified letter explaining why the patient needs to be seen

- Discharge the patient based on a string of missed consecutive appointments

- Schedule future patient appointments at times convenient for the provider, such as at the end of the morning or at the end of the day

The provider should also document the missed appointment in the patient's record, or if the medical practice has an electronic appointments system, missed appointments can be tracked electronically. Finally, another way the practice can manage the number of missed appointments would be to have the patient sign a contract outlining the patient's responsibilities for

Figure 8.3. Medical appointment cancellation policy

Medical Appointment Cancellation Policy

Dear Patient:

We strive to render excellent medical care to you and the rest of our patients. In an attempt to be consistent with this, we have a Medical Appointment Cancellation Policy that allows us to schedule appointments for all patients. When an appointment is scheduled, that time has been set aside for you and when it is missed, that time cannot be used to treat another sick patient.

Our policy is as follows:

We request that you please give our office a 24 hour notice in the event that you need to reschedule your appointment with the physician. This allows other sick patients to be scheduled into that appointment. It also makes it possible to reschedule your appointment more efficiently. If a patient misses an appointment without contacting our office, this is considered a missed appointment ("No-Show, No-Call.") A fee of $ _(insert dollar amount)_ will be charged to you for a missed appointment. If a patient accumulates a total of three (3) missed appointments within a twelve-month period, the patient may not be rescheduled for future appointments and will be asked to leave the practice.

Additionally, if a patient is more than 15 minutes late to his/her appointment, the appointment will be cancelled and considered a "No-Show, No Call" appointment.

If you have any questions regarding this policy, please let our staff know and we will be glad to clarify any questions you have.

We thank you for your patronage.

I have read and understand the Medical Appointment Cancellation Policy of the practice and I agree to be bound by its terms. I also understand and agree that such terms may be amended from time to time by the practice.

I, _____ (print name), have received a copy of _Name of medical practice_ Medical Appointment Cancellation Policy.

_____   _____
Printed Name of the Patient Relationship to Patient (if patient is a minor)   Date

_____   _____
Signature of Patient or Responsible Party if a Minor   Date

keeping appointments and the ramifications of missed appointments. Figure 8.3 provides a sample policy for missed appointments.

Release of Information

Protecting the privacy and rights of patient health information is paramount when discussing release of patient health information. One of the main functions of the HIM department involves compliance in the release of information function. "Many laws and regulations govern how, what, when, and to whom protected health information may be released" (Bock et al. 2008). The Health Insurance Portability and Accountability Act (HIPAA) Privacy Rule contains specific requirements regarding disclosure of patient health information (PHI) as well as state laws. State laws vary in the requirements and process of releasing PHI. The medical practice should have thorough release of information policies and procedures that are followed by all the individuals authorized to release patient health information.

Receipt of the Request for PHI

When a request to release PHI is received by the medical practice, the HIM department should begin to track the following items to ensure that the request is fulfilled by the medical practice. The request can be tracked on paper, a spreadsheet, or a commercial release of information/

correspondence software package. The following items should be tracked by the medical practice:

- Date the request for information is received by the practice
- Name of the individual/organization requesting the health information
- Valid authorization signed by the patient/legal guardian
- Nature of the information requested
- Due date of the information requested

Upon completion of the release of information by the medical practice, the practice should also collect the following information on the spreadsheet or commercial release of information software:

- Number of pages copied
- Which documents were copied and released
- Name and address of receiver of the health information
- Date the health information was mailed or transmitted

Processing the Request

Processing the request for release of PHI involves the following steps:

1. Read the request from the individual/organization requesting the health information. Note any specifics that need to be addressed as part of the release of information process, such as due dates, the period of time information is being requested, or payment information.

2. Review the authorization for disclosure of PHI for the following components to ensure the authorization is valid:

   - Written request (faxes or copies may be acceptable)
   - Addressed to the medical practice or provider
   - Identifies the patient along with other identifying information, such as date of birth or the patient's address
   - Lists the name of the individual/organization to whom the information will be released
   - Details the information to be released
   - Documents the reason/purpose for disclosure
   - Notes the expiration of the authorization
   - Documents the statement regarding the revocation of the authorization by the patient/legal guardian

- Describes the impact of treatment if the patient refuses to authorize the requested use and disclosure of protected health information. This statement explains that the patient may not be denied treatment if he/she does not authorize the requested use and disclosure of protected health information.

- Documents the statement explaining that information used or disclosed under the authorization may be redisclosed by the individual or party receiving it and that redisclosed information may not be protected by the federal privacy rules (45 CFR 164.508(c))

- Authorization is signed and dated by the patient/legal guardian

If someone other than the patient signs the Permission to Release Information form, their relationship to the patient must be stated on the form. When the Permission to Release Information form does not include all the required elements, the medical practice should return the request along with the form to the entity requesting information. The practice can use a checklist to compare with the received request form to determine whether all the elements are present, as in figures 8.4 and 8.5.

Requests for health information should be prioritized based on when the health information is needed and what is requested.

Authority to Grant Authorization

Authority to grant authorization to disclose health information is held by:

- The patient (competent adult or emancipated minor)

- A legal guardian (usually a parent in the case of a minor)

- An executor or someone with power of attorney when the patient is deceased or incompetent. Figure 8.6 displays a sample health information access and disclosure grid.

A minor is an individual is under the legal age as defined by state law. A parent may grant authorization on behalf of a minor, except when parents are legally separated or divorced. When in doubt as to who can authorize release of information, the parents can provide the medical practice with a legal document that outlines the responsibilities of the parents when healthcare is involved. When in doubt, consult with the medical practice's legal counsel.

Minors are usually defined by state law. A minor who is "emancipated" could be:

- Married

- Self-supporting and living away from home

- Legally declared emancipated by a court of law

- Unmarried and pregnant

- On active duty with the U.S. Armed Forces

- At least 16 years old and living independently from his or her parents or legal guardian

Each medical practice should consult with state law to determine the rights of minors.

Figure 8.4. Authorization checklist for required elements

	AUTHORIZATION CHECKLIST—REQUIRED ELEMENTS	
#	Requirements for Authorization to Disclose Patient Health Information/Records (45 CFR § 164.508(c)—HIPAA)	√
1	Authorization is Written in Plain Language	
2	Authorization Identifies Name of Patient Whose PHI is Being Disclosed	
3	Authorization Identifies Type of Information to be Disclosed	
4	Identifies the Name of/Classes of Persons/Types of Healthcare Providers Authorized to Make the Disclosure	
5	Authorization Identifies the Name of/Classes of Persons/Types of Healthcare Providers Authorized to Whom the Organization May Make the Disclosure	
6	Identifies the Purpose of the Disclosure	
7	Authorization Contains Signature of the Patient/Patient's Authorized Legal Representative	
8	If Signed by Authorized Legal Representative, Relationship of That Person to the Patient	
9	Date on Which the Authorization is Signed	
10	Authorization Identifies Time Period for Which Authorization is Effective/Expiration Date or Event	
11	Authorization Contains a Statement Placing the Individual on Notice of the Right to Revoke the Authorization in Writing and a Description How to Do So	
12	Authorization Contains a Statement Placing Individual on Notice of the Ability or Inability to Condition Treatment, Payment or Enrollment or Eligibility for Benefits	
13	Authorization Contains Statement Placing Individual on Notice of Potential for Information to be Redisclosed and No Longer Protected by the Federal Privacy Rule	
14	Statement if the Organization is Seeking the Authorization, a Copy Must be Provided to the Individual Signing the Authorization	
15	Authorization Contains Statement That the Individual May Inspect or Copy the Health Information Disclosed	
16	Statement Regarding Assessment of Reasonable Fees for Copy Services	
	Additional Requirements for Authorization to Disclose Sensitive or Restricted Health Information (Refer to Applicable Federal and State Laws for Categories Below)	
	Mental Health/Behavioral Health Patient Health Information/Records	
	Alcohol or Other Drug Abuse (AODA) Patient Health Information/Records	
	Developmental Disability Patient Health Information/Records	
	HIV Test Results/Patient Health Information/Records	
	Other: Sexual Abuse, Child Abuse, Elder Abuse, etc.	

The HIPAA Privacy Rule requires that an Authorization contain either an expiration date or an *expiration event* that relates to the individual or the purpose of the use or disclosure. For example, an Authorization may expire "one year from the date the Authorization is signed," "upon the minor's age of majority," or "upon termination of enrollment in the health plan." An Authorization remains valid until its expiration date or event, unless effectively revoked in writing by the individual before that date or event. (http://www.hhs.gov/hipaafaq/use/476.html)

One Authorization form may be used to authorize uses and disclosures by *classes or categories of persons or entities,* without naming the particular persons or entities. For example, it would be sufficient if an Authorization authorized disclosures by "any health plan, physician, health care professional, hospital, clinic, laboratory, pharmacy, medical facility, or other health care provider that has provided payment, treatment or services to me or on my behalf" or if an Authorization authorized disclosures by "all medical sources." A separate Authorization specifically naming each health care provider from whom protected health information may be sought is not required. Similarly, the Rule permits the identification of classes of persons to whom the covered entity is authorized to make a disclosure. Thus, a valid Authorization may authorize disclosures to a particular entity, particular person, or class of persons, such as "the employees of XYZ division of ABC insurance company." (http://www.hhs.gov/hipaafaq/use/473.html)

When a patient is incompetent, the individuals that may serve as the patient's legal representative, in order of priority, are:

- Legal guardian or attorney ad litem
- An individual with power of attorney for healthcare

Figure 8.5. HIPAA Checklist for Patient Authorizations

HIPAA CHECKLIST FOR PATIENT AUTHORIZATIONS

Complete this checklist to ensure that a patient authorization complies with the HIPAA privacy regulations regarding the use and disclosure of our patients' protected health information (PHI). Check off each element that is contained in the patient authorization you have received before accepting the authorization.

Note: The required elements may be listed in a different order from in the checklist, but if any of the required elements are missing, you must deny the request for PHI and give the requesting party the reason for the denial.

❑ The authorization is written in plain language (is easy to read and understand).

❑ The authorization describes in detail the PHI that is being requested (for example, lab reports).

❑ The authorization says who (the name of our organization or a person at our organization) is permitted to make the requested use or disclosure of PHI.

❑ The authorization says to whom (the name of the person or organization and address) the PHI may be disclosed.

❑ The authorization includes an expiration date or expiration event, which has not yet passed.

❑ The authorization states that the individual who signed it has the right to revoke the authorization, in writing.

❑ The authorization describes the exceptions to that revocation right (for example, no revocation if authorization has already been relied upon, or if authorization was obtained as a condition of getting insurance and insurance law gives the right to contest a claim).

❑ The authorization describes how the individual may revoke it.

❑ The authorization states that the PHI, once disclosed to others, may be redisclosed to individuals or organizations not subject to HIPAA and may no longer be protected by HIPAA.

❑ The authorization is either signed by the individual or signed and dated by the individual's personal representative, and describes that person's authority to act for the individual.

❑ The authorization is dated.

Patient Name: _____   Medical Record #_____

Figure 8.6. Authority to grant authorization to release information

Patient Is	Authorizing Individual
Competent adult (age of majority is defined by state law)	Patient
Minor	Parent or legal guardian
Deceased	Legal representative; executor of estate
Legally judged incompetent	Legally appointed guardian
Emancipated minor	Patient
Minor and parent are both minors	Parent

- Next of kin in the following order:
  - Spouse of a current marriage
  - Adult son or daughter
  - Mother or father
  - Adult brother or sister

Each medical practice should review state laws regarding next of kin, because next of kin definitions may vary from state to state.

Verify the Patient

Prior to processing the request, the patient's identification provided in the request must be matched with the information in the patient's record to ensure the correct patient health records are retrieved. Types of information that can be used to establish the patient listed on the request corresponds to the patient health record maintained by the medical practice are: the patient's legal name, date of birth, Social Security number, address, telephone number, guarantor, and next-of-kin, to name a few. The patient's signature on the request should also be matched with the patient's signature contained in the health record.

Exceptions to Required Authorizations

Depending on state statutes, health information may be released without authorization by the patient when it involves statutory reporting. Some of these exceptions may include reporting of abuse or neglect of a minor or an elderly or incompetent adult, contagious disease, vital statistics for birth defects, or registries such as cancer.

Other examples where information may be released without authorization are:

- For treatment, payment, and healthcare operations as described in the medical practice's Notice of Privacy

- When required by law institutions involving victims of abuse, neglect, domestic violence, or crime committed at the medical practice or against the personnel

- When required by health oversight activities

- For judicial proceedings

- For public health purposes

- For law enforcement purposes

- For certain purposes required by coroners, medical examiners, and funeral directors

- For organ donor purposes, relating to cadavers

- For medical research purposes

- When necessary to prevent or lessen a severe or imminent threat to the health or safety of a person or the public

- For certain military and government purposes

- To comply with workers' compensation

Figure 8.7 provides a table of examples that a medical practice might build to facilitate an efficient release of information process. State and federal regulations should be reviewed as they apply to release of information, along with legal counsel for the medical practice. Special attention should be given to subpoenas and whether or not subpoenas are actually valid (Whitney 2007).

Completing a Request to Release Information

Upon verification of a valid authorization form, information shall be prepared to respond to the request for information. Only minimum necessary information required to comply with the request should be provided.

Figure 8.7. Health information access and disclosure grid

Requestor	Authorization Requirement Yes or No	Comments
Accrediting agencies, licensing surveyors, review organizations	No, as long as	Individual patients remain anonymous in survey reports.
Attorneys	Yes	Or a valid subpoena plus a reasonable assurance the patient has been notified. Reasonable assurances could be stated in the subpoena/ request or an additional Permission to Release Information form can be attached to the subpoena.
Attorneys representing the medical practice	No	
Coroner/medical examiner	No, when	Conducting a post-mortem exam on a patient to determine cause of suspicious death.
Courts of law	No, when	Issuing subpoena or court orders; however, there must be reasonable assurance patient has been notified.
Disability determination	Yes	Evaluating a patient's medical condition to support disability benefits.
Employees involved in patient care	No	
Employees accessing health records of family members or patients not under their care	Yes	
Employees needing health information to perform their job and is not related to patient care	No, however	Records accessed shall be only those that are part of their work or as a study.
Employers	Yes, unless	Workers' compensation case with information pertaining to injury upon verification of case.
Family members (parents/legal guardian) when the patient is a minor	No, unless	The patient is an emancipated minor, or in some states when a child consents to treatment without parental involvement or consent, such as sexually transmitted disease and alcohol or substance abuse treatment.
Family members/friends	Yes	
Family members in cases of incompetence or incapacity	Yes, unless	A person has been granted power of attorney to act on behalf of the patient who is now incapacitated.
FBI	No, however	In lieu of authorization, a court order is required.
Food and Drug Administration	No, unless	Information limited to the clinical trial administration.
Government agencies	Yes, unless	Required by law; Office of Inspector (OIG) or Centers for Medicare or Medicaid Services (CMS).
Health department	Yes, unless	Obtaining health information within reasonable scope of their function, for example infectious disease reporting.
Hospitals	Yes, unless	Direct transfer from the medical practice to the hospital or in case of a life threatening situation or patient unable to sign with no other family member present.
Inmate	Yes	
Insurance companies (if not listed as patient's insurance on chart)	Yes, however	Some have a preauthorized consent for claim payment; BC/BS, CHAMPUS, Medicare, Medicaid, and HMOs.
Law enforcement officials	Yes, unless	In compliance of subpoena or court order or documented cases of abuse (child, spouse, vulnerable adult), search warrants and cases involving national security.
Life insurance company	Yes	Evaluate patient's medical condition for issuance of a life insurance policy.
Nursing home	Yes, unless	Transferred from the medical practice directly to their facility.
Home health agency	Yes, unless	Treating the patient based on orders of a provider.
News media	Yes	
Physician offices	No, as long as	Physicians are involved in the patient's care and treatment.
Recruiters (military service)	Yes	

(continued on next page)

Figure 8.7.   Health information access and disclosure grid *(continued)*

Requestor	Authorization Requirement Yes or No	Comments
Researchers	Yes, unless	Written approval from Institutional Review Board (IRB) as long as articles, papers, other products of research do not identify patients.
Schools	Yes, unless	Immunization record (refer to state law for regulations regarding potential disclosures).
Students affiliated with medical practice	No, however	Need verification from their instructor that they can review health records.
Third party reviewers/business associates/ auditors	No	
Treatment of alcohol/drug abuse	Yes	Authorization must specifically request/release information regarding substance abuse and treatment.
Testing and treatment of HIV	Yes	Authorization requires specific disclosure of HIV records.
Treatment of mental health	Yes, unless	It is determined that the life or health of an individual is in danger and that without the information a person's health may be in jeopardy.
Workers' compensation	No, if	Stated as worker's comp in record and only information related to the injury.

According to Bock et al., the final aspect of the quality control process is evaluating the completion of the request. Critical questions include:

- If the content of the request does not meet the organization's required elements, was the request returned to the requestor with an explanation of the additional information required?

- If the content of the request meets the requirements, was the request processed in accordance with the organization's policies and procedures?

- Was the information directed only to the individual or entity designated in the authorization for release of the information?

- Was the information released recorded for internal auditing and recordkeeping?

- If a patient picked up the information in person, was there a process in place to verify that person's identity?

- Was the information delivered to the designated entity in accordance with the organization's policies and procedures? (Bock et al. 2008)

A sample authorization to use or disclose health information may be found in appendix M. Additionally some states have standardized consent forms. Minnesota's standard consent form may be found in the Sample Forms folder on the CD-ROM accompanying this book.

Special Situations

Each medical practice should consult with its legal counsel in the development of policies and procedures related to special situation release of information. Listed below are some special situations in which a practice might consult with its legal advisors when developing policies and procedures. State regulations should also be reviewed because each of the issues listed below may differ from state to state. Finally, any situation that deviates from the general rule that the patient has the right to control access to his or her records should be included in the medical practice's policies and procedures. Examples of some of these special situations are:

- HIV/AIDS
- Adoption
- Alcohol/drug abuse
- Photographs
- Behavioral health records

Accounting of Disclosures

Medical practices should develop policies and procedures related to HIPAA's requirement for accounting of disclosures. The accounting of disclosures requirement allows an individual to request an accounting for disclosures as far back as six years before the time of the request—but to start no earlier than April 14, 2003.

Disclosures *not* requiring accounting include disclosures made:

- For treatment, payment, or healthcare operations (TPO)
- To the individual who is the subject of the PHI
- Incident to an otherwise permitted disclosure
- Based on the individual's signed authorization
- For a facility directory
- For national security or intelligence purposes
- To correctional facilities or law enforcement on behalf of inmates
- As part of a limited data set
- Prior to the compliance date of April 14, 2003 (45 CFR 164.514)

Disclosures that *do* require an accounting of disclosure include those:

- Required by law
- For public health activities
- For victims of abuse, neglect, violence
- For health oversight activities
- For judicial/administrative proceedings
- For law enforcement purposes
- For organ/eye/tissue donations
- For research purposes
- To avert threat to health and safety
- For specialized government functions
- About decedents

- For workers' compensation

- Releases made in error to an incorrect person/entity (that is, breaches)

There are new proposed requirements in the American Recovery and Reinvestment Act (ARRA) that change the accounting of disclosures that physician practices must maintain. The law suggests that covered entities that maintain PHI in electronic health record systems account for disclosures of PHI made for the purposes of TPO, which are currently exempt under HIPAA. Individuals then have the right to obtain an "accounting of disclosures" of PHI created by the covered entity (CEs) over a certain period of time. In addition to addressing the maintenance of PHI through an electronic medical record (EMR), legislation would require that CEs make available copies of PHI in electronic format without charge.

Restriction to Access of Health Information

There are some instances when the patient may be denied access to his or her health information. One example would be if there is concern that the patient may harm himself or herself, or someone else.

Proposed healthcare legislation under ARRA includes provisions that would allow individuals to restrict what PHI may be disclosed to a covered entity for the purposes of payment or healthcare operations if the individual pays out of pocket for a healthcare service.

Redisclosure

When providers receive health records from other facilities or providers and it is determined that these records will be incorporated into the patient's health record, it is recommended that:

- Records from other facilities ordered by the provider be made part of the health record.

- If the information is used to diagnose or treat the patient, copies should be retained in the health record. (If a patient brings the records to the medical practice, copies can be made and the original records returned to the patient.)

- The medical practice may redisclose health information from another provider or healthcare facility that is needed for treatment purposes or authorized by the patient when completing a disclosure to release information form.

Substance Abuse Patient Records

According to the American Health Information Management Association practice brief entitled "Redisclosure of Patient Health Information":

> The Confidentiality of Alcohol and Drug Abuse Patient Records regulations generally prohibit redisclosure of health information. The rules require that a notice accompany each disclosure made with a patient's written consent. The notice must state:

> The information has been disclosed to you from records protected by federal confidentiality rules (42 CFR 2.32). The federal rules prohibit you from making any further disclosure of this information unless further disclosure is expressly permitted by the written consent of the person to whom it pertains or as otherwise permitted by 42 CFR Part 2. A general authorization for the release of medical or other information is not sufficient for this purpose. The federal rules restrict any use of the information to criminally investigate or prosecute any alcohol or drug abuse patient.

The regulations do not prohibit redisclosure:

- To medical personnel to the extent necessary to address a genuine medical emergency.

- If authorized by an appropriate court order of competent jurisdiction granted after an application showing good cause. However, the court is expected to impose appropriate safeguards against unauthorized disclosure. (AHIMA 2009, 51–54)

Charges

Medical practices may charge entities for releasing patient healthcare information, depending on state and federal laws and policies of the medical practice. In regards to charging a patient or his or her personal representative for copies of their healthcare information, HIPAA's Final Rule 164.524(c) states the following regarding copying fees to the patient: "If the individual requests a copy of the protected health information or agrees to a summary or explanation of such information, the covered entity may impose a reasonable, cost-based fee, provided that the fee includes only the cost of: (i) Copying, including the cost of supplies for and labor of copying the protected health information requested by the individual; (ii) postage, when the individual has requested that the copy or the summary or explanation be mailed; and (iii) Preparing an explanation or summary of the protected health information, if agreed to be the individual as required by paragraph (c)(2)(ii) of this section" (Hjort 2004).

The medical practice may charge other entities who request healthcare information such as an attorney, insurance company, workers' compensation, or state disability. One of the first steps in developing a policy in regards to charging for release of information would be to determine whether state law exists that dictates the extent these entities may be charged for healthcare information. Fees that can be charged also vary based on the entity requesting the information. For example, fees charged for workers' compensation typically differ from fees charged for a request from state disability. Hjort (2004) has found that factors that affect the cost of release of information include:

- Labor costs involved with ensuring authorization appropriateness

- Labor costs and software associated with logging requests in a database

- Labor costs and expenses involved in physically retrieving health information from on-site and off-site storage facilities

- Capital costs associated with copying equipment (copy machines, microfilm, and microfiche readers/printers)

- Expense costs for paper, toner, and equipment maintenance involved in copying

- Labor costs associated with the physical copying of health information

- Labor costs associated with re-filing retrieved health information

- Supplies and handling expenses involved in preparing a document for mailing

- Postal expenses

- Expenses associated with invoicing for copies

- Collections and bad debt expenses

- Real estate costs: work space and storage space for the ROI and copying functions (Hjort 2004)

Once research is completed, the medical practice should establish fees that are appropriate, legitimate and customary. The following Web site summarizes different states' regulations and associated charging limits, if available: http://www.lamblawoffice.com/medical-records-copying-charges.html. A best practice is to revisit these established fees on an annual basis, or more frequently if regulations warrant.

Outsourcing

Many medical practices outsource the release of information function to handle some of the routine tasks associated with release of information. Often these functions can be performed more efficiently and at a lower cost to the practice. When these services are performed by another entity, the "HIM professional should oversee the confidentiality, security, and appropriate handling of health information" (Abdelhak et al. 2001, 457).

Management of the ROI Process

Medical practices should monitor the information that is collected, whether manually or electronically, to determine the types of incoming requests, the resources needed to complete the function, and the average turnaround time to process a request by type of requestor. The medical practice needs to set standards for the anticipated turnaround to process a request. Practices should also prioritize request types, so requests of an urgent nature are processed more quickly than a routine request. This can be determined by policy; however, in some states, state law mandates how soon a practice must respond to a request and how. Finally, the medical practice needs to set charges for some request types.

In conclusion, release of information can often be confusing and difficult to manage. The most important aspect of release of information is to maintain and protect the confidentiality of the patient while responding to the request for health information. Many policies and procedures should be documented for proper release of information. Following is a partial list of these policies and procedures:

- Proper release of information
- Unauthorized access to patient information
- Disclosure to law enforcement
- Disclosure to public health agencies
- Reporting of child and adult abuse and neglect
- Disclosures related to judicial and legal actions
- Marketing activities that require an authorization
- Disclosure of PHI after death
- Patient's refusal to sign authorization
- Revoking of an authorization
- Release of information for minors
- Patient access to health information

- Denial of requests to access PHI by patient

- Amendments of health information

- Maintenance of record disclosures

- Copying costs

Finally, along with good medical practice policies and procedures, staff must be properly trained on the rules of release of information as it pertains to their job within the practice. A sample policy on disclosure of patient protected health information may be found in appendix N.

Flow of the Disclosure of Patient Health Information

When a patient requests health information from a medical practice, there is a common flow that should be followed in order to release this information directly to the patient. Figure 8.8 displays the flow of a patient request to a medical practice.

When a medical practice requests health information from another medical practice, the flow for this disclosure is slightly different. Figure 8.9 displays the flow of disclosure of health information from one medical practice to another medical practice.

Record Retention

A records retention program is a written plan that guides the removal of records to inactive storage and possible later destruction. Health records and data types include paper, images, optical disk, computer disk, microfilm, microfiche, CD-ROM, and other electronic media. There are several factors a medical practice needs to consider in the development of a records retention program.

State statutes and regulations—State laws define what constitutes a record and the period of time a record needs to be retained. Medical practices should also consider the statute of limitations when determining the records retention policy. "The statute of limitations determines the period of time in which a legal action can be brought against a facility for injury, improper care, or breach of contract" (Abdelhak et al. 2001, 199). The statue of limitations begins at the time of the event or at the age of majority if the patient was treated as a minor.

Characteristics of a retention program—A legally sound records retention program should have the following characteristics:

- Documented program of retention

- Addresses all types of records and media to inventory

- Compliant with state laws and accreditation and professional practice standards

- Procedures and schedules used for the destruction of records

- Approval by legal counsel, the medical staff, administration, and malpractice insurers

- Ability to maintain, monitor, and audit the retention program

Not only does a well-planned records retention program provide for an organized, methodical removal of inactive records, but it also provides evidence of when health records were

Figure 8.8. Patient request to medical practice for disclosure of patient health information

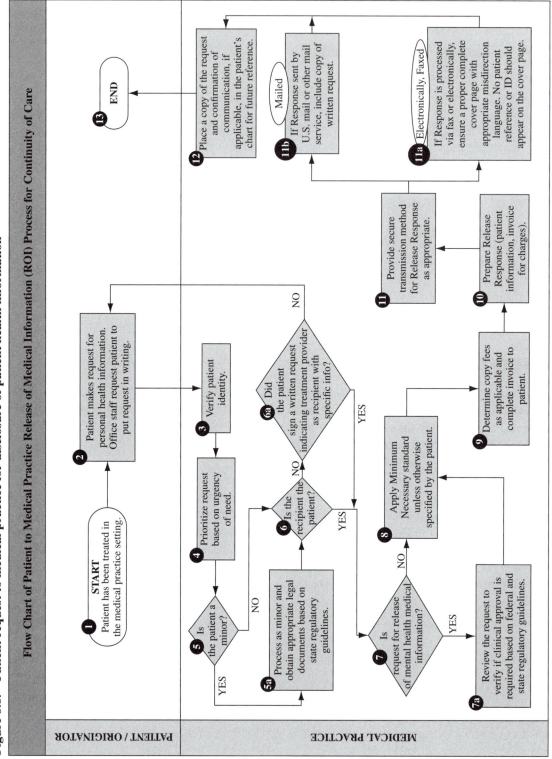

Flow Chart of Patient to Medical Practice Release of Medical Information (ROI) Process for Continuity of Care

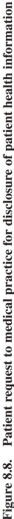

Figure 8.9. One medical practice to another medical practice for disclosure of patient health information

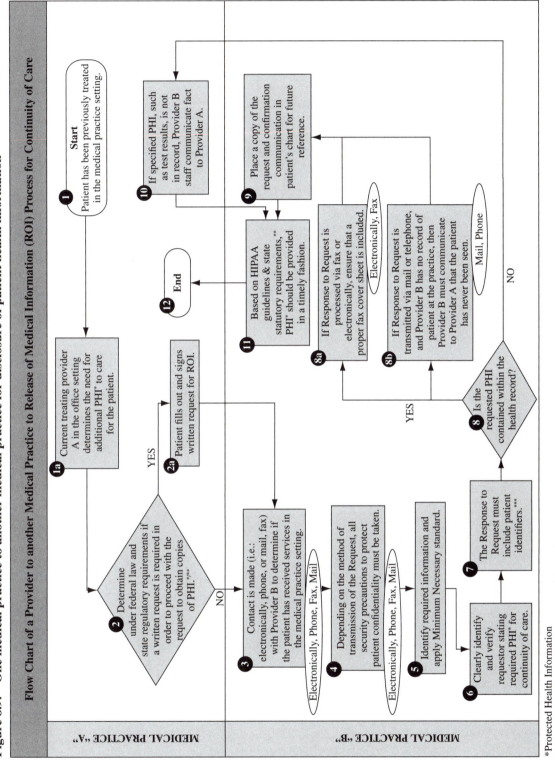

Flow Chart of a Provider to another Medical Practice to Release of Medical Information (ROI) Process for Continuity of Care

*Protected Health Information
**See quick reference grid for state specific requirements.
***The request must include patient identifiers, including, but not limited to, patient's full name, address, date of birth, maiden name, etc.

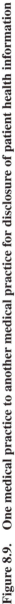

destroyed. The length of time that health records are kept should be guided by the following factors:

- Legal requirements and accreditation standards
- Available filing space
- Patient's age (in relation to statute of limitations)
- Clinical care needs
- Percentage of return visits and length of time between return visits
- Research and teaching needs
- Costs involved in storing, scanning to optical disk, converting to microfilm, or destroying inactive records

According to Abdelhak et al., once a medical practice "has decided what records to place on a retention schedule and how long the records need to be maintained, a schedule should be developed and approved by the medical practice's attorney. The schedule should list all medical and business records that will be retained" (Abdelhak et al. 2001, 199).

When the decision is made to store records, additional factors should be considered:

- Space is an expense and consideration should be made as to which records should be stored and which records should be destroyed.
- The environmental condition of the chosen space should be free from mold, dust, humidity, pests, water, and fire, such as water pipes and flammable materials.
- The ability to preserve the health records in the event of a natural disaster, such as a flood. As documented in the retention program, restoration from a flood may include vacuum freezing as the preferred method.
- When a patient has multiple volumes, a decision needs to be made if all volumes will remain active or if the older volumes, if the time frames documented in the retention program are met, will be stored.
- Additional types of health records must be documented in the retention policies and procedures. These types include, but are not limited to, radiology films, cardiology tracings, ultrasound images, stress test tracings, and photographs, to name a few.

According to Abdelhak et al., "When it is time for destructions of patient health records, these records should only be destroyed when it is determined that all laws, state statutes, regulations, to name a few, have been followed along with approval from the medical practice's administrator and attorney. A record of all patient files destroyed should be kept permanently. The destruction process should take place in the presence of two witnesses who both sign a destruction letter that has the complete manifest as a referenced attachment" (Abdelhak et al. 2001, 199).

The destruction policy and procedure should include, but not be limited to, the following components:

- Key responsible personnel
- Method of destruction, for example shredding or burning

- Destruction schedule, if applicable (a medical practice may destroy records once a year, quarterly, or monthly)

- Outsourced company, if applicable

- Location of destruction, such as on-site or at vendor facility

- Verification of receipt and disposal

- Sample certificate of destruction

- Identity of the responsible party for signature

A certificate of destruction must be completed by the individual performing the destruction and a sample of such a form may be found in figure 8.10 as well as in the Sample Forms folder on the CD-ROM accompanying this book. (AHIMA 2007)

For a detailed look at record retention, please see appendix O for AHIMA's practice brief on the retention of health information (updated). There are four tables accompanying this practice brief that list state laws and regulations pertaining to retention of health information; in addition, federal records retention policies by the site of service are documented in this appendix.

Closing a Medical Practice

Providers who elect to close a practice need to do it right, whether it is turning the practice over to a colleague, selling it, or simply walking away. Planning ensures that the provider gets the maximum value from their medical practice. Providers also need to make sure that patient

Figure 8.10. Sample certificate of destruction

Medical Practice Name
The information described below was destroyed in the normal course of business pursuant to a proper retention schedule and destruction policies and procedures.
Date of destruction: _____
Description of records or record series disposed of: _____
_____
_____
Inclusive dates covered: _____
Method of destruction:
❏ Burning   ❏ Shredding   ❏ Pulping
❏ Demagnetizing   ❏ Overwriting   ❏ Pulverizing
❏ Other: _____
Records destroyed by: _____
Witness signature: _____
Department Manager: _____

Note: This sample form is provided for discussion purposes only. It is not intended for use without advice of legal counsel.

confidentiality is maintained and provisions to handle patient records are managed according to the following, as detailed by Rhodes and Brandt:

- State laws regarding record retention and disposal, as well as statutes of limitation
- State licensing standards
- Medicare and Medicaid requirements
- Federal laws governing treatment of drug and alcohol abuse (if applicable)
- Guidelines issued by professional organizations
- The needs and wishes of patients (Rhodes and Brandt 2003)

Health records can be stored or transferred utilizing the following means:

- Records can be archived at a state health department in some cases.
- Records can be transferred to another healthcare provider.
- Records can be transferred to a new owner or partner.
- Records can be stored with a reputable commercial storage company.

Rhodes and Brandt also have this to say regarding closing a facility:

During the course of treatment, patients share private details of their lives with physicians and other healthcare providers. Patients trust their healthcare providers to respect their privacy, maintain the confidentiality of their health information, protect the integrity of the information, and assure its availability for their continuing care. Because of this trust, healthcare providers must be concerned with the protection of health information when the facility closes. (Rhodes and Brandt 2003)

Further, Weiss deals with the question of when the practice/provider should begin to notify patients.

As a general rule, active patients should be notified a minimum of three months prior to the provider leaving or the clinic closing. Active patients are defined as those currently undergoing treatment or who have been seen in the office within the past two years. Notification should be in writing and include the following information:

- The name of the physician taking over the practice, if applicable
- Names of physicians willing to accept new patients, or other sources of referral
- How copies of medical records can be obtained or transferred to another physician
- An authorization form a patient can fill out, sign and send to the individual/facility who is in custody of the records (Weiss 2004)

Liability Issues

Rhodes and Brandt have this to say regarding liability issues over disclosure:

Generally, a healthcare provider remains liable for accidental or incidental disclosure of health information during or after a closure. Therefore, the provider must make appropriate plans to protect the integrity of the records and the confidentiality of the information they contain, while assuring access for continued patient care. State laws and regulations addressing facility or practice closure should be followed. These are usually available from the state department of health. If state laws and regulations are silent on how to proceed, the provider should consider several other factors. (Rhodes and Brandt 2003)

In the absence of state laws, the provider should consider licensure requirements, Medicare requirements, and federal regulations (such as Alcohol and Drug Abuse Treatment) as they relate to retention issues. Other factors to consider would be advice from legal counsel and recommendations from professional organizations.

Retention Issues for Practice Closings

Providers are bound by applicable federal and state laws, and Medicare requirements. State laws usually dictate the length of time a record must be retained. If state law doesn't specify the length of time records must be kept, the provider must consider the state's malpractice statute of limitations for both adults and minors and assure that records are maintained for at least the period of time specified by those limitations. In the case of a minor, the provider should maintain records until the patient reaches the state's age of majority plus the period of the statute of limitations. Providers should also notify their malpractice insurance carrier of the closure in the event they would need records for a malpractice claim. As noted by Rhodes and Brandt, "If the provider participates in the Medicare program, records must be kept in their original form for at least five years from the date of the settlement of the claim to comply with the Medicare Conditions of Participation" (Rhodes and Brandt 2003).

If the medical practice has an alcohol and/or drug abuse program, these records must meet requirements outlined by federal law regarding these health records. In this case, Rhodes and Brandt offer the following:

When a program discontinues operations or is acquired by another program, this law requires the patient's written authorization for records to be transferred to the acquiring program or any other program named in the patient's authorization. If records are required by law to be kept for a specified period which does not expire until after the discontinuation or acquisition of the program and the patient has not authorized transfer of the records, these records must be sealed in envelopes or other containers and labeled as follows:

Records of [insert name of program] required to be maintained pursuant to [insert citation to law or regulation requiring that records be kept] until a date not later than December 31, [insert appropriate year].

Records marked and sealed as prescribed may be held by any lawful custodian, but the custodian must follow the procedures outlined by law for disclosure. If the patient does not authorize transfer of his records to another program, they may be destroyed after the required retention period. (Rhodes and Brandt 2003)

Other organizations that can be contacted would be professional organizations, medical societies, and legal counsel.

Once the provider or medical practice has reviewed all laws and retention requirements, the practice shall determine the appropriate disposition of the record. If the provider or medical practice decides to destroy records based on the investigation, arrangements may be made for the shredding of all health records that can legally be destroyed to minimize storage or transfer costs.

Budgeting for a Closure

When budgeting for a closure, Rhodes and Brandt offer the following advice:

Regardless of which plan of action your facility institutes to deal with the patient records, resources will need to be allocated to carry out the plan. Some of the resources that need to be budgeted for include:

- labor

- copy equipment and supplies

- postage

- telephone

- utilities

- storage boxes and supplies

- transportation costs (to storage unit)

- storage and retrieval costs for required retention period (Rhodes and Brandt 2003)

Closure/Dissolution with a Sale

"If a healthcare facility or medical practice is sold to another healthcare provider, patient records may be considered assets and included in the sale of the property" (Rhodes and Brandt 2003). The records usually go with the practice and are part of the sales agreement, with the original provider who created the records allowed to access the records and obtain copies if needed in the case of a pending malpractice claim or a regulatory investigation.

Note: The information presented next, until the heading "Conclusion," is quoted from Rhodes and Brandt (2003).

In addition, if the new owner considers a sale to a third party, the original provider should retain the right to reclaim the patient records.

If the facility or medical practice is sold to a non-healthcare entity, patient records should not be included in the assets available for purchase. The provider should make arrangements to either transfer the records to an archive or another provider who agrees to accept responsibility for maintaining them.

Closure/Dissolution without a Sale

If a facility or a practice is closed without a sale, the patient should be notified in advance of closure to allow them enough time to find another physician, along with instructions on how to obtain their records, especially if the patient's current condition requires follow up. The facility or practice will then need to make arrangements to safely store the records for a period of time based on retention requirements.

Facilities or practices may also make other arrangements with another healthcare provider where patients may seek future care, unless otherwise required by state law. That provider should agree to maintain the records, permit access by authorized persons, and destroy the records when applicable time periods have expired.

Health information management professionals at the receiving facility should be familiar with record retention and destruction requirements, as well as confidentiality concerns, and have systems in place to allow patients and other legitimate users to have access to the health information. Prior to transferring the records, a written agreement outlining terms and obligations should be executed. The original provider is responsible for assuring that records are stored safely for an appropriate length of time.

If transfer to another provider is not feasible, records may be archived with a reputable commercial storage firm. Such a firm should be considered only if it:

- has experience in handling confidential patient information

- guarantees the security and confidentiality of the records

- assures that patients and other legitimate requestors will have access to the information

If a storage firm is used, specific provisions should be negotiated and included in the written agreement. Such provisions include but are not limited to:

- agreement to keep all information confidential, disclosing only to authorized representatives of the provider or upon written authorization from the patient/legal representative

- prompt return of all embodiments of confidential information without retaining copies thereof upon the provider's request

- prohibition against selling, sharing, discussing, assigning, transferring, or otherwise disclosing confidential information with any other individuals or business entities

- prohibition against use of confidential information for any purpose other than providing mutually agreed upon services

- agreement to protect information against theft, loss, unauthorized destruction, or other unauthorized access

- return or destruction of information at the end of the mutually agreed upon retention period

- assurance that providers, patients, and other legitimate users will have access to the information

Providers may consider giving original records directly to patients, but only copies should be given to patients unless the required retention period has expired. During the required retention period, the provider may need access to the original records for the provider's own business reasons.

Regardless of the archival method used, the provider must assure that the integrity and confidentiality of the patient health records will be maintained and that the records are accessible to the patient and other legitimate users.

[Appendix P, Practice Brief: Protecting Patient Information after a Facility Closure (Updated), provides additional detail by state regarding retention of health records after closure of facility.]

Conclusion

Protecting the privacy of patients and the confidentiality of their healthcare information can be a difficult task in this day and age when one has to consider all the state and federal laws that govern the maintenance, retention, and disclosure of patient health information. The passage of HIPAA in 1996 brought to the attention of the patient/consumer their rights regarding their health information and increased the attention a medical practice needs to pay to the management and disclosure of these patient records. Impending ARRA legislation should also be watched closely. Provisions that will take effect over the next three years are related to breach notification and disclosure. The medical practice must study all the legal aspects of each section described in this chapter. Policies and procedures need to be developed and approved by the medical practice's administration as well as its legal counsel. Finally, staff needs continuous training on the policies and procedures developed by the practice in regards to the maintenance and legal issues surrounding the patient record.

Check Your Understanding

1. The provider must disclose which of the following to a patient prior to a procedure in which the patient is consenting to the proposed treatment, test, or procedure?

   a. The patient's diagnosis, if known
   b. Information on the proposed treatment, test, or procedure
   c. Risks and benefits of the proposed treatment, test, or procedure
   d. Alternatives to the proposed treatment, test, or procedures and the risks and benefits or risks of not receiving the alternative treatment, test, or procedure
   e. All of the above

2. Which one of the following individuals is not competent to make an informed decision in regards to a proposed treatment, test, or procedure?

   a. Emancipated minor
   b. Patient's spouse in the case of an emergency
   c. Patient with a hearing impairment without an interpreter
   d. None of the above

3. Which of the following documents is not considered an advance directive?

   a. Durable power of attorney
   b. Living will
   c. Family trust
   d. None of the above

4. What types of information are not required to be documented in a patient's health record?

   a. Telephone calls between the provider and the patient
   b. Appointment reminders
   c. Treatment plans when diagnostic tests are abnormal
   d. Patient visits with the provider

5. A computerized chart-tracking system should be capable of which of the following?

   a. Displaying the record's current and historical location
   b. Tracking multiple volumes of a record when they exist
   c. Alerting the user checking in a record that it has a request
   d. All of the above

6. Which of the following describes a centralized recordkeeping system?

    a. Record control is more difficult to maintain when the possibility of multiple volumes exist in multiple locations.
    b. There is increased risk for the patient because the provider may not have access to the entire health record, unless components of the health record are electronic.
    c. There is reduced duplication of effort with regard to record creation, maintenance, and storage.
    d. Retrieval and delivery time is usually decreased.

7. What action might a medical practice take when a patient "no-shows"?

    a. Discharge the patient from the practice
    b. Schedule future appointments with the patient at the end of a day
    c. Send the patient a letter of explanation
    d. All of the above

8. What information is unnecessary to track when a request for information is received by a medical practice?

    a. Patient's Social Security number
    b. Name of the entity requesting information
    c. Date the request is received
    d. Nature of the request

9. What element is not required on a valid authorization to release patient information?

    a. Reason for the disclosure
    b. A listing of every facility the entity is requesting records from
    c. Statement of revocation
    d. Details of the information requested

10. Who has the authority to grant authorization to release information for an unmarried 16-year-old's baby?

    a. The 16-year-old's parents
    b. The 16-year-old mother
    c. Nobody
    d. The baby's father

11. When a medical practice closes, what shouldn't the practice do with the patient health records?

    a. Shred the records
    b. Transfer the records to another provider
    c. Store the records with a reputable commercial storage facility
    d. Give the records to the patient
    e. A and D

12. Which of the following should a medical practice consider when deciding how long to maintain health records?

    a. State laws
    b. Research endeavors
    c. Continued patient care needs
    d. All of the above

References

42 CFR 2: Confidentiality of Alcohol and Drug Abuse (AODA) Patient Records. 2002.

42 CFR 2.32: Confidentiality of Alcohol and Drug Abuse (AODA) Prohibition on Redisclosure. 1987.

45 CFR 164.508(c): Uses and disclosures for which an authorization is required. 2003.

45 CFR 164.514: Other requirements relating to uses and disclosures of protected health information. 2004.

Abdelhak, M., S. Grostick, M.A. Hanken, and E. Jacobs. 2007. *Health Information: Management of a Strategic Resource,* 3rd ed. Philadelphia: W.B. Saunders Co.

American Health Information Management Association. 2007. Online course. Managing HIM in physician practices, lesson 7: Retention and destruction. http://campus.ahima.org.

American Health Information Management Association. 2009. Practice brief: Redisclosure of patient health information (Updated). *Journal of AHIMA* 80(2):51–54.

Bock, L.J., B. Demster, A.K. Dinh, E.R. Gorton, and J.R. Lantis, Jr. 2008. Practice brief: Management practices for the release of information. *Journal of AHIMA* 79(11):77–80.

Burrington-Brown, J., and D.G. Wagg. 2003. Practice brief: Regulations governing research. *Journal of AHIMA* 74(3):56A–56D.

Edwards, K.A. 2008. Informed consent. *Ethics in Medicine.* http://depts.washington.edu/bioethx/topics/consent.html.

Hjort, B. 2004. Practice brief: Release of information reimbursement laws and regulations (Updated March 2004).

Rhodes, H., and M.D. Brandt. 2003. Practice brief: Protecting patient information after a facility closure (Updated November 2003).

Weiss, G. 2004. How to close a practice. *Medical Economics* 81(1):69–72, 77.

Whitney, J.E. 2007. A subpoena by any other name might not be legal. *Journal of AHIMA* 78(5):52–53.

Resources

45 CFR 160, 164: Standards for Privacy of Individually Identifiable Health Information; Final Rule. 2002 (Aug. 14). *Federal Register* 67(157). http://aspe.hhs.gov/admnsimp/.

American Medical Association, Office of the General Counsel. 2008 (March 20). Informed consent. http://www.ama-assn.org/ama/pub/category/4608.html.

Carrier, D. 1999. Best practices: What works? *Journal of AHIMA* 70(7):61–68.

Davis, N., et al. 2006. Practice brief: Facsimile transmission of health information. (Updated August 2006).

Grzybowski, D. 2007. In search of eHIM: A case study of transformation to a centralized HIM record archival and EDMS processing center in a multihospital network. *AHIMA's 79th National Convention and Exhibit Proceedings,* October 2007.

Grzybowski, D. 2008. Storage solution: A plan for paper in the transition to electronic document management. *Journal of AHIMA* 79(5):44–47.

Harford, J.P., and K. Rizzo. 2006. You can't throw IT in the dumpster anymore. *Journal of AHIMA* 77(1):66–67.

Herrin, B.S. 2008. Releasing records from other providers. *Journal of AHIMA* 79(11):55.

Herrin, B.S. 2009. Releasing information of deceased patients. *Journal of AHIMA* 80(1):52–53.

Rhode, D. 2009. Recovery and privacy: Why a law about the economy is the biggest thing since HIPAA. *Journal of AHIMA* 80(5):42–44.

Rhodes, H. 2002. Practice brief: Retention of health information. (Updated June 2002).

Tomes, J.P. 2002. Practice brief: Retaining healthcare business records. *Journal of AHIMA* 73(3):56A–56G.

University of Washington. 1998. Informed consent. http://depts.washington.edu/bioethx/topics/consent.html.

WebMD. 2009. Informed consent. http://www.emedicinehealth.com/informed_consent/article_em.htm.

Chapter 9

Risk Management and Liability

Laurie A. Rinehart-Thompson, JD, RHIA, CHP

Learning Objectives

- Gain an understanding of the concept of the legal health record and its significance to the medical practice

- Appropriately document adverse events in the health record and minimize liability

- Understand the elements of healthcare compliance and develop an effective compliance program that protects the medical practice against government enforcement actions

- Identify HIPAA requirements associated with the medical practice and ensure compliance with those requirements to protect patient privacy and to safeguard against allegations of HIPAA violations

- Explore the significance of appropriate documentation and compliance efforts in the risk management process

Key Terms

Abuse
Adverse event
Affiliated covered entity
American Recovery and
    Reinvestment Act
    (ARRA)
Attorney–client privilege
Business records exception
Centers for Medicare and
    Medicaid Services (CMS)
Compliance
Compliance officer
Covered entity
Department of Justice (DOJ)
Designated record set

e-Discovery
Entity authentication
Federal Bureau of
    Investigation (FBI)
Federal Rules of Civil
    Procedure
Federal Rules of Evidence
Fraud
Health Insurance Portability
    and Accountability Act of
    1996 (HIPAA)
Hearsay
Incident report
Legal health record
Liability

Medical identity theft
Never event
Office of Inspector General
    (OIG)
Office of the National
    Coordinator for Health
    Information Technology
    (ONC)
Organized healthcare
    arrangement
Peer review records
Protected health information
Risk management
Sentinel event
Spoliation

Introduction

As in any healthcare setting, the health record plays an important role in the medical practice. Documentation that is present in, or absent from, the health record can affect medical practice liability as it relates to the provision of care, acceptability of the record as evidence in legal proceedings, appropriateness of billing, and compliance requirements. In addition to the importance of documentation, the protection of patient information is critical. The health record is a key factor in a medical practice's risk management program.

Legal Health Record

The legal health record (LHR) has been defined as "the subset of all patient-specific data created or accumulated by a healthcare provider that may be released to third parties in response to legally permissible requests" (Servais 2008). Such requests may be made by healthcare providers, payers, attorneys, administrative agencies, and court systems, to name a few. Further, the American Health Information Management Association (AHIMA) has suggested that the LHR is an organization's business record (AHIMA e-HIM Work Group on Defining the Legal Health Record 2005). Although the definition of the LHR is relatively straightforward in the context of paper health records maintained in folders, determining what documents and data elements it should include becomes much less clear when considering the electronic health record (EHR). The U.S. government has promoted migration toward EHRs for all Americans since 2004, when Executive Order 13335 was signed by President Bush and, subsequently, the Office of the National Coordinator for Health Information Technology (ONC) was established (ONC 2004). However, with the passage of the American Recovery and Reinvestment Act (ARRA) by President Obama in February 2009, significant financial support for health information technology points toward a paradigm shift. Historically, implementation of the EHR has primarily been seen in the inpatient acute sector and has lagged behind in physician and other independent medical practices. Now, however, it is expected that EHR implementation—and the complexities accompanying it—will become very relevant to the medical practice. This section will discuss, first, the complications associated with defining an LHR, with a focus on the electronic environment. It will then proceed to discuss the significance of the LHR in its role in the legal process and in the risk management function, which seeks to identify and reduce the likelihood of unfavorable outcomes and associated financial loss.

Definitions of the LHR have been provided by numerous sources, but there is no one-size-fits-all definition. Applicable statutes and regulations vary by jurisdiction, and other factors specific to an organization come into play, thus requiring the medical practice to make its own determination about the contents of its LHR. In creating a definition, AHIMA has suggested consideration of common principles. These are outlined in figure 9.1.

As technology advances with the promise of improved documentation and, subsequently, improved patient care, determining the content of the LHR becomes more complex. For example, portions of the record may physically exist in a variety of locations. While this is the case to some extent with paper records, the challenge of multiple locations is much more apparent with EHRs and the storage of data in numerous databases and electronic locations. Because a medical practice possesses a variety of documents relating to a particular patient, a decision must be made regarding the types of documents that constitute the LHR. The medical practice "must determine which data elements, electronic-structured documents, images, audio files, video files, and paper documents do and do not belong in the LHR" (Brodnik et al. 2009).

In addition to serving a vital role in patient care, the health record serves as a key piece of evidence in many types of legal proceedings such as medical malpractice, personal injury

Figure 9.1.   Common principles of the legal health record

- The legal health record is generated at or for a healthcare organization as its business record and is the record that will be disclosed upon request. It does not affect the discoverability of other information held by the organization.

- Legal health records are records of care in any health-related setting used by healthcare professionals while providing patient care services or for administrative, business, or payment purposes. Some types of documentation that comprise the legal health record may physically exist in separate and multiple paper-based, or electronic or computer-based databases.

- The legal health record is the documentation of healthcare services provided to an individual during any aspect of healthcare delivery in any type of healthcare organization. It is consumer- or patient-centric. It contains individually identifiable data stored on any medium and collected and directly used in documenting healthcare or health status.

- The legal health record must meet accepted standards as defined by applicable federal regulations, state laws, and standards of accrediting agencies as well as the policies of the healthcare provider.

- The custodian of the legal health record is usually a health information management professional in collaboration with information technology personnel. Health information and informatics management professionals oversee the operational functions related to collecting, protecting, and archiving the legal health record, while information technology staff manages the technical infrastructure of the electronically stored information.

Source: AHIMA e-HIM Work Group on Defining the Legal Health Record 2005

lawsuits, workers' compensation disputes, and criminal cases, to name a few. During the discovery process, which precedes trial, the parties assess the merits of both sides of the case. Access to the health record, which is critical to this process, is generally more liberal than admissibility of that same record as evidence during trial. Technically, health records are considered to be hearsay because they contain out-of-court statements that are often offered in court to prove the truth of a particular matter in question. The Federal Rules of Evidence (FRE 803) generally provide that hearsay is not admissible as evidence. However, the FRE also provide a number of hearsay exceptions that allow for the admissibility of hearsay that, although deemed inherently trustworthy, would be otherwise excluded. One of these is the "business records exception" (FRE 803(6)), which provides that a record may be admitted into evidence if it meets all of the following conditions:

- It was made at or near the time by, or from information transmitted by, a person with knowledge.

- It was kept in the course of a regularly conducted business activity.

- It was the regular practice of that business activity to make the record. (Brodnik et al. 2009)

Of particular relevance to the medical practice, especially as it becomes increasingly electronic and innovative in the ways that it serves patients, is the creation of information that does not meet the legal definition of a "business record" and is not appropriate for inclusion in a practice's LHR. For example, with a greater emphasis on personalized health and availability of e-mail access by patients, communication between the patient and provider via e-mail is becoming increasingly prominent. Also, the importation of data from patients and other providers into provider-hosted, Web-based portals and the creation of personal health records (PHRs) pose a dilemma. Although the information contained in both types of communications is valuable to the provider–patient relationship, its inclusion in the LHR is discouraged. In this situation, a distinction must be drawn between information that may affect treatment decisions (a broader definition) versus information that would qualify as a business record (a narrower definition). Other types of documents and data that are not appropriate content for an LHR include administrative data and documents (for example, incident reports) and data derived and abstracted from individual health records (for example, aggregated quality assurance data). Figure 9.2 discusses various types of data and presents recommendations regarding their inclusion in the LHR.

Figure 9.2.   Considerations in defining data in the legal health record

1. Sources and Secondary Data—The same information can reside in more than one location, the source system that originally collects and receives patient information, and the secondary system that receives data from the source system. For example, laboratory results may reside in both the laboratory's information system as well as in a clinical repository or results-reporting system. In determining which system will produce the document or data for the LHR, an organization must decide which system will be the "source of truth" or official source of data. Failure to designate a source may result in inconsistent or incomplete information being disclosed.

2. Detail versus Summary Data—Findings of diagnostic studies may exist digitally in both detail and interpretive/summary form in an EHR database. Because the documents containing the findings are not identical, a decision about whether one or both will be included in the LHR must be made.

3. Paper versus Images—Documents may exist both on paper and as images in a document management system. Examples include consents and do-not-resuscitate orders. The Uniform Photographic Copies of Business and Public Records as Evidence Act, which allows originals to be destroyed and reproductions to be used in their place, has been adopted by over half of the states.

4. Data Not to Include—Some documents or data elements, either in electronic or some other form, are not appropriate for inclusion in the content of the LHR because they do not meet the business record hearsay exception established by the Federal Rules of Evidence. For example, incident reports, insurance forms, psychotherapy notes, cancer registry data, and derived data such as accreditation reports, statistical reports, and reports of data on quality measures (for example, the physician quality reporting initiative (PQRI)) would not normally be included as part of an LHR.

5. Decision Support—Many EHR systems contain decision support documentation such as alerts, pop-up notices, and other reminders regarding orders, tests, and treatments. A healthcare organization must decide whether this documentation should be included in the LHR. Although they are not part of the healthcare documentation made in the regular course of business, actions taken in response to these reminders do affect provider treatment decisions that ultimately impact a patient's care.

6. Sources of Communication—Communications with patients and their family members may take place electronically through voice mails, e-mails, and Web-based portals. Whether or not these communications become part of the LHR depends on whether or not the communication provides documentation of the patient's care or justifies treatment or diagnoses. An electronic communication that establishes an appointment would not ordinarily be considered documentation of patient care and would not be considered part of the LHR and subject to disclosure. However, if the electronic communication provides documentation of patient care, treatment, or diagnosis, it would be included in the LHR.

7. Personal Health Records—Patients are becoming much more involved in and educated about their own healthcare decisions. Accordingly, they are being encouraged to maintain their own personal health records (PHRs). Because information in a PHR, particularly documents compiled by patients such as immunization histories, would likely not qualify as a business record, they would not be included in the LHR even though they might affect treatment decisions.

8. Sharing of Data Between Providers—Patient data may be transmitted electronically from one provider to another. Whether data created elsewhere becomes a part of a receiving organization's LHR must be determined by the organization. If the information received is used to make decisions about the patient's care, treatment, or diagnosis, it should be included in the LHR. However, the receiving provider must document that the data were used in the health record for them to be part of the LHR.

Source: Servais 2008.

Another important consideration when defining an LHR is a medical practice's designated record set (DRS). A DRS, defined by the HIPAA Privacy Rule, refers to health records and records involving billing, insurance enrollment and coverage, and other documents "used, in whole or in part . . . to make decisions about individuals" (45 CFR 164.501). It includes records in all formats and records from other providers that are used to make decisions about an individual, including e-mail communications between a patient and provider. The DRS encompasses more information than what is normally considered part of an LHR. Thus, a medical practice needs to determine which elements of the DRS will be part of its LHR and which will not (Brodnik et al. 2009).

Changes to the Federal Rules of Civil Procedure, effective in 2006, address the unique issue of the discovery of electronic documents in all industries, not only healthcare. Referred to as e-discovery, the rules are technically applicable only in the federal court system. However, the e-discovery rules are important because of the various types of health record documentation that exist in an electronic format and because they are expected, over time, to set the standard for the discovery of electronic documentation in state and local jurisdictions as well. Elements relevant to the medical practice include changes to the "any and all" request common to subpoenas in the past. No longer will these requests be construed literally when electronic documents are involved due to the vast amount of information created about a patient. Rather, the parties to a legal proceeding must meet to determine which electronic documents are relevant to the proceeding. The changes also require medical practices to develop expansive retention and destruction policies that include documents unique to an electronic environment. For example, the retention and destruction of electronic drafts of records, e-mails, voice mails, and backup tapes must be documented. Finally, the e-discovery rules address spoliation, which is the intentional destruction, alteration, or concealment of evidence. Although the concept is not unique to electronic records, the concerns associated with spoliation are amplified. The e-discovery rules require providers to demonstrate that efforts are being made to prevent the destruction, tampering, alteration, or concealment of electronic records (Servais 2008).

Managing Adverse Events

Adverse events receive much attention from the standpoint of avoiding medical errors, providing high-quality patient care, and minimizing legal liability. More recently, avoidance of adverse events has been linked to "pay for performance" reimbursement mechanisms.

Adverse events include a wide range of incident types and include phrases commonly understood in the medical profession. The Joint Commission defines an adverse event as "an untoward, undesirable, and usually unanticipated event" (Joint Commission 2009). It gives as examples the death of a patient, employee, or visitor in a healthcare organization. It also includes in its definition incidents that result in no permanent effect on the patient, such as falls or the improper administration of medications. Thus, adverse events encompass situations that result, could result, or do not result in a grave consequence to patients and nonpatients alike. They include sentinel events, defined by the Joint Commission as "unexpected occurrence(s) involving death or serious physical or psychological injury, or the risk thereof, with serious injury specifically including the loss of limb or function" (Joint Commission 2009) and never events, 28 serious medical errors that should never happen and that are defined by the National Quality Forum as "of concern to the public, healthcare professionals and providers; clearly identifiable and measureable; and of a nature such that the risk of occurrence is significantly influenced by the policies and procedures of the healthcare organization" (NQF 2009). Never events include medication errors resulting in death or serious disability, and retention of a foreign object after a procedure (NQF 2009). Although adverse events are most commonly associated with hospitals, they can occur in any healthcare setting, including the medical practice.

Where an adverse event involves a patient (or an individual who becomes a patient as a result of the event), appropriate documentation of the event in the health record is critical for both patient care and risk management (legal) purposes. Although serious adverse events such as sentinel events or never events may subject a medical practice to a heightened risk of liability, their occurrence—although unfavorable—must not be hidden from the record. In a legal action, omitted, incomplete, or improper documentation may result in a jury being permitted to infer negligence or presume provider deceit. Documentation of an adverse event must be objective. Although the health record is the location for documenting an event, it is not the appropriate venue in which to raise red flags that target individual blame or liability. Individuals should not be blamed, and inflammatory words such as "negligent," "wrong," or "mistaken" should not be used.

While a component of managing adverse events is the creation of appropriate documentation in the health record, if a patient is involved, the completion of an incident report is important for all adverse events. Although it is more common to inpatient or residential facilities, the incident report is also useful in a medical practice. Incident reports are not created to treat the patient. Rather, they serve as the basis by which to document and investigate an incident. The main goals of incident reporting are to:

- Describe the unexpected occurrence or incident
- Provide the foundation for an investigation of the occurrence or incident
- Provide information necessary for taking remedial or corrective action
- Provide data useful for identifying risks of future similar occurrences (Brodnik et al. 2009)

Although the health record will virtually always be subject to discovery by opposing parties in a lawsuit and, universally, is likely to be admissible in court, the same does not hold true for incident reports. Therefore, the health record should not refer to the incident report and the incident report should not be placed in the health record. Likewise, further attempts may be made to protect the incident report from discovery by labeling it as "attorney–client communication" and prohibiting its distribution. However, plaintiffs do vigorously seek incident reports because of the critical information they may contain in proving a negligence claim. State statutes vary on the degree to which incident reports are subject to discovery during litigation and, as such, should be consulted.

Peer review records are also generated outside the health record. Peer review, which includes a broad range of activities by a peer review committee to continually ensure high-quality care, also results in documentation that may be of great interest to a plaintiff during the discovery process and as admissible evidence at trial. It has been argued that peer review records should be protected because if they are not, professional candor in identifying and discussing problems will be inhibited and patient care will subsequently suffer. Because the goal of both incident reporting and the peer review process is to eventually use the knowledge obtained from unexpected events to prevent them from reoccurring, there are differing opinions on the degree to which they should be open to inspection for legal purposes.

Other sensitive situations resulting in health record documentation include disagreements among staff members and the treatment of hostile patients. These situations must be handled carefully because they may also prove harmful to patient care and lead to liability.

It is expected that when a patient is treated by more than one practitioner, professional opinions may differ. Because the health record is an instrument by which healthcare practitioners communicate with one another to optimize patient care, differences in opinion may need to be communicated in the record. Further, because health records in medical practices may likely include documentation by various providers (such as physicians, nurse practitioners, physician assistants, and others), their professional standards and medical opinions may differ. As such, the presence of differing opinions in the health record should not be discouraged. However, as with adverse events, when professional opinions differ, documentation should not raise red flags that cause the reader to question the competence of a provider and lead to litigation. Practice policy should establish appropriate documentation of staff disagreements. Documentation should be factual and objective, with words such as "mistaken," "negligent," and other inflammatory language avoided. While inconsistent professional conclusions are inherent in the practice of medicine, bringing attention to those inconsistencies or inserting emotional assertions does not serve the patient's interests or enhance the quality of care provided (Brodnik et al. 2009).

The medical practice will occasionally encounter patients who are hostile or irritable. General documentation principles continue to apply, such as charting complete and objective facts and avoiding the use of personal opinions, particularly if they are critical of the patient. Objectivity is especially important because a hostile patient may be more likely to pursue legal action if dissatisfied with the care received (Brodnik et al. 2009).

Check Your Understanding 9.1

Instructions: Select the phrase that best completes the following statements.

1. The legal health record (LHR) _____.
   a. must be maintained on electronic media
   b. may be released to third parties in response to legally permissible requests
   c. must reside on paper
   d. is the same as an incident report

2. Which of the following is a condition of a record that meets the business records exception?
   a. Pertains to financial records only
   b. Is a summary of discussions held during a meeting
   c. Is kept in the course of a regularly conducted business activity
   d. Is maintained on paper

3. An adverse event pertaining to a patient must _____.
   a. not be documented in the health record
   b. be documented in an incident report, which is made a part of the health record
   c. be documented in the health record
   d. only be documented in the health record if the patient is aware of it

4. A purpose of an incident report is to _____.
   a. assign blame to the wrongdoer
   b. provide the foundation for an investigation of the occurrence or incident
   c. serve as a record of patient treatment encounters
   d. record meeting minutes

5. Differences in opinions among medical professionals _____.
   a. must be omitted from the patient record
   b. should be respectfully documented in the patient record
   c. must be documented as arguments in the patient record
   d. constitute attorney–client privilege

Compliance Considerations

Compliance is adhering to both federal and state laws as well as the program requirements established by federal, state, and private health plans that provide reimbursement for health services (Showalter 2008). This section discusses various aspects of compliance applicable to medical practices. It identifies the principal agencies involved in investigating fraud and abuse activities, describes different types of audits used in determining noncompliance, and discusses compliance plans and the seven major elements that identify an effective compliance program.

As defined by the National Health Care Anti-Fraud Association (NHCAA 2009), *fraud* is the intentional representation of false information as the truth. Such deception or misrepresentation is made with the knowledge that it could result in some unauthorized benefit to the individual or entity making the false representation, or to some other party. *Abuse* is the performance of unsound practices—either medical or business—that may result in unnecessary and increased costs to payers of healthcare services (Showalter 2008). Abusive acts are not committed with intention or knowledge. Every investigation of fraud and abuse in medical practices is different. Figure 9.3 provides examples.

Cooperating Government Components

Many cooperating government components are responsible for investigating and sanctioning fraudulent providers and organizations. The Centers for Medicare and Medicaid Services, the Office of Inspector General, the Federal Bureau of Investigation, and the Department of Justice are among those agencies.

The Centers for Medicare and Medicaid Services (CMS) is a federal agency that ensures that the Medicare, Medicaid, and Children's Health Insurance programs are operated properly. State agencies and contractors are used to operate these programs. CMS also is responsible for contractor claims payment, fiscal audits, payment policies, overpayment prevention, enforcement actions, and research. The agency's mission is to ensure effective, up-to-date healthcare coverage and to promote quality care for beneficiaries (CMS 2009a). CMS improves the quality of healthcare delivery by enforcing regulatory standards, improving care outcomes, and educating both providers and patients. The agency uses its Office of Benefits Integrity to oversee carrier operations related to fraud, audit, overpayment collections, medical review, and the demand on monetary penalties for violations of Medicare law (CMS 2009e).

The Office of Inspector General (OIG) investigates fraud and abuse cases through audits and inspections. The OIG is authorized to enforce civil and criminal monetary penalties and program exclusions as well as to refer cases to the Department of Justice and impose sanctions. The OIG houses a number of different offices. Four components of the OIG assist with the mission of the OIG. The Office of Evaluations and Investigations (OEI) has responsibility for all Department of Health and Human Services (HHS) criminal investigations. The OEI presents cases to the Department of Justice for civil or criminal prosecution. The Office of Audit Services (OAS) performs and oversees comprehensive audits to reduce waste, abuse, and mismanagement and promote efficiency throughout HHS. The Office of Inspections (OI) conducts evaluations and inspections to ensure program improvement. The Office of Counsel to the Inspector General (OCIG) provides general legal services to the OIG and represents the OIG in civil and administrative fraud and abuse cases that involve HHS programs. Additionally, the OCIG negotiates and monitors all corporate integrity agreements, as well as publishes fraud alerts, and issues compliance program guidance and advisory opinions. Additional information about the structure of the OIG can be located at http://oig.hhs.gov and in the Office of Inspector General 2010 Work Plan (http://oig.hhs.gov/publications/docs/workplan/2010/Work_Plan_FY_2010.pdf).

The OIG publishes a variety of documents dealing with compliance in medical practice settings. The OIG's work plans describe the activities and projects planned for each calendar year (OIG 2010). The plan's areas of focus are listed in figure 9.4. Physicians and other

Figure 9.3.   Examples of healthcare fraud and abuse

- Unbundling services, such as laboratory disease panels
- Billing for services that were not performed
- Altering or manipulating claims data for reimbursement purposes
- Billing for noncovered services as covered services, such as preventive care
- Falsifying homebound documents for reimbursement purposes
- Misrepresenting diagnostic information to justify medical necessity
- Submitting duplicate claims to primary and secondary insurance carriers for double payments
- Allowing staff to sign for physicians
- Receiving a kickback for ordering services
- Using invalid Medicare beneficiary data to receive payment
- Allowing staff to assign codes without physician input

Figure 9.4. **2010 OIG work plan focus areas for Medicare and Medicaid**

The Table of Contents was structured as follows:

Medicare Part A and Part B

Hospitals

Home Health Agencies

Nursing Homes

Other Part A and Part B Providers Payments

Other Part A and part B Provider Payments (Physician Billing for Medicare Hospice Beneficiaries; Trends in Medicare Hospice Utilization; Medicare Incentive Payments for E-Prescribing; Place-of-Service Errors; Ambulatory Surgical Center Payment System; Evaluation and Management Services During Global Surgery Periods; Medicare Payments for Part B Imaging Services; Services Performed by Clinical Social Workers; Outpatient Physical Therapy Services Provided by Independent Therapists; Appropriateness of Medicare Payments for Polysomnography; Laboratory Test Unbundling by Clinical Laboratories; Medicare Billings With Modifier GY;

Geographic Areas With a High Density of Independent Diagnostic Testing Facilities; Enrollment Standards for Independent Diagnostic Testing Facilities; Physician Reassignment of Benefits; Medicare Providers' Compliance With Assignment Rules; Payments for Services Ordered or Referred by Excluded Providers; Ambulance Services Used To Transport End-Stage Renal Disease Beneficiaries; Medicare Payments for Transforaminal Epidural Injections; Comprehensive Error Rate Testing Program: FY 2008 Transportation Claims Error Rate;

Comprehensive Error Rate Testing Program: Fiscal Year 2008 Part A and Part B Error Rates;and Medicare Services Billed With Dates of Service After Beneficiaries' Dates of Death

Durable Medical Equipment and Supplies

Part B Payments for Prescription Drugs

Medicare Part A and Part B Contractor Operations

Medicare Part C (Medicare Advantage)

Medicare Part D Prescription Drug Program

Medicaid Program

Medicaid Hospitals

Medicaid Home, Community, and Nursing Home Care

Medicaid Prescription Drugs

Other Medicaid Services

Medicaid Administration

Medicare and Medicaid Information Systems and Data Security

State Children's Health Insurance Program

Investigative and Legal Activities Related to Centers for Medicare and Medicaid Services Programs and Operations

Public Health Programs

Human Service Programs

Departmentwide Issues

healthcare professionals are represented throughout the entire work plan. For example, within the physician area of focus, the OIG evaluates the conditions under which physicians bill "incident-to" services and supplies. Incident-to services, which are paid at 100 percent of the Medicare physician fee schedule, must be provided by an employee of the physician and under the physician's direct supervision (CMS 2009a). The OIG also provides many types of publications. These may be found in figure 9.5. They can be accessed, along with each year's OIG work plan, on the OIG Web site at http://oig.hhs.gov. In addition, the OIG documents a semiannual report for the time periods of April through September and October through March of each year (OIG 2009c). These reports are available online and cite recent findings from investigations. The OIG's semiannual report is another good resource to use in monitoring medical practice compliance.

False Claims Act violations are the most common type of fraud. Claims for services that either were not performed or resulted in misleading prices or costs fall into this category of criminal and/or civil penalties. There is no requirement of intent for a false claim. The Health Insurance Portability and Accountability Act of 1996 (HIPAA), among other requirements (discussed later in this chapter), imposes criminal and civil penalties for improper coding practices and for attempts to gain reimbursement for medically unnecessary services. HIPAA makes healthcare fraud a federal offense with high penalties.

The Federal Bureau of Investigation (FBI) is the primary investigative entity of the Department of Justice (DOJ). The FBI conducts federal investigations of cases that involve criminal and civil penalties. The DOJ is responsible for continuing the fraud investigations for penalties that were referred by the OIG. The DOJ prosecutes proven fraudulent activities.

Quality improvement organizations (QIOs) are private organizations that contract with and work under the control of CMS. With substantial access to Medicare patient records, their role is to monitor the appropriateness and quality of care provided to Medicare beneficiaries. Previously called peer review organizations, they operate on three-year contracts called "Statements of Work" (SOWs). The Medicare Quality Improvement Community (MedQIC), which can be found at http://www.qualitynet.org/dcs/ContentServer?pagename=Medqic/MQPage/Homepage, is an online resource that includes tools, toolkits, presentations, and links to other resources that are associated with the Statement of Work.

The most recent effort by CMS to rein in improper provider billing and government spending for healthcare is reflected through recovery audit contractors (RACs), which are independent organizations that contract with CMS to review Medicare claims. Authorized by the 2003 Medicare Prescription Drug Improvement and Modernization Act (MMA), the detection and correction of improper Medicare billing through RACs began via a three-year demonstration project designed to assess the cost-effectiveness of such a program. The demonstration project, which was carried out in New York, Massachusetts, Florida, South Carolina, California, and Arizona, operated through March 2008. Through the completion of the demonstration project, over $1.03 billion was identified as improper Medicare payments (96 percent, or $992.7 million, was overpayments and 4 percent ($37.8 million) was underpayments repaid to providers). The cost to run the RACs was 20 cents per $1.00 and there were some claims that were

Figure 9.5. Office of Inspector General publications

• Advisory Opinions	• Exclusion Program	• Safe Harbor Regulations
• Compliance Guidance	• Fraud Alerts	• Self Disclosure Information
• Corporate Integrity Agreements	• Open Letters	• Special Advisory Bulletins
• Enforcement Actions	• Other Policy Guidance	• State False Claims Act Reviews

overturned during the appeals process. As a result, there was a total of $693.6 million returned to the Medicare Trust Fund from this demonstration project.

Paid a contingency fee based on the correction of both overpayments and underpayments, RACs possess a strong incentive to locate billing errors. Contingency fees vary by contract and therefore differ from one RAC to another. Because the motives and therefore the validity of RACs have been questioned by healthcare providers, CMS contracted with an independent organization to serve as a RAC validation contractor (RVC). This organization's role is to approve new issues requested by RACs for improper payment review and to review random samples of claims reviewed by RACs, and for which overpayments were collected, for accuracy. The RVC is a mechanism by which CMS provides oversight of RACs, whose intended goal is to provide oversight of healthcare provider billing practices.

With the completion of the demonstration project, CMS is implementing the permanent RAC program nationwide with a completion deadline of January 1, 2010. Expansion to the permanent RAC program included a bidding process for contractors interested in serving as RACs (CMS 2008).

Four RAC regions were developed, with the initial states to be implemented:

- RAC Region A—Maine, New Hampshire, Vermont, Massachusetts, Rhode Island, and New York

- RAC Region B—Michigan, Indiana, and Minnesota

- RAC Region C—South Carolina, Florida, Colorado, and New Mexico

- RAC Region D—Montana, Wyoming, North Dakota, South Dakota, Utah, and Arizona

Although this schedule was shifted slightly forward in February 2009, the permanent RAC phase-in schedule may be found in figure 9.6.

There are many differences between the demonstration and permanent RAC, which may be found in figure 9.7.

Audits for Noncompliance

The government and/or the insurance companies can use various types of reviews or audits to ferret out potentially fraudulent claims. Certain red flags will suggest medical practice non-compliance—for example, complaints from beneficiaries, a medical practice's inability to document the service(s) billed, comparisons with peer groups, and inducements offered in marketing the practice's services (such as advertising that transportation is provided to the medical practice providing the service[s]). The types of audits and reviews used include random one-record prepayment audits, electronic claims submission audits, focused health record reviews, and comprehensive health record reviews.

Random One-Record Prepayment Audits

Health record requests from insurance companies to justify reimbursement for services provided during one patient visit fall into the random style of audits. In this type of audit, the medical practice that provided the services is not paid until the requested medical information has been received, reviewed, and accepted by the insurance company. The entire reimbursement is held until the process is complete. In the medical practice setting, medical necessity, level of evaluation and management (E/M) visit, and frequency of services are some of the justifying factors for correct reimbursement. Indeed, results from a single patient visit may

Figure 9.6.   RAC phase-in schedule as of January 2009

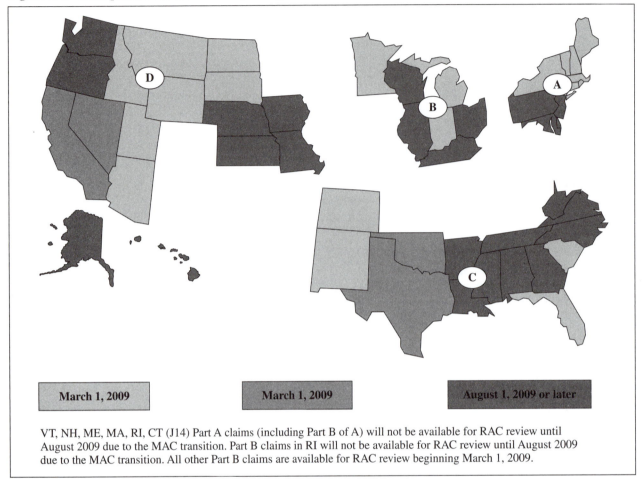

| March 1, 2009 | March 1, 2009 | August 1, 2009 or later |

VT, NH, ME, MA, RI, CT (J14) Part A claims (including Part B of A) will not be available for RAC review until August 2009 due to the MAC transition. Part B claims in RI will not be available for RAC review until August 2009 due to the MAC transition. All other Part B claims are available for RAC review beginning March 1, 2009.

Source: CMS 2009b.

show that the documentation of the E/M level meets the requirements stipulated in a previous version of the American Medical Association's documentation guidelines but does not meet the documentation guidelines for a more recent version.

Electronic Claims Submission Audits

The most common type of audit is an electronic claims submission audit. Along with computerized editing functions at the insurance companies, electronic claims submission audits are conducted in volumes of up to 20 health records at a time. These reviews may pertain to one patient visit/procedure or multiple visits/procedures on the same patient or different patients. Electronic claims submission audits are commonly performed to verify that a medical practice provided a specific service or procedure and that the provider should receive payment.

Focused Health Record Reviews

A focused health record review may be required of a provider who has been identified by the insurance company as having a utilization of services that falls outside the norm of services

Figure 9.7. Comparison of RAC demonstration project and permanent RAC

RAC Demonstration Project	Permanent RAC
Medical Director not required	Medical Director mandatory
Look-back period 4 years	Look-back period 3 years
No maximum look-back date	Can only look for improper claims paid after October 1, 2007
Could not review claims in current fiscal year	Can review claims in the current fiscal year
Certified coders optional	Certified coders mandatory
Minimum claim amount = $10.00 aggregate	Minimum claim amount = $10.00
No Web-based application	Required Web-based application by January 1, 2010 and to include customized addresses, contact information, and status of cases
Optional external validation process, varied by state	Mandatory and uniform process for all states
Contingency fees private	Public disclosure of contingency fees
No requirement of standardized notification to providers	Mandatory standardized notification of overpayment letters to providers
Reason for review not required to be listed on requests for overpayment	Reason for review required to be listed on requests for overpayment
No optimal medical record limit	Mandatory limits set by CMS
Optional discussion with RAC Medical Director if requested by providers	Mandatory
Limited reporting by RAC on problem areas	Mandatory frequent problem area reporting required
No quality assurance/internal control audits required	Mandatory quality assurance/internal control audits
No time frame for paying photocopying vouchers	Payment within 45 days of receipt of medical record
RAC to pay back contingency fee if they lost at first level of appeal	Pay back now applies to all levels of appeals

for another provider of the same specialty within the same geographic region. Ordinarily, after being notified, the provider has a period of time, such as six months, to alter his or her practice patterns. If the pattern of care continues, the provider is subject to corrective action and potentially may be required to submit health records for a comprehensive review.

Comprehensive Health Record Reviews

A comprehensive health record review examines a provider's charges for a period of time, such as the past six months. Evidence of fraud and abuse will result in overpayment penalties and further investigation with the potential of insurance plan exclusions.

The OIG has two offices that may assist in investigation: (1) Office of Audit Services and (2) Office of Investigations. The organizational charts for each of these offices may be found in figures 9.8 and 9.9.

In addition to audits conducted by payer organizations, in 1998 the OIG introduced to providers the option of participating in the Provider Self-Disclosure Protocol (SDP) that encourages provider transparency regarding potentially fraudulent referrals and billing practices. The premise of the SDP is that, by disclosing evidence of self-discovered fraud, providers can avoid the negativity associated with government-initiated investigations. Further, the costs associated with a government investigation can be lessened. As a result, a spirit of cooperation between the provider and the government can be achieved and penalties imposed on the provider can be lessened. The OIG has emphasized that the SDP is not the appropriate venue for

Figure 9.8.   Organizational chart for the OIG's Office of Audit Services

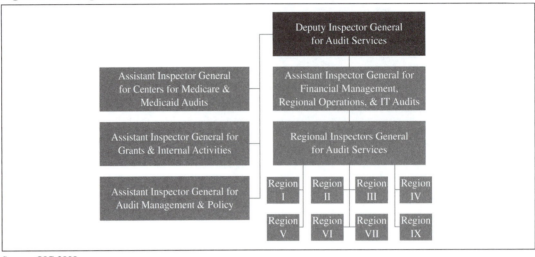

Source: OIG 2009a.

Figure 9.9.   Organizational chart for the OIG's Office of Investigations

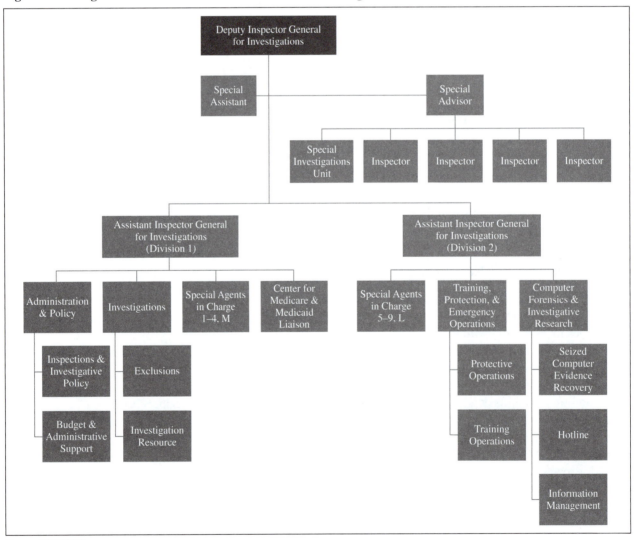

Source: OIG 2009b.

reporting mere billing errors or overpayments that are not believed to be fraudulent. The Open Letter of 2006 encouraged providers to utilize the SDP for matters involving the anti-kickback statute and the physician self-referral or Stark law. In the Open Letter of April 15, 2008, the OIG reported that $120 million had been returned to the Medicare Trust Fund through the SDP program (OIG 2008). The OIG continues to clarify the expectations for providers involved in SDP and to streamline OIG internal processes. Additionally, the OIG stated in an Open Letter issued March 24, 2009:

> To more effectively fulfill our mission and allocate our resources, we are narrowing the SDP's scope regarding the physician self-referral law. OIG will no longer accept disclosure of a matter that involves only liability under the physician self-referral law in the absence of a colorable anti-kickback statute violation. We will continue to accept providers into the SDP when the disclosed conduct involves colorable violations of the anti-kickback statute, whether or not it also involves colorable violations of the physician self-referral law. Although we are narrowing the scope of the SDP for resources purposes, we urge providers not to draw any inferences about the Government's approach to enforcement of the physician self-referral law. (OIG 2009d)

For kickback-related issues, a minimum of $50,000 settlement amount to resolve the matter has been established. This dollar amount is consistent with the OIG's statutory authority to impose a penalty of up to $50,000 for each kickback and an assessment of up to three times the total remuneration.

Compliance Plans and Programs

To help avoid issues of noncompliance, medical practices would be wise to implement a compliance program. The basis of such a program would be the formulation of a compliance plan. Medical practices use compliance plans to document the road maps necessary for identifying and correcting potentially fraudulent scenarios. Compliance plans are not just for large, multidisciplinary medical practices; they also are used by small medical practices and even solo physician practices. A properly written and executed compliance plan can help reduce the risk and number of sanctions. Additionally, the OIG believes that effective compliance plans help providers to reduce fraud and abuse, improve operational quality, enhance the quality of healthcare, and reduce healthcare costs. A compliance program requires more than a written plan; it requires corporate commitment to compliance. To be successful, formal compliance programs depend on organizational structure, thorough communications, and effective implementation.

The OIG publishes model compliance programs that are specific to locations and types of services. Model programs for individual and small group physician practices, hospitals, home healthcare, hospices, nursing facilities, clinical laboratories, third-party medical billing companies, Medicare +Choice, and durable medical equipment, prosthetics, orthotics, and the supply industry have been published and can be found in the *Federal Register* or online at http://www.oig.hhs.gov. Health information management (HIM) professionals lead the way to a successful compliance program. Their expertise and skills are essential to corporate compliance. They are listed in figure 9.10.

Elements of a Compliance Program

According to the OIG, a reasonably designed, implemented, and enforced compliance program will be effective in preventing and detecting criminal activities. Compliance programs

Figure 9.10.   Expertise and skills of HIM professionals relevant to corporate compliance

- A strong knowledge base and experience in appropriate coding and billing practices
- Knowledge of multiple reimbursement systems
- Knowledge of multiple regulations, standards, policies, and requirements pertaining to clinical documentation, coding, and billing
- Knowledge of multiple third-party payer requirements
- The ability to accurately interpret and implement regulatory standards
- The ability to interpret legal requirements
- An established rapport with physicians and other healthcare practitioners
- Strong managerial, leadership, and interpersonal skills
- Strong analytical skills

Source: AHIMA Compliance Task Force 1999.

include at least seven major elements: oversight, policies and procedures, training and education, communication methods and tools, internal audit and controls, enforcement and follow-up, and problem resolution and corrective action (AHIMA Compliance Task Force 1999).

Oversight

Who is responsible for corporate compliance in the medical practice? This question is often asked when a medical practice begins discussions about compliance. For large practices, a dedicated individual—the compliance officer—may oversee the compliance program in conjunction with a compliance committee. In smaller practices, however, the compliance officer may have additional responsibilities. One option is to have the compliance officer oversee the program but use a multidisciplinary team to do the hands-on work. Broadly speaking, all the employees in medical practices share responsibility for compliance.

Compliance activities often involve legal counsel. When conducting interviews, investigations, follow-up meetings, and such, the attorney–client privilege can be advantageous. Commitment of the medical practice's physician leaders also contributes to the success of a corporate compliance program. In medical practices, providers who understand the importance and focus of compliance should be involved in developing the program. In addition to the compliance officer, the physician leader(s) will be instrumental in ensuring the program's acceptance and success among the medical staff.

Policies and Procedures

Written policies and procedures on compliance should include coding, documentation, and billing requirements and be customized to fit the services provided at the medical practice. For example, if the medical practice provides specialized care in obstetrics and gynecology, its policies and procedures should reflect that fact. Attention to chargemaster maintenance, coding completed outside the HIM operations, and medical necessity requirements for services and procedures should not be overlooked. The use of Advanced Beneficiary Notices (ABNs) pertains to medical practices and should be included in the practice's policies.

In addition to policies and procedures, every medical practice should document a compliance mission. The compliance mission statement should incorporate the existing medical practice's mission statement. Customizations of compliance mission statements should address ethical, legal, and quality practices. Additionally, medical practices should adopt a standard of conduct. AHIMA recommends that its Standards of Ethical Coding be used for this purpose (see chapter 6). An annual review of the mission and standard of conduct should be completed and signed by each employee. This gives every employee an opportunity to discuss any potentially fraudulent or abusive activities that may be performed at the medical practice. Moreover, it is each employee's obligation to report potentially fraudulent or abusive activities. Along with employees, physicians and outside contractors should be required to review and sign the standard of conduct.

Training and Education

Training and education is a continuous process and should be highly regarded at the medical practice. Emphasis on coding, documentation, and billing programs should be part of the regular training schedule for physicians and employees alike. The medical practice's training and education efforts should focus primarily on the employees directly involved with the coding and billing process. Training and education should address third-party payer requirements, medical necessity, coding principles, and documentation practices.

Communication Methods and Tools

All medical practices need to analyze the compliance program's communication requirements. Some questions that need to be considered are listed in figure 9.11. Answering these questions and reviewing the pertinent OIG model compliance program will assist a medical practice in creating an effective communication plan.

Figure 9.11.   Compliance program communication considerations

1. Does the medical practice have a formal training program that will promote the newly established policies and procedures?
2. Is there a mechanism to communicate changes in compliance programs?
3. Is there a means by which physicians and employees can report potentially abusive or fraudulent activities anonymously?
4. Does the medical practice have a clear reporting structure?
5. Do physicians and employees know who and how to report potential violations?
6. How will the medical practice address potential issues with outside contractors?
7. Does the medical practice have a formal mechanism for distributing third-party payer newsletters?
8. Is there a tool that can be used to acknowledge that physicians and/or staff have read and understand compliance information that has been distributed to them?
9. Is compliance information given and explained to new hires?
10. Are mechanisms in place to address potential violations when they are reported?
11. Does the medical practice have a well-publicized hotline?
12. Is compliance addressed at staff meetings?
13. Are outside contractors checked on the published sanction list?
14. Do newly hired employees receive continuing education on compliance issues?
15. Is there a method of communication in place to follow up with compliance issues?
16. Does the medical practice provide an orientation program for physicians on coding, documentation, and billing practices?
17. Is there a mechanism for documenting audit procedures?
18. Are there signed attendance records for each educational session?
19. Is there a mechanism for involving legal counsel?
20. Are meetings held monthly to discuss third-party payer requirements?

Internal Audit and Controls

The OIG recommends internal audit and controls in combination with external audits and reviews. Outside consultants may be used to perform external audits and, at a minimum, should be selected based on their knowledge of legislation/regulatory developments, skill set, and communication methods.

A baseline audit should be performed first, with follow-up reviews. The baseline audit should be a larger sample size than follow-up audits. The time frames for follow-up audits should be determined by the medical practice and facilitated by the strategic goals for corporate compliance. For example, the medical practice may decide to perform a baseline audit of each physician using 20 to 30 patient visits/procedures, but the follow-up audit may be completed on a quarterly basis and consist of only 5 to 10 patient visits/procedures. Another method of calculating audit size would be to use a percentage of patient visits/procedures.

The medical practice should decide the areas for potential audit. Medical practices should identify individual areas of risk and use this list in formulating audit criteria and schedules. The OIG publishes a listing of fraud alerts, which is available online at http://www.oig.hhs. gov. Potential monitoring topics are listed in figure 9.12.

Enforcement and Follow-up

The success and validity of the compliance program depends in large part on how well it is enforced. Policies and procedures should identify who has responsibility for completing each step of the corrective action plan. Moreover, noncompliant providers, employees, and outside contractors must be instructed on the various levels of corrective action, which include termination of employment or breach of contract. If compliance team members responsible for enforcing the compliance program are negligent in their duties, they also should be subject to corrective action.

Problem Resolution and Corrective Action

HIM professionals must be actively involved in the corporate compliance effort. Problem resolution with multidisciplinary teams is the ideal proposition for the HIM professional. The HIM skill set discussed above yields the qualities necessary to provide solutions to noncompliance within registration areas, patient financial services, clinical areas, and so on.

Human Resources Compliance

Many compliance directives deal directly with human resources. Medical practices are no exception. Wage and hours laws, employment discrimination, the Occupational Safety and

Figure 9.12.   Potential audit topics

Top CPT services/procedural codes	Bundling and unbundling of services
Top ICD-9-CM diagnosis codes	Appropriate code assignments
Use of modifiers	Use of unspecified codes
Level of E/M service	Use of consultation codes
Use of physician assistants and nurse practitioners	Use of global surgical procedure codes
Simple random sampling	Chargemaster reviews by service
Appropriate linking between diagnosis and procedure	Superbill reviews by specialty
Medical necessity	

Health Administration (OSHA), the Family Medical Leave Act, the Employee Retirement Income Security Act (ERISA), the Immigration Reform and Control Act, and government contracting all are compliance regulations directed toward human resources. Compliance should be a part of every job description, annual evaluation, and exit interview.

Check Your Understanding 9.2

Instructions: Select the phrase that best completes the following statements.

1. _____ is a federal agency that ensures that the Medicare, Medicaid, and Children's Health Insurance programs are operated properly.

   a. Office of Inspector General (OIG)
   b. Centers for Medicare and Medicaid Services (CMS)
   c. Occupational Safety and Health Administration (OSHA)
   d. Medical Review Unit

2. _____ is a practice that is inconsistent with accepted medical practices and directly or indirectly results in unnecessary cost to the Medicare program.

   a. Fraud
   b. Abuse
   c. Compliance
   d. Peer review

3. The ____ publishes model compliance programs that are specific to locations and types of services.

   a. Office of Inspector General (OIG)
   b. Centers for Medicare and Medicaid Services (CMS)
   c. Occupational Safety and Health Administration (OSHA)
   d. Medical Review Unit

4. To ensure compliance within an organization, the Office of Inspector General (OIG) recommends _____.

   a. internal audits and controls
   b. external audits and reviews
   c. both a and b
   d. neither a nor b

5. Compliance _____.

   a. refers only to billing rules and regulations
   b. involves following many types of pertinent laws
   c. is handled only by attorneys
   d. does not require staff training and education

HIPAA Considerations

The privacy and security regulations that were developed as part of the Health Insurance Portability and Accountability Act (HIPAA) have had far-reaching implications for the handling and management of patient-identifiable information in every healthcare setting. The HIPAA Privacy Rule (hereafter referred to as "the Privacy Rule"), which went into effect for most covered entities (CEs) in April 2003, applies to healthcare providers who transmit any health information pertaining to certain transactions (financial or administrative in nature) in electronic form; health plans; and healthcare clearinghouses, which process billing transactions between a healthcare provider and health plan (45 CFR 160.103(3)). Because virtually all healthcare providers conduct electronic transactions, the Privacy Rule applies to virtually all providers. The Privacy Rule also applies to patient-identifiable health information (known as protected health information or PHI) that is under the control of a HIPAA-covered entity, regardless of its format. Thus, the Privacy Rule applies to PHI maintained and communicated in any medium, including electronic, paper, and oral forms. The security regulations, which went into effect for most CEs in April 2005, apply only to patient-identifiable information created, stored, maintained, and communicated electronically. They do not, therefore, apply to paper records or oral communications.

HIPAA Privacy Rule

As noted above, virtually all healthcare providers—and virtually all medical practices—are covered by the Privacy Rule. Its intent is to ensure the consistent protection of healthcare information across the United States. Under the legal theory of preemption, in most cases, where the Privacy Rule conflicts with applicable state laws, the Privacy Rule prevails. Exceptions include situations where state law is more stringent (that is, it provides greater privacy protection or greater individual rights). The Privacy Rule also enumerates certain situations where, although not more stringent, state law will continue to prevail. Examples include the use or disclosure of PHI to prevent fraud and abuse in healthcare payments or to ensure appropriate regulation of insurance and health plans by the state (45 CFR 160.203).

In practical terms, the best way for medical practices to comply with the Privacy Rule is to make the presumption that all patient-identifiable information is PHI and, therefore, covered by the Privacy Rule. Attempting to identify exceptions to the standards would probably prove more costly than handling all patient-identifiable information as though it were covered. The Privacy Rule is complex and covers aspects of operations that are already subject to a number of existing rules, statutes, regulations, and state laws. In most cases, medical practices should enlist assistance from legal counsel to ensure ongoing compliance. Providers in all settings must inform patients of the CE's privacy practices, and that communication must be separate from consent and authorization forms used by the CE. The information may take the form of a brochure, pamphlet, or posted notice. Information required for inclusion in the notice of privacy practices is detailed in figure 9.13. The HIPAA Privacy Rule also mandates staff training and documentation of staff training activities.

The Privacy Rule provides individuals with a number of rights that the medical practice must honor. These rights were designed to give individuals some degree of control over their health information and are described in the following sections.

Figure 9.13. Inclusions for the notice of privacy practices

- A description of the uses and disclosures of health information that are routinely made by the medical practice, along with examples
- A statement about whether the organization uses patient information to issue appointment reminders, to support marketing and fundraising efforts, and/or to report information to the sponsors of the individual's health plan
- A statement of the rights of individual patients
- A description of the mechanism for making complaints about violations of the medical practice's stated privacy policies
- Any other information about the medical practice's use and disclosure of patient information

(Note: The following section, through the heading "Submit Complaints," was adapted from the AHIMA publication *Fundamentals of Law for Health Informatics and Information Management* by Brodnik et al.)

Access

Section 164.524 of the Privacy Rule gives an individual the right of access to inspect and obtain a copy of his or her own PHI contained in a designated record set for as long as the PHI is maintained. There are exceptions to what PHI may be accessed. For example, psychotherapy notes; information compiled in reasonable anticipation of a civil, criminal, or administrative action or proceeding; or PHI that is part of a research study and to which access has been suspended are all exceptions. In other words, individuals do not have a right of access to this information.

Individuals may be required to make their requests in writing. The Privacy Rule specifies time periods for responding. Also, a CE entity must arrange a convenient time and place of inspection with the individual or mail a copy of the PHI at the individual's request. The Privacy Rule allows the CE to impose a reasonable cost-based fee when the individual requests a copy of the PHI or agrees to accept summary or explanatory information. Per ARRA (Subtitle D, section 13405), an individual has the right to receive his or her PHI in electronic format from CEs with EHRs and to have it transmitted directly to a designated person or entity.

Request Amendment

Section 164.526 of the Privacy Rule gives an individual the right to request that a CE amend PHI about the individual in a designated record set. However, there are several situations in which the CE may deny the request. For example, if the PHI was not created by the CE or if it is deemed to be accurate or complete as is, denial is appropriate. The Privacy Rule specifies time requirements for responding to amendment requests.

Accounting of Disclosures

The Privacy Rule imposes requirements about monitoring and tracking PHI disclosures. Section 164.528(a) states that an individual has the right to receive an accounting of certain disclosures that were made by a CE within the six years prior to the request, whether in writing, electronically, by telephone, or orally. Disclosures that must be included in the accounting are limited and there are many exceptions. For example, an accounting is *not* required pursuant to an authorization, for disclosures made to persons involved in the individual's care, or for national security or intelligence requirements. It also is not required for disclosures to carry out treatment, payment, and healthcare operations, although this exception will be discontinued when the HITECH Act, which is a portion of ARRA, goes into effect pursuant to the passage of ARRA. Under ARRA, a CE using or maintaining an EHR will be required to include treatment, payment, and operations (TPO) disclosures from the previous three years in its accounting of disclosures. Effective dates will vary depending on when a CE acquired its EHR. There are many exclusions to the disclosure requirement. So, what *does* have to be included in an accounting? Examples include disclosures pursuant to court orders (without a patient's written authorization); erroneous disclosures (for example, facsimile transmission to the wrong recipient); mandatory public health reporting, which is not considered part of a CE's operations (for example, a report of a patient case of tuberculosis from a medical practice to a public health authority); and, in the future, disclosures for treatment, payment, and health-care operations. Failure by the recipient to read the PHI is immaterial. If a CE discloses PHI that is subject to the accounting of disclosures requirement, but the recipient does not actually review the PHI, the mere right of access must be included in an accounting of disclosures.

An accounting must include the date of disclosure, name and address (when known) of the entity or person who received the information, and the purpose of the disclosure. The Privacy Rule specifies time requirements for responding to accounting of disclosure requests. The first accounting within any 12-month period is free, and subsequent requests in the same period may result in a reasonable, cost-based fee with advance notification. Policies and procedures must be developed to ensure that PHI disclosed from all areas of the medical practice can be tracked and compiled when an accounting request is received. (An example of a request for accounting of disclosures is provided in the Sample Forms folder on the CD-ROM accompanying this book.)

Confidential Communications

Section 164.522(b) requires healthcare providers and health plans to give individuals the opportunity to request that communications of PHI be routed to an alternative location or by an alternative method. Healthcare providers must honor a request, without requiring a reason, if it is reasonable. Health plans must honor such a request if it is reasonable, and if the requesting individual states that disclosure could pose a safety risk. Both healthcare providers and health plans may refuse to accommodate requests if the individual does not provide information as to how payment will be handled or if the individual does not provide an alternative address or method by which he or she can be contacted. An example of a request for confidential communications would be a patient who requests that billing information from her psychiatrist, from whom she is seeking treatment because of domestic violence, be sent to her work address instead of her home.

Request Restrictions

The Privacy Rule (Section 164.522(a)) requires a CE to permit an individual to request that the uses and disclosures of PHI for carrying out treatment, payment, or healthcare operations be restricted. Historically the CE has not been required to agree to the request and, in some cases, has been restricted from doing so (for example, disclosures required by law). A CE is required to inform the individual of consequences of a restriction (for example, a patient's health plan is unlikely to process an incomplete claim for reimbursement). When, however, a CE agrees to a restriction, it must abide by it until terminated by either the individual or the CE. If a CE chooses to terminate a restriction, it must inform the individual of the termination. Termination is only effective with respect to the PHI created or received after the individual has been informed. ARRA (Subtitle D, Section 13405) has changed this individual right. When ARRA is implemented, a CE must comply with requested restrictions that involve disclosure to a health plan for payment or healthcare operations and the PHI pertains to a healthcare service or item paid fully out of pocket by the individual.

Submit Complaints

The CE must enable an individual to file a complaint about the entity's policies and procedures, noncompliance with policies and procedures, or noncompliance with the Privacy Rule.

The CE's notice of privacy practices must contain contact information for an individual at the CE and must inform individuals they can submit complaints of HIPAA violations to the Office of Civil Rights (OCR), Department of Health and Human Services. If individuals choose not to complain to the CE or choose to submit complaints at both the CE and OCR, the OCR maintains regional offices that field complaints from individuals. A CE must document all complaints that it receives and the disposition of each complaint. Complaints are often submitted to the privacy officer, a designee required by the Privacy Rule. This individual is responsible for the development and implementation of privacy policies and procedures. No specific qualifications are stipulated, but because he or she is charged with ensuring the privacy of patients, the privacy officer should be well versed in the requirements of state and federal regulations and accreditation standards that apply to the confidentiality of healthcare information.

Release of Information To and From Affiliated Inpatient Facilities

An understanding of the HIPAA Privacy Rule's stance regarding the sharing of PHI between treatment providers is a prerequisite to a discussion of inpatient facilities that possess an affiliation with a medical practice. The HIPAA Privacy Rule's concept of TPO (45 CFR 164.501) recognizes there are functions necessary in order for a CE to conduct business successfully. Because it was never the intent of the creators of the Privacy Rule to hinder a CE's vital functions, the rule provides a number of exceptions where TPO is involved. For example, the Privacy Rule requires patient authorization for the use or disclosure of a patient's PHI. However, an exception is provided for TPO, and providers may disclose a patients' PHI to other providers without authorization as long as it is for treatment purposes. This exception is permissive, meaning that a CE may opt to require authorization nonetheless either for recordkeeping purposes or simply to protect the PHI being requested and to safeguard itself against liability. Requiring authorization is good practice where the requesting treatment provider is previously unknown or the request is made of the CE some time later, and a "continuity of care" factor is lacking. It behooves the CE to provide an additional level of assurance by obtaining the patient's authorization before sending PHI to any unfamiliar requestor who purports to need the information for treatment purposes.

The Privacy Rule creates additional exceptions for the disclosure of PHI for treatment purposes. One concept, the "minimum necessary" requirement, generally mandates that only the information necessary to fulfill the needs of the user requesting the information should be used or disclosed. For example, when a CE provides supporting documentation to an insurance company to justify a claim, only the PHI necessary to facilitate that claim shall be disclosed. However, this requirement is waived for the use and disclosure of PHI for treatment purposes. Thus, even among treatment providers that are not affiliated in some way, the "minimum necessary" requirement does not apply for treatment purposes. ARRA has also affected the "minimum necessary" concept. Under Subtitle D, section 13405, further guidance is forthcoming from the secretary of HHS, with a potential definition change. Because the Privacy Rule is generously permissive regarding the disclosure of PHI for TPO purposes, it can be expected that this permissiveness will continue among healthcare organizations that are affiliated with one another in some way. Indeed, this is the case. "Affiliated," a HIPAA term of art, cannot be used loosely. Under the Privacy Rule, an "affiliated CE" is a legally separate CE affiliated with the CE by common ownership or control. These legally separate entities may recognize themselves as a single CE as long as this is referenced in writing (45 CFR 164.105). Similar in concept is the term "organized healthcare arrangement," which involves "more than one CE who share PHI to manage and benefit their common enterprise and are recognized by the public as a single entity" (45 CFR 164.103). It is likely that a medical practice may possess either an "affiliated CE" or "organized healthcare arrangement" with one or more inpatient facilities. As such, to foster the exchange of information in furtherance of timely and high-quality patient care, authorization requirements are waived.

Related to the sharing of PHI between treatment providers is the accessibility of health information in the event of a disaster. Initiated by the Veterans Administration, the national Health Data Repository database provides immediate access to local data on a national basis for disaster preparedness purposes. Figure 9.14, a decision tool created by the OCR, addresses the disclosure of health information for emergency preparedness (Odom-Wesley et al. 2009, 273).

HIPAA Security Regulations

HIPAA's information security regulations are technology-neutral and emphasize accountability over technology, including documentation of information security processes and policies. They apply to every healthcare provider, facility, plan, and clearinghouse (that is, CE) that

Figure 9.14. Decision tool

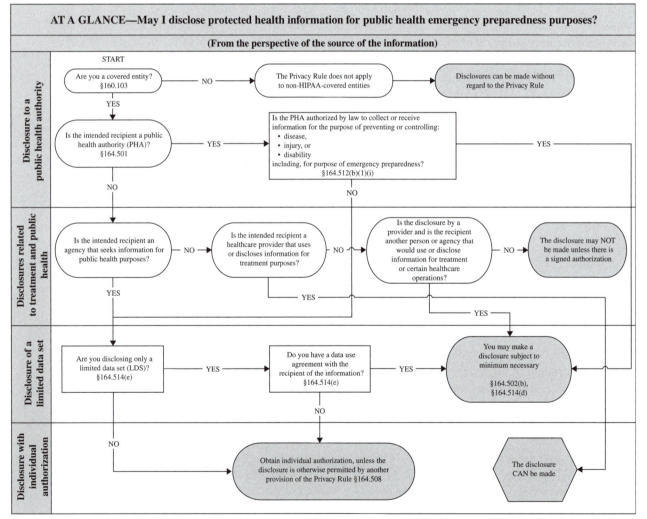

electronically creates, maintains, or transmits individually identifiable healthcare information in the handling of electronic information. The regulations apply specifically to health information and not to marketing- or business-related information unless it contains information about a unique individual. The security regulations apply only to electronic information; however, reports that are printed for storage in a paper-based record are covered by the regulations if they originally were created in a computer-based system (for example, computer-based transcription and imaging systems). Paper-based health records that are not created, stored, or transmitted electronically are not covered by HIPAA security standards (Fuller 2000, 4). Safeguards must be established that are physical, technical, and administrative in nature.

Policy Development

The medical practice must document and follow a specific policy on the processing of electronic records. The policy should address the receipt, manipulation, storage, dissemination, transmission, and destruction of patient-identifiable healthcare information. The organization's policy on record processing should answer the following questions (Fuller 2000, 12):

- Who is responsible for the maintenance of electronic record systems?
- How is the receipt of electronic records documented?
- What records are kept to document the electronic transmittal of information?

Further, every medical practice should have an access control policy that facilitates legitimate access to patient-identifiable information at the same time that it ensures the privacy of patients and the confidentiality of healthcare information. The policy should include information on how authorization is granted and how and when it can be modified or terminated. Healthcare organizations usually create an access grid that delineates the various levels of authorization required to access confidential information, from complete access to read-only access to access prohibited. The grid should clearly indicate the users who are authorized to access the different types of information. The access control policy also should address how the access grid is to be developed and maintained, as well as how users are to be informed about which information and applications they are authorized to access and which information and applications they are not permitted to access. Moreover, the access control policy should describe how access is to be protected (Fuller 2000, 13). It should answer the following questions:

- How will the identity of legitimate users be authenticated?
- How will access to protected applications be limited to authorized users?
- What security and confidentiality training will users receive?
- How will the access control system be maintained and kept up-to-date? (Fuller 2000, 13)

Whatever the procedure for keeping the access control system up-to-date, maintenance procedures should be documented in the access control policy. Organizations must maintain records of all security transactions (for example, modification or termination of access authorizations) and audit logs. Internal audit procedures must be described in the organization's access control policy and must specify who will be responsible for conducting audits and what actions will be taken when security violations are identified.

Contingency Planning

The HIPAA security regulations require contingency planning in three areas to protect the integrity of electronic health information: data backup, emergency mode operation, and disaster recovery. They also emphasize the need to test and revise contingency plans on an ongoing basis.

The first step in contingency planning is to identify the data and applications most critical to the operation of the healthcare organization. With this information, a data backup plan can be developed to ensure that the organization is able to access critical data and applications during times of crisis (for example, computer system failures, power failures, natural disasters, fires, down phone lines, or the aftermath of accidents or vandalism). The data backup plan should stipulate how often the health information system should be backed up, how much information should be backed up, who will perform the backup, and where the backup files will be stored.

A plan for emergency mode operation also should be developed to address how the organization would operate during a crisis:

- Which systems would be supported by emergency power sources? How long would the emergency power last?

- How long would it take to bring up the backup system for accessing critical computer-based data and applications?

- What hardware alternatives would be in place to support the emergency backup information system?

- What would be the process for switching to manual information management procedures, if necessary? Would the resources be adequate (for example, paper forms)?

- Would the staff know how to use the manual system? (Fuller 1999, 39–40)

The disaster recovery plan should address how long it would take vendors to replace damaged hardware and software so that the organization can return to normal operations. After contingency planning is complete, the organization must develop a written process for the periodic testing and revision of the contingency plans.

At some point in the useful life of every information system, the computer hardware will need to be replaced. Information technology is evolving rapidly, and computer systems often become obsolete only a few years after they were implemented. In addition, new and improved versions of software programs are issued every few years. Hardware and software conversions put the integrity of healthcare data at risk, and procedures should be in place to ensure that the data are backed up before the conversion and then tested afterward.

User training for new hardware and software should always be performed on test data and not on live data. The mistakes that inevitably occur during training should never be allowed to affect the quality of the organization's data. Version control for software applications, tables, and data definitions also should be maintained to ensure that data are not corrupted by other features of the system.

Managing the Information Security Program

The HIPAA security regulations require medical practices to assign responsibility for managing its information security program to a specific individual and require the development and maintenance of an information security policy that includes risk analysis, risk management, sanctions against security violations, and system configuration, as well as the contingency plans discussed earlier in this section. Although no specific qualifications for the information security officer are stipulated in the HIPAA regulations, a medical practice should look beyond technical expertise to identify an individual who understands the use and flow of information in the medical practice, as well as the requirements of state and federal regulations and accreditation standards that apply to the confidentiality of healthcare information. Just as important is a demonstrated commitment to the integrity and confidentiality of healthcare information (Fuller 2000, 16). HIPAA recognizes that policy alone cannot adequately protect the integrity and confidentiality of electronic patient-identifiable information. All of the management safeguards instituted to protect paper-based health information must apply equally to electronic health information. Employee training is critical, as are adequate physical security measures, access and authorization controls, and technical security measures specific to computer-based clinical information systems.

Common technical security measures include the use of encryption, password-based access controls, and audit trails. HIPAA security regulations require that health information systems include integrity controls and message authentication mechanisms when the information system is part of a larger network or includes other communications features such as Internet links and e-mail. Integrity controls are technical security mechanisms that ensure messages are not altered during transmission. Message authentication features typically use a code to ensure that the message received matches the message sent (Fuller 2000, 22).

Finally, information systems should include alarm systems and entity authentication features. An *alarm* is any device that can sense an abnormal condition within the system and issue a signal that indicates the nature of the problem. For example, an alarm might signal that the network server has crashed. *Entity authentication* is a network mechanism that confirms that an entity (user, program, or process) is who or what it says it is and then authorizes the entity to transmit electronic information via the network. Entity authentication prevents messages from going to the wrong system or computer via the organization's internal network or an external communications line.

Check Your Understanding 9.3

Instructions: Select the phrase that best completes the following statements.

1. It is best practice for a medical practice to make the presumption that _____.

   a. all patient-identifiable information is protected health information
   b. no patient-identifiable information is protected health information
   c. only a patient's history is protected health information
   d. none of the above

2. Individual rights afforded by the HIPAA Privacy Rule include the right to _____.

   a. change one's health record
   b. request restrictions
   c. receive one's original health record
   d. all of the above

(continued on next page)

> **Check Your Understanding 9.3 (continued)**
>
> 3. Under the HIPAA security regulations, contingency planning includes all of the following *except* _____.
>   a. data backup
>   b. emergency mode operation
>   c. recovery of marketing information
>   d. disaster recovery
>
> 4. Regarding disclosure of PHI for treatment purposes, the HIPAA Privacy Rule _____.
>   a. is permissive
>   b. is very restrictive
>   c. does not articulate a position
>   d. permits disclosure only to affiliated covered entities
>
> 5. An access control policy that facilitates legitimate access only to patient-identifiable information is an example of what type of mechanism?
>   a. Security
>   b. Privacy
>   c. Permissive
>   d. None of the above

Medical Identity Theft

A rapidly evolving threat to health providers, payers, and patients alike is the phenomenon of medical identity theft. Taking elements of both healthcare fraud and identity theft, medical identity theft is defined as the assumption of a person's name and/or other identifiers without the victim's knowledge or consent (a) in order to procure medical services or goods or (b) to falsify claims for medical services. The danger central to medical identity theft is the alteration of one's health information or the insertion of incorrect information in a victim's health record. In a tumultuous economy where the numbers of uninsured are increasing daily, medical identity theft is being committed by the uninsured to receive covered medical services under another's name, either with or without that individual's consent. In any case, both a victim's financial and medical information is negatively impacted. Committed by either individuals external to a medical practice or by individuals working within a medical practice, there are a number of steps that can be taken to prevent, detect, and remediate medical identity theft. However, dealing with the threat of external medical identity theft (for example, verifying the identity of patients who present for service) is different than addressing internal identity theft (for example, conducting appropriate background checks on prospective employees and employing audit trails to detect inappropriate access to electronic health information).

With a planned implementation of June 1, 2010, the Federal Trade Commission's red flag rules mandate that financial institutions and creditors develop and implement procedures that identify, detect, and respond to "red flags" or triggers that may indicate the presence of identity theft. Although the red flag rules are not specific to medical identity theft, they will play an important role in the healthcare arena as many providers meet the "creditor" definition by regularly extending, renewing, or continuing credit to individuals or organizations. The Federal Trade Commission has identified five categories that would trigger action. These categories are: (1) alerts, notification, or warnings from a consumer reporting agency; (2) suspicious documents; (3) suspicious personally identifying information such as a suspicious address; (4) unusual use of, or suspicious activity relating to, a covered account; and (5) notices from customers, victims of identity theft, law enforcement authorities, or other businesses about possible identity theft in connection with an account.

These steps, in addition to changes to the HIPAA Privacy Rule (pursuant to the HITECH Act of the American Recovery and Reinvestment Act) that will require payment disclosures to be included in an accounting of disclosures, will begin to identify instances of medical identity theft. However, continued measures will have to be taken to address those incidents that remain undetected despite these changes in the law.

A medical identity theft checklist, which offers consumer guidance in the event of a medical identity theft, may be found in the Sample Forms folder on the CD-ROM accompanying this book.

Conclusion

Like all other types of healthcare organizations, medical practices are subject to liability for improper health record maintenance and documentation. Defining the elements of the legal health record and ensuring appropriate documentation practices are key components in a risk management program that effectively minimizes organizational liability.

Medical practices also risk consequences for failure to adequately follow rules and regulations established by the government with regard to Medicare billing and health information privacy and security. A number of government agencies, including the Department of Health and Human Services and the Federal Bureau of Investigation, are charged with investigating fraud and abuse activities within the healthcare industry. The Department of Health and Human Services, Office of Civil Rights is also responsible for investigating alleged violations of HIPAA. Medical practices can help avoid sanctions by establishing compliance programs that enable them to self-regulate their efforts in appropriate billing and the development of policies and procedures that protect patient information, while continuing to operate at the highest possible level of service.

References

45 CFR 160.103(3): Definitions. 2008 (Jan. 1).

45 CFR 160.203: General rule and exceptions. 2008 (Jan. 1).

45 CFR 164.103: Definitions. 2008 (Jan. 1).

45 CFR 164.105: Organizational requirements. 2008 (Jan. 1).

45 CFR 164.501: Definitions. 2008 (Jan. 1).

AHIMA Compliance Task Force. 1999. Practice brief: Seven steps to corporate compliance: The HIM role. *Journal of AHIMA* 70(9):84A–84F.

AHIMA e-HIM Work Group on Defining the Legal Health Record. 2005. Practice brief: The legal process and electronic health records. *Journal of AHIMA* 76(9):96A–96D.

American Recovery and Reinvestment Act (ARRA) of 2009. Public Law 111-5.

Brodnik, M., M. McCain, L. Rinehart-Thompson, and R. Reynolds. 2009. *Fundamentals of Law for Health Informatics and Information Management.* Chicago: AHIMA.

Centers for Medicare and Medicaid Services. 2008. The Medicare recovery audit contractor (RAC) program: An evaluation of the 3-year demonstration. http://www.cms.gov/RAC/Downloads/RACEvaluationReport.pdf.

Centers for Medicare and Medicaid Services. 2009a. Mission, vision & goals: Overview. http://www.cms.gov/MissionVisionGoals.

Centers for Medicare and Medicaid Services. 2009b. Office of Benefits Integrity. http://cms.gov.

Centers for Medicare and Medicaid Services. 2009c. RAC expansion schedule. http://www.cms.gov/RAC/Downloads/RAC%20Expansion%20Schedule%20Web.pdf.

Federal Rules of Evidence (803). 2008 (Dec. 1). http://judiciary.house.gov/hearings/printers/110th/evid2008.pdf.

Fuller. 1999. Implementing HIPAA security standards: Are you ready? *Journal of AHIMA* 70(9):39–44.

Fuller. 2000. *Information Security: HIPAA Sets the Standard.* Chicago: AHIMA.

Joint Commission. 2009. Sentinel event. http://www.jointcommission.org/SentinelEvents.

National Health Care Anti-Fraud Association. 2009. http://www.nhcaa.org.

National Quality Forum. 2009. http://www.qualityforum.org.

Odom-Wesley, B., D. Brown, and C.L. Meyers. 2009. *Documentation for Medical Records.* Chicago: AHIMA.

Office of Inspector General. 2008. An Open Letter to Health Care Providers, April 15, 2008. http://oig.hhs.gov/fraud/docs/openletters/OpenLetter4-15-08.pdf.

Office of Inspector General. 2009a. Office of Audit Services. http://www.oig.hhs.gov/organization/oas.

Office of Inspector General. 2009b. Office of Investigations. http://www.oig.hhs.gov/organization/oi.

Office of Inspector General. 2009c (March 31). *OIG Semiannual Report to Congress.*

Office of Inspector General. 2009d. An Open Letter to Health Care Providers, March 24, 2009. http://oig.hhs.gov/fraud/docs/openletters/OpenLetter3-24-09.pdf.

Office of Inspector General. 2009e. OIG's 2010 Work Plan. http://oig.hhs.gov/publications/docs/workplan/2010/Work_Plan_FY_2010.pdf.

Office of the National Coordinator for Health Information Technology. 2004 (July 21). The decade of health information technology: Delivering consumer-centric and information-rich health care. Washington, DC.

Servais, C. 2008. *The Legal Health Record.* Chicago: AHIMA.

Showalter, J.S. 2008. *The Law of Healthcare Administration,* 5th ed. Chicago: Health Administration Press.

Resources

45 CFR 160 Subpart B: Preemption of state law. 2008 (Jan. 1).

American Health Information Management Association. 2010. *Pocket Glossary for HIM and Technology,* 2nd ed. Chicago: AHIMA.

Health Information Technology for Electronic and Clinical Health (HITECH) Act (ARRA): Public Law 111-5, Subtitle D, section 13405.

Chapter 10

Consumer-Driven Implications

Bryon D. Pickard, MBA, RHIA

Learning Objectives

- Describe the consumer's role in healthcare decision making

- Explain how key stakeholders contribute to healthcare decisions impacting consumers

- Discuss and explain how consumers can utilize health information in the home

- Describe the methodology for determining medical practice prices, and the impact of pricing on consumer decision making

- Identify medical practice policy considerations for responding to uninsured customers

- Understand the opportunities and challenges associated with personal health records

- Name several examples of retail medical centers and some of the benefits of retail healthcare

- Understand and discuss the essential core elements making up the medical home

Key Terms

Actuarial model
Allowable amount
American Recovery and
    Reinvestment Act of 2009
    (ARRA)
Beneficiary
Benefit level
Benefits
Capitation
Centers for Medicare and
    Medicaid Services (CMS)
Charge
Coinsurance
Consolidated Omnibus
    Budget Reconciliation Act
    of 1975 (COBRA)

Consumer
Consumer-directed (driven)
    healthcare
Consumer-directed (driven)
    healthcare plan (CDHP)
Conversion factor
Copayment
Coverage
Current Procedural
    Terminology (CPT)
Customer
Deductible
Electronic health record
    (EHR)
Evaluation and management

Fair Debt Collections
    Practices Act (FDCPA)
Federal poverty level (FPL)
Fee
Fee schedule
Flexible spending account
    (FSA)
Geographic practice cost
    index (GPCI)
Global fee
Group practice
Healthcare provider
Health maintenance
    organization (HMO)
Health plan

Health reimbursement account (HRA)

Health savings account (HSA)

High deductible health plan (HDHP)

Hospital-based practice

Insurance

Legal health record

Managed care organization (MCO)

Medical home

Open enrollment

Out-of-pocket costs

Personal health record (PHR)

Physician-office based

Place of service

Point-of-service collections

Point-of-service plan

Preferred provider organization (PPO)

Premium

Pricing transparency

Primary care

Professional component (PC)

Provider

Relative value unit (RVU)

Retail healthcare

Retail medical center

Solo practice

State Children's Health Insurance Program (SCHIP)

Technical component (TC)

Third-party payer

Visit

Introduction

It is perhaps not surprising that to a great extent, healthcare and healthcare decisions begin and occur in the home. Consumer expectations and perception of care can have a great influence on the type and level of healthcare provided. At least that is the manner in which consumer-driven healthcare is supposed to function, placing greater decision-making power in the hands of individual consumers.

What You Should Know

Throughout history, U.S. society offers a number of valuable examples of effective home routines, treatments, and self-help systems to improve and perpetuate individual consumer healthcare. In many households it is commonplace for mothers and other family caregivers to stress the importance of preventive care at an early age, making sure children brush their teeth and visit the dentist and family doctor for a checkup every six to twelve months. It is common for mothers to be a source of trusted healthcare guidance, and quick to offer a warm blanket and a hot bowl of soup to make their children feel better whenever they are sick or feeling under the weather. Turning to sympathetic caregivers or trusted medical providers for their expertise, guidance, and comfort is just the way it is. This kind of paternalistic approach to healthcare decision making illustrates the manner in which consumers have historically acquiesced and taken a backseat role when making healthcare choices.

Growing up, healthy behaviors are often stressed and the familiar saying *an apple a day keeps the doctor away* is a regular expression in many consumer households. While adding an apple a day to our daily menu may not necessarily circumvent the need to see a doctor, this simple well-known phrase nonetheless offers sage advice to consumers in regards to the importance of including fresh fruits and vegetables for maintaining a healthy balanced and nutritional diet.

In addition to such preventive measures, there are literally thousands of alternative medicine techniques and natural treatments looked upon by consumers to alleviate and cure the most common of ailments. There are individual self-care home remedies for such things as headaches, various aches and pains, fevers, the common cold, and even hiccups. In fact, in today's information-rich environment, consumers can very easily get hold of an array of self-help guidance to most health concerns or questions by simply logging onto the nearest computer. All it takes is to point and click and any user can launch an inquiry in relation to any sign or symptom on any number of easy-to-access Internet search engines. Nowadays, consumers can even research the difference between those exasperating hiccups and a trained clinician's professional diagnosis of synchronous diaphragmatic flutter (even if abbreviated as SDF, and even if specified alternatively as singulitis). Today, the list of available options consists of a multitude of reliable resources and Web sites, with smart tools, hyperlinked blogs, online health guides, and in-home testing devices available to consumers.

While making use of accessible informational resources may sound like a simple enough task, with so many health information resources available and so many choices to consider, it is easy to observe how consumers might feel anxious and uncomfortable in this role. Throw in the demanding schedules experienced in so many of today's hectic consumer households, and it is quite understandable that consumers could become distracted or overwhelmed. There is little debate that health information tools, technology improvements, and increased involvement of consumers offer tremendous opportunity for individuals to become more effective in managing their personal health and healthcare. At the same time, this can quickly sprout new demands and additional responsibilities on top of everything else that fills our lives.

Significant research exists offering insight into the interconnectedness of health information and consumer behavior, as well as some of the challenges consumers face associated with organizing, storing and effectively utilizing this information. A report in the *Journal of the American Medical Informatics Association* summarizes various goals and individual uses of personal health information in consumer households (Moen and Brennan 2005). Some of the more frequent goals for managing health information in the household include but are not limited to the following:

- Prevention—dental exams, flu shots, immunizations, fitness, screenings, to name a few

- Health issues—arthritis, cancer, diabetes, cardiovascular disease and other chronic illness, respiratory problems, nutritional concerns, mental health, and so forth

- Self-assessment—identifying and securing appropriate healthcare services given constraints of access, insurance coverage, ability to pay, and language skills

Certainly the activities and do-it-yourself way of managing personal healthcare will carry consumers far toward better understanding diagnoses and treatments, and becoming better overall stewards of their own healthcare. With that said, even the most savvy well-versed consumers gain value and have need of professional medical advice and the services of physicians, hospitals, emergency departments, medical clinics, and the like. Informed consumers are wise to seek out physicians or other professional healthcare providers whenever in doubt about personal health and specific medical conditions—and of course, when becoming seriously ill. A relationship with a professional healthcare provider is advantageous not only for treating life-threatening illnesses, but for recommending good preventative care as well.

What's Next

The healthcare landscape of the 21st century is on course to transform right before our eyes, and is dramatically changing healthcare from what we as consumers are accustomed to. National and worldwide factors such as economic upheaval and recession, rapidly soaring and uncontrolled healthcare costs, growing ranks of the uninsured, aging populations, and continual advances in technology are creating a perfect storm. The federal government is exploring alternatives to reform healthcare to expand coverage and reduce costs, and attempting to do so without completely restraining free market innovation. The unknowns are plentiful and the outlook is uncertain.

We are at a unique point in history and the success or failure of the future of U.S. healthcare places the consumer and the ability to manage, understand, and effectively use health information right in the middle—the proverbial eye of the storm. At the same time, a number of emerging forces and trends are enabling consumers to take a more active role in decision making, to ask the right questions, and affect the choices made about their own health and healthcare rather than just being passive participants of the past.

Establishing a Menu of Services

In general, the more active role consumers take in their own personal healthcare, the better likelihood for favorable healthcare outcomes and overall improved health over a lifetime. So what goes into the decision-making process for taking on a more active role and becoming more engaged? What information do consumers need, and what are some of the implications?

A Big-Picture Perspective

First, let's be very clear about something, and that is, healthcare is big business. Healthcare in the United States is extraordinarily expensive, and costs are steadfastly rising, now representing over 17 percent of the gross national product, and in 2009 the National Coalition on Health Care reported that national health spending for that year was expected to reach $2.5 billion (NCHC 2009). What's more, there are also wide disparities in both the actual quantity and quality of healthcare provided. In addition to the choices made by individual consumers themselves, a number of other key stakeholders contribute to healthcare decisions impacting consumers. Some of the other primary stakeholders referred to include a broad spectrum of physicians, specialists, and other nonphysician medical professionals, as was fully described in chapter 2. Other chief participants impacting consumer preferences and subsequent choices comprise insurance companies, employers, various government entities, and countless others. The actual menu of services and buffet of options to be had and shared by each of these stakeholders are quite interrelated, yet contrast to a great extent depending on the individual motivations and viewpoints of each. Let's take a closer look at some of these individual stakeholder perspectives.

Consumer Perspective

Earlier we stated that individual expectations and perceptions are key drivers for consumers in making healthcare choices. That is to say, individual consumers are ultimately responsible for making decisions about their own health. Oftentimes socioeconomic standing and employment status can also influence healthcare decision making, and ultimately may be a considerable predictor of one's current and long-term health status. Because of the manner in which healthcare is paid for, whoever foots the bill often has a deciding factor in the menu of services offered to consumers, as well as what amount of healthcare is ultimately consumed.

Today, employer-sponsored health coverage represents approximately 60% of the total U.S. population. Add in federal and state government insurance coverage and this figure shoots up to 85%. The other 15% of the population that remains corresponds to those individuals not covered by formal health insurance, a sizable figure approximating upwards of 46 million U.S. citizens (DeNavas et al. 2007). The combination of such aspects as employment status and healthcare coverage has been a common association for years. Even workers who lose their job or find themselves between jobs frequently seek to maintain the lower-cost group health coverage made accessible to consumers during periods of personal unemployment. Unemployed workers may accomplish this by seeking COBRA (Consolidated Omnibus Budget Reconciliation Act) insurance coverage. COBRA is a health insurance benefit mandated by federal law that provides continued health coverage that otherwise would be discontinued when a worker terminates employment. An economic stimulus plan designated as the American Recovery and Reinvestment Act (ARRA) of 2009, passed by the federal government, expands COBRA benefits and reduces premium costs for unemployed workers (EBSA 2009).

Open Enrollment

Over the past several years, the months making up the latter part of the year have become a point on the calendar marked as open enrollment season for large numbers of insured consumers. This is the time of year when scores of employees and other eligible participants look over their employer's benefit offerings and make decisions as to which health insurance plan best meets their individual needs. For those with dependents, the annual drill is much the same when considering family coverage. In most cases, when evaluating employer benefit offerings, there is usually a wide range of health plan options presented. Deciphering the menu of available services and confirming which selections make the most sense has become an annual event, regardless of the actual point in the year it occurs.

Table 10.1 provides a comparison of two health plan options an employee might be faced with in selecting health benefits for an upcoming year. Note the actual coverage for medical services and prescription drug coverage is quite similar for each health insurance plan. Although some differences exist, the primary distinction between the two benefit plan options presented in the example center on the dollar amounts for premiums and annual deductibles.

Table 10.1. Health benefit plan comparison

Description of Coverage	Benefit Plan Option A	Benefit Plan Option B
Premium (Annual)		
Individual	$492	$768
Family	$2,112	$3,540
Deductible (Annual)		
Individual	$750	$300
Family	$1,500	$600
Out-of-Pocket Maximum (Annual)		
Individual	$3,500	$2,500
Family	$7,000	$5,000
Medical Services:		
Preventive Visit	$30 copay	$30 copay
Physician Office Visit	$30 copay	$30 copay
Mental Health Visit	$30 copay	$30 copay
Emergency Room Visit	$100 copay; then 30% after deductible	$100 copay; then 20% after deductible
Hospital Inpatient	30% after deductible	20% after deductible
Prescription Drugs	$15–$50	$15–$50
Generic	$15	$15
Formulary	$35	$35
Non-Formulary	$50	$50

When selecting a benefit plan, employees must decide how much they can afford and how much they are willing to pay in monthly health insurance premiums. As you can see from table 10.1, these amounts vary a great deal, depending on whether single or family coverage is being considered. Premiums are the upfront amount paid in order to enroll and receive health insurance coverage. Deductibles are the out-of-pocket dollar amount consumers pay each year for medical services prior to a health plan beginning to pay. The deductible amount must be met in each 12-month cycle.

A challenge for consumers is predicting the amount of health services necessary in an upcoming year. Consumers must decide whether it makes sense to select lower premiums in the short term in hopes that minimal healthcare services will occur with the higher deductible plan option. Also, dental and vision benefit plans are often carved out as separate benefit options and may or may not be included in an employer's standard package. Selecting benefit plan options is often a case of making a choice of paying a high or low upfront premium and levels of risk associated with known or unknown health expenses that lie ahead.

The same annual election period described holds true for various government-sponsored health coverages as well. Each year Medicare-eligible beneficiaries must also carry out the task of considering the many choices and deciding amongst the assortment of healthcare coverage plans offered. Medicare advantage plans, supplemental insurance, and prescription drug plans often follow the similar annual timeframes for making coverage selections. While Medicare Part A and Part B provide basic coverage for respective categories of care, Medicare advantage plans offer an expanded menu of available options for beneficiaries to select.

Understanding healthcare processes, the funding of healthcare services, and the many coverage choices available is becoming more and more complex, but this understanding is becoming increasingly necessary to effectively navigate the healthcare system. Informed consumers are better able to become partners in the healthcare decision-making process throughout a lifetime. Knowledgeable individuals and professionals who can decipher all this information are nicely positioned to provide valuable assistance to consumers in a number of roles and work settings.

Employer Perspective

As stated earlier, companies make healthcare benefits available for their employees to choose. Providing healthcare benefits to workers is a cost of doing business for U.S. companies, and to be profitable, organizations must strike a balance of providing competitive healthcare benefits while effectively managing costs. During tough economic times, the cost of healthcare can become an excessive burden on an organization's bottom line and its ability to meet workforce expectations. As we see in figure 10.1, the annual premium an employer pays to a health plan averaged $12,700 in 2008 for workers with dependents selecting family coverage. Of that amount, employed workers contributed $3,400 on average, or approximately a quarter of the annual premium amount necessary to receive insurance coverage (NCHC 2008). Note the premium amount for family coverage is actually higher than the annual pay of a minimum

Figure 10.1.   Employer and employee health insurance costs

Annual Premiums—U.S. Average for 2008	
Family Coverage	$12,700
Single Coverage	$4,700
Full-time Minimum Wage—Annual Gross Pay	$10,712

Source: NCHC 2008.

wage worker. Just like employees who must manage their own personal bank accounts and expenses, companies seek to achieve the most benefit out of their limited healthcare dollars. By the same token, proactive employers also understand that employees who lead healthier lifestyles are more apt to be further productive on the job.

In an effort to beat the rising cost of healthcare and avoid dropping health benefits altogether, many employers have increasingly sought out new strategies to achieve cost-sharing plans with employees to balance organization costs with workforce coverage expectations. With the increasing popularity and expansion of consumer-directed healthcare products, the thought is that as employees contribute more and more out of pocket, they are more apt to be conservative and will turn out to be better consumers and more engaged participants in their own healthcare. In other words, provide shared incentives to employees for accomplishing mutual goals directed at becoming more active with exercise, eating healthier foods, and initiating steps to take care of themselves.

We already discussed some of the factors consumers utilize in their selection of employer health benefit options and deciding on levels of health coverage. Traditional coverage plans designed to reimburse for healthcare expenditures have given way to several innovative and emerging types of insurance products. Many of the more contemporary health insurance products employers are now making available to their workers include alternative types of consumer-directed health plan options. These plans offer numerous tax advantages, and are designed and marketed with the intent to increase transparency and cost sharing with consumers. Some of the more common consumer-directed health plan products are described as follows:

- Flexible spending account (FSA)—employer- or employee-funded accounts using pretax contributions that can be used to pay for various healthcare and dependent care expenses. Savings are achieved by reducing taxable income and the amount of taxes paid.

- Health reimbursement account (HRA)—employer-funded accounts that pay employees for medical expenses not covered by the employer's health plan. Employees gain an advantage from the additional funds made available to cover medical expenses, and employers benefit since the distributions are considered tax deductible.

- Health savings account (HSA)—employer- or consumer-funded accounts using pretax contributions that are used to pay deductible and other health expenses. The HSA may also be referred to as a health spending account. Savings are achieved by reducing taxable income and the amount of taxes paid.

- High deductible health plan (HDHP)—an insurance coverage option offering lower premiums and higher deductibles in comparison to traditional health plan options. Refer back to Option A in table 10.1 as an example HDHP. This option is also commonly referred to as a consumer-directed health plan. Participation in these plans is a requirement for health savings accounts and other tax-advantaged programs.

While many advocates of consumer-directed health plans contend these products achieve savings by placing greater responsibility for decision making with the consumer, others argue that the primary reason and subsequent impact is to shift greater percentages of the cost from the employer back to the consumer. Regardless of individual perspectives, it is indeed true that these plans encourage consumers to assume greater financial responsibility for their healthcare. Conversely, some industry experts express concerns these plans may incentivize individual consumers to forgo beneficial healthcare services. The jury is still out and time will tell if this holds true, as well as whether there is an overall satisfaction with these plans.

In addition to healthcare coverage, some businesses go even further by offering innovative means to actively encourage behavioral changes and improved personal health habits of employees. Some organizations offer added incentives and targeted messages to workers, aimed at improving overall health and wellness, along with mechanisms to better utilize health services more efficiently. Annual health risk assessments, smoking cessation programs, healthy food options, walking programs, on-site fitness centers, and wellness reimbursements have become the norm for many employers. These businesses believe they can achieve more of a return on their investment with greater focus directed toward keeping employees well, rather than strictly focusing on healthcare coverage expenditures for treating employees after they become ill.

Health Plan Perspective

For the most part, employers look to health plans and the insurance payer community to administer their healthcare coverage benefit programs for employees and covered dependents. Self-employed individuals and other consumers who are not covered by an employer's group healthcare coverage plan may seek out an individual policy. Because of the high price tag associated with healthcare premiums, many individuals and small businesses find this to be cost prohibitive. Just like other businesses and organizations, health insurance companies come in many alternative shapes, sizes, and corporate structures.

The various types of insurance products and levels of service offered by health plans are dependent upon sophisticated actuarial models and subsequent premium dollars collected. Behind-the-scenes probability modeling and detailed statistical analysis by professional actuaries enable health plans to evaluate assorted consumer risk scenarios to make future financial projections. Again, the actual fees employers and individual consumers pay for health plan services are referred to as health insurance premiums. Over the years, escalating levels of healthcare services to consumers have resulted in much increased costs and higher levels of premiums being charged by health plans.

Most health insurance companies today are commonly structured as a preferred provider organization (PPO), a health maintenance organization (HMO), a point of service (POS) plan, or some other hybrid. The customers of these health plans include both employer groups and individual consumers, and each are commonly referred to as enrollees or members. Some of the principal differences and similarities of these health plans are described as follows:

- Preferred provider organization (PPO)—managed care entity with contractual arrangements between physicians, hospitals, and other healthcare providers offering services to defined employer groups and health plan enrollees at reduced rates. PPO network providers are reimbursed based on the actual services provided, and consumers who receive services from noncontracted providers may usually do so at an added out-of-network expense.

- Health maintenance organization (HMO)—managed care entity that combines the provision of health insurance and the delivery of care by assigning each enrollee a primary care physician (PCP) to serve as a gatekeeper for healthcare services. PCPs are paid predetermined periodic fixed capitation payments for member coverage and are responsible for coordinating all healthcare services, including referrals for specialist care as needed. Unless prior approval is given, HMO members receiving healthcare services out-of-network usually must do so at their own expense. HMO membership is most always a lower-cost option for consumers, and because of the fixed method of reimbursement, HMO providers are incentivized to keep members healthy.

- Point of service (POS) plan—a form of managed care that may often be referred to as a hybrid between HMO and PPO options. Similar to HMOs, enrollees are obliged to select a primary care physician (PCP) who must complete a referral when specialist care becomes necessary. Like the PPO alternative, consumers may choose to see an out-of-network healthcare provider; however, most always this will be at additional out-of-pocket expense to the consumer.

There are many trade-offs to be considered when evaluating the various managed care organization (MCO) alternatives. The menu of services health insurance plans offer employers and consumers most always centers attention on such categories as ability to manage costs and financial well-being of the company or capacity for administering claims. Overall customer service, enrollee health management, and available technology offerings are important considerations as well. In fact, the accuracy and timeliness of claims administration is often considered by employers as the single most important deciding factor when selecting a health plan. Figure 10.2 lists several basic functions and specific features employers consider foremost when seeking to partner with a health plan or MCO (PricewaterhouseCoopers 2008).

Selecting a health insurance plan to associate with can have numerous short-term and long-term implications, both for employers and consumers. The role of health plans and the services they provide are certain to continue evolving to conform to any future healthcare reform movements, and to reduce costs and improve efficiencies in the overall U.S. healthcare industry. Data integrity and other health information principles play a key role for the insurance payer community and, once again, offer significant opportunities for those who invest in understanding the services health plans provide.

Physician Practice Perspective

Let's step back for a moment and glance at the menu of services through the eyes of the actual healthcare provider. Again, when we speak of healthcare providers we are not just talking about physicians. Rather, individual professionals, practices, or entities supplying healthcare services, medical equipment, or other health products are referred to as a healthcare provider. For the purposes of this chapter, however, we will continue to focus our attention on physicians and medical practices.

Figure 10.2.   What employers want from health plans

• Financial administrative fees	• Debit card interfaces at point of service
• Performance guarantees	• Disease management programs
• Provider discounts	• Wellness programs
• Accuracy & timeliness of claims	• Reporting capabilities
• Ability to view payments and eligibility online	• Preparation of risk profiles of certain populations
• Offering personal health records	
• Online tools to obtain pricing and quality information about physicians	

Source: PricewaterhouseCoopers 2008.

To be sure, physicians and other medical practices offering healthcare services also come in many sizes and legal business structures. A medical practice may run the gamut, from an individual solo practitioner or small group practice offering primary or specialty care, to large multispecialty group practices, to even larger multimillion dollar medical practice management corporations. While different forms of legal business structures may exist, medical practices generally fall into one of the following basic types of medical practice entities:

- Solo practice
- Group practice
- Large multispecialty group practice
- Medical practice management company

Each form of medical practice may provide no more than one unique clinical specialty service, or there may be a broad selection of diverse healthcare services and treatments made available. Again, the menu of services that exists will depend on the type and composition of providers making up a medical practice. So how does a medical practice or physician organization determine exactly what menu of services to offer?

It does not take a brain surgeon to understand that there are many factors that go into analyzing and then identifying the types of services to be provided by physicians. The more difficult challenge is cutting through all the details and making the right decisions in defining the precise menu of services. As an example, a recent medical school graduate embarking on a new career in medicine as a pediatric physician would probably not want to establish a practice in a retirement community. By the same token, establishing a geriatric medical practice in a community dominated with young families may lack for sought after patient volumes and probably will not be sustainable. Yet another example: while setting up a medical practice in a community experiencing job loss and economic decline may offer healing and comfort to the local population, it would certainly be advantageous to understand any potential monetary ramifications upfront rather than scrambling to deal with unexpected dire financial results after the fact.

A thorough market analysis is a good place to start when evaluating services to be rendered. It is essential to understanding basic consumer needs and potential opportunities of the healthcare marketplace. Understanding the environment and characteristics of a market service area and defining the consumer population—including the socioeconomic classes and median household incomes, as well as targeted consumer populations—are all essential elements in completing a market analysis. Equally important, is the need to consider the existence and strength of would-be competitors providing similar healthcare services, as well as potential payer mix and managed care penetration throughout the defined geographic target market area. For many physicians, employing the services of a professional consultant familiar with medical practices to complete a thorough analysis of market forces and other influential factors may be warranted.

A primary source of comparative demographic data for medical practices is readily available from the U.S. Census Bureau and includes a variety of pertinent social and economic indicators (U.S. Census Bureau 2009). Several of the most common market characteristics useful in evaluating consumer demographics are summarized in figure 10.3.

The National Center for Health Statistics, through the Department of Health and Human Services, Centers for Disease Control, offers a number of additional data tools and informational surveys useful for completing a market analysis. Numerous statistics and benchmark

Figure 10.3. Consumer market characteristics

• Population size	• Educational levels	• Occupations
• Age patterns	• Ethnic and racial makeup	• Poverty rate
• Sex ratios	• Housing characteristics	

Source: U.S. Census Bureau 2009.

information are readily available to medical practices, ranging from the most common symptoms of consumers by geographic area to the principle reasons consumers visit the doctor (Cherry et al. 2007).

Once the need for healthcare services has been defined and final practice location settled upon, a medical practice needs to determine hours of operation. Will services be provided by scheduled appointment, Monday through Friday, 9:00 a.m. to 5:00 p.m., or will walk-in patients be accepted 24 hours a day, seven days a week, including holidays? Medical practices must determine if they will also be operating a pharmacy for dispensing drugs and injections, or providing lab services or x-ray services. Some practices that perform procedures may even consider developing an ambulatory surgery center.

When all is said and done, and it is time to open the doors and hang out the shingle, Current Procedural Terminology and assigned CPT codes best describe the precise menu of services or treatments available. The actual services and treatments provided will be determined by the provider's expertise and training. We will discuss the role of CPT coding in describing services later in the chapter.

Check Your Understanding 10.1

1. Please name three (3) common goals of a consumer responsible for managing health information in the household.

   a. Check-ups and self-care, copayments, certification
   b. Deductibles, diet, healthcare purchasing decisions
   c. Insurance coverage, disease management, CPT coding
   d. Prevention, managing health issues, self-assessment

2. The dollar amount consumers pay in order to enroll and receive health insurance coverage with a health plan.

   a. Health reimbursement account
   b. Medical savings account
   c. Healthcare premium
   d. Coinsurance

3. Please name a common method health insurance plans utilize to evaluate consumer risk scenarios when establishing premium levels.

   a. Offer performance guarantees
   b. Develop actuarial models
   c. Evaluate practice expense
   d. Complete market analysis

(continued on next page)

Check Your Understanding 10.1 *(continued)*

4. When selecting a managed care organization to provide health coverage for employees, specific plan features considered most important might include
_____.

   a. provider discounts
   b. performance guarantees
   c. administration of claims
   d. all of the above

5. A course of action or mechanism undertaken to expand healthcare benefits and reduce premium costs for unemployed workers.

   a. American Recovery and Reinvestment Act
   b. Health savings account
   c. Supplemental insurance
   d. All of the above

Pricing Considerations

Back in chapters 2 and 6 we talked about the importance of documentation for professional services, along with several additional factors capable of impacting practice reimbursement and profitability. In this section, we will break pricing down a bit further and be more specific; namely, how does a medical practice go about determining what prices to charge? And also, what impact does medical practice pricing have on consumer decision making?

Historically, a lot of consumers have paid little attention to individual practice prices because of the manner in which healthcare services are reimbursed. Although a medical practice may charge everyone the same amount for a particular service, the actual cash payment received can be very different. The truth is, very few consumers, health plans, or other stakeholders actually pay the full prices that are charged. To better comprehend how prices are determined and how pricing information may be used, consumers and other stakeholders are well served by taking steps to better understand the terminology of pricing professional services. Even then, it remains difficult to get hold of much more than a ballpark estimate, as opposed to an exact price, when making decisions about healthcare. Price transparency is not a hallmark of the traditional healthcare environment within the United States, but speaking the same language is a good place to start.

Pricing Transparency

When we mention pricing transparency we are really referring to placing greater power into the hands of consumers by making information more readily available. The information we are talking about is not limited to price alone, but rather, more complete information enabling consumers to better understand what they are purchasing. In healthcare, greater transparency results in consumers being better able to evaluate cost in comparison to quality of care and expected outcomes as part of the decision-making process. Of course, just as in any industry or any other purchasing decision, there are numerous factors that can influence the actual consumer decision process and the eventual choice that is made.

For instance, let's share another example most are familiar with. Have you ever driven down the street in your automobile and noticed how each gas station you pass along the way broadly displays their fuel prices on full-size, eye-catching signs, totally transparent for all passers-by to see? Every so often gasoline stations sitting side-by-side on a roadway or on adjacent street corners may display an identical price. At other times the prices will be markedly different. Either way, now imagine you drive your car across town to yet another street corner, or return to the original gas station later in the same day, and you may even notice a different price posted openly on the huge signs. As a consumer, when you fill up the gas tank of your car or sports utility vehicle, you always know in advance the price you pay. Just like when consumers visit the grocery store or go shopping at the mall, prices are most always advertised and readily available. As we stated previously, such pricing transparency has not always been the case in healthcare.

Continuing with our gasoline pricing example, do you ever wonder if those big, openly displayed numbers with the dollar signs at the gas station are just pulled out of the air? Often it might seem that way; that there is little rhyme or reason to how gasoline prices are determined. Just ask the average consumer of healthcare how a physician or medical practice determines the price for services and you just might draw a similar perplexing look and glazed eyes.

The good news is this lack of pricing transparency in healthcare is beginning to change. Health insurance plans, government entities, and other third-party payers are making increased amounts of cost and quality information available to the public for various types of healthcare services. Later in the chapter we will also see how pricing transparency is changing as new entrants to the healthcare marketplace become more prevalent in providing services to consumers.

Determining Medical Practice Prices

So, let's get down to business and answer the question—how are prices established for the menu of services provided in a medical practice? As we alluded, Current Procedural Terminology and unique CPT codes are an essential element for pricing medical services. CPT codes represent the common denominator for describing the complete menu of services or treatments to be provided by a medical practice. The actual range of services may consist of a short list of CPT codes for a single physician, or the list might be quite extensive for a larger multispecialty medical group practice. While the services provided and actual prices (fees) charged for medical services may vary greatly from physician to physician and geographically from community to community, CPT codes represent a standard—a common language for documenting each service performed. An understanding of health record documentation and advanced knowledge of CPT coding rules are indispensible skills when it comes to developing and managing physician fee schedules.

To gain a better understanding and to further explain how physician services can be priced, let's spend a few moments talking about a second important ingredient: relative value units (RVUs). Most physician services are described by a descriptive numerical CPT code, and each CPT code in turn is assigned a corresponding relative value unit (RVU). Of course, there is an exception to every rule, so let's just note that for certain types of services such as anesthesia, dentistry, and orthodontics, and others there may be different mechanisms. For example, unique dental codes are utilized in dentistry and time units may be used in establishing anesthesia prices. Conversely, for the vast majority of descriptive CPT services, RVUs afford a basic framework for establishing prices.

There are three notable components making up an RVU, and the assigned values for each of these components are based on the amount of work, practice costs, and malpractice expense associated with each singular CPT code. For a novice, or the untrained eye of a consumer, this may seem like a complicated concept; however, the formula is really quite straightforward:

Work RVU + Practice Cost + Malpractice Expense = Total RVU

Table 10.2 offers an example of how this formula translates to assign RVU values for select services and CPT codes commonly found in medical practices. Note that each service carries its own distinctive RVU.

Once an RVU value is established for a particular service or CPT code, applying a conversion factor times the total RVU amount will result in a designated price. This price is generally referred to as the physician fee schedule amount for a particular CPT code. Make certain to note that a change in either RVU or the conversion factor will result in increasing or decreasing a set price:

Total RVUs × Conversion Factor (CF) = Price (Fee Schedule)

Using this RVU pricing formula, you will notice in table 10.3 that a separate price or fee schedule amount is produced for each of the matching CPT codes used in the prior example.

In fact, health plans and managed care organizations often utilize the very same methodology for calculating the contract price, or allowable amount physicians are reimbursed for each CPT code. The contracted price or allowed amount will vary depending on whether prenegotiated rates have been agreed upon and at what dollar amount between the physician and the payer. The dollar value applied to the conversion factor will be a determining factor in the contracted price. In the case of Medicare, Medicaid, and other government payers, there is usually little or no opportunity for negotiation of a conversion factor and the resulting contracted price is offered on a take it or leave it basis.

CPT codes are organized into separate groupings, such as Evaluation & Management, Surgery, Radiology, Pathology, Medicine, and so forth. As a point of reference, tables 10.4–10.6 provide examples of pricing methodologies for alternative groupings of physician services. Again, make a note of the impact that changing the conversion factor has on establishing a price.

Table 10.2. Select CPT codes: Work RVU + Practice Cost + Malpractice Expense = Total RVU

CPT Code	Description of Service	Work RVU	Practice Cost	Malpractice Expense	Total RVU
10060	Drainage of skin abscess	1.19	1.48	0.12	2.79
92004	Eye exam, new patient	1.82	1.62	0.04	3.48
99203	Office or other outpatient visit, new patient	1.34	1.12	0.09	2.55

Source: CMS 2009b.

Table 10.3. Select CPT codes: Total RVUs × Conversion Factor (CF) = Price (Fee Schedule)

CPT Code	Description of Service	Total RVU	Conversion Factor	Price
10060	Drainage of skin abscess	2.79	70	$195.30
92004	Eye exam, new patient	3.48	70	$243.60
99203	Office or outpatient visit, new patient	2.55	70	$178.50

Source: CMS 2009b.

Table 10.4. RVU examples—evaluation and management services

CPT Code	Description of Service	RVU	CF	Price
99201	Office or outpatient visit, new patient (Level 1)	0.65	70	$45.50
99202	Office or outpatient visit, new patient (Level 2)	1.25	70	$87.50
99203	Office or outpatient visit, new patient (Level 3)	1.89	70	$132.30
99204	Office or outpatient visit, new patient (Level 4)	3.16	70	$221.20
99205	Office or outpatient visit, new patient (Level 5)	4.11	70	$287.70

Source: CMS 2009b.

Table 10.5. RVU examples—radiology services

CPT Code	Description of Service	RVU	CF	Price
70450	Ct head/brain w/o dye	1.21	80	$96.80
70486	Ct maxillofacial w/o dye	1.61	80	$128.80
71010	Chest x-ray	0.25	80	$20.00
71020	Chest x-ray	0.31	80	$24.80
72100	X-ray exam of lower spine	0.31	80	$24.80

Source: CMS 2009b.

Table 10.6. RVU examples—surgery services

CPT Code	Description of Service	RVU	CF	Price
10060	Drainage of skin abscess	2.35	110	$258.50
11730	Removal of nail plate	1.56	110	$171.60
11750	Removal of nail bed	4.44	110	$488.40
17000	Destruct premalg lesion	1.35	110	$148.50
17003	Destruct premalg les, 2-14	0.12	110	$13.20

Source: CMS 2009b.

The Centers for Medicare and Medicaid Services (CMS) evaluates RVUs annually to determine the weighting and values given for each RVU, as well as an overall conversion factor. Also, because costs of practice may vary in different locales throughout the nation, RVU values may be adjusted regionally by way of a geographic practice cost index (GPCI). It is important to consider the impact of the GPCI toward increasing or lowering the values for each of the components making up an RVU when establishing fees (CMS 2009b).

Another important factor in determining a price is whether a medical practice will be considered as a hospital-based practice or physician-office practice. The place of service and whether procedures and services are classified as occurring in a facility or nonfacility setting are important elements in establishing prices. Because of the differences in practice expense for providing services in a hospital versus a nonfacility setting such as a physician office, RVU values may vary greatly. As a rule of thumb, if the place of service is a physician office, the RVU value for a particular procedure or service can be expected to be higher due the greater practice expense of providing that service. Conversely, similar services provided in a hospital or facility setting would result in a lower RVU due to not having to incur the full practice expense of providing the service, such as utility expenses and staff costs.

For each fee, the question needs to be answered whether the physician will be charging and billing for just the professional component (PC) fee or the technical component (TC) as well.

When both the professional component and the technical component are combined together, this is referred to as a global fee (GF).

Professional Component + Technical Component = Global Fee

When all is said and done, we need to keep in mind that for a majority of consumers with insurance coverage through their employer or by a government payer, the implications and final amount paid will be dependent upon a precontracted price to be paid for each service. Out-of-pocket expenses are determined by this contracted rate, or allowable amount, and not by the entire amount charged. Actual price differences between physicians have traditionally become less relevant to the consumer because of the payment methodologies, such as allowable amounts. In some cases, differing prices may have no material impact at all for those possessing insurance.

Having said that, increased movements toward greater pricing transparency and emerging reimbursement products, such as the high-deductible coverage plans, in response to the higher costs of healthcare have resulted in increased out-of-pocket portions being passed on to the consumer. This offers the potential of motivating consumers to become more active participants in evaluating physician services based on costs. Market competition and pricing sensitivity for certain procedures can play a role in how prices are established.

Policies Concerning Uninsured Customers

Earlier in the chapter we stated that approximately 85% of consumers are covered under some form of employer-based or various federal and state government-sponsored healthcare insurance programs. Even so, in 2008 there were still 46 million individuals throughout the country, representing approximately 15% of the U.S. population, who remain uninsured (DeNavas et al. 2007). In some states such as Texas and other southern states, as many as one out of four individuals are without health coverage. Given uncertainties in the economy and financial projections over the next several years, one can only surmise that the number of uninsured consumers will continue to grow. A number of industry experts and government forecasts expect this figure to continue to climb over the next decade without some form of additional government intervention.

Increased uninsured consumers coupled with rising out-of-pocket costs for the insured, create an environment where having formal policies and procedures is essential for a medical practice. Equivalent to the concern of the uninsured, are the class of consumers who do have health insurance, though still may be truly underinsured given the level and type of care needed. Increased amounts for deductibles, copayments, and coinsurance, along with possible spending caps, intensify the need for sound policies to oversee medical practice collection processes for all consumers—not just the uninsured. It is important to realize that out-of-pocket healthcare costs can add up to significant layers of additional expense for consumers and potential financial risk to physician practices.

The single largest factor resulting in personal bankruptcy is unmet healthcare expenses, often caused by unplanned accidents or illnesses. Even employed individuals covered by insurance may have every right to be concerned about financial security and might delay seeking needed treatments. Other consumers may possibly put off seeing a physician altogether, which could further worsen an existing medical condition.

Prioritizing patient care decisions, provider schedules, and potentially conflicting values of extending needed services while conserving economic resources and sustaining financial revenues of a practice can be especially challenging. Some medical practices may institute policies to deny providing services other than emergency care, while other practices may treat all consumers regardless of ability to pay. There are multiple circumstances that may result in a consumer being discharged or terminated from a medical practice, with nonpayment for services possibly being one such justification. Ending a physician–consumer relationship is usually an action of last resort after all other efforts have been exhausted. If terminating the relationship becomes necessary, good documentation and administering well thought out and approved policies in a consistent way can minimize potential legal implications.

It is also important for medical practices to know what is acceptable versus unacceptable practice when it comes to collection of self-pay balances from consumers. The Fair Debt Collections Practices Act (FDCPA) provides guidance to medical practices, professional collection agencies, and other third-party contractors on acceptable practices for collecting consumer debts (FTC 2006). This longstanding legislation was enacted to protect consumers from unreasonable collection activities, and there has been a number of other state and federal laws to protect consumers since. It is important for medical practice employees to incorporate and follow these guidelines as part of practice policies and procedures.

Point-of-Service Collections

A strategy gaining increased acceptance is the concept of point-of-service collections. The best opportunity for a medical practice to secure payment is either by prepayment in advance of providing a service or ensuring payment is received at the time a consumer is seen. This can be especially important when seeing consumers who lack insurance coverage. There are important lessons learned from having an effective point-of-service collection policy in place, and beyond just for the uninsured, too. First, increased numbers of health insurance plans are now able to provide just-in-time benefit eligibility determination and residual benefit levels such as unmet deductible amounts. Medical practices have been able to communicate with health plans by telephone or via payer Web sites to verify insurance coverage for some time. Nowadays, new technologies, transaction standards, and streamlined processes can make it easier to confirm actual benefit eligibility levels in order to provide more timely up-to-date financial information to consumers.

It is always better for consumers to know in advance when a particular procedure may not be covered or what payment is expected from unmet deductibles, copayments, and coinsurance. The more information made available upfront, the greater chance of making the best decision for both the consumer and the medical practice. If a practice can get their hands on this information in advance of providing treatment, they can communicate an expected payment amount to the consumer ahead of providing the actual service. This offers the added benefit to the consumer of informing them prior to performing the service what their expected out-of-pocket expense will total.

In some cases where services will not be covered by insurance, it might be appropriate for consumers to delay nonurgent treatment until a later date. Procedure eligibility based on age appropriateness, routinely found in consumer benefit program guidelines, could be just such a case. For instance, a typical example of this might include a mammogram for breast cancer screening for a 38-year old woman when the insurance authorized preventive eligibility age is 40. Another example might be the true necessity of a screening colonoscopy for a 49-year old. Even though suggested by a physician, it may be appropriate to hold off until a 50th birthday if that is the age eligibility requirement to obtain full coverage in a consumer's health benefit plan. Again, the best time to communicate financial policies or collect from a consumer is prior to the service being rendered or when the consumer is face-to-face with the medical practice staff.

Evaluating Financial Need

Another policy decision to consider is whether to expend practice resources to evaluate consumer financial situations to make sure consumers aren't eligible for one of the many state or federal government programs, such as Medicare, Medicaid, or the State Children's Health Insurance Program (SCHIP). Many states provide expanded coverage for consumers with incomes frequently ranging from 200 to 300 percent of the federal poverty level (HHS 2009). Some providers may also have policies in place offering discounts to uninsured patients, additional financial assistance, or charity care. These services are often based on these poverty guidelines. Figure 10.4 describes potential assistance eligibility for various income levels based on family size. Initiating conversations with consumers about their financial responsibility and education on any available options as early as possible is the best plan.

Some states even mandate an uninsured discount based on a variety of formulas using a weighted average of common managed care discounts. Still other medical practices may offer additional prompt pay discounts to secure quicker payments and reduce the added cost and delay of extended payment arrangements. Given the state of the economy in 2009, it only stands to reason that the ranks of the uninsured will continue to increase in the months and years before us. All the more reason for medical practices and other healthcare providers to have up-to-date policies in place for handling uninsured and out-of-pocket expenses of consumers.

Figure 10.4. 2009 Poverty guidelines

Persons in family	Poverty guideline	200% of Poverty guideline	300% of Poverty guideline
1	$10,830	$21,660	$32,490
2	$14,570	$29,140	$43,710
3	$18,310	$36,620	$54,930
4	$22,050	$44,100	$66,150
5	$25,790	$51,580	$77,370
6	$29,530	$59,060	$88,590
7	$33,270	$66,540	$99,810
8	$37,010	$74,020	$111,030

For families with more than 8 persons, add $3,740 for each additional person.
Source: HHS 2009.

Check Your Understanding 10.2

1. When a medical practice creates a fee schedule and determines what prices to charge for services, it is important to consider all but the following:

   a. Place of service and practice expense
   b. Access and convenience
   c. RVU for each CPT
   d. Professional and technical component

2. The Medicare fee for 99203 – new patient office visit is $91.80, and assigned RVUs for this same CPT are 1.34 (work RVUs), 1.12 (practice cost) and 0.09 (malpractice cost). What conversion factor is used for 2009?

   a. $81.96
   b. $36.00
   c. $68.51
   d. None of the above

3. Relative value units are an important component in establishing which of the following:

   a. Medicare reimbursement
   b. Physician fee schedule
   c. Practice and malpractice expense
   d. All of the above

4. A method for medical practices to provide greater decision-making control and purchasing power to consumers?

   a. Establish prices as a physician-office based practice
   b. Establish prices as a hospital-based practice
   c. Open enrollment
   d. Pricing transparency

5. When reviewing medical practice collection policies and procedures it is a prudent idea to consider all but the following:

   a. Copayments, coinsurance, and deductibles
   b. Individual and family premiums
   c. Out-of-pocket expenses
   d. Point of service collection strategy

Personal Health Records (PHRs)

In an age of consumer-driven healthcare and greater empowerment, the longtime saying *knowledge is power* could not be more applicable than right now when it comes to considering consumer expectations and perspectives on healthcare. The point is clear: The more engaged and knowledgeable a consumer becomes, the greater control they will have over decisions impacting their health and healthcare. Without a doubt, more well-informed consumers raise the value of each variable in the *knowledge is power* equation.

Knowledge = Power

Let's step back and define this exact formula for relating consumer healthcare decision making. Adding the proposition that knowledge in fact equates to greater control and power, it only stands to reason that information is a vital resource for sustaining and advancing consumer knowledge. Put another way, the more data and health information put into the hands of consumers as stewards of their own health, the more knowledgeable consumers become. This results in even greater decision-making power:

Information + Knowledge = **Power**

One of the most promising trends unfolding to make information more readily accessible and engage all stakeholders in the consumer healthcare movement is the advent of the personal health record (PHR). Physicians and other healthcare providers have long maintained and utilized provider-based health records, documenting patient health status, course of treatment, and medical decision making. Advances in health information technology and the expansion of interoperable health records over the past several years have helped facilitate a growing interest and evolution to the PHR. A comprehensive up-to-date PHR assists in placing consumers in the driver's seat, giving them the information they need to more effectively communicate with providers. A PHR also benefits consumers by expanding their knowledge and understanding of their own health status. This in turn enhances their decision-making power when making choices about their own healthcare.

$$PHR + Information + Knowledge = \textbf{Power}$$

A PHR enables consumers to have detailed personal health information readily available to assist in describing historical health status, as well as facilitating future decisions about their own healthcare. The principal difference between the personal health record (PHR) and the electronic medical record (EMR) (or its paper equivalent), used by healthcare givers, is the actual control over the information. Medical practices and healthcare providers own the actual legal health record of consumers in their practice. The information in the legal health record is customarily shared with individual consumers and other stakeholders according to appropriate legal guidelines and institutional policies and procedures. Individual consumers own and control the information in a PHR. Consumers are in charge of what information goes into the PHR and determine who gains access rights to the information contained in the PHR.

As with all healthcare issues, consumers ask questions. When concerning the selection of a PHR, AHIMA Personal Health Record Practice Council developed a summation of basic questions that may be asked by consumers. This list of questions may be found in figure 10.5 (AHIMA Personal Health Record Practice Council 2006).

What to Include

Since consumers own and oversee what information is contained in a PHR, it is important that they understand what elements to include. Information making up a consumer's health history can generate from a variety of sources and it is important that the PHR be accurate and as up-to-date as possible. The American Health Information Management Association (AHIMA) recommends the following key pieces of information that should be incorporated into a consumer's PHR:

- Personal identification, including name and birth date

- People to contact in case of emergency

- Names, addresses, and phone numbers of your physician, dentist, and specialists

- Health insurance information

- Living wills, advance directives, or medical power of attorney

- Organ donor authorization

- A list and dates of significant illnesses and surgical procedures

- Current medications and dosages

Figure 10.5.   Twelve questions consumers should ask when choosing a PHR

Content

- Will the PHR provide all the information I need for a complete health history?

- Will information be automatically added to the PHR from any other records (for example, insurance, employment, or care)? If so, what information will be added, and how will it be added? Is the information transfer audited?

- Do I have the opportunity to delete, correct, or add information? How will I do this?

Ownership

- Does the PHR sponsor have any ownership rights to the collected information?

- Can the PHR sponsor sell my information to anyone or for any reason? If so, how can I protect my privacy? Can I specify that my information not be sold?

- Will my information be used for employment or insurance coverage decisions (for example, to determine insurance eligibility)?

Access and Security

- Who has access to the information in my PHR?

- Can I choose to give my doctor, dentist, and other caregivers access? How do I control the sharing of my information?

- How will my information be protected from unauthorized use?

Portability

- If I am no longer employed/insured by you, can I still continue to use the PHR?

- How can I transfer my information to another PHR sponsor (for example, new insurer or new vendor)?

Cost

- Will there be any cost for me to have a PHR with you? (For instance, are there fees if I give my doctor, dentist, or other caregivers access to my PHR)?

Source: AHIMA Personal Health Record Practice Council 2006.

- Immunizations and their dates

- Allergies or sensitivities to drugs or materials, such as latex

- Important events, dates, and hereditary conditions in your family history

- Results from a recent physical examination

- Opinions of specialists

- Important tests results; eye and dental records

- Correspondence between you and your provider(s)

- Current educational materials (or appropriate Web links) relating to your health

- Any information you want to include about your health—such as your exercise regimen, any herbal medications you are taking, and any counseling you may receive

- Dietary practices, such as whether you are vegetarian or on a temporary diet (especially if changes in your diet have produced changes in your health in the past) (AHIMA 2009)

Samples of personal health record forms for an adult and a child may be found in the Sample Forms folder on the CD-ROM accompanying this book.

Additionally, the Centers for Disease Control (CDC) recommends records that are necessary for travel. Appendix Q provides information regarding tips for traveling abroad or within the United States, insurance issues, medication refills, and traveling with pets, along with a sample personal health record form (Wolter 2009).

A PHR Challenge

One of the central advantages consumers gain by making use of a PHR is that it offers the potential to provide a complete longitudinal picture of an individual's health. This is quite different from the episodic and incompatible nature true of many traditional medical office health records. Consolidating a consumer's personal health information in one place will make it more accessible to retrieve and share throughout a lifetime. Stop for a moment and imagine one central system that stores and organizes everything about your health status and that you can easily access whenever you need it. Information may come from a variety of sources, including physician documentation, hospital records, outpatient clinic encounters, labs, and even personal logs and entries from consumers themselves. Therein presents one of the utmost challenges for broadly implementing PHRs.

In a nutshell, consumers often may lack the wherewithal to compile pertinent and complete information, let alone responding to the additional chore of keeping current all pieces of information concerning their health status. Although we like to think of ourselves as organized and prepared most of the time, many consumers are already wrapped up in day-to-day activities or can become disorganized at one point or another. One need only look at the stacks of mail or numbers of e-mail messages clogging the in-boxes of many consumers to recognize the enormous amount of information consumers are already bombarded with. Of course, some consumers will have less difficulty keeping a PHR current.

Secondly, it's one thing to put additional information and decision-making power into the hands of consumers; it's another point to declare with confidence that consumers will effectively make use of this information to make better choices that improve their health. As a nation, it is characteristic for a large portion of the American public to become complacent and resist change even when the potential benefits are understood. Case in point, for years warnings have been issued concerning the hazards of smoking, and yet hundreds of thousands of U.S. citizens die each year due to tobacco-related causes. We know heart disease is a leading cause of death, but we don't change our lifestyles. We recognize how to stay on top of our blood sugar with diet and exercise, yet the prevalence of diabetes is increasing dramatically. Many of us, most of us, if not all of us would like six-pack abs, but we continue to put on weight and add to our body mass index (BMI). Obesity is a national epidemic. Unfortunately, these chronic diseases are being diagnosed in children at astonishing levels, which may result in severe drains to the healthcare systems as these children reach adulthood.

Incentives and creative alternatives must be put in place to encourage consumers to utilize the information in PHRs for adults as well as children. Consumers must become convinced to believe that it's actually worth their while to put healthy behaviors into practice. PHR developers and other key stakeholders must offer clever innovations to engage consumers to support behavior change and prevention. This includes giving consumers the ability to populate PHRs seamlessly and with little effort.

The expansion of PHR tools offers tremendous opportunities for medical practices to strengthen the physician–consumer relationship. Medical practices should takes steps to evaluate their own internal policies and procedures for handling and releasing health information related to PHR usage. AHIMA and the American Medical Informatics Association (AMIA) jointly developed Position Statement for Consumers of Health Care. This document is an excellent resource for medical practices during their internal policies and procedures review and can be found on the CD-ROM accompanying this book. As PHR applications continue to develop and spring up in response to growing consumer interest toward viewing and managing their own personal health information, this is sure to accelerate new roles for serving as consumer educators, advocates, PHR implementers, analysts, and more.

Check Your Understanding 10.3

1. A principle advantage to consumers for making use of a personal health record (PHR) includes which of the following?

   a. A PHR is the legal health record
   b. Ownership and control of information
   c. Reduced practice expense
   d. All of the above

2. Important pieces of information to include in a personal health record (PHR) might be which of the following?

   a. Physician notes from an electronic medical record
   b. Emergency contact information
   c. Daily exercise log
   d. All of the above

3. Key challenges for broadly implementing personal health records to consumers include all but which of the following?

   a. Episodic nature of a PHR compared to medical practice records
   b. Potential difficulty to keep PHR information current
   c. Effective use of information contained in a PHR
   d. Capability for consumers to populate PHR seamlessly

Retail Medical Centers

The retail option for offering medical services has entered the healthcare arena as one more trend whose time has come. In many cases, retail healthcare presents the potential for offering consumers a more convenient, rational, and lower-cost alternative. Over the past several years retail businesses have assumed a dramatically expanded role in U.S. healthcare.

Earlier in this chapter, we stated that a good deal of healthcare, and to a great extent healthcare decision making, occurs right in the home. In fact, outside the household, most people still obtain a majority of their healthcare through conventional institutions such as medical practices, hospitals, emergency departments, ambulatory care centers, clinics, and the like. That being said, times are rapidly changing and there is a growing trend toward shopping for healthcare much in the same manner as consumers go shopping at the mall. Entrepreneurs and innovative retail companies are getting in the business of healthcare, and at the same time, increased numbers of traditional healthcare providers are assessing how best to get into the business of retail.

Defining Retail Healthcare

Let me ask a couple of questions. Exactly what is retail healthcare? What is the best way to describe a retail medical center? The truth is there are many ways to express this phenomenon, and attempting to define, once again, depends on consumer perspectives. Simply put, retail healthcare is market driven by the specific needs of individual consumers; and in turn, the medical providers and institutions offering services to satisfy those needs. In the case of retail healthcare, it is quite appropriate for the terms "consumer," "patient," and "customer" to be used interchangeably.

Retailers recognize that not all consumers share the same needs, goals, and motivations when it comes to making purchasing decisions. Successful retail companies from other industries take great pains to research and fully grasp the attitudes and preferences of various consumer groups. These companies tailor their products and services based on individual targeted consumer segments. Retail healthcare takes advantage of this notion and employs such techniques as competitive pricing, marketing promotion, convenient location, and targeted service strategies to gain a competitive edge.

The growth of the retail concept in the healthcare environment and development of retail medical centers is still a relatively new model for delivering healthcare services. However, the basic fundamentals driving the retail trend are not new at all. Basic economic forces and market competition driven by demand and supply are the primary motivations behind this concept.

Retail medical centers focus on strategies directed at consumer decision-making perspectives, rather than strictly from a provider or wholesale payer-centered point of view. Looking back at traditional healthcare models consumers are accustomed to, most are structured in a manner that leaves little in the way of free choice by individual consumers. They are really provider-centered, and most often choices are driven by providers or by predetermined employer health plan reimbursement contracts—again, a return to the paternalistic approach to decision making we mentioned at the beginning of the chapter.

The breadth and scope of retail medical centers can be as varied as the range of consumer segments considered. Examples of the retail healthcare market may range from customers purchasing convenient primary care services in an easy-to-access clinic, grocery store, or big-box department store, to other consumers seeking particular specialty healthcare services. Still others target those consumers willing to pay extra for increased levels of personalized boutique or concierge services. Individual preferences and attitudes vary greatly by demographic group or life stages.

Some of the earliest retailers to enter the healthcare market were retail pharmacies located in drug stores. Figure 10.6 offers further examples of today's more common retail medical centers, spas, and clinics available to consumers.

The most successful retail medical centers not only know how to effectively deliver a product or service, they excel in identifying and satisfying customer needs; that is, paying attention to how potential consumers view price, quality, accessibility, and convenience. With access to greater amounts of information, consumers can shop for healthcare services based on value, cost, quality, and service. Medical practices today should expect increasing numbers of consumers to ask about prices up front, and possibly to be shopping around for the best deals on specific services.

Figure 10.6. Retail medical centers

• Optical eyeglass stores	• Sleep labs	• Fitness spas
• Dental care offices	• Cosmetic care services	• Health and wellness centers
• Convenient care clinics	• Lasik vision centers	
• Concierge care centers	• Fertility centers	

In some cases, medical services are provided on a cash-only basis, although many retail medical centers will accept insurance plans as well. Again, this depends on the scope of services and targeted customer base. This coupled with the advent of consumer-driven healthcare creates a situation where consumers are incentivized to become more cost-conscious in evaluating healthcare choices. As deductibles and copayments continue to rise, resulting in greater out-of-pocket expenses, consumers are more apt to consider competitive price levels. At the same time, for those consumers who are unemployed or do not have the funds to pay for health coverage, the retail option may provide a more affordable alternative for basic healthcare services.

The important point here is that it is not just the physical facilities and location of retailers, but the increased supply and demand market forces at work and the increased competition that comes with it. In the retail environment, advertised prices are readily available and consumers know in advance what a visit or service is going to cost out of their own pockets. This increased pricing transparency places greater decision-making control back into the hands of consumers.

Check Your Understanding 10.4

1. The most successful retail medical centers recognize which of the following?

   a. All consumers have the same needs, goals, and motivations
   b. Employer relations are most important for obtaining purchasing decisions
   c. Importance of linking consumers to a primary care physician (PHP)
   d. Importance of price, quality, accessibility, and convenience

2. A retail medical practice offering healthcare services to a targeted consumer segment on a cash-only basis would be wise to promote which of the following?

   a. Flexible spending accounts
   b. Transparency in pricing
   c. Extended payment arrangements for the uninsured
   d. All of the above

3. Which of the following strategies might a retail medical center consider in order to gain a competitive edge over other healthcare providers?

   a. Marketing promotion
   b. Competitive pricing
   c. Convenient location and service
   d. All of the above

Medical Home

Over the past several decades there has been an increased realization that the system of healthcare in the United States is not achieving the greatest outcomes for the price being paid. Not only is healthcare unaffordable, but more importantly, it is unsustainable over the long haul. Some would argue whether the U.S. healthcare system is truly a system at all, but rather, is an array of disconnected subsystems and competing goals amongst different stakeholders. In many respects the United States lags other countries in achieving an effective model that brings all consumers, providers, and payers of healthcare together in a unified fashion. This is perhaps most evident as documented in a 2008 Commonwealth Fund report, signaling that the United States continues to fall further behind when compared to accepted best practice standards and equivalent international performance benchmarks (Commonwealth Fund Commission on a High Performance Health System 2008).

In 2006, federal legislation in the form of the Tax Relief and Health Care Act, charged the Department of Health and Human Services with establishing a demonstration of the medical home care model designed to target high-need populations with chronic conditions (CMS 2009a). The Centers for Medicare and Medicaid Services conducted the Physician Group Practice (PGP) Demonstration to improve the quality of care delivered to patients with congestive heart failure, coronary artery disease, and diabetes mellitus during a two-year period as announced in the press release dated August 14, 2008 (CMS 2008). Ten medical groups earned $16.7 million in incentive payments under the demonstration that rewards healthcare providers for improving health outcomes and coordinating the overall healthcare needs of Medicare patients assigned to the groups. There were benchmarks or target performance on at least 25 out of 27 quality markers for patients with diabetes, coronary artery disease, and congestive heart failure.

To take part in the medical home demonstration, participating personal physicians are required to be board certified, along with providing documented evidence of possessing the capability to contribute necessary support staff and resources to manage the comprehensive and coordinated care of targeted beneficiaries. Participating medical practices were also charged with identifying and encouraging individual participation of eligible beneficiaries, as well as additional detailed responsibilities for each of the following:

- Safe and secure information technology—to promote beneficiary access to personal health information
- Health assessment tool—to be completed and utilized for each participating beneficiary
- Training programs—for all supporting staff involved in coordination of care activities

A second phase of the CMS demonstration project scheduled for 2010 to 2012 reimburses qualified medical practices based on ability to meet designated basic core elements of a medical home. Medical practices, meeting expanded requirements and documented evidence of further enhanced qualifications of electronic health records, coordination of inpatient and outpatient care follow-up, measures of performance, and physician reporting are eligible for a higher-tiered level of reimbursement from CMS.

Bringing it Home

The Institute of Medicine (IOM) and the World Health Organization (WHO) have long regarded the medical home model of healthcare as a comprehensive and well-organized approach for providing acute, chronic, and preventive healthcare services (AAFP 2007). Not only is care all-inclusive, but it is more complete when it comes to improving consumer health and recognizing the substantial benefits of a reliable consumer–provider connection. In fact, the medical home is a widely accepted model of healthcare and embraced by many nations around the globe, as shown in figure 10.7.

Defining the Medical Home

When describing the medical home, we are talking about timely access to care, regardless of background or where consumers live. Put another way, it is the type of care that benefits and strengthens the relationship amongst all stakeholders—consumers, physicians, payers,

Figure 10.7. Medical home—around the globe

China	医学首页
Denmark	Medicinsk Home
France	Medical Accueil
Korea	의료 홈
Saudi Arabia	الطبية الرئيسية الصفحة
Slovenia	Medicinska Domov
Spain	Hogar Médico
Sweden	Medicinsk Hem
Taiwan	醫學首頁
Thailand	แพทย์หน้าแรก
United States	Medical Home

employers, and others. The medical home can best be described as a comprehensive, coordinated and continuous model of healthcare which many believe improves access, enhances quality and safety, and offers the added prospect of achieving much sought after cost savings.

In the medical home model of healthcare, consumers are linked to primary care providers in a relationship designed to offer longitudinal healthcare and guidance specific to their unique personal circumstances. All care and coordination of care, be it preventive, acute care services, complex chronic conditions, or palliative care, are monitored and facilitated by a primary care physician. This type of partnership differs greatly from the traditional approach to healthcare delivery experienced in the United States, which is typically episodic and uncoordinated. On the other hand, the medical home is quite consistent in many respects with other emerging trends that encourage individual decision making and active participation by consumers in their own healthcare.

Engaging consumers in their own care and enhanced access to primary care services as a regular source of care are common themes of the medical home. The American Academy of Family Physicians and several other medical specialty organizations have outlined important characteristics as fundamental to the medical home concept (AAFP 2007). Figure 10.8 offers

Figure 10.8. Basic features of the medical home

• Personal physician	• Quality and safety
• Physician-directed medical practice	• Enhanced access
• Whole person orientation	• Payment reform
• Care is coordinated and/or integrated	

Source: AAFP 2007.

an outline of these central attributes. Let's take a closer examination of each of these core medical home features and discuss them individually.

Personal Physician

The medical home model emphasizes that each consumer will have an ongoing relationship with a primary care physician (PCP). In short, a comprehensive and consistent consumer–physician partnership exists in this model with intent being that the relationship be sustained over time. It is widely believed that having a personal physician is one of the greatest influences toward overall consumer satisfaction. A continuing relationship with a physician for primary care also enhances two-way accountability, as well as greater probability for achieving better quality and healthier outcomes.

Physician-Directed Medical Practice

As was stated, interpersonal continuity with a personal physician offers the distinct advantage of ensuring the needs and preferences of individual consumers are being met. Of course, not all primary care services require the level of expertise of a physician. In the medical home model, a primary care physician guides a team of health professionals who collectively assume oversight for the immediate or ongoing healthcare of individual consumers. The team often includes other nonphysician primary care providers and specialists, pharmacists, home health, nursing homes, educators, and others brought in as necessary. A key success factor in the physician-directed medical practice is that all care coordination is planned, purposeful, and understood by the consumer. Effective processes and tools to communicate amongst providers, as well as to guide discussions with consumers, are essential. Physicians and other team members use EHRs to reinforce treatment plans between office visits and promote adherence to instructions regarding medications, monitoring, and timely response to symptoms.

Whole Person Orientation

One of the distinct advantages of the medical home is that it is a longitudinal model. What this means for consumers is that healthcare advice and treatments include all of life's circumstances: preventive care, acute care, chronic conditions, and end-of-life needs. By taking a whole person approach, both the physical health and mental well-being of consumers are taken into consideration so that the right care is consistently offered at the right time and in the best setting. Again, this is very different than the episodic problem-focused care consumers are historically accustomed to. The consumer–physician partnership mentioned earlier is built on trust and strengthened by ongoing mutual sharing of information and knowledge.

Coordinated and Integrated Care

A medical home provides an integrated network of healthcare providers to meet the needs of individual consumers, along with the education and support necessary for consumers to be active participants in their care. Enabling consumers to partner in monitoring their conditions and managing the complexities of care helps navigate referrals and transitions to other nonprimary care specialty services when necessary. The many alternative types of health services encountered and actual historical sequence of healthcare events over time can be a demanding exercise to properly capture, let alone ask consumers to recall. This is one of the explicit advantages for longitudinal electronic health records and individual personal health records. Health information exchange helps facilitate the coordinated care requirements in a medical home model. Having information in the right location, in the right amount, and at the right time significantly impacts efficient coordination of care, not to mention the potential of reducing costly duplication of services.

Quality and Safety

Possibly one of the biggest benefits resulting from the medical home concept is the ability to decrease unwanted variability in the system. Because the care of each consumer is fully integrated, the risk of undertreatment and overtreatment is significantly reduced. This in turn offers the potential for reduced chance of medical errors and greatly improved overall quality and safety of care. We already stated how essential it is to make use of EHRs and interoperable health information exchange for coordinating the care of providers. These tools are equally important for communicating directly with consumers. Keep in mind that consumers are partners in decision making of the medical home model. Utilizing available decision support tools and evidence-based medicine to bring in line the most appropriate care and medical decision making are important features of the medical home.

Enhanced Access

An objective of providing access anywhere anytime emphasizes the value added of the medical home in providing care in the most appropriate location. The medical home concept goes a step further in focusing on what care is most appropriate to avoid providing excessive services, or conversely, undertreating a condition because of a lack of access. Enhanced access for consumers doesn't always result in an appointment to see a physician, yet may include telephone calls, e-mail, or other forms of communication. Similar to other emerging modes of healthcare delivery, the enhanced access medical home places greater control in the hands of consumers. The key is 24/7 access for consumers to obtain answers to any question or concern whenever the need arises.

Payment Reform

Earlier in the chapter we stated that whoever foots the bill often has a deciding factor in what amount of healthcare is provided and ultimately is consumed. To some degree, this remains true in the medical home model as well, and because of this, expansion of the concept on a broader scale is not a trivial undertaking. To be most successful, it will require a fundamental rethinking of how healthcare is reimbursed, and away from the more prevalent fee-for-service model that exists today. Instead of reimbursement based on each encounter or number of services and treatments provided, the medical home reimburses healthcare providers based on specific performance measures. Incentives might target preventive care measures, such as the number of screenings and immunizations, chronic disease management, decreased hospital utilization, and overall consumer health. In essence, this means a financing system that considers the accountability and value added of enhanced integration, coordination, and communications with consumers.

Check Your Understanding 10.5

1. Which of the following best describes enhanced access in a patient-centered medical home?

   a. Open scheduling, expanded hours, and expanded communication options
   b. Pay for performance
   c. Retail convenient care clinics
   d. All of the above

2. The use of EHRs and health information technology is a requirement in the medical home model in order to achieve what?

   a. Enable surveillance of each eligible beneficiary by multiple assigned primary care physicians
   b. Ensure continuing care is properly overseen and coordinated by multiple specialty providers
   c. Engage consumers in accessing and utilizing their personal health information
   d. All of the above

3. The medical home approach to healthcare is best suited for overseeing which of the following?

   a. Complex chronic conditions
   b. Emergent and acute care services
   c. Health and wellness services
   d. All of the above

4. The medical home offers enhanced access to integrated healthcare services for consumers in what way?

   a. Ensuring access to a primary care physician for every appointment
   b. Offering discounted services by all participating primary care and specialist medical home providers
   c. Providing greater control for healthcare services in the hands of the consumer
   d. All of the above

5. Which healthcare trend is seen as a lower-cost alternative and at the same time enables consumers to take a more active role in their own healthcare?

   a. Medical home
   b. Retail healthcare
   c. High deductible health plans
   d. All of the above

Final Consumer Implications

In this chapter we have acknowledged that healthcare and healthcare decisions are frequently based on consumer expectations and perception of care. And at the same time, it is widely recognized that healthcare in the United States is significantly encumbered with numerous complexities, disparities, excessive costs, and intricate reimbursement issues. We have also touched on a number of the dynamics and most important trends impacting healthcare for the 21st century—the implications for consumers, medical practices, and other stakeholders in this transformation are undeniably linked.

Increasingly, consumer-driven healthcare is happening, and the implications are far-reaching. It's not hard to imagine, the consumer–physician relationship will continue to evolve as more and more consumers accept personal responsibility to see that their preferences and needs are fulfilled. Greater amounts of information in the hands of consumers, advanced information technologies, continued treatment breakthroughs, and changing market dynamics all suggest greater decision-making control in support of consumers.

One thing is for certain: educating and engaging consumers to take an active role to better understand their own health, healthcare, health coverage, and health information are all essential elements to any future system of healthcare. Clearly, consumer-driven healthcare holds great promise and opportunity. The question is: what choice will consumers make?

References

AHIMA Personal Health Record Practice Council. 2006. Helping consumers select PHRs: Questions and considerations for navigating an emerging market. *Journal of AHIMA* 77(10):50–56.

American Academy of Family Physicians. 2007. The patient centered medical home: History, seven core features, evidence and transformational change. http://www.graham-center.org/PreBuilt/PCMH.pdf.

American Health Information Management Association. 2009. MyPHR. http://www.myphr.com.

Centers for Medicare and Medicaid Services. 2008. Physician groups earn performance payments for improving quality of care for patients with chronic illnesses. http://www.cms.gov/apps/media/press_releases.asp.

Centers for Medicare and Medicaid Services. 2009a. Medical home demonstration fact sheet. http://www.cms.hhs.gov/DemoProjectsEvalRpts/downloads/MedHome_FactSheet.pdf.

Centers for Medicare and Medicaid Services. 2009b. National physician fee schedule relative value file. http://www.cms.hhs.gov/PhysicianFeeSched/PFSRVF/list.asp.

Cherry, D., D. Woodwell, and E. Rechtsteiner. 2007. National ambulatory medical care survey. *Advance Data from Vital and Health Statistics.* 387:1–40. http://www.cdc.gov/nchs/data/ad/ad387.pdf.

Commonwealth Fund Commission on a High Performance Health System. 2008. Why not the best? Results from the national scorecard on U.S. health system performance. http://www.commonwealthfund.org/Content/Publications/Fund-Reports/2008/Jul/Why-Not-the-Best--Results-from-the-National-Scorecard-on-U-S--Health-System-Performance--2008.aspx.

DeNavas, W., B. Proctor, and J. Smith. 2007. Economics and Statistics Administration. Income, poverty, and health insurance coverage in the United States. http://www.census.gov/prod/2008pubs/p60-235.pdf.

Department of Health and Human Services. 2009 (Jan. 23). The 2009 HHS poverty guidelines. Federal Register 74(14):4200. http://aspe.hhs.gov/poverty/09poverty.shtml.

Employee Benefits Security Administration. 2009. COBRA continuation coverage assistance under ARRA. http://www.dol.gov/ebsa/cobra.html.

Federal Trade Commission. 2006. Fair Debt Collections Practices Act. Public Law 109–351. http://www.ftc.gov/bcp/edu/pubs/consumer/credit/cre27.pdf.

Moen, A. and P. Brennan. 2005. Health@Home: The work of health information management in the household (HIMH): Implications for consumer health informatics (CHI) innovations. *Journal of the American Medical Informatics Association* 12(6):648–656, 651. http://www.pubmedcentral.nih.gov/articlerender.fcgi?tool=pubmed&pubmedid=16049230.

National Coalition on Health Care. 2009. Health care facts: Costs. http://nchc.org/sites/default/files/resources/Fact%20Sheet%20-%20Cost.pdf.

PricewaterhouseCoopers. 2008. Health Research Institute. What employers want from health insurers—now. http://www.pwc.com/extweb/pwcpublications.nsf/docid/E903DC27B947DE2D852574D3007F767C.

U.S. Census Bureau. 2009. http://www.census.gov.

Wolter, J., ed. 2009. *The Personal Health Record.* Chicago: AHIMA.

Resources

American Medical Association. 2008. *Current Procedural Terminology (CPT) 2009.* Chicago: AMA.

Centers for Medicare and Medicaid Services. 2009. National physician fee schedule relative value file. http://www.cms.hhs.gov/PhysicianFeeSched/.

National Committee on Quality Assurance. 2009. Physician Practice Connections®—Patient-centered medical home.™ http://www.ncqa.org/tabid/631/Default.aspx.

Chapter 11

New Opportunities for HIM Professionals

Cheryl Gregg Fahrenholz, RHIA, CCS-P

Learning Objectives

- Identify the diversity of skills of the health information management (HIM) professional

- Recognize the multitude of positions in a medical practice that may be accomplished by the HIM professional

Key Terms

Accreditation coordinator
AHIMA certified professional
American Recovery and Reimbursement Act (ARRA)
Appeal
Audit
Baseline
Benchmarking
Best practice
Certification
Chief executive officer (CEO)
Chief financial officer (CFO)
Chief information officer (CIO)

Chief medical informatics officer (CMIO)
Chief operating officer (COO)
Chief privacy officer
Chief security officer (CSO)
Coder
Compliance
Content and records management
C-suite positions
Denial management
Electronic health record (EHR)
Health information management (HIM)

ICD-9-CM
ICD-10-CM
Medical informatician
Personal health record (PHR)
Physician Quality Reporting Initiative (PQRI)
Record completion
Recovery audit contractor (RAC)
Reimbursement
Release of information (ROI)
Request for proposal (RFP)
Revenue cycle management
Terminology asset manager

Introduction

This book has documented many aspects of health record documentation in medical practices. The health information management (HIM) professional plays an active role in many, if not all, of these aspects. Whether it is from the role of executive leadership, auditing the documentation, coding, and reimbursement of professional services, or implementing an electronic health record, the HIM professional has the educational foundation and many have the wealth of experience to lead medical practices into a successful business while assuring regulatory compliance.

This detail-oriented, yet global perspective, skill set of the HIM professional results in a leader for medical practices seeking success. The expertise in financial, regulatory, compliance, electronic health records, documentation, coding, billing, privacy, security, communications, project management, as well as the revenue cycle, operational management, and best practices for all aspects of practice management is well suited for medical practices.

Roles for Health Information Management Professionals

Executive Leadership

The experienced HIM professional has the education and knowledge to fulfill one of the C-suite positions within a medical practice network. At the corporate level, the HIM professional may operate in the capacity of the chief executive officer (CEO), chief operating officer (COO), chief financial officer (CFO), chief information officer (CIO), or chief medical informatics officer (CMIO). Additional corporate positions may be the vice presidents of revenue cycle, health informatics, compliance, information systems, business development, payer contracting, professional billing, or quality management, to name a few. In multi-location practices, the HIM professional may function as a regional director over many locations or a practice administrator over one large location. In smaller practices where corporate positions do not exist, the HIM professional may be titled as office manager and/or business office manager.

Revenue Cycle

Revenue cycle management encompasses every phase of the finances for a medical practice. Details of the revenue cycle may be found in chapter 6. The opportunities for HIM professionals most often fall into positions where coding is the focus of the role; however, HIM professionals have the financial background to perform business analyses to assist with trending, identification of baselines, and conducting benchmark comparisons of best practices. Monitoring the financial opportunities and implementing solutions to identified roadblocks or issues may also be efficiently completed by the HIM professional.

With the clinical background, HIM professionals may combine the expertise of regulatory compliance with documentation standards, which is helpful when implementing financial incentive programs, such as the Physician Quality Reporting Initiative (PQRI). As with all new programs, the project planning, education and training, evaluating, monitoring, and continuous attention to the project's unique needs are prime tasks for an HIM professional.

Proper coding for professional services and the internal auditing of the documentation and coding process have traditionally been roles for HIM professionals; however, not all medical practices have taken advantage of the expertise offered by credentialed HIM professionals. Some practices continue to have the coding completed by noncredentialed individuals, which may result in uncaptured revenue or worse. The use of noncredentialed coders exposes the practice to a multitude of compliance vulnerabilities, such as inaccurate coding, upcoding, and fraudulent claim submissions, to name a few. Unfortunately, these compliance issues may be unknown to the physicians, providers, and practice leadership until an audit (internal or external) discovers them. The utilization of AHIMA credentialed coders continues to be in the spotlight and will increase over the next years as the transition and implementation from ICD-9-CM to ICD-10-CM occurs and is effective October 2013.

In the business office, many functions may be completed by HIM professionals. These functions begin with credentialing and continue throughout the billing process into analyzing the financials and trending payer reimbursements. The detailed nature of HIM professionals is a perfect fit for leadership of the business office. Denials management, appeals processing, as well as a multitude of auditing and analyzing functions may be completed. Although this area of the medical practice has been minimally tapped by HIM professionals, the opportunities are endless and the benefits to the medical practice are exceptional.

Information Systems

As the American Recovery and Reimbursement Act (ARRA) advances the nation in the electronic capture and exchange of health information, HIM professionals play key roles.

The information systems (IS) area of a small medical practice is sometimes outsourced to an external company; however, larger medical practices or networks may have corporate IS departments where HIM professionals may offer a wealth of knowledge when implementing electronic health records. Even though the steps of implementing an electronic health record may appear daunting at the beginning, the HIM professional may assist in the planning, request for proposal (RFP), system evaluation and selection, preimplementation, implementation, training, and postimplementation processes. The development of a personal health record (PHR) also presents challenges for medical practices, and HIM professionals may serve as excellent resources.

Some of the potential positions in the IS arena may be medical informatician, internal health IS consultant, health information engineer, health data administrator, enterprise content and information manager, health information analyst and designer, terminology asset manager, and clinical information manager, to list a few. As movement toward the national health information infrastructure occurs, the roles that support the development and implementation of the electronic health record in medical practices are prime roles for HIM professionals.

In October 2008, the American Health Information Management Association and American Medical Informatics Association developed a document entitled "Health Information Management and Informatics Core Competencies for Individuals Working With Electronic Health Records." This 20-page document outlines:

1. Health information literacy and skills

2. Health informatics skills using the EHR and PHR

3. Privacy and confidentiality of health information skills

4. Health information/data technical security skills

5. Basic computer literacy skills

This document may be useful to medical practices when establishing the necessary skill set that best fits the unique needs of medical practices.

More information on the potential tasks for HIM professionals in information systems may be found in chapter 5.

Regulatory Compliance

With the formation of recovery audit contractors (RACs), the need for qualified staff in the medical practice to monitor and address the RAC requests could clearly be fulfilled with the HIM professional. Depending upon the size of the medical practice, there may be a need to have a RAC coordinator to be responsible for all of the RAC activities.

As with governmental payers, commercial payers also conduct audits that require monitoring. Hand in hand with the auditing function are provider education and training on documentation and coding. These duties provide additional opportunities for HIM professionals.

Although ARRA addresses the needs for electronic health information, there are many changes for privacy and security. Historically, the HIM professional has always protected the privacy and security of health information. HIM professionals complement medical practices in their quest for compliance.

In addition to RAC coordinator, potential positions in the medical practice may be chief compliance officer, chief privacy officer, chief information security officer, education and training director, and accreditation coordinator.

There may be times when a new medical practice is opened, an existing medical practice joins another medical practice, or a medical practice closes. Similarly, there will be scenarios when a new provider enters an existing practice, an established provider moves to another medical practice, or a provider retires. These scenarios result in detailed processes that require oversight and follow-through. The HIM professional has the diverse skill set to perform the tasks required for each of these business development scenarios.

Health Information Management

Traditionally known HIM functions of release of information and record completion, along with record conversion projects and health record content projects continue to remain responsibilities for some HIM professionals in medical practices. As with the transition to the electronic health records, project management for any medical practice initiative may be completed by the HIM professional. More information on traditional HIM functions may be found in chapters 4 and 8.

HIM in Medical Practices

"The emergence of quality improvement initiatives that rely on the medical record and the increase in physician practices use of EHRs makes the HIM consultant role more important than ever" (Dimick 2008, 28). For many large medical practice networks, the opportunity to hire HIM professionals is a must for a successful strategic plan. However, many smaller practices may not recognize the asset of an employed HIM professional. As with other services in the medical practice, there is an alternative to permanently hiring the HIM professional, namely known as outsourcing or contracting. There are HIM consultants available to medical practices for many, if not all, of the areas discussed in this chapter. Perhaps the project requiring an HIM professional has a short time frame associated and hence, would be better suited for an external HIM consultant rather than a full-time HIM employee. For many such circumstances, the medical practice may quickly acknowledge the expertise and diverse skill set of HIM professionals.

Whether the HIM professional is internal or external to the medical practice, the extensive knowledge and experience offer a wealth of opportunity to medical practices. Regardless of the level of electronic health information, HIM professionals may lead the medical practice into each step of the transition from the paper-based to the electronic world. The HIM professional may direct the proper data and charge capture to result in appropriate payer reimbursement, as well as ensure regulatory compliance and correct coding and billing processes. Operational leadership is inherent to the HIM professional as are the many other skills noted in this chapter. It is the HIM professional who will be most valued during the initiatives of ARRA and future financial and operational advances in medical practices. A sample position description for the HIM professional in a small physician practice may be found in appendix R.

Check Your Understanding 11.1

Instructions: Select the phrase that best completes the following statements.

1. Which of the following statements is false?
   a. The HIM professional has the educational foundation for a multitude of positions within a medical practice.
   b. The HIM professional does not have the skill set to fulfill the C-suite positions.
   c. The HIM professional may lead the revenue cycle process within a medical practice.
   d. The HIM profession is well suited to monitor the RAC activities, as well as payer audits.

2. In what department would the following positions (medical informatician, internal health IS consultant, health information engineer, health data administrator, enterprise content and information manager, health information analyst and designer, terminology asset manager, and clinical information manager) be found?
   a. Executive leadership
   b. Revenue cycle
   c. Information systems
   d. Regulatory compliance

3. The HIM professional has the educational background to perform which of the following duty/duties?
   a. Revenue cycle management
   b. Denials management
   c. Revenue audit contractor activity responses, monitoring, and follow-up
   d. All of the above

4. Which of the following is true?
   a. The HIM professional has a diverse educational foundation.
   b. The HIM professional is not a detail-oriented individual.
   c. The HIM professional should be limited to single tasks with little responsibility.
   d. The HIM professional does not have the ability to communicate well with medical practice staff.

5. According to the sample position description for the HIM professional in a small physician practice, the HIM professional may effectively perform which of the following responsibilities?
   a. Daily operations
   b. Information systems and revenue cycle management
   c. Compliance, confidentiality, privacy, and security
   d. All of the above

Conclusion

As can be read in this chapter along with other chapters of this book, HIM professionals play a vital role in the operational and financial success, as well as regulatory compliance and information systems of medical practices. This unique skill set resulting from the educational foundation and experience results in a win-win scenario for medical practices. To evaluate the skill set of HIM professionals, the American Health Information Management Association (AHIMA) offers *Self-Assessment: Health Information Management Professional in the Small Physician Practice,* which is available to AHIMA members for a nominal fee.

References

Dimick, C. 2008. HIM jobs of tomorrow: Eleven new and revised jobs illustrate the trends changing HIM and the opportunities that lie ahead. *Journal of AHIMA* 79(10):26–34.

Resources

AHIMA and AMIA Joint Workforce Task Force. 2008. Health information management and informatics core competencies for individuals working with electronic health records. Chicago: AHIMA. http://www.ahima.org/infocenter/whitepapers/workforce_2008.pdf.

Centers for Medicare and Medicaid Services. 2009. Physician Quality Reporting Initiative. http://www.cms.hhs.gov/PQRI.

Centers for Medicare and Medicaid Services. 2009. Recovery audit contractors. http://www.cms.hhs.gov/RAC.

Appendix A

Contents of the CD-ROM

1. Web Links
2. 1995 CMS Documentation Guidelines for Evaluation and Management
3. 1997 CMS Documentation Guidelines for Evaluation and Management
4. Fair Debt Collection Practices Act
5. 2009 PQRI Measures List
6. Family Medicine Data Collection Tool
7. PHR Position Papers

Sample Forms (folder)

1. Registration Form, Premier HealthNet
2. Registration Form, PriMed Physicians
3. Pediatric Registration Form, PriMed Physicians
4. Consent to Treat, PriMed Physicians
5. Problem List
6. Medication List
7. Child Immunization Record
8. Facesheet (EHR), Greenway
9. Vital Signs Flow Sheet (EHR), Greenway
10. Prenatal Flow Sheet, Obstetrix Medical Group
11. Preventive Care Flow Sheets, Wesley Medical Center
12. Adult Health Questionnaire
13. Medical History Questionnaire
14. Pediatric Family History, PriMed Physicians
15. Neurology Medical Review of Symptoms, PriMed Physicians
16. Obstetric History, Obstetrix Medical Group
17. Genetic/Family History, Obstetrix Medical
18. Obstetrical Review of Systems, Obstetrix Medical Group
19. Progress Note (EHR), Greenway
20. Initial Visit, Cardiology, PriMed
21. Asthma Visit Form, Child, American Academy of Pediatrics
22. Prenatal Record, University of Minnesota Physicians
23. Postpartum Examination, University of Minnesota Physicians

Appendix B

CLIA Listing of State Agencies

Alabama Department of Public Health
Division of Health Care Facilities
CLIA Program
P.O. Box 303017
Montgomery, AL 36130-3017
(334) 206-5120
Contact: Brenda Furlow
E-mail: bfurlow@adph.state.al.us

Public Health Laboratory Anchorage
4500 Boniface Parkway
Anchorage, AK 99507
(206) 615-2379
FAX: (206) 615-2088
Contact: Keith Scott
E-mail: keith.scott@cms.hhs.gov

Arizona Department of Health Services
Division of Public Health Services
Office of Laboratory Services
250 N. 17TH Avenue
Phoenix, AZ 85007
(602) 364-0741
FAX: (602) 364-0759
Contact: Odalys Hinds

Health Facility Services Slot H9
Arkansas Department of Health and Human
Services
5800 West 10th Street, Suite 400
Little Rock, AR 72204-9916
(501) 661-2201
Contact: Laura Moody

Department of Public Health
Division of Laboratory Science

Laboratory Field Services
320 West 4th Street, Suite 890
Los Angeles, CA 90013
(213) 620-6160
FAX: (213) 620-6565
Contact: Donna McCallum, Examiner III

**Colorado Department of Public Health &
Environment**
Laboratory Services Division
8100 Lowry Blvd.
Denver, CO 80230-6928
(303) 692-3681
FAX: (303) 344-9965
Contact: Jeff Groff
E-mail: Jeff.Groff@state.co.us

CLIA Laboratory Program
Department of Public Health
P.O. Box 340308
410 Capitol Avenue, MS#12 HSR
Hartford, CT 06134-0308
(860) 509-7400
FAX: (860) 509-7535
Contact: John J. Murphy

Delaware State Public Health Laboratory
Donna Phillips-DiMaria
30 Sunnyside Road
Smyrna, DE 19977
(302) 223-1392
FAX: (302) 653-2877
Contact: Donna Phillips-DiMaria
E-mail: Donna.phillips-dimar@state.de.us

DC Department of Health
Health Regulations and Licensing
Administration
Health Facilities Division
Laboratory Services
717 14th Street NW Suite 600
Washington DC 20005
Office: (202) 727-1740
Cell: (202) 494-4917
FAX: (202) 442-9431
Contact: Semret Tesfaye
Email: semret.tesfaye@dc.gov

State of Florida
Agency for Health Care Administration
Laboratory Licensing Unit
2727 Mahan Drive, Mail Stop 32
Tallahassee, FL 32308
(850) 487-3109
FAX: (850) 410-1511
Contact: Karen Rivera
E-mail: LABSTAFF@ahca.myflorida.com

Georgia Department of Human Resources
Office of Regulatory Services
Diagnostic Service Unit
2 Peachtree Street, N.W. 31.447
Atlanta, GA 30303-3142
(404) 657-5447
Contact: Sheela E. Puthumana
E-mail: seputhumana@dhr.ga.gov

****
**FOR LABS IN GUAM, AMERICAN
SAMOA OR SAIPAN CONTACT THE
HAWAII State Agency.**
****

Hawaii Department of Health
CLIA Program
601 Kamokila Boulevard, Room 395
Kapolei, HI 96707
(808) 692-7420
FAX: (808) 692-7447
Contact: Susan O. Naka

Laboratory Improvement Section
Bureau of Laboratories
2220 Old Penitentiary Road
Boise, ID 83712-8299
(208) 334-2235 x245
FAX: (208) 334-2382

Contact: David Eisentrager
E-mail: eisentra@dhw.idaho.gov

Illinois Department of Public Health
Division of Health Care Facilities &
Programs
525 W. Jefferson Street
Fourth Floor
Springfield, IL 62761
(217) 782-6747
FAX: 217-782-0382
Contact: William Garrett
E-mail: william.garrett@illinois.gov

Indiana State Department of Health
Division of Acute Care Services
2 North Meridian Street, Room 4A
Indianapolis, IN 46204
(317) 233-7502
FAX: (317) 233-7157
Contact: Wanda Proffitt
E-mail: wproffit@isdh.in.gov

University of Iowa Hygienic Laboratory
Iowa CLIA Laboratory Program
102 Oakdale Campus, H101 OH
Iowa City, IA 52242
(319) 335-4500
Contact: Nancy Grove

**Kansas Department of Health &
Environment**
Laboratory Certification Building
740 Forbes Field
Topeka, KS 66620-0001
(785) 296-3811
Contact: Ruby Brower

Kentucky CLIA Program
Office of Inspector General
275 East Main Street, 5E-A
Frankfort, KY 40601
(502) 564-7963
Contacts: Jason Bishop, Ext. 3298
             Connie Barker, Ext. 3280

Department of Health & Hospitals
Health Standards Section
500 Laurel Street, Suite 100
Baton Rouge, LA 70821
(225) 342-9324
Contact: Staci Glueck

CLIA Program
Division of Licensing & Regulatory Services
41 Anthony Avenue, Station #11
Augusta, ME 04333-0011
(207) 287-9339
FAX: (207) 287-9304
Contact: Alelia Hilt-Lash

Maryland Department of Health & Mental Hygiene
Office of Health Care Quality—Labs
Bland Bryant Building
Spring Grove Hospital Center
55 Wade Avenue
Catonsville, MD 21228
(410) 402-8025
FAX: (410) 402-8213
Contact: Sarah Bennett

Division of Health Care Quality
Clinical Laboratory Program
99 Chauncy Street, 3rd floor
Boston, MA 02111
(617) 753-8438 or 8439
FAX: (617) 753-8240
Contact: Roberta Teixeira

Michigan Department of Community Health
Laboratory Improvement Section
P.O. Box 30664
611 W. Ottawa Street, First Floor
Lansing, MI 48909
(517) 241-2648
FAX: (517) 241-3354
Contact: Pamela Diebolt
E-mail: pjdiebo@michigan.gov

Minnesota Department of Health
Licensing and Certification
CLIA Program
85 E. 7th Place
P.O. Box 64900
St. Paul, MN 55164-0900
(651) 201-4120
FAX: (651) 215-9697
Contact: Roxanne Beyer
E-mail: roxanne.beyer@state.mn.us

Licensure and Certification
Mississippi Department of Public Health
P.O. Box 1700
Jackson, MS 39215-1700

(601) 364-1115
Contact: Theresa Irwin
E-mail: theresa.irwin@msdh.state.ms.us

Missouri Department of Health and Senior Services
CLIA Section
PO Box 570
Jefferson City, MO 65102
(573) 751-6318
Contact: William Nugent

Montana CLIA Program
Division of Quality Assurance
Department of Public Health & Human Services
2401 Colonial Drive, 2nd Floor
P.O. Box 202953
Helena, MT 59620-2953
(406) 444-1451
FAX: (406) 444-3456
Contact: Ed Adams
E-mail: eadams@mt.gov

Nebraska State Health & Human Services
Licensure Unit—Division of Public Health
Office of Acute Care Facilities
P.O. Box 94986
Lincoln, NE 68509-4986
(402) 471-3484
Contact: Joann Erickson
E-mail: Joann.Erickson@dhhs.ne.gov

State of Nevada Department of Health and Human Services
Health Division
Bureau of Health Care Quality and Compliance
Medical Laboratory Services
1550 E. College Parkway, #158
Carson City, NV 89706
(775) 687-4475
FAX: (775) 687-6588
Contact: Vickie Estes, MT(ASCP)

Health Facilities Administration
Department of Health & Human Services
129 Pleasant Street
Concord, NH 03301
(603) 271-4832
FAX: (603) 271-4968
Contact: Rodney Bascom

Clinical Laboratory Improvement Service
State of New Jersey
Department of Health & Senior Services
P.O. Box 361
Trenton, NJ 08625-0361
(609) 292-0016
FAX: (609) 633-9601
Contact: Marilou Mallada
E-mail: Marilou.Mallada@doh.state.nj.us

Health Facility Licensing & Certification Bureau
Bank of the West Building
5301 Central Avenue NW, Suite 400
Albuquerque, NM 87108
(505) 222-8646
FAX: (505) 841-5834
Contact: Julie Aragon

For Physician Office Laboratories in New York:
State of New York Department of Health
Physician Office Laboratory Evaluation Program
Empire State Plaza
P.O. Box 509
Albany, NY 12201-0509
(518) 485-5352
Contact: Thomas Heckert

For All Other Laboratory Facility Types in New York:
Clinical Laboratory Evaluation Program
Empire State Plaza
P.O. BOX 509
Albany, NY 12201-0509
(518) 485-5378
Contact: Deirdre Astin

North Carolina Department of Health and Human Services
Division of Health Service Regulation/CLIA Certification
2713 Mail Service Center
Raleigh, NC 27699-2713
(919) 855-4620
FAX: (919) 733-0176
Contact: Azzie Conley
E-mail: azzie.conley@NCmail.net

Health Resources Section
North Dakota Department of Health
State Capitol
600 East Boulevard Avenue/Dept. 301
Bismarck, ND 58505-0200
(701) 328-2352
FAX: (701) 328-1890
Contact: Bridget Weidner
E-mail: bweidner@nd.gov

Ohio Department of Health
CLIA Laboratory Program
246 N. High Street, 3rd Floor
Columbus, OH 43215
(614) 644-1845
FAX: (614) 387-2762
Contact: Nancy Spence
E-mail: CLIA@odh.ohio.gov

Oklahoma State Department of Health
Protective Health Services
Medical Facilities
1000 NE 10th Street
Oklahoma City, OK 73117-1299
(405) 271-6576
Contact: Dean Bay
E-mail: medicalfacilities@health.state.ok.us

Department of Human Services
Oregon State Public Health Division
Laboratory Compliance Section (LCS)
3150 NW 229th Avenue, Suite 100
Hillsboro, OR 97124-6536
(503) 693-4121
FAX: (503) 693-5602
Contact: Rita A. Youell
E-mail: rita.a.youell@state.or.us

Pennsylvania Department of Health
Bureau of Laboratories
110 Pickering Way
Lionville, PA 19353
(610) 280-3464
FAX: (610) 594-9763
Contact: Clerical Support Section
Internet: http://www.health.state.pa.us/labs

Commonwealth of Puerto Rico
Puerto Rico Health Department
Office of Certification & Licensure
Former-Ruiz Soler Hospital

Road No. 2
Bayamon, PR 00619
(787) 782-0120 Ext. 2214
Contact: Ricardo Santiago

Division of Facilities Regulation

Department of Health
3 Capitol Hill
Providence, RI 02908
(401) 222-4526
FAX: (401) 222-3999
Contact: Nancy Hines

South Carolina Department of Health & Environmental Control

Bureau of Certification/Health Regulation
2600 Bull Street
Columbia, SC 29201
(803) 545-4291
FAX: (803) 545-4563
Contact: Denise L. Abbott
E-mail: abbottdl@dhec.sc.gov

South Dakota Department of Health

Office of Health Care Facilities Licensure &
Certification
615 E. 4th Street
Pierre, SD 57501-1700
(605) 773-3694
FAX: (605) 773-6667
Contact: Connie Richards
E-mail: Connie.Richards@state.sd.us

Tennessee Health Care Facilities

227 French Landing, Suite 501
Heritage Place Metro Center
Nashville, TN 37243
(615) 741-7023
FAX: (615) 532-2700
Contact: Sandra Bogard

Health Facility Compliance Division

Patient Quality Care Unit
Texas Department of State Health Services
1100 West 49th Street
Austin, TX 78756-3199
(512) 834-6792
Internet: http://www.dshs.state.tx.us

Utah Department of Health

Bureau of Laboratory Improvement
46 North Medical Drive
Salt Lake City, UT 84113-1105
(801) 584-8471
FAX: (801) 584-8501
Contact: Rebecca Christiansen
E-mail: rchristiansen@utah.gov

****

LABORATORIES LOCATED IN THE VIRGIN ISLANDS SHOULD CONTACT THE NEW YORK REGIONAL OFFICE.

****

Virginia Department of Health

Office of Licensure and Certification
9960 Mayland Drive, Suite 401
Richmond, VA 23233
(804) 367-2107
FAX: (804) 527-4504
Contact: Sarah Pendergrass

CLIA Laboratory Program

Vermont Department of Health
108 Cherry Street
Burlington VT 05401
(802) 652-4145
FAX: (802) 865-7701
Contact: Carol Drawbaugh

Office of Laboratory Quality Assurance

Department of Health
1610 NE 150th Street
Shoreline, WA 98155-9701
(206) 418-5418
FAX: (206) 418-5505
Contact: Susan Walker
E-mail: susan.walker@doh.wa.gov

West Virginia Department of Health

Office of Laboratory Services
167 11th Avenue
South Charleston, WV 25303-1137
(304) 558-3530, Ext. 2103
FAX: (304) 558-2006
Contact: Jerry Gross
E-mail: jerry.w.gross@wv.gov

Department of Health Services
Division of Quality Assurance
Clinical Laboratory Section
1 W. Wilson Street, Room 1151
Madison, WI 53701-2969
(608) 261-0653
FAX: (608) 264-9847
Contact: Barbara Saar
E-mail: barbara.saar@dhs.wisconsin.gov

Office of Healthcare Licensing and Surveys
400 Qwest Building
6101 North Yellowstone Road
Cheyenne, WY 82002
Contact: Russ Forney
(307) 777-7123
FAX: (307) 777-7127
Email: russ.forney@health.wyo.gov

Appendix C

Specialty Codes

Medicare Claims Processing Manual, Chapter 26 Completing and Processing Form CMS-1500 Data Set

10.8.2—Physician Specialty Codes

Code	Physician Specialty	Code	Physician Specialty
01	General Practice	25	Physical Medicine and Rehabilitation
02	General Surgery	26	Psychiatry
03	Allergy/Immunology	27	Available
04	Otolaryngology	28	Colorectal Surgery (formerly proctology)
05	Anesthesiology	29	Pulmonary Disease
06	Cardiology	30	Diagnostic Radiology
07	Dermatology	31	Available
08	Family Practice	32	Anesthesiologist Assistants
09	Interventional Pain Management	33	Thoracic Surgery
10	Gastroenterology	34	Urology
11	Internal Medicine	35	Chiropractic
12	Osteopathic Manipulative Therapy	36	Nuclear Medicine
13	Neurology	37	Pediatric Medicine
14	Neurosurgery	38	Geriatric Medicine
15	Available	39	Nephrology
16	Obstetrics/Gynecology	40	Hand Surgery
17	Available	41	Optometry
18	Ophthalmology	44	Infectious Disease
19	Oral Surgery (dentists only)	46	Endocrinology
20	Orthopedic Surgery	48	Podiatry
21	Available	66	Rheumatology
22	Pathology	70	Single or Multispecialty Clinic or Group Practice
23	Available	72	Pain Management
24	Plastic and Reconstructive Surgery	73	Mass Immunization Roster Biller

Code	Physician Specialty	Code	Physician Specialty
74	Radiation Therapy Center	85	Maxillofacial Surgery
75	Slide Preparation Facilities	86	Neuropsychiatry
76	Peripheral Vascular Disease	90	Medical Oncology
77	Vascular Surgery	91	Surgical Oncology
78	Cardiac Surgery	92	Radiation Oncology
79	Addiction Medicine	93	Emergency Medicine
81	Critical Care (Intensivists)	94	Interventional Radiology
82	Hematology	98	Gynecological/Oncology
83	Hematology/Oncology	99	Unknown Physician Specialty
84	Preventive Medicine		

10.8.3—Nonphysician Practitioner, Supplier, and Provider Specialty Codes

(Rev. 1552, Issued: 07-18-08, Effective: 01-01-09, Implementation: 01-05-09)

The following list of 2-digit codes and narrative describe the kind of medicine nonphysician practitioners or other healthcare providers/suppliers practice.

Code	Nonphysician Practitioner/Supplier/Provider Specialty
32	Anesthesiologist Assistant
42	Certified Nurse Midwife (effective July 1, 1988)
43	Certified Registered Nurse Anesthetist (CRNA)
45	Mammography Screening Center
47	Independent Diagnostic Testing Facility (IDTF)
49	Ambulatory Surgical Center
50	Nurse Practitioner
51	Medical supply company with orthotic personnel certified by an accrediting organization
52	Medical supply company with prosthetic personnel certified by an accrediting organization
53	Medical supply company with prosthetic/orthotic personnel certified by an accrediting organization
54	Medical supply company not included in 51, 52, or 53
55	Individual orthotic personnel certified by an accrediting organization
56	Individual prosthetic personnel certified by an accrediting organization
57	Individual prosthetic/orthotic personnel certified by an accrediting organization
58	Medical Supply Company with registered pharmacist
59	Ambulance Service Supplier (e.g., private ambulance companies, funeral homes)
60	Public Health or Welfare Agencies (Federal, State, and local)
61	Voluntary Health or Charitable Agencies (e.g., National Cancer Society, National Heart Association, Catholic Charities)
62	Clinical Psychologist (Billing Independently)
63	Portable X-Ray Supplier (Billing Independently)
64	Audiologist (Billing Independently)
65	Physical Therapist in Private Practice
67	Occupational Therapist in Private Practice
68	Clinical Psychologist
69	Clinical Laboratory (Billing Independently)
71	Registered Dietician/Nutrition Professional

Code	Nonphysician Practitioner/Supplier/Provider Specialty
73	Mass Immunization Roster Billers (Mass Immunizers have to roster bill assigned claims and can only bill for immunizations)
74	Radiation Therapy Centers
75	Slide Preparation Facilities
80	Licensed Clinical Social Worker
87	All other suppliers, e.g., Drug Stores
88	Unknown Supplier/Provider
89	Certified Clinical Nurse Specialist
95	Available
96	Optician
97	Physician Assistant
A0	Hospital
A1	Skilled Nursing Facility
A2	Intermediate Care Nursing Facility
A3	Nursing Facility, Other
A4	Home Health Agency
A5	Pharmacy
A6	Medical Supply Company with Respiratory Therapist
A7	Department Store
A8	Grocery Store
B2	Pedorthic Personnel
B3	Medical Supply Company with Pedorthic Personnel
B4	Rehabilitation Agency

Note: Specialty Code Use for Service in an Independent Laboratory. For services performed in an independent laboratory, show the specialty code of the physician ordering the x-rays and requesting payment. If the independent laboratory requests payment, use type of supplier code "69."

Appendix D

1995, 1997, and New Framework Table of Risk

Level of Risk	Presenting Problem(s)	Diagnostic Procedure(s)	Management Options Selected
Minimal	• One self-limited or minor problem, ie, cold, insect bite, tinea corporis	• Laboratory tests requiring venipuncture • Chest x-rays • EKG/EEG • Urinalysis • Ultrasound, ie, echocardiography • KOH prep	• Rest • Gargles • Elastic Bandages • Superficial dressing
Low	• Two or more self-limited or minor problems • One stable chronic illness, ie, well controlled hypertension or non-insulin dependent diabetes, cataract, BPH • Acute uncomplicated illness or injury, ie, cystitis, allergic rhinitis, simple sprain	• Physiologic tests not under stress, ie, pulmonary function tests • Non-cardiovascular imaging studies with contrast, ie, barium enema • Superficial needle biopsy • Clinical laboratory tests requiring arterial puncture • Skin biopsies	• Over-the-counter drug • Minor surgery with no identified risk factors • Physical therapy • Occupational therapy • IV fluids without additives
Moderate	• One or more chronic illnesses with mild exacerbation, progression, or side effects of treatment • Two or more stable chronic illnesses • Undiagnosed new problem with uncertain prognosis, ie, lump in breast • Acute illness with systemic systems, ie, pyelonephritis, pneumonitis, colitis • Acute complicated injury, ie, head injury with brief loss of consciousness	• Physiologic tests under stress, ie, cardiac stress test, fetal contraction stress test • Diagnostic endoscopies with no identified risk factors • Deep needle or incisional biopsy • Cardiovascular imaging studies with contract and no identified risk factors, ie, arteriogram, cardiac catheterization • Obtain fluid from body cavity, ie, lumbar puncture, thoracentesis, culdocentesis	• Prescription drug management • Minor surgery with identified risk factors • Elective major surgery (open, percutaneous, or endoscopic) *with no* identified risk factors • Therapeutic nuclear medicine • IV fluids with additives • Closed treatment of fracture or dislocation without manipulation
High	• One or more chronic illnesses with severe exacerbation, progression, or side effects of treatment • Acute or chronic illnesses or injuries that pose a threat to life or bodily function, ie, multiple trauma, acute MI, pulmonary embolus, severe respiratory distress, progressive severe rheumatoid arthritis, psychiatric illness with potential threat to self or others, peritonitis, acute renal failure • An abrupt change in neurologic status, ie, seizure, TIA, weakness, or sensory loss	• Cardiovascular imaging studies with contrast with identified risk factors • Cardiac electrophysiologic tests • Diagnostic endoscopies with identified risk factors • Discography	• Elective major surgery (open, percutaneous, or endoscopic) *with* identified risk factors • Emergency major surgery (open, percutaneous or endoscopic) • Parenteral controlled substances • Drug therapy requiring intensive monitoring for toxicity • Decision not to resuscitate or to de-escalate care because of poor prognosis

Appendix E

AAPA Summary of Co-signature Requirements

Summary of State Laws and Regulations Requiring Physicians to Review or Co-Sign PA Medical Record Entries

Alabama

For hospitalized patients, physician assistants may enter verbal admission orders and verbal subsequent orders for medications from the physician. All such orders must be validated by the ordering physician within 24 hours or within the time period specified in the hospital bylaws or policies.

Alabama Administrative Code §540-X-7.28 (8)

Countersignature by supervising physician must conform to established policy and/or applicable legal regulations and accreditation standards.

Alabama Administrative Code §540-X-7.23

Alaska

No co-signature requirement.

Arizona

A supervising physician shall develop a system for recordation and review of all instances in which the physician assistant prescribes 14-day prescriptions of schedule II or schedule III controlled substances. The board shall approve this system.

Arizona Revised Statutes §32-2533 D

Arkansas

No co-signature requirement.

California

The supervising physician and surgeon shall review, countersign, and date a sample consisting of, at a minimum, 5% of the medical records of patients treated by the physician assistant functioning under the protocols within 30 days of the date of treatment by the physician assistant. The physician and surgeon shall select for review those cases that by diagnosis, problem, treatment, or procedure represent, in his or her judgment, the most significant risk to the patient.

Annotated Code of California, Business and Professions Chapter 7.7, §3502(c)(2)

Any schedule II drug order that has been issued or carried out shall be reviewed, countersigned and dated by a supervising physician and surgeon within 7 days.

Annotated Code of California, Business and Professions Chapter 7.7, §3502.1(e)

A physician assistant and the supervising physician must establish written guidelines for adequate supervision, which include one or more of the following:

(1) same day examination of patient by physician

(2) countersignature and dating of all medical records within 30 days

(3) adoption of protocols to govern a physician assistant's performance

(4) other mechanisms approved by PAC

The supervising physician must review, countersign and date at least 10% of medical records within 30 days for patients treated by physician assistants working under protocols.

If the physician assistant is operating under interim approval, the supervising physician must review, sign and date medical records of all patients within 7 days if the physician was on the premises when the physician assistant diagnosed or treated the patient. If the physician was not on the premises, this shall be done within 48 hours.

California Administrative Code, Title 16, §1399.545*

*Regulatory change to implement 2007 statute change has not yet been adopted.

Colorado

When a physician assistant performs a medical function in an acute care hospital where the supervising physician regularly practices or in a designated health manpower shortage area, the supervising physician does not have to be present, but will review the medical records of the physician assistant every 2 working days.

Colorado Revised Statutes, §12-36-106(5)(b)

"Reviewing the medical records" means review and signature by the primary physician supervisor or a secondary physician supervisor.

New physician assistant graduates:
For the first 6 months of employment and a minimum of 500 patient encounters, a physician supervisor shall review the chart for every patient seen by the physician assistant no later than 7 days after the physician assistant has performed an act defined as the practice of medicine. The physician supervisor shall document the performance of such review by signing the chart in a legible manner. In lieu of signing the chart, the physician supervisor may document the performance of such review by the use of an electronically generated signature provided that reasonable measures have been taken to prevent the unauthorized use of the electronically generated signature.

Experienced Physician Assistants New to a Practice Setting:

For the first 3 months of employment and a minimum of 500 patient encounters, a physician supervisor shall review the chart for every patient seen by an experienced physician assistant new to a practice setting no later than 14 days after the physician assistant has performed an act defined as the practice of medicine. The physician supervisor shall document the performance of such review by signing the chart in a legible manner. In lieu of signing the chart, the physician supervisor may document the performance of such review by the use of an electronically generated signature provided that reasonable measures have been taken to prevent the unauthorized use of the electronically generated signature.

All other PAs must meet with supervising physician twice yearly and physician must conduct performance assessment (to include review and initialing of selected charts).

Colorado State Board of Medical Examiners, Rule 400, §2

Connecticut

The supervising physician must co-sign a physician assistant's order for Schedule II or III drugs within 24 hours.

Connecticut General Statutes, Chapter 370 §20-12d

Supervision includes, but is not limited to:

(i) Continuous availability of direct communication either in person or by radio, telephone or telecommunications between the physician assistant and the supervising physician;

(ii) active and continuing overview of the physician assistant's activities to ensure that the supervising physician's directions are being implemented and to support the physician assistant in the performance of his or her services;

(iii) personal review by the supervising physician of the physician assistant's services through a face-to-face meeting with the physician assistant, at least weekly or more frequently as necessary to ensure quality patient care, at a facility or practice location where the physician assistant or supervising physician performs services;

(iv) review of the charts and records of the physician assistant on a regular basis as necessary to ensure quality patient care and written documentation by the supervising physician of such review at the facility or practice location where the physician assistant or supervising physician performs services

Connecticut General Statutes, Chapter 370 §20-12a(7)

Delaware

The relaying, transcribing, or executing specific diagnostic or therapeutic orders must be countersigned by the physician within 24 hours.

Delaware Code Annotated, Title 24, Chapter 17, §1770A(a)(3)

District of Columbia

A licensed physician assistant employed or extended privileges by a hospital may, if permissible under the bylaws, rules and regulations of the hospital, write medical orders, including those for controlled substances, for patients under the care of the physician responsible for his/her supervision. Countersignature by the supervising physician shall not be required prior to the execution of any orders, but shall be accomplished within 30 days of the execution of the order.

District of Columbia Municipal Regulations, §4916.3

Physician assistants may write orders and progress notes in outpatient settings. Countersignature by the supervising physician shall not be required prior to the execution, but shall be accomplished within 10 days of the execution of the order and within 10 days of any progress note.

District of Columbia Municipal Regulations, §4916.4

Florida

No co-signature requirement.

Georgia

Except in facilities operated by the Division of Public Health of the Department of Human Resources, the supervising physician shall review the prescription drug or device order copy and medical record entry for prescription drug or device orders issued within the past 30 days by the physician assistant. Such review may be achieved with a sampling of no less than 50 percent of such prescription drug or device order copies and medial record entries.

Georgia Code Annotated, §43-34-103

A copy of the prescription is maintained in the patient's medical file and the supervising physician must countersign the prescription or medical record entry for prescription within 7 working days.

Rules and Regulations of the State of Georgia, §360-5.12

In a remote site (physician is present at least 25% of the time) in an area with a shortage and maldistribution of health care services a supervising physician must be physically present at least twice a week and review patient records daily and all entries made by a physician assistant in patient medical records must be co-signed by a supervising physician within 7 days.

Rules and Regulations of the State of Georgia, §360-5-.08

Hawaii

Medical record of controlled substance prescription must be reviewed and initialed by the supervising physician within 7 working days.

Hawaii Revised Statutes, §329-38

Idaho

Delegation agreement shall include:

. . .

iii. Periodic review of a representative sample of records and a periodic review of the patient services being provided by the licensee. This review shall also include an evaluation of adherence to the delegation of services.

Idaho Administrative Code, §22.01.03 - 030.03(c)

Illinois

The supervising physician shall periodically review medication orders issued by a physician assistant.

Illinois Compiled Statutes, Chapter 225 ILCS 95, §7.5

It is the responsibility of the supervising physician to direct and review the work, records and practice of the physician assistant on a timely basis.

Illinois Administrative Code, Title 68, Chapter VII(b), §1350.80(f)

Indiana

The supervising physician shall review all patient encounters not later than 24 hours after the physician assistant has seen the patient.

Indiana Code, §25-27.5-6-1

Direction and supervision must be personally rendered by supervising physician, who must be physically present or immediately available at all times. Supervising physician shall review medical services provided by a physician assistant within a reasonable time, not to exceed 24 hours.

Indiana Administrative Code, Title 844, §2.2-2-2(6)

Iowa

Although every chart need not be signed nor every visit reviewed, nor does the supervising physician need to be physically present at each activity of the physician assistant, it is the responsibility of the supervising physician and physician assistant to ensure that each patient has received the appropriate medical care.

Patient care provided by the physician assistant may be reviewed with a supervising physician in person, by telephone or by other telecommunicative means.

When signatures are required, electronic signatures are allowed if: (1) The signature is transcribed by the signer into an electronic record and is not the result of electronic regeneration; and (2) A mechanism exists allowing confirmation of the signature and protection from unauthorized reproduction.

Iowa Administrative Code, §645-326.8(4)

A physician assistant may provide medical services in a remote medical site if one of the following three conditions is met:

(a)   The physician assistant has a permanent license and at least one year of practice as a physician assistant; or

(b)   The physician assistant with less than one year of practice has a permanent license and meets the following criteria:

    (1)   The physician assistant has practiced as a physician assistant for at least six months; and

    (2)   The physician assistant and supervising physician have worked together at the same location for a period of at least three months; and

    (3)   The supervising physician reviews patient care provided by the physician assistant at least weekly; and

(4) The supervising physician signs all patient charts unless the medical record documents that direct consultation with the supervising physician occurred; or

(c) The physician assistant and supervising physician provide a written statement sent directly to the board that the physician assistant is qualified to provide the needed medical services and that the medical care will be unavailable at the remote site unless the physician assistant is allowed to practice there. In addition, for three months the supervising physician must review patient care provided by the physician assistant at least weekly and must sign all patient charts unless the medical record documents that direct consultation with the supervising physician occurred.

Iowa Administrative Code, §645-327.4(1)

Kansas

Direction and supervision of the physician assistant shall be considered to be adequate if the responsible physician meets all of the following requirements:

. . .

(g) at least every 14 days, reviews all records of patients treated by the physician assistant and authenticates this review in the patient record;

(h) reviews patient records and authenticates the review in each patient record within 48 hours of treatment provided by the physician assistant if the treatment provided in an emergency exceeded the authority granted to the physician assistant by the responsible physician request form required

Kansas Administrative Regulations, §100-28a-10

Kentucky

A supervising physician shall:

. . .

(10) Sign all records of service rendered by a physician assistant in a timely manner as certification that the physician assistant performed the services as delegated.

Kentucky Revised Statutes, §311.856

Louisiana

A physician assistant may administer medication to a patient, or transmit orally, electronically, or in writing on a patient's record, a prescription from his or her supervising physician to a person who may lawfully furnish such medication or medical device. The supervising physician's prescription, transmitted by the physician assistant, for any patient cared for by the physician assistant, shall be based on a patient-specific order by the supervising physician. . . . [T]he medical record of any patient cared for by the physician assistant for whom the physician's prescription has been transmitted or carried out shall be reviewed, countersigned and dated by a supervising physician within 72 hours, or as otherwise required by law.

Louisiana Administrative Code, Title 46, Part 45, §4505(D)

The physician assistant and supervising physician shall:

. . .

(4)   insure that, with respect to each direct patient encounter, all activities, functions, services, treatment measures, medical devices or medication prescribed or delivered to the patient by the physician assistant are properly documented in written form in the patient's record by the physician assistant and that each such entry is countersigned by the supervising physician within 24 hours with respect to inpatients in an acute care setting and patients in a hospital emergency department; within 48 hours with respect to patients of nursing homes and other sub-acute settings and within 72 hours in an office, clinic and all other practice settings

Louisiana Administrative Code, Title 46, Part 45, §4511(A)

Maine

No co-signature requirement.

Maryland

No co-signature requirement.

Massachusetts

Any prescription or medication order issued by a physician assistant for a Schedule II controlled substance, as defined in 105 CMR 700.002, shall be reviewed by his or her supervising physician, or by a temporary supervising physician designated pursuant to 263 CMR 5.05(4)(g), within 96 hours after its issuance.

263 Code of Massachusetts Regulations, §5.07(3)

Michigan

A physician is not required to countersign orders written in a patient's clinical record by a physician assistant to whom the physician has delegated the performance of medical care services for a patient.

*Michigan Compiled Laws, §333.17049(6) and §333.17549(6)**

*identical language appears in laws governing the practice of osteopathic medicine

Minnesota

No co-signature requirement.

Mississippi

The supervising physician shall, on at least a monthly basis, conduct a review of the records/charts of at least ten percent (10%) of the patients treated by the physician assistant, said records/charts selected on a random basis. During said review, the supervising physician shall note the medical and family histories taken, results of any and all examinations and tests, all diagnoses, orders given, medications prescribed, and treatments rendered. The review shall be evidenced by the supervising physician placing his or her signature or initials next to each of the above areas of review, and shall submit proof of said review to the Board upon request.

Mississippi State Board of Medical Licensure, Rules and Regulations, Chapter 11, §705

Missouri

Supervision is defined as control exercised over a physician assistant working within the same facility as the supervising physician sixty-six percent of the time a physician assistant provides patient care, except that a physician assistant may make follow-up patient examinations in hospitals, nursing homes and correctional facilities, each such exam being reviewed, approved and signed by the supervising physician.

Missouri Revised Statutes, §334.735(1)(8)

It is the responsibility of the supervising physician and licensed physician assistant to jointly review and document the work, records, and practice activities of the licensed physician assistant at least once every two (2) weeks. The supervising physician must review a minimum of ten percent (10%) of the physician assistant's patients' records every two (2) weeks and have documentation supporting the review. For nursing home practice, such review shall occur at least once a month. The documentation of this review shall be available to the Board of Registration for the Healing Arts for review upon request.

Missouri Code of State Regulations, Title 20, §2150-7.135(12)

Montana

(1) The supervising physician shall review a minimum of 10 percent of the physician assistant charts on at least a monthly basis.

(2) Chart review for a physician assistant having less than one year of full time practice experience from the date of initial licensure must be 100 percent for the first three months of practice, and then may be reduced to not less than 25 percent for the next three months, on a monthly basis, for each supervision agreement.

(3) The supervising physician shall countersign and date all written entries that have been chart reviewed and shall document any amendments, modifications, or guidance provided.

(4) Chart review for a physician assistant who has been issued a probationary license must be 100 percent on a monthly basis, unless the board terminates the probationary period.

Administrative Rules of the State of Montana, §24.156.1623

Nebraska

A physician assistant may not practice at a secondary site without the personal presence of the supervising physician unless approval has been granted on an individual basis by the Board. Such approval must be granted when the following conditions are met:

. . .

(4) The supervising physician, as a method of regular reporting, must review 100% of the charts of the patients seen by the physician assistant. A systematic documentation of these reviews must be established and maintained by the supervising physician.

Nebraska Administrative Code, Title 172, §90-006.01H

Nevada

The supervising physician shall review and initial selected charts of the patients of the physician assistant.

Nevada Administrative Code, §630.370(2)

A physician who supervises a physician assistant shall develop and carry out a program to ensure the quality of care provided by a physician assistant. The program must include, without limitation:

. . .

(b)   A review and initialing of selected charts

Nevada Administrative Code, §630.370(5)

New Hampshire

A physician assistant may write orders for patients as delegated by the supervising physician or alternate. Such orders shall be countersigned by the RSP or ARSP as required by institutional policy, however, such countersignature shall not be required prior to the order being executed.

New Hampshire Code of Administrative Rules, Chapter MED §603.01(c)

New Jersey

In an inpatient setting, direct supervision of a physician assistant shall include, but not be limited to:

. . .

(3)   personal review by a physician of all charts and records of patients and countersignature by a physician of all medical orders, including prescribing and administering medication, within 24 hours of their entry by the physician assistant.

New Jersey Revised Statutes §45:9-27.18(b)

In an outpatient setting, direct supervision of a physician assistant shall include, but not be limited to:

. . .

(3)   personal review by a physician of the charts and records of patients and countersignature by a physician of all medical orders, within seven days of their entry by the physician assistant, except that in the case of any medical order prescribing or administering medication, a physician shall review and countersign the order within 48 hours of its entry by the physician assistant.

New Jersey Revised Statutes §45:9-27.18(c)

New Mexico*

The supervising physician must review the quality of medical services rendered by the physician assistant by reviewing at least 10% of each months medical records generated by the physician assistant.

New Mexico Adminstrative Code, §18.6.8(B)

The supervising physician will review and countersign each patient's chart in which the physician assistant has prescribed more than 72 hours of Schedule II drugs in a 30 day period for that patient.

New Mexico Administrative Code, §18.7.9(A)(2)

*These regulations apply only to PAs licensed by the NM Board of Osteopathic Medical Examiners

New York

A registered physician assistant employed or extended privileges by a hospital may, if permissible under the bylaws, rules and regulations of the hospital, write medical orders, including those for controlled substances, for inpatients under the care of the physician responsible for his supervision. Countersignature of such orders may be required if deemed necessary and appropriate by the supervising physician or the hospital, but in no event shall countersignature be required prior to execution.

New York Codes, Rules and Regulations, Title 10, §94.2(e)(6)

North Carolina

Entries by a physician assistant into patient charts of inpatients (hospital, long term care institutions) must comply with the rules and regulations of the institution.

North Carolina Administrative Code, Title 21, §32S.0110(c)

North Dakota

No co-signature requirement.

Ohio

During the course of the provisional period*, each supervising physician who supervises the physician assistant in the exercise of physician-delegated prescriptive authority shall review and evaluate the physician assistant's competence, knowledge, and skill in pharmacokinetic principles and the application of these principles to the physician assistant's area of practice. The review and evaluation shall be documented by the supervising physician's signing of patient charts in a legible manner. In lieu of signing the patient charts, the supervising physician may document the review and evaluation by the use of an electronically generated signature provided that reasonable measures have been taken to prevent the unauthorized use of the electronically generated signature.

(1) During the first five hundred hours of the provisional period, the review and evaluation shall be completed and documented on every chart by each supervising physician who provided supervision within a reasonable period of time after the physician assistant rendered service to a patient.

(2) During the remainder of the provisional period, the review and evaluation shall be completed and documented on at least fifty percent of the patient charts by each supervising physician who provided supervision within a reasonable period of time after the physician assistant rendered service to a patient.

Ohio Administrative Code, §4730-2-04(D)

*The provision period shall be, at minimum, 1,000 hours during at least six months and no longer than 1,800 hours during a one year period, but may be extended by the supervising physician for up to one additional year

Oklahoma

In all patient care settings, the supervising physician shall provide appropriate methods of supervising the health care services provided by the physician assistant including:

. . .

(b) regularly reviewing the health care services provided by the physician assistant and any problems or complications encountered

Oklahoma Statutes Annotated, Title 59, §519.6(b)

Physician supervision shall be conducted in accordance with the following standards:

. . .

(2) The supervising physician regularly reviews the health care services provided by the physician assistant and any problems or complications encountered.

Oklahoma Administrative Code, §435:15-9-2(b)

(a) Office setting

. . .

(2) It is assumed that the physician regularly and systematically checks the charts and notes of the patients seen by the physician assistant, checking for accuracy and completeness of such records, and in particular, the suitability of the plan of management. It is assumed that this type of review is conducted within 48 hours of the care being delivered.

. . .

(b) Hospital setting

. . .

(3) Initial workup of patients upon admission is often delegated to the physician assistant. This is an appropriate function if checked and countersigned by the supervising physician on his/her next visit to the hospital, which should usually occur within 24 hours.

(4) Initial orders may be delegated to a physician assistant. These activities are very important in that they involve the function of others, such as the R.N. and L.P.N. assigned to the ward. Copies of all standing orders that the physician has delegated to the physician assistant to order on his/her behalf should be on file in the hospital and available to the nurse accepting such orders as a means of assurance that these orders are emanating from the responsible physician and that they are within the authority which the physician has delegated to the physician assistant. All orders should be checked and countersigned by the responsible physician at his/ her next visit to the hospital, which should usually occur within 24 hours.

Oklahoma Administrative Code, §435:15-9-4

Oregon

No co-signature requirement.

Pennsylvania

A separate statement shall be made for each satellite location. The statement must demonstrate that:

. . .

(4) The supervising physician will visit the satellite location at least once every 10 days and devote enough time onsite to provide supervision and personally review the records of selected patients seen by the physician assistant in this setting. The supervising physician shall notate those patient records as reviewed.

Pennsylvania Code, Title 49, §18.155(b)

Recordkeeping requirements are as follows:

. . .

(3) The physician assistant shall report, orally or in writing, to the supervising physician within 36 hours, a drug prescribed or medication dispensed by the physician assistant while the supervising physician was not physically present, and the basis for each decision to prescribe or dispense in accordance with the written agreement.

(4) The supervising physician shall countersign the patient record within 10 days.

Pennsylvania Code, Title 49, §18.158(d)

An appropriate degree of supervision includes:

. . .

(C) Personal and regular review within 10 days by the supervising physician of the patient records upon which entries are made by the physician assistant.

Pennsylvania Code, Title 49, §18.122

(a) A physician assistant may execute a written or oral order for a medical regimen or may relay a written or oral order for a medical regimen to be executed by a health care practitioner subject to the requirements of this section.

. . .

(c) The physician assistant shall record, date and authenticate the medical regimen on the patient's chart at the time it is executed or relayed. . . . The supervising physician shall countersign the patient record within a reasonable amount of time not to exceed 10 days, unless countersignature is required sooner by regulation, policy within the medical care facility or the requirements of a third-party payor.

Pennsylvania Code, Title 49, §18.153

An appropriate degree of supervision includes:

. . .

    (iii)   Personal and regular—at least weekly—review by the supervising physician of the patient records upon which entries are made by the physician assistant.

Pennsylvania Code, Title 49, §25.141*

*This provision applies only to PAs licensed by the State Board of Osteopathic Medicine

No physician assistant may be permitted to be utilized in an office or clinic separate and apart from the supervising physician's primary place for meeting patients unless the supervising physician has obtained specific approval from the Board. . . . The criteria for granting approval is that the supervising physician demonstrate the following to the satisfaction of the Board:

. . .

    (4)   That the supervising physician will visit the remote office at least weekly and spend enough time on-site to provide supervision and personally review the records of each patient seen by the physician assistant in this setting.

Pennsylvania Code, Title 49, §25.175(a)*

*This provision applies only to PAs licensed by the State Board of Osteopathic Medicine

Rhode Island

No co-signature requirement.

South Carolina

For off-site practice ... [t]he supervising physician or alternate must review, initial, and date the off-site physician assistant's charts not later than 5 working days from the date of service if not sooner as proportionate to the acuity of care and practice setting.

South Carolina Code of Laws, §40-47-955(C)

South Dakota

No co-signature requirement.

Tennessee

    (1)   Supervision requires active and continuous overview of the physician assistant's activities to ensure that the physician's directions and advice are in fact implemented, but does not require the continuous and constant physical presence of the supervising physician. The board and the committee shall adopt, by September 19, 1999, regulations governing the supervising physician's personal review of historical, physical and therapeutic data contained in the charts of patients examined by the physician assistant.

Tennessee Code, §63-19-106

(7) Within ten (10) business days after the physician assistant has examined a patient who falls in one of the following categories, the supervising physician shall make a personal review of the historical, physical, and therapeutic data gathered by the physician assistant on that patient and shall so certify in the patient's chart within thirty (30) days:

(a) when medically indicated;

(b) when requested by the patient;

(c) when prescriptions written by the physician assistant fall outside the protocols;

(d) when prescriptions are written by a physician assistant who possesses a temporary license; and

(e) when a controlled drug has been prescribed.

(8) In any event, a supervising physician shall personally review at least twenty percent (20%) of charts monitored or written by the physician assistant every thirty (30) days.

Rules and Regulations of the State of Tennessee, §0880-2-.18

Texas

(b) At an alternate site, a physician licensed by the board may delegate to an advanced practice nurse or physician assistant, acting under adequate physician supervision, the act of administering, providing, or carrying out or signing a prescription drug order as authorized through a physician's order, a standing medical order, a standing delegation order, or another order or protocol as defined by the board.

(c) Physician supervision is adequate for the purposes of this section if

. . .

(2) the delegating physician reviews at least 10 percent of the medical charts, including through electronic review of the charts from a remote location, for each advanced practice nurse or physician assistant at the site

Texas Statutes, Occupations Code, Chapter 157, §157.0541 Prescribing at alternate sites

Utah

A physician assistant, in accordance with a delegation of services agreement, may prescribe or administer an appropriate controlled substance if:

. . .

(c) the supervising physician cosigns any medical chart record of a prescription of a Schedule 2 or Schedule 3 controlled substance made by the physician assistant.

Utah Code Annotated, §58-70a-501(2)

The [delegation of services] agreement defines the working relationship and delegation of duties between the supervising physician and the physician assistant as specified by division rule and shall include:

. . .

(iii)   the frequency and mechanism of chart review

Utah Code Annotated, §58-70a-102(2)(b)

The supervising physician shall review and co-sign sufficient numbers of patient charts and medical records to ensure that the patient's health, safety, and welfare will not be adversely compromised. The Delegation of Services Agreement, maintained at the site of practice, shall outline specific parameters for review that are appropriate for the working relationship.

Utah Administrative Code, §R156-70a-501(3)

Vermont

The scope of practice document shall cover at least the following:

(b)   Supervision:

(5) Provisions for retrospective review of PA charts:

(A) the frequency with which these reviews will be conducted

(B) the methods to be used to document this review

Vermont Rules of the Board of Medical Practice, Section II Rules for Physician Assistants, §7.3

Virginia

Prior to initiation of practice, a physician assistant and his supervising physician shall submit a written protocol which spells out the roles and functions of the assistant. Any such protocol shall take into account such factors as the physician assistant's level of competence, the number of patients, the types of illness treated by the physician, the nature of the treatment, special procedures, and the nature of the physician availability in ensuring direct physician involvement at an early stage and regularly thereafter. The protocol shall also provide an evaluation process for the physician assistant's performance, including a requirement specifying the time period, proportionate to the acuity of care and practice setting, within which the supervising physician shall review the record of services rendered by the physician assistant.

Virginia Administrative Code, Title 18, §85-50-101

Washington

A physician assistant and supervising physician shall ensure that, with respect to each patient, all activities, functions, services and treatment measures are immediately and properly documented in written form by the physician assistant. Every written entry shall be reviewed and countersigned by the supervising physician within two working days unless a different time period is authorized by the commission.

*Washington Administrative Code, §246-918-130(4)**

*This provision applies only to PAs who are not certified

It shall be the responsibility of the certified physician assistant and the sponsoring physician to ensure that appropriate consultation and review of work are provided.

Washington Administrative Code, §246-918-140(3)*

*This provision applies only to PAs who are certified (PA-C)

    (5) The osteopathic physician assistant and supervising osteopathic physician shall ensure that:

. . .

        (d) The supervising osteopathic physician provides adequate supervision and review of the osteopathic physician assistant's practice. The supervising osteopathic physician or designated alternate physician shall review and countersign:

           (i) All charts of the licensed osteopathic physician assistant within seven working days for the first thirty days of practice and thereafter ten percent of their charts, including clinic, emergency room, and hospital patients within seven working days.

           (ii) Every chart entry of an interim permit holder within two working days

Washington Administrative Code, §246-854-015*

*This provision applies to PAs who are supervised by osteopathic physicians, whether the PA is certified or not.

West Virginia

A physician assistant may sign orders to be countersigned later by his or her supervising physician.

West Virginia Code of State Rules, § 11-1B-7.6

No physician assistant may be utilized in an office or clinic separate and apart from the supervising physician's primary place for meeting patients unless the supervising physician has obtained specific approval from the Board. . . . The criteria for granting the approval is that the supervising physician demonstrate the following to the satisfaction of the Board:

. . .

    (d)   That the supervising physician visits the remote office at least once every fourteen (14) days and demonstrate that he or she spends enough time on site to provide supervision and personal and regular review of the selected records upon which entries are made by the physician assistant. Patient records shall be selected on the basis of written criteria established by the supervising physician and the physician assistant and shall be of sufficient number to assure adequate review of the physician assistant's scope of practice.

West Virginia Code of State Rules, § 11-1B-13.8

An appropriate degree of supervision includes:

. . .

(3) Personal and regular (at least monthly) review by the supervising physician of selected patient records upon which entries are made by the physician assistant. The supervising physician shall select patient records for review on the basis of written criteria established by the supervising physician and the physician assistant and shall be of sufficient number to assure adequate review of the physician assistant's scope of practice

West Virginia Code of State Rules, § 11-1B-2.1(f)

Supervision requires the availability of the supervising osteopathic physician. An appropriate degree of supervision includes:

. . .

c. Personal and regular (at least monthly) review by the supervising osteopathic physician of selected patient records upon which entries are made by the osteopathic physician assistant. The supervising osteopathic physician shall select patient records for review on the basis of written criteria established by the supervising osteopathic physician and the osteopathic physician assistant and these records shall be of sufficient number to assure adequate review of the osteopathic physician assistant's scope of practice

West Virginia Code of State Rules, §24-2-2.5.2*

*This provision applies only to PAs supervised by osteopathic physicians

Wisconsin

No co-signature requirement

Wyoming

No co-signature requirement

11/09

Appendix F

AHIMA Code of Ethics

Preamble

The ethical obligations of the health information management (HIM) professional include the protection of patient privacy and confidential information; disclosure of information; development, use, and maintenance of health information systems and health records; and the quality of information. Both handwritten and computerized medical records contain many sacred stories—stories that must be protected on behalf of the individual and the aggregate community of persons served in the healthcare system. Healthcare consumers are increasingly concerned about the loss of privacy and the inability to control the dissemination of their protected information. Core health information issues include what information should be collected, how the information should be handled, who should have access to the information, and under what conditions the information should be disclosed.

Ethical obligations are central to the professional's responsibility, regardless of the employment site or the method of collection, storage, and security of health information. Sensitive information (genetic, adoption, drug, alcohol, sexual, and behavioral information) requires special attention to prevent misuse. Entrepreneurial roles require expertise in the protection of the information in the world of business and interactions with consumers.

Professional Values

The mission of the HIM profession is based on core professional values developed since the inception of the Association in 1928. These values and the inherent ethical responsibilities for AHIMA members and credentialed HIM professionals include providing service; protecting medical, social, and financial information; promoting confidentiality; and preserving and securing health information. Values to the healthcare team include promoting the quality and advancement of healthcare, demonstrating HIM expertise and skills, and promoting interdisciplinary cooperation and collaboration. Professional values in relationship to the employer include protecting committee deliberations and complying with laws, regulations, and policies. Professional values related to the public include advocating change, refusing to participate or conceal unethical practices, and reporting violations of practice standards to the proper authorities. Professional values to individual and professional associations include obligations to be honest; bringing honor to self, peers, and profession; committing to continuing education and lifelong learning; performing Association duties honorably; strengthening professional membership; representing the profession to the public; and promoting and participating in research.

These professional values will require a complex process of balancing the many conflicts that can result from competing interests and obligations of those who seek access to health information and require an understanding of ethical decision making.

Purpose of the American Health Information Management Association Code of Ethics

The HIM professional has an obligation to demonstrate actions that reflect values, ethical principles, and ethical guidelines. The American Health Information Management Association (AHIMA) Code of Ethics sets forth these values and principles to guide conduct. The code is relevant to all AHIMA members and credentialed HIM professionals and students, regardless of their professional functions, the settings in which they work, or the populations they serve.

The AHIMA Code of Ethics serves six purposes:

- Identifies core values on which the HIM mission is based.

- Summarizes broad ethical principles that reflect the profession's core values and establishes a set of ethical principles to be used to guide decision-making and actions.

- Helps HIM professionals identify relevant considerations when professional obligations conflict or ethical uncertainties arise.

- Provides ethical principles by which the general public can hold the HIM professional accountable.

- Socializes practitioners new to the field to HIM's mission, values, and ethical principles.

- Articulates a set of guidelines that the HIM professional can use to assess whether they have engaged in unethical conduct.

The code includes principles and guidelines that are both enforceable and aspirational. The extent to which each principle is enforceable is a matter of professional judgment to be exercised by those responsible for reviewing alleged violations of ethical principles.

The Use of the Code

Violation of principles in this code does not automatically imply legal liability or violation of the law. Such determination can only be made in the context of legal and judicial proceedings. Alleged violations of the code would be subject to a peer review process. Such processes are generally separate from legal or administrative procedures and insulated from legal review or proceedings to allow the profession to counsel and discipline its own members although in some situations, violations of the code would constitute unlawful conduct subject to legal process.

Guidelines for ethical and unethical behavior are provided in this code. The terms "shall and shall not" are used as a basis for setting high standards for behavior. This does not imply that everyone "shall or shall not" do everything that is listed. For example, not everyone participates in the recruitment or mentoring of students. A HIM professional is not being unethical if this is not part of his or her professional activities; however, if students are part of one's professional responsibilities, there is an ethical obligation to follow the guidelines stated in the code. This concept is true for the entire code. If someone does the stated activities, ethical behavior is the standard. The guidelines are not a comprehensive list. For example, the statement "protect all confidential information to include personal, health, financial, genetic, and outcome information" can also be interpreted as "shall not fail to protect all confidential information to include personal, health, financial, genetic, and outcome information."

A code of ethics cannot guarantee ethical behavior. Moreover, a code of ethics cannot resolve all ethical issues or disputes or capture the richness and complexity involved in striving to make responsible choices within a moral community. Rather, a code of ethics sets forth values and ethical principles, and offers ethical guidelines to which professionals aspire and by which their actions can be judged. Ethical behaviors result from a personal commitment to engage in ethical practice.

Professional responsibilities often require an individual to move beyond personal values. For example, an individual might demonstrate behaviors that are based on the values of honesty, providing service to others, or demonstrating loyalty. In addition to these, professional values might require promoting confidentiality, facilitating interdisciplinary collaboration, and refusing to participate or conceal unethical practices. Professional values could require a more comprehensive set of values than what an individual needs to be an ethical agent in their personal lives.

The AHIMA Code of Ethics is to be used by AHIMA and individuals, agencies, organizations, and bodies (such as licensing and regulatory boards, insurance providers, courts of law, agency boards of directors, government agencies, and other professional groups) that choose to adopt it or use it as a frame of reference. The AHIMA Code of Ethics reflects the commitment of all to uphold the profession's values and to act ethically. Individuals of good character who discern moral questions and, in good faith, seek to make reliable ethical judgments, must apply ethical principles.

The code does not provide a set of rules that prescribe how to act in all situations. Specific applications of the code must take into account the context in which it is being considered and the possibility of conflicts among the code's values, principles, and guidelines. Ethical responsibilities flow from all human relationships, from the personal and familial to the social and professional. Further, the AHIMA Code of Ethics does not specify which values, principles, and guidelines are the most important and ought to outweigh others in instances when they conflict.

Code of Ethics 2004

<u>Ethical Principles:</u> The following ethical principles are based on the core values of the American Health Information Management Association and apply to all health information management professionals.

Health information management professionals:

I.   *Advocate, uphold, and defend the individual's right to privacy and the doctrine of confidentiality in the use and disclosure of information.*

II. *Put service and the health and welfare of persons before self-interest and conduct themselves in the practice of the profession so as to bring honor to themselves, their peers, and to the health information management profession.*

III. *Preserve, protect, and secure personal health information in any form or medium and hold in the highest regard the contents of the records and other information of a confidential nature, taking into account the applicable statutes and regulations.*

IV. *Refuse to participate in or conceal unethical practices or procedures.*

V. *Advance health information management knowledge and practice through continuing education, research, publications, and presentations.*

VI. *Recruit and mentor students, peers, and colleagues to develop and strengthen professional workforce.*

VII. *Represent the profession accurately to the public.*

VIII. *Perform honorably health information management association responsibilities, either appointed or elected, and preserve the confidentiality of any privileged information made known in any official capacity.*

IX. *State truthfully and accurately their credentials, professional education, and experiences.*

X. *Facilitate interdisciplinary collaboration in situations supporting health information practice.*

XI. *Respect the inherent dignity and worth of every person.*

How to Interpret the Code of Ethics

The following ethical principles are based on the core values of the American Health Information Management Association and apply to all health information management professionals. Guidelines included for each ethical principle are a noninclusive list of behaviors and situations that can help to clarify the principle. They are not to be meant as a comprehensive list of all situations that can occur.

I. *Advocate, uphold, and defend the individual's right to privacy and the doctrine of confidentiality in the use and disclosure of information.*

Health information management professionals **shall**:

1.1. Protect all confidential information to include personal, health, financial, genetic, and outcome information.

1.2. Engage in social and political action that supports the protection of privacy and confidentiality, and be aware of the impact of the political arena on the health information system. Advocate for changes in policy and legislation to ensure protection of privacy and confidentiality, coding compliance, and other issues that surface as advocacy issues as well as facilitating informed participation by the public on these issues.

1.3. Protect the confidentiality of all information obtained in the course of professional service. Disclose only information that is directly relevant or necessary to achieve the purpose of disclosure. Release information only with valid consent from a patient or a person legally authorized to consent on behalf of a patient or as authorized by federal or state regulations. The need-to-know criterion is essential when releasing health information for initial disclosure and all redisclosure activities.

1.4. Promote the obligation to respect privacy by respecting confidential information shared among colleagues, while responding to requests from the legal profession, the media, or other non-healthcare-related individuals, during presentations or teaching and in situations that could cause harm to persons.

II. ***Put service and the health and welfare of persons before self-interest and conduct themselves in the practice of the profession so as to bring honor to themselves, their peers, and to the health information management profession.***

Health information management professionals **shall**:

2.1. Act with integrity, behave in a trustworthy manner, elevate service to others above self-interest, and promote high standards of practice in every setting.

2.2. Be aware of the profession's mission, values, and ethical principles, and practice in a manner consistent with them by acting honestly and responsibly.

2.3. Anticipate, clarify, and avoid any conflict of interest, to all parties concerned, when dealing with consumers, consulting with competitors, or in providing services requiring potentially conflicting roles (for example, finding out information about one facility that would help a competitor). The conflicting roles or responsibilities must be clarified and appropriate action must be taken to minimize any conflict of interest.

2.4. Ensure that the working environment is consistent and encourages compliance with the AHIMA Code of Ethics, taking reasonable steps to eliminate any conditions in their organizations that violate, interfere with, or discourage compliance with the code.

2.5. Take responsibility and credit, including authorship credit, only for work they actually perform or to which they contribute. Honestly acknowledge the work of and the contributions made by others verbally or written, such as in publication.

Health information management professionals **shall not**:

2.6. Permit their private conduct to interfere with their ability to fulfill their professional responsibilities.

2.7. Take unfair advantage of any professional relationship or exploit others to further their personal, religious, political, or business interests.

III. ***Preserve, protect, and secure personal health information in any form or medium and hold in the highest regards the contents of the records and other information of a confidential nature obtained in the official capacity, taking into account the applicable statutes and regulations.***

Health information management professionals **shall**:

3.1. Protect the confidentiality of patients' written and electronic records and other sensitive information. Take reasonable steps to ensure that patients' records are stored in a secure location and that patients' records are not available to others who are not authorized to have access.

3.2. Take precautions to ensure and maintain the confidentiality of information transmitted, transferred, or disposed of in the event of a termination, incapacitation, or death of a healthcare provider to other parties through the use of any media. Disclosure of identifying information should be avoided whenever possible.

3.3. Inform recipients of the limitations and risks associated with providing services via electronic media (such as computer, telephone, fax, radio, and television).

IV. *Refuse to participate in or conceal unethical practices or procedures.*

Health information management professionals **shall**:

4.1. Act in a professional and ethical manner at all times.

4.2. Take adequate measures to discourage, prevent, expose, and correct the unethical conduct of colleagues.

4.3. Be knowledgeable about established policies and procedures for handling concerns about colleagues' unethical behavior. These include policies and procedures created by AHIMA, licensing and regulatory bodies, employers, supervisors, agencies, and other professional organizations.

4.4. Seek resolution if there is a belief that a colleague has acted unethically or if there is a belief of incompetence or impairment by discussing their concerns with the colleague when feasible and when such discussion is likely to be productive. Take action through appropriate formal channels, such as contacting an accreditation or regulatory body and/ or the AHIMA Professional Ethics Committee.

4.5. Consult with a colleague when feasible and assist the colleague in taking remedial action when there is direct knowledge of a health information management colleague's incompetence or impairment.

Health information management professionals **shall not**:

4.6. Participate in, condone, or be associated with dishonesty, fraud and abuse, or deception. A noninclusive list of examples includes:

- Allowing patterns of retrospective documentation to avoid suspension or increase reimbursement

- Assigning codes without physician documentation

- Coding when documentation does not justify the procedures that have been billed

- Coding an inappropriate level of service

- Miscoding to avoid conflict with others

- Engaging in negligent coding practices

- Hiding or ignoring review outcomes, such as performance data

- Failing to report licensure status for a physician through the appropriate channels

- Recording inaccurate data for accreditation purposes

- Hiding incomplete medical records

- Allowing inappropriate access to genetic, adoption, or behavioral health information

- Misusing sensitive information about a competitor

- Violating the privacy of individuals

V. *Advance health information management knowledge and practice through continuing education, research, publications, and presentations.*

Health information management professionals **shall**:

5.1. Develop and enhance continually their professional expertise, knowledge, and skills (including appropriate education, research, training, consultation, and supervision). Contribute to the knowledge base of health information management and share with colleagues their knowledge related to practice, research, and ethics.

5.2. Base practice decisions on recognized knowledge, including empirically based knowledge relevant to health information management and health information management ethics.

5.3. Contribute time and professional expertise to activities that promote respect for the value, integrity, and competence of the health information management profession. These activities may include teaching, research, consultation, service, legislative testimony, presentations in the community, and participation in their professional organizations.

5.4. Engage in evaluation or research that ensures the anonymity or confidentiality of participants and of the data obtained from them by following guidelines developed for the participants in consultation with appropriate institutional review boards. Report evaluation and research findings accurately and take steps to correct any errors later found in published data using standard publication methods.

5.5. Take reasonable steps to provide or arrange for continuing education and staff development, addressing current knowledge and emerging developments related to health information management practice and ethics.

Health information management professionals **shall not**:

5.6. Design or conduct evaluation or research that is in conflict with applicable federal or state laws.

5.7. Participate in, condone, or be associated with fraud or abuse.

VI. *Recruit and mentor students, peers, and colleagues to develop and strengthen professional workforce.*

Health information management professionals **shall**:

6.1. Evaluate students' performance in a manner that is fair and respectful when functioning as educators or clinical internship supervisors.

6.2. Be responsible for setting clear, appropriate, and culturally sensitive boundaries for students.

6.3. Be a mentor for students, peers and new health information management professionals to develop and strengthen skills.

6.4. Provide directed practice opportunities for students.

Health information management professionals **shall not**:

6.5. Engage in any relationship with students in which there is a risk of exploitation or potential harm to the student.

VII. *Accurately represent the profession to the public.*

Health information management professionals **shall**:

7.1. Be an advocate for the profession in all settings and participate in activities that promote and explain the mission, values, and principles of the profession to the public.

VIII. Perform honorably health information management association responsibilities, either appointed or elected, and preserve the confidentiality of any privileged information made known in any official capacity.

Health information management professionals **shall**:

8.1. Perform responsibly all duties as assigned by the professional association.

8.2. Resign from an Association position if unable to perform the assigned responsibilities with competence.

8.3. Speak on behalf of professional health information management organizations, accurately representing the official and authorized positions of the organizations.

IX. State truthfully and accurately their credentials, professional education, and experiences.

Health information management professionals **shall**:

9.1. Make clear distinctions between statements made and actions engaged in as a private individual and as a representative of the health information management profession, a professional health information organization, or the health information management professional's employer.

9.2. Claim and ensure that their representations to patients, agencies, and the public of professional qualifications, credentials, education, competence, affiliations, services provided, training, certification, consultation received, supervised experience, and other relevant professional experience are accurate.

9.3. Claim only those relevant professional credentials actually possessed and correct any inaccuracies occurring regarding credentials.

X. Facilitate interdisciplinary collaboration in situations supporting health information practice.

Health information management professionals **shall**:

10.1. Participate in and contribute to decisions that affect the well-being of patients by drawing on the perspectives, values, and experiences of those involved in decisions related to patients. Professional and ethical obligations of the interdisciplinary team as a whole and of its individual members should be clearly established.

XI. Respect the inherent dignity and worth of every person.

Health information management professionals **shall**:

11.1. Treat each person in a respectful fashion, being mindful of individual differences and cultural and ethnic diversity.

11.2. Promote the value of self-determination for each individual.

Acknowledgement

Adapted with permission from the Code of Ethics of the National Association of Social Workers.

Resources

AHIMA Code of Ethics, 1957, 1977, 1988, and 1998.

Harman, L.B. (ed.). 2001. *Ethical Challenges in the Management of Health Information*. Gaithersburg, MD: Aspen.

National Association of Social Workers. 1999. Code of Ethics. http://www.naswdc.org.

Revised and adopted by AHIMA House of Delegates—July 1, 2004.

_____

Appendix G

CMS-1500 Claim Example

CMS-1500 Claim [Detailed Measures Group] – Sample 1 (continues on next pg)

The following is a claim sample for reporting the Rheumatoid Arthritis (RA) Measures Group on a CMS-1500 claim and it continues on the next page. Two samples are included: one is for reporting of individual measures for the RA measures group; the second sample shows reporting performance of all measures in the group using a composite G-code.
See http://www.cms.hhs.gov/PQRI/15_MeasuresCodes.asp#TopOfPage for more information.

For group billing, the rendering NPI number of the individual Eligible Professional (EP) who performed the service will be used from each line-item in the PQRI calculations.

Quality-Data Codes (QDCs) must be submitted with a line-item charge of $0.00. Charge field cannot be blank.

24D. Procedures, Services, or Supplies – CPT/HCPCS, Modifier as needed

21. Review and determine if ANY diagnosis (Dx) listed in Item 21 meets the patient sample criteria for the RA measures group.

The NPI of the billing provider is entered here. If a solo practitioner, then enter the individual NPI; if a Group is billing, enter the NPI of the group here. This is a required field.

Rheumatoid Arthritis (RA)

Report ALL applicable measures' QDCs within the RA measures group

Patient encounter during reporting period

RA Measures Group Intent G-code

RA–PQRI #108
RA–PQRI #176 code 1
AND
RA–PQRI #176 code 2
RA–PQRI #177

Identifies claim line-item

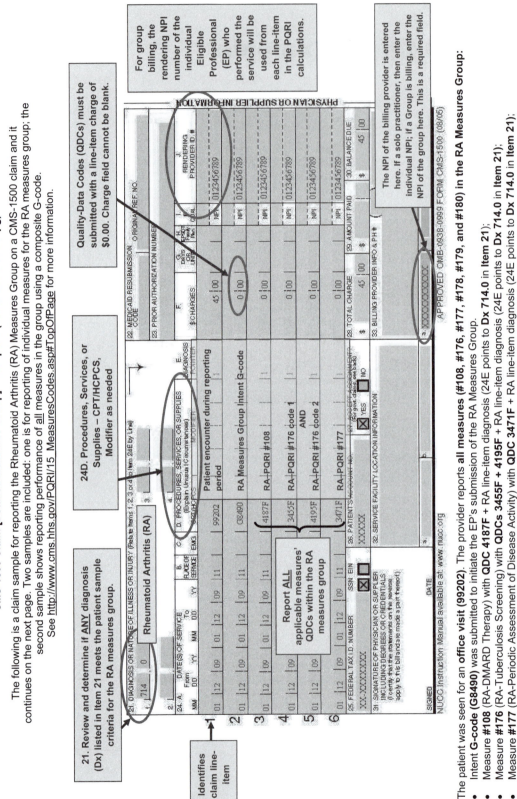

The patient was seen for an **office visit (99202)**. The provider reports **all measures (#108, #176, #177, #178, #179, and #180) in the RA Measures Group**:

- Intent **G-code (G8490)** was submitted to initiate the EP's submission of the RA Measures Group.
- Measure **#108** (RA-DMARD Therapy) with **QDC 4187F** + RA line-item diagnosis (24E points to **Dx 714.0** in **Item 21**);
- Measure **#176** (RA-Tuberculosis Screening) with **QDCs 3455F + 4195F** + RA line-item diagnosis (24E points to **Dx 714.0** in **Item 21**);
- Measure **#177** (RA-Periodic Assessment of Disease Activity) with **QDC 3471F** + RA line-item diagnosis (24E points to **Dx 714.0** in **Item 21**);

RA Measures Group Sample 1 continues on the next page.

Version 2.1

CMS-1500 Claim [Detailed Measures Group] – Sample 1 (cont.)

If billing software limits the line items on a claim, you may add a nominal amount such as a penny to one of the QDC line items on that second claim for a total charge of $0.01

For group billing, the rendering NPI number of the individual EP who performed the service will be used from each line-item in the PQRI calculations.

QDC(s) must be submitted with a line-item charge of $0.00 or $0.01. Charge field cannot be blank.

24D. Procedures, Services, or Supplies – CPT/HCPCS, Modifier as needed

21. Review and determine if ANY diagnosis (Dx) listed in Item 21 meets the patient sample criteria for the RA measures group.

Rheumatoid Arthritis (RA)

Report ALL applicable measures' QDCs within the RA measures group

Solo practitioner - Enter individual NPI here

Identifies claim line-item

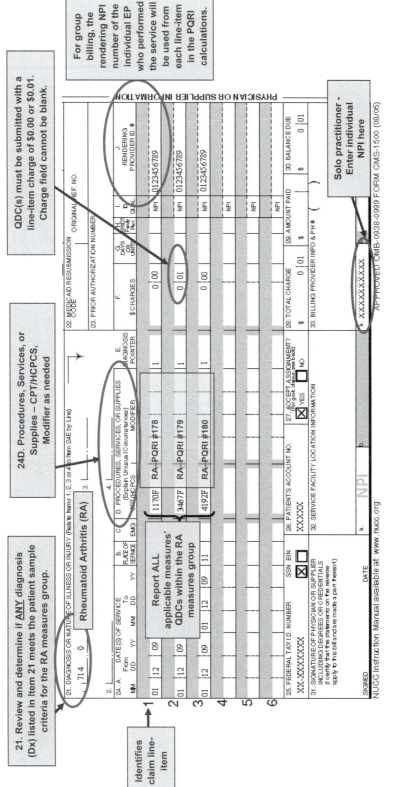

NUCC Instruction Manual available at: www.nucc.org

- Measure #178 (RA-Functional Status Assessment) with **QDC 1170F** + RA line-item diagnosis (24E points to **Dx 714.0** in **Item 21**);
- Measure #179 (RA-Assessment & Classification) with **QDC 3476F** + RA line-item diagnosis (24E points to **Dx 714.0** in **Item 21**); and
- Measure #180 (RA-Glucocorticoid Management) with **QDC 4192F** + RA line-item diagnosis (24E points to **Dx 714.0** in **Item 21**).
- **Note:** All diagnoses listed in **Item 21** will be used for PQRI analysis. (Measures that require the reporting of two or more diagnoses on a claim will be analyzed as submitted in Item 21.)
- **NPI placement: Item 24J must** contain the NPI of the individual provider that rendered the service when a group is billing.

Version 2.1

4/9/09
Page 2 of 3

375

CMS-1500 Claim [Sample Measures Group] – Sample 2

A detailed sample of an individual NPI reporting the RA Measures Group on a related CMS-1500 claim is shown below. This sample shows reporting performance of all measures in the group using a composite G-code.

See http://www.cms.hhs.gov/PQRI/15_MeasuresCodes.asp#TopOfPage for more information.

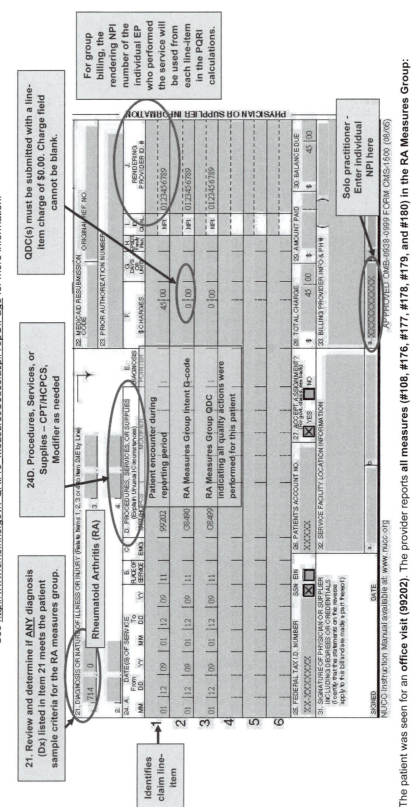

21. Review and determine if **ANY** diagnosis (Dx) listed in Item 21 meets the patient sample criteria for the RA measures group.

24D. Procedures, Services, or Supplies – CPT/HCPCS, Modifier as needed

QDC(s) must be submitted with a line-item charge of $0.00. Charge field cannot be blank.

For group billing, the rendering NPI number of the individual EP who performed the service will be used from each line-item in the PQRI calculations.

Solo practitioner - Enter individual NPI here

Identifies claim line-item

The patient was seen for an **office visit (99202)**. The provider reports **all measures (#108, #176, #177, #178, #179, and #180) in the RA Measures Group**:

- Intent **G-code (G8490)** was submitted to initiate the EP's submission of the RA Measures Group.
- Measures Group **QDC G8499** (indicating all quality actions related to the RA Measures Group were performed for this patient) + RA line-item diagnosis (24E points to **Dx 714.0** in **Item 21**). The composite G-code G8499 may not be used if performance modifiers (1P, 2P, 3P, or G-code equivalent) or the 8P reporting modifier apply.
- **Note:** All diagnoses listed in **Item 21** will be used for PQRI analysis. (Measures that require the reporting of two or more diagnoses on claim will be analyzed as submitted in Item 21.)
- **NPI placement: Item 24J** must contain the NPI of the individual provider that rendered the service when a group is billing.

Version 2.1

Appendix H

Getting Started with 2009 PQRI

Getting Started with 2009 PQRI Reporting of Measures Groups

Introduction:

This document contains general guidance for reporting 2009 Physician Quality Reporting Initiative (PQRI) Measures Groups. Measures groups include reporting on a group of clinically-related measures either through claims-based or registry-based submission mechanisms. Seven (7) measures groups have been created for 2009 PQRI which include Diabetes Mellitus, Chronic Kidney Disease (CKD), Preventive Care, Coronary Artery Bypass Graft (CABG), Rheumatoid Arthritis, Perioperative Care and Back Pain.

Eligible professionals (EPs) can choose to participate under more than one 2009 PQRI reporting option. Professionals who satisfactorily report under more than one reporting option will receive a maximum of one incentive payment, which will be equivalent to 2.0% of Medicare Physician Fee Schedule (PFS) allowed charges for all covered professional services furnished during the longest reporting period for which he or she has satisfied reporting criteria.

The 2009 PQRI Measures Groups reporting alternative is available for the 12-month reporting period from January 1 through December 31, 2009 or the six-month reporting period from July 1 through December 31, 2009. Individual participating EPs who satisfactorily report under measures groups may receive an incentive payment equivalent to 2.0% of total allowed PFS charges for covered professional services furnished to patients enrolled in Medicare Part B Fee-For-Service during either the January 1 through December 31, 2009 reporting period or the July 1 through December 31, 2009 reporting period. This document provides strategies and information to facilitate satisfactory reporting by each EP who wishes to pursue this alternative.

The *2009 PQRI Measures Groups Specifications Manual*, which can be found at http://www.cms.hhs.gov/PQRI/15_MeasuresCodes.asp#TopOfPage, contains detailed descriptions for each quality measure within each measures group. Denominator coding has been modified from the original measure as specified by the measure developer to allow for implementation as a measures group. To get started, review the *2009 PQRI Measures Groups Specifications Manual* to determine if a particular measures group is applicable to Medicare services the practice provides.

Measures Groups Participation Strategy:

1. Plan and implement processes within the practice to ensure satisfactory reporting of measures groups.

2. Become familiar with the methods for satisfactory reporting of measures groups. The two methods for measures groups are:

    Consecutive Patient Sample Method: For claims-based submissions, 30 consecutive Medicare Part B Fee-For-Service enrolled patients meeting patient sample criteria (see Patient Sample Criteria Table below) for the measures group. **Counting will begin on the date of service that the measures group-specific G-code is submitted.** For example, an EP can indicate intent to begin reporting the Diabetes Mellitus Measures Group by submitting G8485 on the first patient claim in the series of consecutive diabetic patients. For registry-based submissions, EPs must report on all applicable measures within the selected measures group for a minimum of 30 consecutive patients (which may include non-Medicare Part B Fee-For-Service patients) who meet patient sample criteria for the measures group. For both claims-based and registry-based submissions, all *applicable* measures within the group must be reported at least once during the reporting period (January 1 through December 31, 2009) for each of the 30 consecutive patients.

Getting Started with 2009 PQRI Reporting of Measures Groups

OR

80% Patient Sample Method: All Medicare Part B Fee-For-Service enrolled patients seen during the reporting period (either January 1 through December 31, 2009 **OR** July 1 through December 31, 2009) and meeting patient sample criteria (see Patient Sample Criteria Table below) for the measures group. For claims-based submissions, PQRI analysis will be initiated when the measures group-specific G-code is submitted on a claim but all claims meeting patient sample criteria in the selected reporting period will be included regardless of the date of service the measures group-specific G-code is submitted. A minimum of 80% of this patient sample must be reported for all applicable measures within the group according to the individual measures group reporting instructions. For the 12-month reporting period, a minimum of 30 patients must meet the measures group patient sample criteria to report satisfactorily. For the six-month reporting period, a minimum of 15 patients must meet the measures group patient sample criteria to report satisfactorily.

3. Determine the patient sample based on the patient sample criteria, which is used for both the Consecutive Patient Sample Method and the 80% Patient Sample Method. The following table contains patient sample criteria (common codes) that will qualify an EP's patient for inclusion in the measures group analysis. For claims-based submissions, claims must contain a line-item ICD-9-CM diagnosis code (where applicable) accompanied by a specific CPT patient encounter code. All diagnoses included on the base claim are considered in PQRI analysis.

Patient Sample Criteria Table		
Measures Group	**CPT Patient Encounter Codes**	**ICD-9-CM Diagnosis Codes**
Diabetes Mellitus 18–75 years	97802, 97803, 97804, 99201, 99202, 99203, 99204, 99205, 99212, 99213, 99214, 99215, 99304, 99305, 99306, 99307, 99308, 99309, 99310, 99324, 99325, 99326, 99327, 99328, 99334, 99335, 99336, 99337, 99341, 99342, 99343, 99344, 99345, 99347, 99348, 99349, 99350, G0270, G0271	250.00, 250.01, 250.02, 250.03, 250.10, 250.11, 250.12, 250.13, 250.20, 250.21, 250.22, 250.23, 250.30, 250.31, 250.32, 250.33, 250.40, 250.41, 250.42, 250.43, 250.50, 250.51, 250.52, 250.53, 250.60, 250.61, 250.62, 250.63, 250.70, 250.71, 250.72, 250.73, 250.80, 250.81, 250.82, 250.83, 250.90, 250.91, 250.92, 250.93, 357.2, 362.01, 362.02, 362.03, 362.04, 362.05, 362.06, 362.07, 366.41, 648.00, 648.01, 648.02, 648.03, 648.04
Chronic Kidney Disease (CKD) 18 years and older	99201, 99202, 99203, 99204, 99205, 99212, 99213, 99214, 99215, 99241, 99242, 99243, 99244, 99245	585.4, 585.5
Preventive Care 50 years and older	99201, 99202, 99203, 99204, 99205, 99212, 99213, 99214, 99215	
Coronary Artery Bypass Graft (CABG) 18 years and older	33510, 33511, 33512, 33513, 33514, 33516, 33517, 33518, 33519, 33521, 33522, 33523, 33533, 33534, 33535, 33536	

Getting Started with 2009 PQRI Reporting of Measures Groups

Patient Sample Criteria Table		
Measures Group	**CPT Patient Encounter Codes**	**ICD-9-CM Diagnosis Codes**
Rheumatoid Arthritis 18 years and older	99201, 99202, 99203, 99204, 99205, 99212, 99213, 99214, 99215, 99241, 99242, 99243, 99244, 99245, 99341, 99342, 99343, 99344, 99345, 99347, 99348, 99349, 99350, 99455, 99456	714.0, 714.1, 714.2, 714.81
Perioperative Care 18 years and older	19260, 19271, 19272, 19301, 19302, 19303, 19304, 19305, 19306, 19307, 19361, 19364, 19366, 19367, 19368, 19369, 22558, 22600, 22612, 22630, 27125, 27130, 27132, 27134, 27137, 27138, 27235, 27236, 27244, 27245, 27269, 27440, 27441, 27442, 27443, 27445, 27446, 27447, 39545, 39561, 43045, 43100, 43101, 43107, 43108, 43112, 43113, 43116, 43117, 43118, 43121, 43122, 43123, 43124, 43130, 43135, 43300, 43305, 43310, 43312, 43313, 43320, 43324, 43325, 43326, 43330, 43331, 43340, 43341, 43350, 43351, 43352, 43360, 43361, 43400, 43401, 43405, 43410, 43415, 43420, 43425, 43496, 43500, 43501, 43502, 43510, 43520, 43605, 43610, 43611, 43620, 43621, 43622, 43631, 43632, 43633, 43634, 43640, 43641, 43653, 43800, 43810, 43820, 43825, 43830, 43832, 43840, 43843, 43845, 43846, 43847, 43848, 43850, 43855, 43860, 43865, 43870, 44005, 44010, 44020, 44021, 44050, 44055, 44120, 44125, 44126, 44127, 44130, 47420, 47425, 47460, 47480, 47560, 47561, 47570, 47600, 47605, 47610, 47612, 47620, 47700, 47701, 47711, 47712, 47715, 47720, 47721, 47740, 47741, 47760, 47765, 47780, 47785, 47800, 47802, 47900, 48020, 48100, 48120, 48140, 48145, 48146, 48148, 48150, 48152, 48153, 48154, 48155, 48500, 48510, 48520, 48540, 48545, 48547, 48548, 48554, 48556, 49215, 50320, 50340, 50360, 50365, 50370, 50380, 60521, 60522, 61313, 61510, 61512, 61518, 61548, 61697, 61700, 62230, 63015, 63020, 63047, 63056, 63081, 63267, 63276	

Getting Started with 2009 PQRI Reporting of Measures Groups

Patient Sample Criteria Table		
Measures Group	**CPT Patient Encounter Codes**	**ICD-9-CM Diagnosis Codes**
Back Pain 18-79 years	Diagnosis codes with CPT codes: 98940, 98941, 98942, 99201, 99202, 99203, 99204, 99205, 99212, 99213, 99214, 99215, 99241, 99242, 99243, 99244, 99245 OR 22210, 22214, 22220, 22222, 22224, 22226, 22532, 22533, 22534, 22548, 22554, 22556, 22558, 22585, 22590, 22595, 22600, 22612, 22614, 22630, 22632, 22818, 22819, 22830, 22840, 22841, 22842, 22843, 22844, 22845, 22846, 22847, 22848, 22849, 63001, 63003, 63005, 63011, 63012, 63015, 63016, 63017, 63020, 63030, 63035, 63040, 63042, 63043, 63044, 63045, 63046, 63047, 63048, 63055, 63056, 63057, 63064, 63066, 63075, 63076, 63077, 63078, 63081, 63082, 63085, 63086, 63087, 63088, 63090, 63091, 63101, 63102, 63103 , 63170, 63172, 63173, 63180, 63182, 63185, 63190, 63191, 63194, 63195, 63196, 63197, 63198, 63199, 63200	Diagnosis codes for CPT 9XXXX codes: 721.3 721.41, 721.42, 721.90, 722.0, 722.10, 722.11, 722.2, 722.30, 722.31, 722.32, 722.39, 722.4, 722.51, 722.52, 722.6, 722.70, 722.71, 722.72, 722.73, 722.80, 722.81, 722.82, 722.83, 722.90, 722.91, 722.92, 722.93, 723.0, 724.00, 724.01, 724.02, 724.09, 724.2, 724.3, 724.4, 724.5, 724.6, 724.70, 724.71, 724.79, 738.4, 738.5, 739.3, 739.4, 756.12, 846.0, 846.1, 846.2, 846.3, 846.8, 846.9, 847.2

4. For claims-based submissions, initiate reporting of measures groups by using measures group-specific G-codes. Indicate your intention to begin reporting a measures group by submitting a measures group-specific G-code on a patient claim. It is not necessary to submit the measures group-specific G-code on more than one claim. If the G-code for a given group is submitted multiple times during the reporting period, only the submission with the earliest date of service will be included in the PQRI analyses; subsequent submissions of that code will be ignored. It is not necessary to submit the measures group-specific G-code for registry-based submissions.

    G8485: I intend to report the Diabetes Mellitus Measures Group
    G8487: I intend to report the Chronic Kidney Disease (CKD) Measures Group
    G8486: I intend to report the Preventive Care Measures Group
    G8490: I intend to report the Rheumatoid Arthritis Measures Group
    G8492: I intend to report the Perioperative Care Measures Group
    G8493: I intend to report the Back Pain Measures Group

Measures group-specific G-code line items on the claim must be complete, including accurate coding, date of service, diagnosis pointer, and individual National Provider Identifier (NPI) in the rendering provider field. The diagnosis pointer field on the claim links the patient diagnosis to the service line. A G-code specific to a condition-specific measures group (e.g., Diabetes Mellitus Measures Group) should be linked to the diagnosis for the condition to which it pertains; a G-code for the Preventive Care Measures Group may be linked to any diagnosis on the claim.

Getting Started with 2009 PQRI Reporting of Measures Groups

Measures group-specific G-code line items should be submitted with a charge of zero dollars ($0.00). Measures group-specific G-code line items will be denied for payment, but are then passed through the claims processing system for PQRI analysis. EPs should check their Remittance Advice ("Explanation of Benefits" or "EOB") for a denial code (e.g., N365) for the measures group-specific G-code, confirming the code passed through their local carrier to the National Claims History file. The N365 denial indicates that the code is not payable and is used for reporting/informational purposes only. Other services/codes on the claim will not be affected by the addition of measures group-specific G-codes. The N365 remark code does **NOT** indicate whether the QDC is accurate for that claim or for the measure the EP is attempting to report.

5. For patients to whom measures groups apply, report all applicable individual measures for the measure group. Report quality-data codes (QDCs) as instructed in the *2009 PQRI Measures Groups Specifications Manual* on all applicable measures within the measures group for each patient included in the sample population for each individual EP. For claims-based submissions, EPs may choose to submit QDCs either on a current claim or on a claim representing a subsequent visit, particularly if the quality action has changed. For example, a new laboratory value may be available at a subsequent visit. Only one instance of reporting for each patient included in the sample population will be used when calculating reporting and performance rates for each measure within a group.

   If all quality actions for the applicable measures in the measures group have been performed for the patient, one G-code may be reported in lieu of the individual quality-data codes for each of the measures within the group. Refer to the *2009 PQRI Measures Groups Specifications Manual* for detailed instructions to report quality-data codes for each of the measures group at http://www.cms.hhs.gov/PQRI/15_MeasuresCodes.asp#TopOfPage.

   An EP is only required to report QDCs on those individual measures in the measures group that meet the criteria (age or gender) according to the *2009 PQRI Measures Groups Specifications Manual*. For example, if an EP is reporting the Preventive Care Measures Group for a 52 year old female patient, only six measures out of nine apply. See the Preventive Measures Group Demographic Criteria table below:

Preventive Measures Group Demographic Criteria		
Age	**Measures for Male Patients**	**Measures for Female Patients**
<50 years	Patient does not qualify for measures group analysis	Patient does not qualify for measures group analysis
50-64 years	110, 113, 114, 115, 128	110, 112, 113, 114, 115, 128
65-69 years	110, 111, 113, 114, 115, 128	39, 48, 110, 111, 112, 113, 114, 115, 128
70-80 years	110, 111, 113, 114, 115, 128	39, 48, 110, 111, 113, 114, 115, 128
≥81 years	110, 111, 114, 115, 128	39, 48, 110, 111, 114, 115, 128

Getting Started with 2009 PQRI Reporting of Measures Groups

Reporting Measures Groups - Common Clinical Scenarios:

The following clinical scenarios are offered as examples describing the quality data that should be reported on claims using a measures groups method:

Diabetes Mellitus Example

Primary care office visit for a new patient with newly diagnosed diabetes mellitus: A1c = lab drawn, result unknown, prior result not available (3046F-8P); LDL-C=110 (3049F); today's BP = 140/80 (3077F and 3079F); referred to eye care professional (optometrist or ophthalmologist) for dilated eye exam (2022F-8P); urine protein screening performed = negative (3061F); foot exam performed (2028F)

Dx 1: 250.00

Measure No.	Date of Service	CPT/HCPCS	Modifier	Diagnosis Pointer	Charges	NPI
	07/01/2008	99201		1	$60.00	0123456789
	07/01/2008	G8485		1	$0.00	0123456789
	07/01/2008	83036		1	$15.00	0123456789
	07/01/2008	81000		1	$6.00	0123456789
1	07/01/2008	3046F	8P	1	$0.00	0123456789
2	07/01/2008	3049F		1	$0.00	0123456789
3	07/01/2008	3077F		1	$0.00	0123456789
3	07/01/2008	3079F		1	$0.00	0123456789
117	07/01/2008	2022F	8P	1	$0.00	0123456789
119	07/01/2008	3061F		1	$0.00	0123456789
163	07/01/2008	2028F		1	$0.00	0123456789

The above is an example of satisfactory reporting in PQRI. The EP included G-code G8485 on the claim form to initiate reporting of the Diabetes Measures Group. In this example, the EP has chosen to report measures 1 and 117 with an 8P modifier indicating that performance of the measure was not met on this visit. An EP may choose whether to report these two measures on the current claim or wait to report them on a claim for a subsequent visit during the reporting period after the results of the test/exam are available.

CKD Example

Stage 5 CKD patient, not receiving RRT, office visit: lab tests ordered on last visit and results documented in the chart (3278F); known hypertensive with documented plan of care for hypertension (G8477 and 0513F); Hgb = 14 and patient is receiving ESA and has a plan of care documented for elevated hemoglobin level (3279F and 0514F and 4171F); record indicates influenza immunization at a previous visit in January of this year (4037F); referred for AV fistula (4051F)

Getting Started with 2009 PQRI Reporting of Measures Groups

Dx 1: 585.5; Dx 2: 401.0; Dx 3: 791.0

Measure No.	Date of Service	CPT/HCPCS	Modifier	Diagnosis Pointer	Charges	NPI
	07/01/2008	99213		1	$50.00	0123456789
	07/01/2008	G8487		1	$0.00	0123456789
121	07/01/2008	3278F		1	$0.00	0123456789
122	07/01/2008	G8477		1	$0.00	0123456789
122	07/01/2008	0513F		1	$0.00	0123456789
123	07/01/2008	3279F		1	$0.00	0123456789
123	07/01/2008	0514F		1	$0.00	0123456789
123	07/01/2008	4171F		1	$0.00	0123456789
135	07/01/2008	4037F		1	$0.00	0123456789
153	07/01/2008	4051F		1	$0.00	0123456789

Preventive Care Example
Primary care office visit for a 67 year old female, established patient presenting with mild cold symptoms. Record indicates patient had a DXA done at age 62, with results documented as within normal limits (G8399); denies urinary incontinence (1090F); record indicates influenza vaccination at a previous visit in January of this year (G8482); pneumonia vaccination administered last year (4040F); results of last month's mammogram (3014F) and last week's FOBT (3017F) reviewed with patient; denies tobacco use (1000F and 1036F and G8457); today's BMI measurement = 24 (G8420)

Dx 1: Use any visit-specific diagnosis for the measures in this group

Measure No.	Date of Service	CPT/HCPCS	Modifier	Diagnosis Pointer	Charges	NPI
	07/01/2008	99212		1	$45.00	0123456789
	07/01/2008	G8486		1	$0.00	0123456789
39	07/01/2008	G8399		1	$0.00	0123456789
48	07/01/2008	1090F		1	$0.00	0123456789
110	07/01/2008	G8482		1	$0.00	0123456789
111	07/01/2008	4040F		1	$0.00	0123456789
112	07/01/2008	3014F		1	$0.00	0123456789
113	07/01/2008	3017F		1	$0.00	0123456789
114	07/01/2008	1000F		1	$0.00	0123456789
114	07/01/2008	1036F		1	$0.00	0123456789
115	07/01/2008	G8457		1	$0.00	0123456789
128	07/01/2008	G8420		1	$0.00	0123456789

Rheumatoid Arthritis Example
Rheumatoid arthritis patient, office visit: prescribed DMARD therapy (4187F); documentation of TB screen performed and results interpreted 2 months ago (3455F and 4195F); disease activity assessed and documented as moderate (3471F); functional status assessed (1170F); disease prognosis assessed and documented as good (3476F); documented glucocorticoid use is for less than 6 months (4193F)

Getting Started with 2009 PQRI Reporting of Measures Groups

Dx 1: 714.0

Measure No.	Date of Service	CPT/HCPCS	Modifier	Diagnosis Pointer	Charges	NPI
	07/01/2008	99213		1	$50.00	0123456789
	07/01/2008	G8490		1	$0.00	0123456789
108	07/01/2008	4187F		1	$0.00	0123456789
176	07/01/2008	3455F		1	$0.00	0123456789
176	07/01/2008	4195F		1	$0.00	0123456789
177	07/01/2008	3471F		1	$0.00	0123456789
178	07/01/2008	1170F		1	$0.00	0123456789
179	07/01/2008	3476F		1	$0.00	0123456789
180	07/01/2008	4193F		1	$0.00	0123456789

Perioperative Care Example

Patient has surgery for resection of small intestine (Enterectomy): documentation of order for prophylactic antibiotic to be given within one hour prior to surgical incision (4047F); the order for the prophylactic antibiotic was for cefazolin (4041F); prophylactic antibiotics were given one hour prior to surgical incision and there is an order to discontinue within 24 hours of surgery end time (4049F and 4046F); documentation there was an order to give VTE prophylaxis within 24 hours of surgery end time (4044F)

Dx 1: Use any visit-specific diagnosis for the measures in this group

Measure No.	Date of Service	CPT/HCPCS	Modifier	Diagnosis Pointer	Charges	NPI
	07/01/2008	44120		1	$1500.00	0123456789
	07/01/2008	G8492		1	$0.00	0123456789
20	07/01/2008	4047F		1	$0.00	0123456789
21	07/01/2008	4041F		1	$0.00	0123456789
22	07/01/2008	4049F		1	$0.00	0123456789
22	07/01/2008	4046F		1	$0.00	0123456789
23	07/01/2008	4044F		1	$0.00	0123456789

Back Pain Example

Initial office visit for a new patient with newly diagnosed back pain: back pain and function assessed including pain assessment, functional status, patient history with notation of no "red flags", prior treatment and response assessment and employment status (1130F); physical exam performed (2040F); patient counseled to resume normal activities (4245F); patient advised against bed rest lasting four days or longer (4248F)

Dx 1: 724.2

Measure No.	Date of Service	CPT/HCPCS	Modifier	Diagnosis Pointer	Charges	NPI
	07/01/2008	99203		1	$60.00	0123456789
	07/01/2008	G8493		1	$0.00	0123456789
148	07/01/2008	1130F		1	$0.00	0123456789
149	07/01/2008	2040F		1	$0.00	0123456789
150	07/01/2008	4245F		1	$0.00	0123456789
151	07/01/2008	4248F		1	$0.00	0123456789

Appendix I
CMS-R-131

(A) **Notifier(s):**

(B) **Patient Name:** _____ *(C)* **Identification Number:** _____

ADVANCE BENEFICIARY NOTICE OF NONCOVERAGE (ABN)

NOTE: If Medicare doesn't pay for *(D)*_____ below, you may have to pay.

Medicare does not pay for everything, even some care that you or your health care provider have good reason to think you need. We expect Medicare may not pay for the *(D)*_____ below.

*(D)*_____	*(E)* Reason Medicare May Not Pay:	*(F)* Estimated Cost:

WHAT YOU NEED TO DO NOW:

- Read this notice, so you can make an informed decision about your care.
- Ask us any questions that you may have after you finish reading.
- Choose an option below about whether to receive the *(D)*_____ listed above.
  Note: If you choose Option 1 or 2, we may help you to use any other insurance that you might have, but Medicare cannot require us to do this.

(G) OPTIONS:	Check only one box. We cannot choose a box for you.

❑ **OPTION 1.** I want the *(D)*_____ listed above. You may ask to be paid now, but I also want Medicare billed for an official decision on payment, which is sent to me on a Medicare Summary Notice (MSN). I understand that if Medicare doesn't pay, I am responsible for payment, but **I can appeal to Medicare** by following the directions on the MSN. If Medicare does pay, you will refund any payments I made to you, less co-pays or deductibles.

❑ **OPTION 2.** I want the *(D)*_____ listed above, but do not bill Medicare. You may ask to be paid now as I am responsible for payment. **I cannot appeal if Medicare is not billed.**

❑ **OPTION 3.** I don't want the *(D)*_____ listed above. I understand with this choice I am **not** responsible for payment, and **I cannot appeal to see if Medicare would pay.**

(H) **Additional Information:**

This notice gives our opinion, not an official Medicare decision. If you have other questions on this notice or Medicare billing, call **1-800-MEDICARE** (1-800-633-4227/**TTY:** 1-877-486-2048).

Signing below means that you have received and understand this notice. You also receive a copy.

(I) Signature:	*(J)* Date:

According to the Paperwork Reduction Act of 1995, no persons are required to respond to a collection of information unless it displays a valid OMB control number. The valid OMB control number for this information collection is 0938-0566. The time required to complete this information collection is estimated to average 7 minutes per response, including the time to review instructions, search existing data resources, gather the data needed, and complete and review the information collection. If you have comments concerning the accuracy of the time estimate or suggestions for improving this form, please write to: CMS, 7500 Security Boulevard, Attn: PRA Reports Clearance Officer, Baltimore, Maryland 21244-1850.

Form CMS-R-131 (03/08)   Form Approved OMB No. 0938-0566

Appendix J

RAC Phase-in Schedule

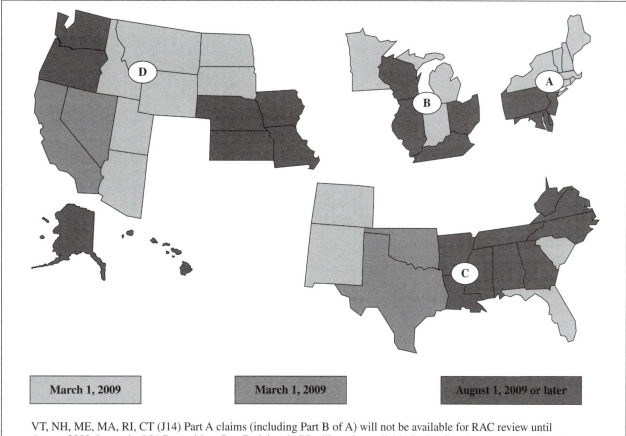

| March 1, 2009 | March 1, 2009 | August 1, 2009 or later |

VT, NH, ME, MA, RI, CT (J14) Part A claims (including Part B of A) will not be available for RAC review until August 2009 due to the MAC transition. Part B claims in RI will not be available for RAC review until August 2009 due to the MAC transition. All other Part B claims are available for RAC review beginning March 1, 2009.

Source: Centers for Medicare and Medicaid Services. 2009d. RAC Expansion Schedule.
http://www.cms.hhs.gov/RAC/Downloads/RAC%20Expansion%20Schedule%20Web.pdf.

Appendix K

NQF Standard Measures

National Quality Forum—National Voluntary Consensus Standards for Ambulatory Care 8/3/2009

NQF#	Title	Date	Description
71	Acute Myocardial Infarction (AMI): Persistence of Beta-Blocker Treatment After a Heart Attack	12/1/2006	Percentage of patients whose day's supply of beta blockers dispensed is >=135 days in the 180 days following discharge
108	ADHD: Follow-Up Care for Children Prescribed Attention-Deficit/ Hyperactivity Disorder (ADHD) Medication.	12/1/2006	a. Initiation Phase: Percentage of children 6–12 years of age as of the Index Prescription Episode Start Date with an ambulatory prescription dispensed for and ADHD medication and who had one follow-up visit with a practitioner with prescribing authority during the 30-Day Initiation Phase. b. Continuation and Maintenance (C&M) Phase: Percentage of children 6–12 years of age as of the Index Prescription Episode Start Date with an ambulatory prescription dispensed for ADHD medication who remained on the medication for at least 210 days and who in addition to the visit in the Initiation Phase had at least two additional follow-up visits with a practitioner within 270 days (9 months) after the Initiation Phase ends.
406	Adolescent and adult clients with AIDS who are prescribed potent ART (PROCESS MEASURE)	7/31/2008	Percentage of patients who were prescribed potent antiretroviral therapy
488	Adoption of Health Information Technology	8/29/2008	Documents whether provider has adopted and is using health information technology. To qualify, the provider must have adopted and be using a certified/ qualified electronic health record (EHR).
486	Adoption of Medication e-Prescribing	8/29/2008	Documents whether provider has adopted a qualified e-Prescribing system and the extent of use in the ambulatory setting
283	Adult asthma (PQI 15)	11/15/2007	This measure is used to assess the number of admissions for asthma in adults per 100,000 population.
326	Advance Care Plan	11/5/2007	Percentage of patients aged 65 years and older who have an advance care plan or surrogate decision maker documented in the medical record or documentation in the medical record that an advance care plan was discussed but the patient did not wish or was not able to name a surrogate decision maker or provide an advance care plan
87	Age-Related Macular Degeneration: Dilated Macular Examination	5/1/2007	Percentage of patients aged 50 years and older with a diagnosis of age-related macular degeneration that had a dilated macular examination performed which included documentation of the presence or absence of macular thickening or hemorrhage AND the level of macular degeneration severity during one or more office visits within 12 months
515	Ambulatory surgery patients with appropriate method of hair removal	9/25/2008	Percentage of ASC admissions with appropriate surgical site hair removal

NQF#	Title	Date	Description
454	Anesthesiology and Critical Care: Perioperative Temperature Management	7/31/2008	Percentage of patients, regardless of age, undergoing surgical or therapeutic procedures under general or neuraxial anesthesia of 60 minutes duration or longer for whom either active warming was used intraoperatively for the purpose of maintaining normothermia, OR at least one body temperature equal to or greater than 36 degrees Centigrade (or 96.8 degrees Fahrenheit) was recorded within the 30 minutes immediately before or the 30 minutes immediately after anesthesia end time
2	Appropriate testing for children with pharyngitis	6/1/2006	Percentage of patients who were diagnosed with pharyngitis, prescribed an antibiotic, and who received a group A streptococcus test for the episode
69	Appropriate treatment for children with upper respiratory infection (URI)	5/1/2006	Percentage of children who were given a diagnosis of URI and were not dispensed an antibiotic prescription on or three days after the episode date
54	Arthritis: disease modifying antirheumatic drug (DMARD) therapy in rheumatoid arthritis	12/1/2006	Percentage of patients 18 years and older diagnosed with rheumatoid arthritis who have had at least one ambulatory prescription dispensed for a DMARD
234	Assessment of Mental Status for Community Acquired Bacterial Pneumonia	5/1/2007	Percentage of patients aged 18 years and older with the diagnosis of community-acquired bacterial pneumonia with mental status assessed
233	Assessment of Oxygen Saturation for Community Acquired Bacterial Pneumonia	5/1/2007	Percentage of patients aged 18 years and older with the diagnosis of community-acquired bacterial pneumonia with oxygen saturation documented and reviewed
94	Assessment of Oxygen Saturation for Community-Acquired Bacterial Pneumonia	5/1/2007	Percentage of patients aged 18 years and older with the diagnosis of community-acquired bacterial pneumonia with oxygen saturation assessed
1	Asthma assessment	5/1/2006	Percentage of patients who were evaluated during at least one office visit for the frequency (numeric) of daytime and nocturnal asthma symptoms
47	Asthma: pharmacologic therapy	5/1/2006	Percentage of all patients with mild, moderate, or severe persistent asthma who were prescribed either the preferred long-term control medication (inhaled corticosteroid) or an acceptable alternative treatment
109	Bipolar Disorder and Major Depression: Assessment for Manic or hypomanic behaviors	12/1/2006	Percentage of patients treated for depression who were assessed, prior to treatment, for the presence of current and/or prior manic or hypomanic behaviors
110	Bipolar Disorder and Major Depression: Appraisal for alcohol or chemical substance use	12/1/2006	Percentage of patients with depression or bipolar disorder with evidence of an initial assessment that includes an appraisal for alcohol or chemical substance use
111	Bipolar Disorder: Appraisal for risk of suicide	12/1/2006	Percentage of patients with bipolar disorder with evidence of an initial assessment that includes an appraisal for risk of suicide
3	Bipolar Disorder: Assessment for diabetes	12/1/2006	Percentage of patients treated for bipolar disorder who are assessed for diabetes within 16 weeks after initiating treatment with an atypical antipsychotic agent
112	Bipolar Disorder: Level-of-function evaluation	12/1/2006	Percentage of patients treated for bipolar disorder with evidence of level-of-function evaluation at the time of the initial assessment and again within 12 weeks of initiating treatment
13	Blood pressure measurement	5/1/2006	Percentage of patient visits with blood pressure measurement recorded among all patient visits for patients aged >18 years with diagnosed hypertension
23	Body Mass Index (BMI) in adults > 18 years of age	5/1/2006	Percentage of adults with BMI documentation in the past 24 months
24	Body Mass Index (BMI) 2 through 18 years of age	5/1/2006	Percentage children, 2 through 18 years of age, whose weight is classified based on BMI percentile for age and gender
391	Breast Cancer Resection Pathology Reporting- pT category (primary tumor) and pN category (regional lymph nodes) with histologic grade	7/31/2008	Percentage of breast cancer resection pathology reports that include the pT category (primary tumor), the pN category (regional lymph nodes), and the histologic grade
31	Breast Cancer Screening	5/1/2006	Percentage of eligible women 50–69 who receive a mammogram in a two year period
66	CAD: ACE inhibitor/angiotensin receptor blocker (ARB) Therapy	12/1/2006	Percentage of patients with CAD who also have diabetes and/or LSVD who were prescribed ACE inhibitor or ARB therapy
67	CAD: Antiplatelet Therapy	12/1/2006	Percentage of patients with CAD who were prescribed antiplatelet therapy

NQF#	Title	Date	Description
70	CAD: Beta-Blocker Therapy-Prior myocardial infarction (MI)	7/1/2005	Percentage of patients with prior MI at any time who were prescribed beta-blocker therapy
72	CAD: Beta-Blocker Treatment after a Heart Attack	12/1/2006	Percentage of patients who have a claim indicating beta blocker therapy or who received an ambulatory prescription for beta-blockers rendered within 7 days after discharge
74	CAD: Drug Therapy for Lowering LDL-Cholesterol	12/1/2006	Percentage of patients with CAD who were prescribed a lipid-lowering therapy (based on current ACC/AHA guidelines)
76	CAD: optimally managed modifiable risk	12/1/2006	Percentage of members who have optimally managed modifiable risk factors (LDL, tobacco non-use, blood pressure control, aspirin usage)
5	CAHPS Clinician/Group Surveys (Adult Primary Care, Pediatric Care, and Specialist Care Surveys)	7/1/2007	Adult Primary Care Survey: 37 core and 64 supplemental question survey of adult outpatient primary care patients. Pediatric Care Survey: 36 core and 16 supplemental question survey of outpatient pediatric care patients. Specialist Care Survey: 37 core and 20 supplemental question survey of adult outpatients specialist care patients. Level of analysis for each of the 3 surveys: group practices, sites of care, and/or individual clinicians.
9	CAHPS Health Plan Survey v 3.0 children with chronic conditions supplement	7/1/2007	31 questions that supplement the CAHPS Child Survey v 3.0 Medicaid and Commercial Core Surveys, that enables health plans to identify children who have chronic conditions and assess their experience with the health care system. Level of analysis: health plan, HMO, PPO, Medicare, Medicaid, commercial.
6	CAHPS Health Plan Survey v 4.0— Adult questionnaire	7/1/2007	30-question core survey of adult health plan members that assesses the quality of care and services they receive. Level of analysis: health plan, HMO, PPO, Medicare, Medicaid, commercial.
404	CD4+ Cell Count	7/31/2008	Percentage of patients, regardless of age, with a diagnosis of HIV/AIDS with a CD4+ cell count or CD4+ cell percentage performed at least once every 6 months
32	Cervical Cancer Screening	5/1/2006	Percentage of women 18–64 years of age, who received one or more Pap tests during the measurement year or the two years prior to the measurement year
429	Change in Basic Mobility as Measured by the AM-PAC	7/31/2008	The Activity Measure for Post Acute Care (AM-PAC) is a functional status assessment instrument developed specifically for use in facility and community dwelling post acute care (PAC) patients.
430	Change in Daily Activity Function as Measured by the AM-PAC	7/31/2008	The Activity Measure for Post Acute Care (AM-PAC) is a functional status assessment instrument developed specifically for use in facility and community dwelling post acute care (PAC) patients.
38	Childhood Immunization Status	5/1/2006	Percentage of children 2 years of age who had four DtaP/DT, three IPV, one MMR, three H influenza type B, three hepatitis B, one chicken pox vaccine (VZV), and four pneumococcal conjugate vaccines by their second birthday. The measure calculates a rate for each vaccine and two separate combination rates.
33	Chlamydia screening in women	5/1/2006	Percentage of eligible women who were identified as sexually active who had at least one test for chlamydia during the measurement year
379	Chronic Lymphocytic Leukemia (CLL) Baseline Flow Cytometry	7/31/2008	Percentage of patients aged 18 years and older with a diagnosis of CLL who had baseline flow cytometry studies performed
80	Chronic Obstructive Pulmonary Disease (COPD): assessment of oxygen saturation	5/1/2006	Percentage of patients with COPD with oxygen saturation assessed at least annually
34	Colorectal Cancer Screening	5/1/2006	Percentage of adults 50–80 years of age who had appropriate screening for colorectal cancer (CRC) including fecal occult blood test during the measurement year or, flexible sigmoidoscopy during the measurement year or the four years prior to the measurement year or, double contrast barium enema during the measurement year or the four years prior to the measurement year or, colonoscopy during the measurement year or the nine years prior to the measurement year
18	Controlling High Blood Pressure	5/1/2006	Percentage of patients with last BP <140/80 mm Hg
102	COPD: inhaled bronchodilator therapy	5/1/2006	Percentage of symptomatic patients with COPD who were prescribed an inhaled bronchodilator
91	COPD: spirometry evaluation	5/1/2006	Percentage of patients with COPD who had a spirometry evaluation documented
65	Coronary Artery Disease (CAD): Symptom and Activity Assessment	12/1/2006	Percentage of patients with CAD who were evaluated for both level of activity and anginal symptoms during one or more office visits

NQF#	Title	Date	Description
29	Counseling on physical activity in older adults—a. Discussing Physical Activity, b. Advising Physical Activity	5/1/2006	Percentage patients 65 years of age and older who reported: discussing their level of exercise or physical activity with a doctor or other health provider in the last 12 months. Percentage patients 65 years of age and older who reported receiving advice to start, increase, or maintain their level of exercise or physical activity from a doctor or other health provider in the last 12 months
64	Diabetes Measure Pair: A Lipid management: low density lipoprotein cholesterol (LDL-C) <130, B Lipid management: LDL-C <100	12/1/2006	Percentage of adult patients with diabetes aged 18–75 years with most recent (LDL-C) <130 mg/dL B: Percentage of patients 18–75 years of age with diabetes whose most recent LDL-C test result during the measurement year was <100 mg/dL
61	Diabetes: Blood Pressure Management	12/1/2006	Percentage of patient visits with blood pressure measurement recorded among all patient visits for patients aged >18 years with diagnosed hypertension
55	Diabetes: Eye exam	12/1/2006	Percentage of adult patients with diabetes aged 18–75 years who received a dilated eye exam or seven standard field stereoscopic photos with interpretation by an ophthalmologist or optometrist or imaging validated to match diagnosis from these photos during the reporting year, or during the prior year, if patient is at low risk for retinopathy. Patient is considered low risk if the following criterion is met: has no evidence of retinopathy in the prior year.
56	Diabetes: Foot exam	12/1/2006	Percentage of adult patients with diabetes aged 18–75 years who received a foot exam (visual inspection, sensory exam with monofilament, or pulse exam)
63	Diabetes: Lipid profile	12/1/2006	Percentage of adult patients with diabetes aged 18–75 years receiving at least one lipid profile (or ALL component tests)
62	Diabetes: Urine protein screening	12/1/2006	Percentage of adult diabetes patients aged 18–75 years with at least one test for microalbumin during the measurement year or who had evidence of medical attention for existing nephropathy (diagnosis of nephropathy or documentation of microalbuminuria or albuminuria)
417	Diabetic Foot & Ankle Care, Peripheral Neuropathy, and Neurological Evaluation	7/31/2008	Percentage of patients, 18 years or older, with diabetes who had a lower extremity neurological exam with risk catorization performed and a treatment plan established at least once within 12 months of diagnosis of diabetes mellitus who had a neurological examination of their lower extremities during one or more office visits within 12 months
416	Diabetic Foot & Ankle Care, Ulcer Prevention, and Evaluation of Footwear	7/31/2008	Percentage of patients aged 18 years and older with a diagnosis of diabetes mellitus who were evaluated for proper footwear and sizing during one or more office visits within 12 months
519	Diabetic Foot Care and Patient Education Implemented	3/31/2009	Percent of diabetic patients for whom physician-ordered monitoring for the presence of skin lesions on the lower extremities and patient education on proper foot care were implemented during their episode of care
89	Diabetic Retinopathy: Communication with the Physician Managing Ongoing Diabetes Care	5/1/2007	Percentage of patients aged 18 years and older with a diagnosis of diabetic retinopathy who had a dilated macular or fundus exam performed with documented communication to the physician who manages the ongoing care of the patient with diabetes regarding the findings of the macular or fundus exam at least once within 12 months
88	Diabetic Retinopathy: Documentation of Presence or Absence of Macular Edema and Level of Severity of Retinopathy	5/1/2007	Percentage of patients aged 18 years and older with a diagnosis of diabetic retinopathy who had a dilated macular or fundus exam performed which included documentation of the level of severity of retinopathy AND the presence or absence of macular edema during one or more office visits within 12 months
106	Diagnosis of attention deficit hyperactivity disorder (ADHD) in primary care for school age children and adolescents	12/1/2006	Percentage of patients newly diagnosed with attention deficit hyperactivity disorder (ADHD) whose medical record contains documentation of Diagnostic and Statistical Manual of Mental Disorders, Fourth Edition (DSM-IV) or Diagnostic and Statistical Manual for Primary Care (DSM-PC) criteria being addressed
369	Dialysis Facility Risk-adjusted Standardized Mortality Ratio (32) Level	5/15/2008	Risk-adjusted standardized mortality ratio for dialysis facility patients
325	Discharged on Antiplatelet Therapy	5/1/2007	Percentage of patients aged 18 years and older with the diagnosis of ischemic stroke or transient ischemic attack (TIA) who were prescribed antiplatelet therapy at discharge

NQF#	Title	Date	Description
`	Discontinuation of Prophylactic Antibiotics (Non-Cardiac Procedures)	7/31/2008	Percentage of non-cardiac surgical patients aged 18 years and older undergoing procedures with the indications for prophylactic antibiotics AND who received a prophylactic antibiotic, who have an order for discontinuation of prophylactic antibiotics within 24 hours of surgical end time
20	Documentation of allergies and adverse reactions in the outpatient record	5/1/2006	Percentage of patients having documentation of allergies and adverse reactions in the medical record
378	Documentation of Iron Stores in Patients Receiving Erythropoietin Therapy	7/31/2008	Percentage of patients aged 18 years and older with a diagnosis of MDS who are receiving erythropoietin therapy with documentation of iron stores prior to initiating erythropoietin therapy
19	Documentation of medication list in the outpatient record	5/1/2006	Percentage of patients having a medication list in the medical record.
22	Drugs to be avoided in the elderly: a. Patients who receive at least one drug to be avoided, b. Patients who receive at least two different drugs to be avoided.	5/1/2006	a. Percentage of patients ages 65 years and older who received at least one drug to be avoided in the elderly in the measurement year. b. Percentage of patients 65 years of age and older who received at least two different drugs to be avoided in the elderly in the measurement year.
487	EHR with EDI prescribing used in encounters where a prescribing event occurred.	8/29/2008	Of all patient encounters within the past month that used an electronic health record (EHR) with electronic data interchange (EDI) where a prescribing event occurred, how many used EDI for the prescribing event.
96	Empiric Antibiotic for Community-Acquired Bacterial Pneumonia	5/1/2007	Percentage of patients aged 18 years and older with the diagnosis of community-acquired bacterial pneumonia with an appropriate empiric antibiotic prescribed
8	Experience of Care and Health Outcomes (ECHO) Survey (behavioral health, managed care versions)	7/1/2007	52 questions including patient demographic information. The survey measures patient experiences with behavioral health care (mental health and substance abuse treatment) and the organization that provides or manages the treatment and health outcomes. Level of analysis: health plan, HMO, PPO, Medicare, Medicaid, commercial.
35	Fall risk management in older adults: a. Discussing fall risk, b.Managing fall risk	5/1/2006	a. Percentage of patients aged 75 and older who reported that their doctor or other health provider talked with them about falling or problems with balance or walking. b. Percentage of patients aged 75 and older who reported that their doctor or other health provider had done anything to help prevent falls or treat problems with balance or walking
101	Falls: Screening for Fall Risk	5/1/2007	Percentage of patients aged 65 years and older who were screened for fall risk (2 or more falls in the past year or any fall with injury in the past year) at least once within 12 months
40	Flu Shot for Older Adults	5/1/2006	Percentage of patients age 65 and over who received an influenza vaccination from September through December of the year
39	Flu shots for Adults Ages 50-64	5/1/2006	Percentage of patients age 50–64 who report having received an influenza vaccination during the past influenza vaccination season
447	Functional Communication Measure: Motor Speech	7/31/2008	This measure describes the change in functional communication status subsequent to speech-language pathology treatment of patients who exhibit deficits in speech-production.
445	Functional Communication Measure: Spoken Language Comprehension	7/31/2008	This measure describes the change in functional communication status subsequent to speech-language pathology treatment related to spoken language comprehension.
444	Functional Communication Measure: Spoken Language Expression	7/31/2008	This measure describes the change in functional communication status subsequent to speech-language pathology treatment related to spoken language expression.
442	Functional Communication Measure: Writing	7/31/2008	This measure describes the change in functional communication status subsequent to speech-language pathology treatment related to writing.
449	Functional Communicaton Measure: Attention	7/31/2008	This measure describes the change in functional communication status subsequent to speech-language pathology treatment of patients who have attention deficits.
448	Functional Communicaton Measure: Memory	7/31/2008	This measure describes the change in functional communication status subsequent to speech-language pathology treatment of patients with memory deficits.
446	Functional Communicaton Measure: Reading	7/31/2008	This measure describes the change in functional communication status subsequent to speech-language pathology treatment of patients with reading disorders.

NQF#	Title	Date	Description
443	Functional Communicaton Measure: Swallowing	7/31/2008	This measure describes the change in functional communication status subsequent to speech-language pathology treatment of patients who exhibit difficuty in swallowing.
427	Functional status change for patients with elbow, wrist or hand impairments	7/31/2008	Percentage of patients aged 18 or older with an elbow, wrist, or hand impairment associated with a functional deficit that had their functional status assessed at the beginning and end of rehabilitation
424	Functional status change for patients with foot/ankle impairments	7/31/2008	Functional status change in patients aged 18 or older with a foot/ankle impairment associated with a functional deficit that had their functional status assessed at the beginning and end of rehabilitation
428	Functional status change for patients with general orthopedic impairments	7/31/2008	Functional status change in patients aged 18 or older with a general orthopedic impairment associated with a functional deficit that had their functional status assessed at the beginning and end of rehabilitation
423	Functional status change for patients with hip impairments	7/31/2008	Percentage of patients aged 18 or older with a hip impairment associated with a functional deficit that had their functional status assessed at the beginning and end of rehabilitation.
422	Functional status change for patients with knee impairments	7/13/2008	Functional status change in patients aged 18 or older with a knee impairment associated with a functional deficit that had their functional status assessed at the beginning and end of rehabilitation
425	Functional status change for patients with lumbar spine impairments	7/31/2008	Percentage of patients aged 18 or older with a lumbar spine impairment associated with a functional deficit that had their functional status assessed at the beginning and end of rehabilitation
426	Functional status change for patients with shoulder impairments	7/31/2008	Percentage of patients aged 18 or older with a shoulder impairment associated with a functional deficit that had their functional status assessed at the beginning and end of rehabilitation
81	Heart Failure (HF): ACEI/ARB Therapy	12/1/2006	Percentage of patients with HF who also have left ventricular systolic dysfunction (LVSD) who were prescribed ACE inhibitor or ARB therapy
78	Heart Failure (HF): Assessment of Clinical Symptoms of Volume Overload (Excess)	12/1/2006	Percentage of patient visits or patients with HF with assessment of clinical symptoms of volume overload (excess)
83	Heart Failure (HF): Beta-blocker therapy	12/1/2006	Percentage of patients with HF who also have LVSD who were prescribed beta-blocker therapy
79	Heart Failure (HF): Left Ventricular Function Assessment	12/1/2006	Percentage of patients with HF with quantitative or qualitative results of left ventricular function (LVF) assessment recorded
82	Heart Failure (HF): Patient Education	12/1/2006	Percentage of patients who were provided with patient education on disease management and health behavior changes during one or more visit(s)
84	Heart Failure (HF): Warfarin Therapy Patients with Atrial Fibrillation	12/1/2006	Percentage of patients with HF who also have paroxysmal or chronic atrial fibrillation who were prescribed warfarin therapy
85	Heart Failure (HF): Weight Measurement	12/1/2006	Percentage of patient visits for patients with HF with weight measurement recorded
77	Heart Failure (HF): Assessment of Activity Level	12/1/2006	Percentage of patient visits or patients with HF with assessment of activity level
323	Hemodialysis Adequacy/Plan of Care	11/15/2007	Percentage of patient calendar months during the 12 month reporting period in which patients aged 18 years and older with a diagnosis of ESRD and receiving hemodialysis have a Kt/V >=1.2 AND have a Kt/V <1.2 with a documented plan of care
59	Hemoglobin A1c management	12/1/2006	Percentage of adult patients with diabetes aged 18–75 years with most recent A1c level greater than 9.0% (poor control)
60	Hemoglobin A1c test for pediatric patients	12/1/2006	Percentage of pediatric patients with diabetes with a HBA1c test in a 12-month measurement period
57	Hemoglobin A1c testing	12/1/2006	Percentage of adult patients with diabetes aged 18–75 years receiving one or more A1c test(s) per year
411	Hepatitis B Screening	7/31/2008	Percentage of patients for whom Hepatitis B screening was performed at least once since the diagnosis of HIV infection or for whom there is documented immunity
412	Hepatitis B Vaccination	7/31/2008	Percentage of patients, regardless of age, with a diagnosis of HIV/AIDS who have received at least one hepatitis B vaccination, or who have documented immunity

NQF#	Title	Date	Description
401	Hepatitis C: Counseling Regarding Risk of Alcohol Consumption	7/31/2008	Percentage of patients aged 18 years and older with a diagnosis of hepatitis C who received counseling regarding the risk of alcohol consumption at least once within the 12 month reporting period
394	Hepatitis C: Counseling Regarding Use of Contraception Prior to Antiviral Treatment	7/31/2008	Percentage of female patients aged 18 to 44 years and all men aged 18 years and older with a diagnosis chronic hepatitis C who are receiving antiviral treatment who were counseled regarding contraception prior to the initiation of antiviral treatment
398	Hepatitis C: HCV RNA Testing at Week 12 of Treatment	7/31/2008	Percentage of patients aged 18 years and older with a diagnosis of chronic hepatitis C who are receiving antiviral treatment for whom quantitative HCV RNA testing was performed at 12 weeks from initiation of antiviral treatment
397	Hepatitis C: Prescribed Antiviral Therapy	7/31/2008	Percentage of patients aged 18 years and older with a diagnosis of chronic hepatitis C who were prescribed peginterferon and ribavirin therapy within the 12 month reporting period
393	Hepatitis C: Testing for Chronic Hepatitis C Confirmation of Hepatitis C Viremia	7/31/2008	Percentage of patients aged 18 years and older with a diagnosis of hepatitis C seen for an initial evaluation who had HCV RNA testing ordered or previously performed
407	HIV RNA control after six months of potent antiretroviral therapy	7/31/2008	Percentage of patients with viral load below limits of quantification OR patients with viral load not below limits of quantification who have a documented plan of care
414	HIV/AIDS: Hepatitis C	7/31/2008	Percentage of patients for whom Hepatitis C (Hep C) screening was performed at least once since the diagnosis of HIV infection or for whom there is documented immunity
265	Hospital Transfer/Admission	11/15/2007	Percentage of ASC admissions requiring a hospital transfer or hospital admission prior to being discharged from the ASC
17	Hypertension Plan of Care	5/1/2006	Percentage of patient visits during which either systolic blood pressure >=140 mm Hg or diastolic blood pressure >=90 mm Hg, with documented plan of care for hypertension
58	Inappropriate antibiotic treatment for adults with acute bronchitis	5/1/2006	Percentage of patients who were diagnosed with bronchitis and were dispensed an antibiotic on or within three days after the episode date
508	Inappropriate use of probably benign assessment category in mammography screening	10/24/2008	Percentage of final reports for screening mammograms that are classified as probably benign
227	Influenza Immunization	11/15/2007	Percentage of patients aged 18 years and older with a diagnosis of ESRD and receiving dialysis who received the influenza immunization during the flu season (September through February)
41	Influenza Vaccination	5/1/2006	Percentage of patients who received an influenza vaccination
431	Influenza Vaccination Coverage among Healthcare Personnel	7/31/2008	Percentage of healthcare personnel (HCP) who receive the influenza vaccination
226	Influenza Vaccination in the ESRD Population—Facilities	11/5/2007	Percentage of all ESRD patients aged 18 years and older receiving hemodialysis and peritoneal dialysis during the flu season (October 1 to March 31) who receive an influenza vaccination during the October 1 to March 31 reporting period
4	Initiation and Engagement of Alcohol and Other Drug Dependence Treatment: a. Initiation, b. Engagement	12/1/2006	a. Percentage of adults aged 18 and over diagnosed with AOD abuse or dependence and receiving a related service who initiate treatment. b. Assessment of the degree to which members engage in treatment with two additional AOD treatments within 30 days after initiating treatment.
68	Ischemic Vascular Disease (IVD): Use of Aspirin or another Antithrombotic	12/1/2006	Percentage of patients who have documentation of use of aspirin or another antithrombotic during the 12-month measurement period
73	IVD: Blood Pressure Management	12/1/2006	Percentage of patients who, at their most recent blood pressure reading during the 12-month measurement period, had a bloodpressure result of <140/90 mm Hg.
75	IVD: Complete Lipid Profile and LDL Control <100	12/1/2006	Percentage of patients with a full lipid profile completed during the 12-month measurement period with date of each component of the profile documented; LDL-C <100
313	LBP: Advice Against Bedrest	11/15/2007	Percentage of patients with medical record documentation that a physician advised them against bed rest lasting four days or longer.

NQF#	Title	Date	Description
314	LBP: Advice for Normal Activities	11/15/2007	Percentage of patients with medical record documentation that a physician advised them to maintain or resume normal activities
315	LBP: Appropriate Imaging for Acute Back Pain	11/15/2007	Percentage of patients with a diagnosis of back pain for whom the physician ordered imaging studies during the 6 weeks after pain onset, in the absence of red flags (overuse measure, lower performance is better)
309	LBP: Appropriate Use of Epidural Steroid Injections	11/15/2007	Percentage of patients with back pain who have received an epidural steroid injection in the absence of radicular pain AND those patients with radicular pain who received an epidural steroid injection without image guidance (overuse measure, lower performance is better)
308	LBP: Evaluation of Patient Experience	11/15/2007	Percentage of physician mechanisms used to evaluate patient experience based on evidence of the following. An ongoing system for obtaining feedback about patient experience with care. A process for analyzing the data and a plan for improving patient experience. Note: This standard is assessed as a process that applies to all patients. Evaluation is not based on documentation in individual medical records.
322	LBP: Initial Assessment Initial Assessment	11/16/2007	Percentage of patients with a diagnosis of back pain who have medical record documentation of all of the following on the date of the initial visit to the physician: 1. Pain assessment 2. Functional status 3. Patient history, including notation of presence or absence of red flags 4. Assessment of prior treatment and response, and 5. Employment status.
316	LBP: Mental Health Assessment	11/15/2007	Percentage of patients with a diagnosis of back pain for whom documentation of a mental health assessment is present in the medical record prior to intervention or when pain lasts more than 6 weeks
307	LBP: Patient Education	11/15/2007	Percentage of patients provided with educational materials that review the natural history of the disease and treatment options, including alternatives to surgery, the risks and benefits, and the evidence. Note: This standard is assessed as a process that applies to all patients. Evaluation is not based on documentation in individual medical records.
306	LBP: Patient Ressessment	11/15/2007	Percentage of patients with documentation that the physician conducted reassessment of both of the following: Pain and functional status
319	LBP: Physical Exam	11/15/2007	Percentage of patients with documentation of a physical examination on the date of the initial visit with the physician
311	LBP: Post-surgical Outcomes	11/15/2007	Percentage of post-surgical outcomes examined by a physician's system that includes the following. Tracking specific complications of back surgery; Periodic analysis of surgical complications data and a plan for improving outcomes. Note: This standard is assessed as a process that applies to all patients. Evaluation is not based on documentation in individual medical records. This standard is applicable only for physicians who perform surgery.
317	LBP: Recommendations for Exercise	11/15/2007	Percentage of patients with back pain lasting more than 12 weeks, with documentation of physician advice for supervised exercise
312	LBP: Repeat Imaging Studies	11/15/2007	Percentage of patients who received inappropriate repeat imaging studies in the absence of red flags or progressive symptoms (overuse measure, lower performance is better)
310	LBP: Shared Decision Making	11/15/2007	Percentage of patients with whom a physician or other clinician reviewed the range of treatment options, including alternatives to surgery prior to surgery. To demonstrate shared decision making, there must be documentation in the patient record of a discussion between the physician and the patient that includes all of the following: Treatment choices, including alternatives to surgery; risks and benefits; evidence of effectiveness. Note: This measure is applicable only for physicians who perform surgery.
305	LBP: Surgical Timing	11/15/2007	Percentage of patients without documentation of red flags who had surgery within the first 6 weeks of back pain onset (overuse measure, lower performance is better). Note: This measure is applicable only for physicians who perform surgery.
52	LBP: use of imaging studies	12/1/2006	Percentage of patients with new low back pain who received an imaging study (plain x-ray, MRI, CT scan) conducted on the episode start date or in the 28 days following the episode start date

NQF#	Title	Date	Description
103	Major Depressive Disorder: Diagnostic Evaluation	12/1/2006	Percentage of patients with a diagnosis of major depressive disorder who met the DSM IV criteria during the visit in which the new diagnosis or recurrent episode was identified
104	Major Depressive Disorder: Suicide Risk Assessment	12/1/2006	Percentage of patients who had a suicide risk assessment completed at each visit
107	Management of attention deficit hyperactivity disorder (ADHD) in primary care for school age children and adolescents	12/1/2006	Percentage of patients diagnosed with attention deficit hyperactivity disorder (ADHD) and on first-line medication whose medical record contains documentation of a follow-up visit twice a year
25	Management plan for people with asthma	5/1/2006	Percentage of patients for whom there is documentation that a written asthma management plan was provided either to the patient or the patient's caregiver OR, at a minimum, specific written instructions on under what conditions the patient's doctor should be contacted or the patient should go to the emergency room
26	Measure pair: a. Tobacco use prevention for infants, children, and adolescents, b. Tobacco use cessation for infants, children, and adolescents	5/1/2006	a. Percentage of patients' charts showing either that there is no tobacco use/ exposure or (if a user) that the current use was documented at the most recent clinic visit. b. Percentage of patients with documented tobacco use or exposure at the latest visit who also have documentation that their cessation interest was assessed or that they received advice to quit.
28	Measure pair: a. Tobacco Use Assessment, b. Tobacco Cessation Intervention	5/1/2006	a. Percentage of patients who were queried about tobacco use one or more times during the two-year measurement period. b. Percentage of patients identified as tobacco users who received cessation intervention during the two-year measurement period.
403	Medical visit	7/31/2008	Percentage of patients, regardless of age, with a diagnosis of HIV/AIDS with at least one medical visit in each 6 month period with a minimum of 60 days between each visit
97	Medication Reconciliation	5/1/2007	Percentage of patients aged 65 years and older discharged from any inpatient facility (for example, hospital, skilled nursing facility, or rehabilitation facility) and seen within 60 days following discharge in the office by the physician providing ongoing care who had a reconciliation of the discharge medications with the current medication list in the medical record documented
370	Monitoring hemoglobin levels below target minimum	5/15/2008	Percentage of all adult (>=18 years old) hemodialysis or peritoneal dialysis patients with ESRD >=3 months and who had Hb values reported for at least 2 of the 3 study months, who have a mean Hb <10.0 g/dL for a 3 month study period, irrespective of ESA use
514	MRI Lumbar Spine for Low Back Pain	10/28/2008	This measure estimates the percentage of people who had an MRI of the Lumbar Spine with a diagnosis of low back pain without claims based on evidence of antecedent conservative therapy. Studies are limited to the outpatient place of service. This measure looks at the proportion of Lumbar MRI for low back pain performed in the outpatient setting where conservative therapy was utilized prior to the MRI. Lumbar MRI is a common study to evaluate patients with suspected disease of the lumbar spine. The most common, appropriate, indications for this study are low back pain accompanied by a measurable neurological deficit in the lower extremity(s) unresponsive to conservative management. The use of Lumbar MRI for low back pain (excluding operative, acute injury or tumor patients) is not typically indicated unless the patient has received a period of conservative therapy and serious symptoms persist. A Lumbar MRI claim for low back pain without the presence of prior Evaluation and Management codes (E/M codes) or claims suggesting conservative therapy (which would include the administration of injectable analgesic care, physical therapy, or chiropractic evaluation and manipulative treatment within specified time periods), suggests that the MRI was likely obtained on the first visit without a trial of conservative therapy.
380	Multiple Myeloma Treatment with Bisphosphonates	7/31/2008	Percentage of patients aged 18 years and older with a diagnosis of multiple myeloma, not in remission, who were prescribed or received intravenous bisphosphonates within the 12 month reporting period
377	Myelodysplastic Syndrome (MDS) and Acute Leukemias. Baseline Cytogenetic Testing Performed on Bone Marrow	7/31/2008	Percentage of patients aged 18 years and older with a diagnosis of MDS or an acute leukemia who had baseline cytogenic testing performed on bone marrow

NQF#	Title	Date	Description
7	NCQA Supplemental items for CAHPS® 4.0 Adult Questionnaire (CAHPS 4.0H)	7/1/2007	20-question supplement to the CAHPS Health Plan Survey v 4.0 adult questionnaire that assesses the health plan's role in offering information and care management to members. Level of analysis: health plan, HMO, PPO, Medicare, Medicaid, commercial.
105	New Episode of Depression: (a) Optimal Practitioner Contacts for Medication Management, (b) Effective Acute Phase Treatment, (c) Effective Continuation Phase Treatment	12/1/2006	a. Percentage of patients who were diagnosed with a new episode of depression and treated with antidepressant medication, and who had at least three follow-up contacts with a practitioner during the 84-day (12-week) Acute Treatment Phase. b. Percentage of patients who were diagnosed with a new episode of depression, were treated with antidepressant medication and remained on an antidepressant drug during the entire 84-day Acute Treatment Phase. c. Percentage of patients who were diagnosed with a new episode of depression and treated with antidepressant medication and who remained on an antidepressant drug for at least 180 days.
385	Oncology: Chemotherapy for Stage IIIA through IIIC Colon Cancer Patients	7/31/2008	Percentage of patients aged 18 years and older with Stage IIIA through IIIC colon cancer who are prescribed or who have received adjuvant chemotherapy within the 12 month reporting period
387	Oncology: Hormonal therapy for stage IC through IIIC, ER/PR positive breast cancer	7/31/2008	Percentage of female patients aged 18 years and older with Stage IC through IIIC, estrogen receptor (ER) or progesterone receptor (PR) positive breast cancer who were prescribed tamoxifen or aromatase inhibitor (AI) within the 12 month reporting period
384	Oncology: Pain Intensity Quantified Medical Oncology and Radiation Oncology (paired with 0383)	7/31/2008	Percentage of visits for patients with a diagnosis of cancer currently receiving intravenous chemotherapy or radiation therapy in which pain intensity is quantified
383	Oncology: Plan of Care for Pain Medical Oncology and Radiation Oncology (paired with 0384)	7/31/2008	Percentage of visits for patients with a diagnosis of cancer currently receiving intravenous chemotherapy or radiation therapy who report having pain with a documented plan of care to address pain
382	Oncology: Radiation Dose Limits to Normal Tissues	7/31/2008	Percentage of patients with a diagnosis of cancer receiving 3D conformal radiation therapy with documentation in medical record that normal tissue dose constraints were established within five treatment days for a minimum of one tissue
381	Oncology: Treatment Summary Documented and Communicated Radiation Oncology	7/31/2008	Percentage of patients with a diagnosis of cancer who have undergone brachytherapy or external beam radiation therapy who have a treatment summary report in the chart that was communicated to the physician(s) providing continuing care within one month of completing treatment
386	Oncology: Cancer Stage Documented Cancer Stage Documented	7/31/2008	Percentage of patients with a diagnosis of breast, colon, or rectal cancer seen in the ambulatory setting who have a baseline AJCC cancer stage or documentation that the cancer is metastatic in the medical record at least once during the 12 month reporting period
51	Osteoarthritis: assessment for use of anti-inflammatory or analgesic over-the-counter (OTC) medications	12/1/2006	Percentage of patient visits with assessment for use of anti-inflammatory or analgesic OTC medications
50	Osteoarthritis: functional and pain assessment	12/1/2006	Percentage of patients with osteoarthritis who were assessed for function and pain
53	Osteoporosis management in women who had a fracture	12/1/2006	Percentage of women 65 years and older who suffered a fracture and who had either a bone mineral density (BMD) test or prescription for a drug to treat or prevent osteoporosis in the 6 months after the date of fracture
37	Osteoporosis testing in older women	5/1/2006	Percentage of female patients aged 65 and older who reported receiving a bone density test (BMD) to check for osteoporosis
45	Osteoporosis: Communication with the Physician Managing Ongoing Care Post-Fracture	5/1/2007	Percentage of patients aged 50 years and older treated for a hip, spine, or distal radial fracture with documentation of communication with the physician managing the patient's ongoing care that a fracture occurred and that the patient was or should be tested or treated for osteoporosis
48	Osteoporosis: Management Following Fracture	5/1/2007	Percentage of patients aged 50 years or older with fracture of the hip, spine, or distal radius that had a central DXA measurement ordered or performed or pharmacologic therapy prescribed
49	Osteoporosis: Pharmacologic Therapy	5/1/2007	Percentage of patients aged 50 years and older with a diagnosis of osteoporosis who were prescribed pharmacologic therapy within 12 months

NQF#	Title	Date	Description
46	Osteoporosis: Screening or Therapy for Women Aged 65 Years and Older	5/1/2007	Percentage of female patients aged 65 years and older who have a central DXA measurement ordered or performed at least once since age 60 or pharmacologic therapy prescribed within 12 months
420	Pain Assessment Prior to Initiation of Patient Therapy	7/31/2008	Percentage of patients with documentation of a pain assessment (if pain is present, including location, intensity and description) through discussion with the patient including the use of a standardized tool on each initial evaluation prior to initiation of therapy and documentation of a follow up plan
395	Paired Measure: Hepatitis C RNA Testing Before Initiating Treatment (paired with 0396)	7/31/2008	Percentage of patients aged 18 years and older with a diagnosis of chronic hepatitis C who are receiving antiviral treatment for whom quantitative HCV RNA testing was performed within 6 months prior to initiation of antiviral treatment
396	Paired Measure: HCV Genotype Testing Prior to Treatment (paired with 0395)	7/31/2008	Percentage of patients aged 18 years and older with a diagnosis of chronic hepatitis C who are receiving antiviral treatment for whom HCV genotype testing was performed within 6 months prior to initiation of antiviral treatment
400	Paired Measure: Hepatitis C: Hepatitis B Vaccination (paired with 0399)	7/31/2008	Percentage of patients aged 18 years and older with a diagnosis fo hepatitis C who have received hepatitis B vaccination, or who have documented immunity
399	Paired Measure: Hepatitis C: Hepatitis A Vaccination (paired with 0400)	7/31/2008	Percentage of patients aged 18 years and older with a diagnosis of hepatitis C who have received hepatitis A vaccination, or who have documented immunity
263	Patient Burn	11/15/2007	Percentage of ASC admissions experiencing a burn prior to discharge
324	Patient Education Awareness—Facilities	11/15/2007	Percentage of all ESRD patients 18 years and older with documentation regarding a discussion of renal replacement therapy modalities (including hemodialysis, peritoneal dialysis, home hemodialysis, transplants and identification of potential living donors, and no treatment). Measured once a year.
320	Patient Education Awareness—Physician	11/15/2007	Percentage of all ESRD patients 18 years and older with documentation regarding a discussion of renal replacement therapy modalities (including hemodialysis, peritoneal dialysis, home hemodialysis, transplants and identification of potential living donors, and no treatment). Measured once a year.
266	Patient Fall	11/15/2007	Percentage of ASC admissions experiencing a fall in the ASC.
405	PCP prophylaxis	7/31/2008	Percentage of patients aged 1 month or older who were prescribed Pneumocystis jiroveci pneumonia (PCP) prophylaxis
465	Perioperative Anti-platelet Therapy for Patients undergoing Carotid Endarterectomy	7/31/2008	Percentage of patients undergoing carotid endarterectomy (CEA) who are taking an anti-platelet agent (aspirin or clopidogrel) within 48 hours prior to surgery and are prescribed this medication at hospital discharge following surgery
318	Peritoneal Dialysis Adequacy—Delivered Dose of peritoneal dialysis above minimum	11/15/2007	Percentage of all adult (>=18 years old) peritoneal dialysis patients whose delivered peritoneal dialysis dose was a weekly Kt/Vurea of at least 1.7 (dialytic + residual) during the four month study period
321	Peritoneal Dialysis Adequacy/Plan of Care	11/15/2007	Percentage of patients aged 18 years and older with a diagnosis of ESRD receiving peritoneal dialysis who have a Kt/V >=1.7 AND patients who have a Kt/V <1.7 with a documented plan of care 3 times a year (every 4 months) during the 12 month reporting period
42	Pneumococcal vaccine needed for all adults aged 65 years or older	5/1/2006	Percentage of adults aged 65 to 67 years who have not received a pneumococcal vaccine
43	Pneumonia vaccination status for older adults	5/1/2006	Percentage of patients 65 years of age and older who ever received a pneumococcal vaccination
44	Pneumonia Vaccination	5/1/2006	Percentage of patients who ever received a pneumococcal vaccination
14	Prenatal Anti-D Immune Globulin	12/1/2006	Percentage of D-negative, unsensitized patients who gave birth during a 12-month period who received anti-D immune globulin at 26–30 weeks gestation
16	Prenatal Blood Group Antibody Testing	12/1/2006	Percentage of patients who gave birth during a 12-month period who were screened for blood group antibodies during the first or second prenatal care visit
15	Prenatal Blood Groups (ABO), D (Rh) Type	12/1/2006	Percentage of patients who gave birth during a 12-month period who had a determination of blood group (ABO) and D (Rh) type by the second prenatal care visit
12	Prenatal Screening for Human Immunodeficiency Virus (HIV)	12/1/2006	Percentage of patients who gave birth during a 12-month period who were screened for HIV infection during the first or second prenatal care visit

NQF#	Title	Date	Description
86	Primary Open Angle Glaucoma: Optic Nerve Evaluation	5/1/2007	Percentage of patients aged 18 years and older with a diagnosis of primary open-angle glaucoma (POAG) who have an optic nerve head evaluation during one or more office visits within 12 months
11	Promoting Healthy Development Survey (PHDS)	7/1/2007	43-item survey given to parents of children ages 3 to 48 months that assesses parent's experience with care for the provision of preventive and developmental services consistent with American Academy of Pediatrics and Bright futures practice guidelines. Level of analysis: Physician, office, medical group, health plan, community, state, national, and by child and parent health and social economic characteristics
264	Prophylactic Intravenous (IV) Antibiotic Timing	11/15/2007	Percentage of ASC patients who received IV antibiotics ordered for surgical site infection prophylaxis on time
390	Prostate Cancer: Adjuvant Hormonal Therapy for High-Risk Patients	7/31/2008	Percentage of patients with a diagnosis of prostate cancer, at high risk of recurrence, receiving external beam radiotherapy to the prostate who were prescribed adjuvant hormonal therapy (GnRH agonist or antagonist)
389	Prostate Cancer: Avoidance of Overuse Measure Isotope Bone Scan for Staging Low-Risk Patients	7/31/2008	Percentage of patients with a diagnosis of prostate cancer, at low risk of recurrence, receiving interstitial prostate brachytherapy, OR external beam radiotherapy to the prostate, OR radical prostatectomy, OR cryotherapy who did not have a bone scan performed at any time since diagnosis of prostate cancer
388	Prostate Cancer: Three-Dimensional Radiotherapy	7/31/2008	Percentage of patients with prostate cancer receiving external beam radiotherapy to the prostate only who receive 3D-CRT (three-dimensional conformal radiotherapy) or IMRT (intensity modulated radiation therapy)
509	Reminder system for mammograms	10/28/2008	Percentage of patients aged 40 years and older undergoing a screening mammogram whose information is entered into a reminder system with a target due date for the next mammogram
418	Screening for Clinical Depression	7/31/2008	Percentage of patients aged 18 years and older screened for clinical depression using a standardized tool and follow up plan documented.
413	Screening for High Risk Sexual Behaviors	7/31/2008	Percentage of patients, aged 13 years and older, who were screened at least once in a 12-month measurement period for high risk sexual behavior
415	Screening for Injection Drug Use	7/31/2008	Percentage of patients, aged 13 years and older, who were screened, at least once in a 12-month measurement period, for injection drug use
402	Screening foreign-born adults for chronic hepatitis B	7/31/2008	Percentage of adults aged 18 years and above born in an HBV-endemic country and tested for hepatitis B surface antigen and antibody
268	Selection of Prophylactic Antibiotic: First OR Second Generation Cephalosporin	7/31/2008	Percentage of surgical patients aged 18 years and older undergoing procedures with the indications for a first OR second generation cephalosporin prophylactic antibiotic, who had an order for cefazolin OR cefuroxime for antimicrobial prophylaxis
27	Smoking Cessation, Medical assistance: a. Advising Smokers to Quit, b. Discussing Smoking Cessation Medications, c. Discussing Smoking Cessation Strategies	5/1/2006	a. Percentage of patients who received advice to quit smoking. b. Percentage of patients whose practitioner recommended or discussed smoking cessation medications. c. Percentage of patients whose practitioner recommended or discussed smoking cessation methods or strategies.
409	STD—Chlamydia and Gonorrhea Screenings	7/31/2008	Percentage of patients screened for chlamydia and gonorrhea at least once since the diagnosis of HIV infection
410	STD—Syphilis Screening	7/31/2008	Percentage of patients aged 13 years and older with a diagnosis of HIV/AIDS for whom syphilis screening was performed in the last 12 months
507	Stenosis measurement in carotid imaging studies	10/28/2008	Percentage of final reports for carotid imaging studies (neck MR angiography [MRA], neck CT angiography [CTA], neck duplex ultrasound, carotid angiogram) performed that include direct or indirect reference to measurements of distal internal carotid diameter as the denominator for stenosis measurement
408	TB Screening	7/31/2008	Percentage of patients for whom there was documentation that a tuberculosis (TB) screening test was placed and read at least once since the diagnosis of HIV infection

NQF#	Title	Date	Description
489	The Ability for Providers with HIT to Receive Laboratory Data Electronically Directly into their Qualified/Certified EHR System as Discrete Searchable Data Elements	8/29/2008	Documents the extent to which a provider uses certified/qualified electronic health record (EHR) system that incorporates an electronic data interchange with one or more laboratories allowing for direct electronic transmission of laboratory data into the EHR as discrete searchable data elements
490	The Ability to use Health Information Technology to Perform Care Management at the Point of Care	8/29/2008	Documents the extent to which a provider uses a certified/qualified electronic health record (EHR) system capable of enhancing care management at the point of care. To qualify, the facility must have implemented processes within their EHR for disease management that incorporate the principles of care management at the point of care which include: a. The ability to identify specific patients by diagnosis or medication use; b. The capacity to present alerts to the clinician for disease management, preventive services and wellness; c. The ability to provide support for standard care plans, practice guidelines, and protocol.
21	Therapeutic monitoring: Annual monitoring for patients on persistent medications	5/1/2006	Percentage of patients 18 years and older who received at least 180-day supply of medication therapy for the selected therapeutic agent and who received annual monitoring for the therapeutic agent. Percentage of patients on ACE inhibitors or ARBs with at least one serum potassium and either a serum creatinine or a blood urea nitrogen therapeutic monitoring test in the measurement year. Percentage of patients on digoxin with at least one serum potassium and either a serum creatinine or a blood urea nitrogen therapeutic monitoring test in the measurement year. Percentage of patients on a diuretic with at least one serum potassium and either a serum creatinine or a blood urea nitrogen therapeutic monitoring test in the measurement year. Percentage of patients on any anticonvulsant for phenytoin, phenobarbital, valproic acid or carbAMA/zepine with at least one drug serum concentration level monitoring test for the prescribed drug in the measurement year. The sum of the four numerators divided by the sum of the five denominators.
270	Timing of Antibiotic Prophylaxis: Ordering Physician	7/31/2008	Percentage of surgical patients aged 18 years and older undergoing procedures with the indications for prophylactic parenteral antibiotics, who have an order for prophylactic antibiotic to be given within one hour (if fluoroquinolone or vancomycin, two hours) prior to the surgical incision (or start of procedure when no incision is required)
269	Timing of Prophylactic Antibiotics— Administering Physician	11/15/2007	Percentage of surgical patients aged >18 years with indications for prophylactic parenteral antibiotics for whom administration of the antibiotic has been initiated within one hour (if vancomycin, two hours) prior to the surgical incision or start of procedure when no incision is required
242	Tissue Plasminogen Activator (t-PA) Considered	5/1/2007	Percentage of patients aged 18 years and older with the diagnosis of ischemic stroke whose time from symptom onset to arrival is less than 3 hours who were considered for t-PA administration (given t-PA or documented reasons for patient not being a candidate for therapy)
491	Tracking of Clinical Results Between Visits	8/29/2008	Documentation of the extent to which a provider uses a certified/qualified electronic health record (EHR) system to track pending laboratory tests, diagnostic studies (including common preventive screenings) or patient referrals. The Electronic Health Record includes provider reminders when clinical results are not received within a predefined timeframe.
419	Universal Documentation and Verification of Current Medications in the Medical Record	7/31/2008	Percentage of patients aged 18 years and older with a list of current medications with dosages (includes prescription, over-the-counter, herbals, vitamin/mineral/ dietary [nutritional] supplements) and verified with the patient or authorized representative documented by the provider
30	Urinary Incontinence Management in Older Adults—a. Discussing urinary incontinence, b. Receiving urinary incontinence treatment	5/1/2006	a. Percentage of patients 65 years of age and older who reported having a urine leakage problem in the last 6 months and who discussed their urinary leakage problem with their current practitioner. b. The percentage of patients 65 years of age and older who reported having a urine leakage problem in the last 6 months and who received treatment for their current urine leakage problem.
98	Urinary Incontinence: Assessment of Presence or Absence of Urinary Incontinence in Women	5/1/2007	Percentage of female patients aged 65 years and older who were assessed for the presence or absence of urinary incontinence within 12 months

NQF#	Title	Date	Description
99	Urinary Incontinence: Characterization of Urinary Incontinence in Women	5/1/2007	Percentage of female patients aged 65 years and older with a diagnosis of urinary incontinence whose urinary incontinence was characterized at least once within 12 months
100	Urinary Incontinence: Plan of Care for Urinary Incontinence in Women	5/1/2007	Percentage of female patients aged 65 years and older with a diagnosis of urinary incontinence with a documented plan of care for urinary incontinence at least once within 12 months.
36	Use of appropriate medications for people with asthma	5/1/2006	Percentage of patients who were identified as having persistent asthma during the measurement year and the year prior to the measurement year and who were dispensed a prescription for either an inhaled corticosteroid or acceptable alternative medication during the measurement year
513	Use of Contrast: Thorax CT	10/28/2008	Thorax CT use of combined studies (with and without contrast). Estimate the ratio of combined (with and without) studies to total studies performed. A high value would indicate a high use of combination studies (71270). Results to be segmented based upon data availability by rendering provider, rendering provider group and facility. This measure calculates the percentage of thorax studies that are performed with and without contrast out of all thorax studies performed (those with contrast, those without contrast, and those with both). Current literature clearly defines indications for the use of combined studies, that is, examinations performed without contrast followed by contrast enhancement. The intent of this measure is to assess questionable utilization of contrast agents that carry an element of risk and significantly increase examination cost. While there may be a direct financial benefit to the service provider for the use of contrast agents due to increased reimbursements for combined studies, this proposed measure is directed at the identification of those providers who typically employ interdepartmental/facility protocols that call for its use in nearly all cases. The mistaken concept is that more information is always better than not enough. The focus of this measure is one of the specific body parts where the indications for contrast material are more specifically defined.
232	Vital Signs for Community-Acquired Bacterial Pneumonia	5/1/2007	Percentage of patients aged 18 years and older with a diagnosis of community-acquired bacterial pneumonia with vital signs (temperature, pulse, respiratory rate, and blood pressure) documented and reviewed
267	Wrong Site, Wrong Side, Wrong Patient, Wrong Procedure, Wrong Implant	11/15/2007	Percentage of ASC admissions experiencing a wrong site, wrong side, wrong patient, wrong procedure, or wrong implant
10	Young Adult Health Care Survey (YAHCS)	7/1/2007	54-item survey given to teenagers that assesses whether young adults (age 14 and older) are receiving nationally-recommended preventive services. Level of analysis: health, state, national.

Appendix L

Ambulatory Care Documentation Standards

Standards General	AAAHC Ambulatory 2009	Joint Commission 2009	Medicare/ Medicaid 2009	NCQA 2009
2009 AAAHC Accreditation Handbook for Ambulatory Health Care, Chapter 6, Clinical Records and Health Information				
An accreditable organization maintains clinical records and a health information system from which information can be retrieved promptly. Clinical records are complete, comprehensive, legible, documented accurately in a timely manner, and readily accessible to health care professionals. Such an organization has the following characteristics.	Chapter 6			
The organization develops and maintains a system for the proper collection, processing, maintenance, storage, retrieval and distribution of patient records.	6.A			
An individual medical record is established for each person receiving care.	6.B			
Reports, histories and physicals, progress notes, and other patient information (such as laboratory reports, x-ray readings, operative reports, and consultations) are reviewed and incorporated into the record in a timely manner.	6.H			
Clinical record entries are legible and easily accessible within the record by the organization's personnel.	6.M			
Any notation in a patient's clinical record indicating diagnostic or therapeutic intervention as part of clinical research is clearly contrasted with entries regarding the provision of non-research-related care.	6.N			
All clinical information relevant to a patient is readily available to authorized health care practitioners any time the organization is open to patients.	6.C			
The organization is responsible for ensuring a patient's continuity of care. If a patient's primary or specialty care provider(s) or health care organization is elsewhere, the organization ensures that timely summaries or pertinent records necessary for continuity of patient care are: 1. Obtained from the other (external) provider(s) or organization and incorporated into the patient's clinical record 2. Provided to the other (external) health care professional(s) or consultant and, as appropriate, to the organization where future care will be provided	6.O			
Entries in a patient's record for each visit include, but are not limited to: 1. Date, department (if departmentalized), and physician or other health care professional's name and credential (for example, PT, RN, CRNA)	6.K-1			
The organization has policies and procedures that address the following information, and distributes the policies and procedures to practice sites: 1) confidentiality of medical records, 2) medical record documentation standards, and 3) an organized medical record keeping system and standards for the availability of medical records.	6.D, E			QI 12 A

| Standards

General (continued)	AAAHC Ambulatory 2009	Joint Commission 2009	Medicare/ Medicaid 2009	NCQA 2009
Contracts with practitioners specifically require that the organization has access to practitioner medical records, to the extent permitted by state and federal law.				QI 3A
The ASC must maintain complete, comprehensive, and accurate medical records to ensure adequate patient care.

(a) Standard: Organization. The ASC must develop and maintain a system for the proper collection, storage, and use of patient records. | Chapter 6, 6.A | | ASC 416.47(a) | |
| The ESRD facility maintains complete medical records on all patients (including self-dialysis patients within the self-dialysis unit and home dialysis patients whose care is under the supervision of the facility) in accordance with accepted professional standards and practices. A member of the facility's staff is designated to serve as a supervisor of medical records services, and ensures that all records are properly documented, completed, and preserved. The medical records are completely and accurately documented, readily available, and systematically organized to facilitate the compilation and retrieval of information. | | | RD 405.2139 | |
| Protection of medical record information. The ESRD facility safeguards medical record information against loss, destruction, or unauthorized use. The ESRD facility has written policies and procedures which govern the use and release of information contained in medical records. Written consent of the patient, or of an authorized person acting in behalf of the patient, is required for release of information not provided by law. Medical records are made available under stipulation of confidentiality for inspection by authorized agents of the Secretary, as required for administration of the ESRD program under Medicare. | | | RD 405.2139(b) | |
| For each patient in need of outpatient physical therapy or speech pathology services there is a written plan of care established and periodically reviewed by a physician, or by a physical therapist or speech pathologist respectively. The organization has a physician available to furnish necessary medical care in case of emergency.

(a) Standard: Medical history and prior treatment. The following are obtained by the organization before or at the time of initiation of treatment:

(1) The patient's significant past history.

(2) Current medical findings, if any.

(3) Diagnosis(es), if established.

(4) Physician's orders, if any.

(5) Rehabilitation goals, if determined.

(6) Contraindications, if any.

(7) The extent to which the patient is aware of the diagnosis(es) and prognosis.

(8) If appropriate, the summary of treatment furnished and results achieved during previous periods of rehabilitation services or institutionalization.

(b) Standard: Plan of care. (1) For each patient there is a written plan of care established by the physician or by the physical therapist or speech-language pathologist who furnishes the services.

(2) The plan of care for physical therapy or speech pathology services indicates anticipated goals and specifies for those services the--

(i) Type;

(ii) Amount;

(iii) Frequency; and

(iv) Duration.

(3) The plan of care and results of treatment are reviewed by the physician or by the individual who established the plan at least as often as the patient's condition requires, and the indicated action is taken. (For Medicare patients, the plan must be reviewed by a physician, nurse practitioner, clinical nurse specialist, or physician assistant at least every 30 days, in accordance with Sec. 410.61(e) of this chapter.)

(4) Changes in the plan of care are noted in the clinical record. If the patient has an attending physician, the therapist or speech-language pathologist who furnishes the services promptly notifies him or her of any change in the patient's condition or in the plan of care. | | | PT/SP 485.711 | |

Standards General (continued)	AAAHC Ambulatory 2009	Joint Commission 2009	Medicare/ Medicaid 2009	NCQA 2009
Consent for treatment	6.P, 9.E, 10.I.R		ASC 416.48(a)(1), 416.47(b)(7)	

Standards Content	AAAHC Ambulatory 2009	Joint Commission 2009	Medicare/ Medicaid 2009	NCQA 2009
The organization effectively manages the collection of health information.		IM 02.01.01		
Entries in a patient's record for each visit include, but are not limited to:	6.B, K			
Date	6.K-1			
Name	6.B-1			
Identification number (if appropriate)	6.B-2			
Date of birth	6.B-3			
Gender	6.B-4			
Responsible party, if applicable	6.B-5			
Department (if organization is departmentalized)	6.K-1			
Physician or other health care professional's name and credential (for example, PT, RN, CRNA)	6.K-1			
Chief complaint or purpose of visit	6.K-2			
Clinical findings	6.K-3			
Diagnosis or impression	6.K-4			
Studies ordered, such as laboratory or x-ray studies	6.K-5			
Care rendered and therapies administered	6.K-6			
Except when otherwise required by law, the content and format of clinical records, including the sequence of information, are uniform. Records are organized in a consistent manner that facilitates continuity of care. Any abbreviations and dose designations must be standardized according to a list approved by the organization.	6.G			
Reports, histories and physicals, progress notes, and other patient information (such as laboratory reports, x-ray readings, operative reports, and consultations) are reviewed and incorporated into the record in a timely manner.	6.H			
If a patient had multiple visits/admissions, and the clinical record is complex and lengthy, a summary of past and current diagnoses or problems, including past procedures, is documented in that patient's record to facilitate the continuity of care.	6.I			
The presence or absence of allergies and untoward reactions to drugs and materials is recorded in a prominent and uniform location in all patient records. This is verified at each patient encounter and updated whenever new allergies or sensitivities are identified.	6.J			
Entries in a patient's record for each visit include: Disposition, recommendations and instructions given to the patient.	6.K-7			
Entries in a patient's record for each visit include: Missed and canceled appointments should have follow-up documentation.	6.K-9			
The organization facilitates the provision of high-quality health care as demonstrated by: Appropriate and timely referrals	4.E-8			
When the need arises, patients are transferred from the care of one health care professional to another with: 1. Adequate specialty consultation services being available by prior arrangement 2. Referral to a health care professional that is clearly outlined to the patient and arranged with the accepting health care professional prior to transfer	4.J			
Entries in a patient's record for each visit include: Authentication and verification of contents by health care professionals	6.K-8			

Standards Content (continued)	AAAHC Ambulatory 2009	Joint Commission 2009	Medicare/ Medicaid 2009	NCQA 2009
Significant medical advice given to a patient by telephone is entered in the patient's record and appropriately signed or initialed, including medical advice provided by after-hours telephone patient information or triage telephone services.	6.L			
Clinical record entries are legible and easily accessible within the record by the organization's personnel.	6.M			
Any notation in a patient's clinical record indicating diagnostic or therapeutic intervention as part of clinical research is clearly contrasted with entries regarding the provision of non-research-related care.	6.N			
Discussions with the patient concerning the necessity, appropriateness and risks of proposed care, surgery or procedure, as well as discussions of treatment alternatives and advance directives, as applicable, are incorporated into the patient's medical record.	6.P			
2009 AAAHC Accreditation Handbook for Ambulatory Health Care, Chapter 16, Health Education and Health Promotion				
Health education and health promotion programs should include, but may not be limited to: 1. Clearly defined educational goals and objectives 2. Evaluation of whether the goals or objectives have been met	16.C-1, 2			
When appropriate, health education and health promotion services, whether they occur within the context of a clinical visit or not, should be referenced or documented in the patient's clinical record.	16.G			
Health education and disease prevention programs should be comprehensive and consider the medical, psychological, social and cultural needs of the population. Topics that should be considered include: 1. Disease-specific screening and educational programs 2. Substance abuse prevention and education, including programs related to alcohol, tobacco, and other drugs 3. Promotion of healthy eating 4. Promotion of physical fitness 5. Sexuality education and skill building for healthy relationships 6. Sexual, physical, and emotional violence prevention 7. Promotion of and education about stress management and relaxation	16.I-1 to 7			
2009 AAAHC Accreditation Handbook for Ambulatory Health Care, Chapter 17, Behavioral Health Services				
The written and signed informed consent of the client is obtained and incorporated into the treatment plan, which may include but is not limited to procedures, therapies, medication management, and other modalities of care and treatment.	17.H			
2009 AAAHC Accreditation Handbook for Ambulatory Health Care, Chapter 24, Radiation Oncology Treatment Services				
Radiation oncology services appropriate to the organization's function include, but are not limited to: 1. Consultation services 2. Treatment planning 3. Simulation of treatment 4. Maintenance of reports of services and radiographic images appropriate to the therapy for the time required by applicable laws and policy of the organization 5. Clinical treatment management including, but not limited to, the use of teletherapy and brachytherapy 6. Appropriate follow-up care of all patients	24.B-1 to 6			

Standards Content (continued)	AAAHC Ambulatory 2009	Joint Commission 2009	Medicare/ Medicaid 2009	NCQA 2009
In addition to the applicable Clinical Records and Health Information requirements found in Chapter 6 of the *2009 AAAHC Accreditation Handbook for Ambulatory Health Care,* the following characteristics indicate good-quality patient care in the radiation oncology setting and are documented: 1. Confirmation of the presence of malignancy by histopathology or a statement of benign condition 2. Definition of tumor location, extent and stage 3. Definition of treatment volume 4. Selection of dose 5. Selection of treatment modality 6. Selection of treatment technique 7. Dosimetry calculations 8. Supervision of treatment and record of patient progress and tolerance 9. Summary of completion with statement of follow-up plan	24.I-1 to 9			
1—The organization defines the components of a complete clinical record.		RC 01.01.01		
5—The clinical record contains the information needed to support the patient's diagnosis and condition.		RC 01.01.01		
6—The clinical record contains the information needed to justify the patient's care, treatment, or services.		RC 01.01.01		
7—The clinical record contains information that documents the course and result of the patient's care, treatment, or services.		RC 01.01.01		
8—The clinical record contains information about the patient's care, treatment, or services that promotes continuity of care among providers.		RC 01.01.01		
9—The organization uses standardized formats to document the care, treatment, or services it provides to patients.		RC 01.01.01		
11—All entries in the clinical record are dated.		RC 01.01.01		
12—The organization tracks the location of all components of the clinical record.		RC 01.01.01		
13—The organization assembles or makes available in a summary in the clinical record all information required to provide patient care, treatment, or services. (See also MM.01.01.01, EP 1)		RC 01.01.01		
14—When needed to provide care, summaries of treatment and other documents provided by the organization are forwarded to other care providers.		RC 01.01.01		
1—Only authorized individuals make entries in the clinical record.		RC 01.02.01		
2—The organization defines the types of entries in the clinical record made by nonindependent practitioners that require countersigning, in accordance with law and regulation.		RC 01.02.01		
3—The author of each clinical record entry is identified in the clinical record.		RC 01.02.01		
4—Entries in the clinical record are authenticated by the author. Information introduced into the clinical record through transcription or dictation is authenticated by the author. Note 1: Authentication can be verified through electronic signatures, written signatures or initials, rubber-stamp signatures, or computer key. Note 2: For paper-based records, signatures entered for purposes of authentication after transcription or for verbal orders are dated when required by law or regulation or organization policy. For electronic records, electronic signatures will be date-stamped.		RC 01.02.01		
5—The individual identified by the signature stamp or method of electronic authentication is the only individual who uses it.		RC 01.02.01		
1—The organization has a written policy that requires timely entry of information into the clinical record. (See also PC.01.02.03, EP 1)		RC 01.03.01		
2—The organization defines the time frame for completion of the clinical record.		RC 01.03.01		

Standards Content (continued)	AAAHC Ambulatory 2009	Joint Commission 2009	Medicare/ Medicaid 2009	NCQA 2009
3—The organization implements its policy requiring timely entry of information into the patient's clinical record. (See also PC.01.02.03, EP 2)		RC 01.03.01		
1—According to a time frame it defines, the organization reviews its clinical records to confirm that the required information is present, accurate, legible, authenticated, and completed on time.		RC 01.04.01		
1—The clinical record contains the following demographic information: • The patient's name, address, phone number, date of birth, and the name of any legally authorized representative • The patient's sex, height, and weight (See also MM.01.01.01, EP 3) • The legal status of any patient receiving behavioral health care services • The patient's language and communication needs		RC 02.01.01		
2—The clinical record contains the following clinical information: • The patient's initial diagnosis, diagnostic impression(s), or condition(s) • Any findings of assessments and reassessments (See also PC.01.02.01, EP 1; PC.03.01.03, EPs 1 and 8) • Any allergies to food • Any allergies to medications • Any conclusions or impressions drawn from the patient's medical history and physical examination • Any diagnoses or conditions established during the patient's course of care, treatment, or services • Any consultation reports • Any progress notes • Any medications ordered or prescribed • Any medications administered, including the strength, dose, and route • Any access site for medication, administration devices used, and rate of administration • The patient's response to any medication administered • Any adverse drug reactions • Plans for care and any revisions to the plan for care (See also PC.01.03.01, EP 1) • Orders for diagnostic and therapeutic tests and procedures and their results		RC 02.01.01		
4—As needed to provide care, treatment, or services, the clinical record contains the following additional information: • Any advance directives • Any informed consent, when required by organization policy (See also RI.01.03.01, EP 13) • Any documentation of clinical research interventions distinct from entries related to regular patient care, treatment, or services (See also RI.01.03.05, EPs 4–6) • Any records of communication with the patient, such as telephone calls or e-mail • Any referrals or communications made to internal or external care providers and community agencies • Any patient-generated information		RC 02.01.01		
21—The clinical record of a patient who receives urgent or immediate care, treatment, or services contains the following: • The times and means of arrival • Indication that the patient left against medical advice, when applicable • Conclusions reached at the termination of care, treatment, or services, including the patient's final disposition, condition, and instructions given for follow-up care, treatment, or services • A copy of any information made available to the practitioner or medical organization providing follow-up care, treatment, or services		RC 02.01.01		

Standards Content (continued)	AAAHC Ambulatory 2009	Joint Commission 2009	Medicare/ Medicaid 2009	NCQA 2009
1—The organization identifies, in writing, the staff who are authorized to receive and record verbal orders, in accordance with law and regulation.		RC 02.03.07		
2—Only authorized staff receive and record verbal orders.		RC 02.03.07		
3—Documentation of verbal orders includes the date and the names of individuals who gave, received, recorded, and implemented the orders.		RC 02.03.07		
4—Verbal orders are authenticated within the time frame specified by law and regulation.		RC 02.03.07		
The clinical record contains documentation of the use of restraint.		RC 02.01.05		
The organization assesses and reassesses its patients.		PC.01.02.01		
1—The organization defines, in writing, the scope and content of screening, assessment, and reassessment information it collects. (See also RC.02.01.01, EP 2) Note 1: The scope and content are dependent on whether the patient is making an initial or follow-up visit and whether the assessment is focused or comprehensive. Note 2: In defining the scope and content of the information it collects, the organization may want to consider information that it can obtain, with the patient's consent, from the patient's family and the patient's other care providers, as well as information conveyed on any medical jewelry.		PC.01.02.01		
2—The organization defines, in writing, criteria that identify when additional, specialized, or more in-depth assessments are performed. (See also PC.01.02.07, EP 1) Note: Examples of criteria could include those that identify when a nutritional, functional, or pain assessment should be performed for patients who are at risk.		PC.01.02.01		
4—Based on the patient's condition, information gathered in the initial assessment includes the following: • Physical, psychological, and social assessment • Nutrition and hydration status • Functional status • For patients who are receiving end-of-life care, the social, spiritual, and cultural variables that influence the patient's and family members' perception of grief		PC.01.02.01		
23—During patient assessments and reassessments, the organization gathers the data and information it requires.		PC.01.02.01		
The organization assesses and reassesses the patient and his or her condition according to defined time frames.		PC.01.02.03		
1—The organization defines, in writing, the time frame(s) within which it conducts the patient's initial assessment, in accordance with law and regulation. (See also RC.01.03.01, EP 1)		PC.01.02.03		
2—The organization performs initial patient assessments within its defined time frame. (See also RC.01.03.01, EP 3)		PC.01.02.03		
3—Each patient is reassessed as necessary based on his or her plan for care or changes in his or her condition. Note: Reassessments may also be based on the patient's diagnosis; desire for care, treatment, or services; response to previous care, treatment, or services; and/or his or her setting requirements.		PC.01.02.03		
9—At each patient's visit, the organization documents updates to the patient's condition.		PC.01.02.03		

411

Standards Content (continued)	AAAHC Ambulatory 2009	Joint Commission 2009	Medicare/ Medicaid 2009	NCQA 2009
(b) Standard: Form and content of record. The ASC must maintain a medical record for each patient. Every record must be accurate, legible, and promptly completed. Medical records must include at least the following: (1) Patient identification. (2) Significant medical history and results of physical examination. (3) Pre-operative diagnostic studies (entered before surgery), if performed. (4) Findings and techniques of the operation, including a pathologist's report on all tissues removed during surgery, except those exempted by the governing body. (5) Any allergies and abnormal drug reactions. (6) Entries related to anesthesia administration. (7) Documentation of properly executed informed patient consent. (8) Discharge diagnosis.	4.E-3, 4.E-9 6.B, E, H, J, K-3-5, K-7, P 9.E, I 10.I.E, K, L, R		ASC 416.47(b)	
(a) Standard: medical record. Each patient's medical record contains sufficient information to identify the patient clearly, to justify the diagnosis and treatment, and to document the results accurately. All medical records contain the following general categories of information: Documented evidence of assessment of the needs of the patient, whether the patient is treated with a reprocessed hemodialyzer, of establishment of an appropriate plan of treatment, and of the care and services provided (see Sec. 405.2137(a) and (b)); evidence that the patient was informed of the results of the assessment described in Sec. 405.2138(a)(5); identification and social data; signed consent forms referral information with authentication of diagnosis; medical and nursing history of patient; report(s) of physician examination(s); diagnostic and therapeutic orders; observations, and progress notes; reports of treatments and clinical findings; reports of laboratory and other diagnostic tests and procedures; and discharge summary including final diagnosis and prognosis.			RD 405.2139(a)	
Completion of medical records and centralization of clinical information: Current medical records and those of discharged patients are completed promptly. All clinical information pertaining to a patient is centralized in the patient's medical record. Provision is made for collecting and including in the medical record medical information generated by self-dialysis patients. Entries concerning the daily dialysis process may either be completed by staff, or be completed by trained self-dialysis patients, trained home dialysis patients, or trained assistants and countersigned by staff.			RD 405.2139(d)	
Documentation of items on the NCQA Medical Record Review Summary Sheet demonstrates that medical records are in conformity with good professional medical practice and appropriate health management. Guidelines for Medical Record Review contain:				QI 13C*
1. Each and every page in the record contains the patient's name or ID number.				QI 13C*
2. Personal/biographical data includes address, employer, home and work telephone numbers, marital status.				QI 13C*
3. All entries in the medical record contain author identification.				QI 13C*
4. All entries are dated.				QI 13C*
5. The record is legible to someone other than the writer. Any record judged illegible by one physician reviewer should be evaluated by a second reviewer.				QI 13C*
6. Significant illnesses and medical conditions are indicated on the problem list. If the patient has no known medical illness or conditions, the chart includes a flow sheet for health maintenance.				QI 13C*
7. Medication allergies and adverse reactions are prominently noted in the record.				QI 13C*
8. Past medical history (for patient seen three or more times) is easily identified and includes serious accidents, operations, illnesses. For children and adolescents (18 years and younger), past medical history relates to prenatal care, birth, operations, and childhood illnesses.				QI 13C*
10. The history and physical documents subjective and objective information for presenting complaints.				QI 13C*

Standards Content (continued)	AAAHC Ambulatory 2009	Joint Commission 2009	Medicare/ Medicaid 2009	NCQA 2009
11. All lab and other studies ordered are appropriate.				QI 13C*
12. Working diagnoses are consistent with findings.				QI 13C*
13. Plans of action/treatment are consistent with diagnoses.				QI 13C*
14. Encounter forms or notes have a notation, when indicated, regarding follow-up care, calls, or visits. The specific time of return is noted in weeks, months or PRN.				QI 13C*
15. Unresolved problems from previous office visits are addressed in subsequent visits.				QI 13C*
16. There is evidence of appropriate use of consultants.				QI 13C*
17. If a consultation is requested, there is a note from the consultant in the record.				QI 13C*
18. Consultation, lab, and x-ray reports filed in the record are initialed by the primary care physician, or some other electronic method is used to signify review. Consultation and abnormal lab and imaging study results have an explicit notation in the record of follow-up plans.				QI 13C*
19. There is no evidence that the patient is placed at inappropriate risk by a diagnostic or therapeutic problem.				QI 13C*
20. For pediatric (ages 10 and under) records, there is a completed immunization record or a notation that "immunizations are up-to-date."				QI 13C*
21. There is evidence that preventive screening and services are offered in accordance with the organization's practice guidelines.				QI 13C*

Standards Surgical and Anesthesia Services	AAAHC Ambulatory 2009	Joint Commission 2009	Medicare/ Medicaid 2009	NCQA 2009
2009 AAAHC Accreditation Handbook for Ambulatory Health Care, Chapter 10, Surgical and Related Services, Subchapter I—General Requirements	10.I			
Surgical procedures performed in the facilities owned and operated by the organization are limited to those procedures that are approved by the governing body upon the recommendation of qualified medical personnel.	10.I.A			
Surgical procedures to be performed in a solo office-based surgical practice are externally reviewed periodically as part of the peer review portion of the organization's quality improvement program.	10.I.D			
An appropriate and current health history must be completed, with a list of current medications and dosages, physical examination, and pertinent pre-operative diagnostic studies incorporated into the patient's clinical record within thirty (30) days prior to the scheduled surgery/procedure.	10.I.E			
With the exception of those tissues exempted by the governing body after medical review, tissues removed during surgery are examined by the pathologist, whose signed report of the examination is made a part of the patient's record.	10.I.K			
The findings and techniques of a procedure are accurately and completely documented immediately after the procedure by the health care professional who performed the procedure. This description is immediately available for patient care and becomes a part of the patient's record.	10.I.L			
Protocols have been developed for obtaining and administering blood and blood products on a timely basis, as determined by the governing body, as necessary and appropriate for the type of surgery/procedure performed at the organization.	10.I.O			
Periodic calibration and/or preventive maintenance of equipment is provided.	10.I.Q			
The informed consent of the patient or, if applicable, of the patient's representative, is obtained before the procedure is performed.	10.I.R			
The organization utilizes a process to identify and/or designate the surgical procedure to be performed and the surgical site, and involves the patient in that process. The person performing the procedure marks the site. For dental procedures, the operative tooth may be marked on a radiograph or a dental diagram.	10.I.S			

Standards Surgical and Anesthesia Services (continued)	AAAHC Ambulatory 2009	Joint Commission 2009	Medicare/ Medicaid 2009	NCQA 2009
Immediately prior to beginning a procedure, the operating team verifies the patient's identification, intended procedure, and correct surgical site, and that all equipment routinely necessary for performing the scheduled procedure, along with any implantable devices to be used, are immediately available in the operating/ procedure room. The provider performing the procedure is personally responsible for ensuring that all aspects of this verification have been satisfactorily completed immediately prior to beginning the procedure.	10.I.T			
A process is in place for the observation, care and communication of such care in all peri-procedural areas of the patient's facility experience. The organization must define and implement a process in which information about the patient's care is communicated consistently. The process must include means to educate the staff and medical care providers about the process and support implementation consistently throughout the organization.	10.I.U			
The organization follows established protocols for instructing patients in self-care after surgery, including the provision of written instructions to patients who receive moderate sedation/analgesia, deep sedation/analgesia, regional anesthesia or general anesthesia.	10.I.V			
2009 AAAHC Accreditation Handbook for Ambulatory Health Care, Chapter 10, Surgical and Related Services, Subchapter II—Laser, Light-Based Technologies and Other Energy-Emitting Equipment	10.II			
Policies and procedures should be established and implemented for these devices, which include, but are not limited to: 1. Safety programs 2. Education and training of personnel, including a requirement for all personnel working with these devices to be adequately trained in the safety and use of each type of device utilized in patient care.	10.II.A			
Documenting that maintenance logs are present that confirm the inspection and testing of these devices.	10.II.B-9			
2009 AAAHC Accreditation Handbook for Ambulatory Health Care, Chapter 9, Anesthesia Services				
A physician, dentist, or qualified individual supervised by a physician or dentist, approved by the governing body, examines the patient immediately prior to the anesthetic to evaluate the risks of anesthesia relative to the procedure to be performed and develops and documents a plan of anesthesia.	9.D			
The informed consent of the patient or, if applicable, of the patient's representative, is obtained before the procedure is performed. One consent form may be used to satisfy the requirements of this standard and AAAHC Standard 10.I.R.	9.E			
At a minimum, all settings in which sedation or anesthesia is administered should have the following equipment for resuscitation purposes: appropriate monitoring equipment for the intended anesthesia care.	9.G-4			
Clinical records include entries related to anesthesia administration.	9.I			
The organization maintains a written policy with regard to assessment and management of acute pain.	9.K			
Before medical discharge from the facility, each patient must be evaluated by a physician, dentist, or delegated qualified individual supervised by a physician or dentist, approved by the governing body to assess recovery. If medical discharge criteria have previously been set by the treating physician or dentist, and approved by the governing body, a delegated qualified individual may determine if the patient meets such discharge criteria, and if so, may discharge when those criteria are met.	9.M-2			
A safe environment for providing anesthesia services is assured through the provision of adequate space, equipment, supplies, medications, and appropriately trained personnel. Written policies must be in place for safe use of injectables and single-use syringes and needles. All equipment should be maintained, tested and inspected according to the manufacturer's specifications. A log is kept of regular preventive maintenance.	9.P			

Standards Surgical and Anesthesia Services (continued)	AAAHC Ambulatory 2009	Joint Commission 2009	Medicare/ Medicaid 2009	NCQA 2009
Having written protocols for the treatment of malignant hyperthermia immediately available in each location where triggering agents may potentially be used	9.R-1			
Having documentation of staff education, training, and practice drills on malignant hyperthermia treatment protocols.	9.R-2			
The organization has a written protocol in place for the safe and timely transfer of patients to a predetermined alternate care facility when extended or emergency services are needed to protect the health or well-being of the patient. AAAHC Standard 4.K addresses medical emergencies that arise in connection with surgical procedures.	9.S			
The organization has a written protocol that explains how the organization will respond in the event that a deeper-than-intended level of sedation occurs.	9.W			
1—The organization documents in the patient's clinical record any operative or other high-risk procedure and/or the administration of moderate or deep sedation or anesthesia.		RC 02.01.03		
2—A licensed independent practitioner involved in the patient's care documents the provisional diagnosis in the clinical record before an operative or other high-risk procedure is performed.		RC 02.01.03		
4—For ambulatory surgical centers that elect to use The Joint Commission deemed status option: The patient's clinical record contains the results of preoperative diagnostic studies.		RC 02.01.03		
5—An operative or other high-risk procedure report is written or dictated upon completion of the operative or other high-risk procedure and before the patient is transferred to the next level of care. Note 1: The exception to this requirement occurs when an operative or other high-risk procedure progress note is written immediately after the procedure, in which case the full report can be written or dictated within a time frame defined by the organization. Note 2: If the practitioner performing the operation or high-risk procedure accompanies the patient from the operating room to the next unit or area of care, the report can be written or dictated in the new unit or area of care.		RC 02.01.03		
6—The operative or other high-risk procedure report includes the following information: • The name(s) of the licensed independent practitioner(s) who performed the procedure and his or her assistant(s) • The name of the procedure performed • A description of the procedure • Findings of the procedure • Any estimated blood loss • Any specimen(s) removed • The postoperative diagnosis		RC 02.01.03		
7—When a full operative or other high-risk procedure report cannot be entered immediately into the patient's clinical record, a note is entered immediately. This note includes the name(s) of the primary surgeon(s) and his or her assistant(s), procedure performed and a description of each procedure finding, estimated blood loss, specimens removed, and postoperative diagnosis.		RC 02.01.03		
8—The clinical record contains the following postoperative information: • The patient's vital signs and level of consciousness (See also PC.03.01.05, EP 1; PC.03.01.07, EP 1) • Any medications, including intravenous fluids and any administered blood, blood products, and blood components • Any unanticipated events or complications (including blood transfusion reactions) and the management of those events		RC 02.01.03		

Standards **Surgical and Anesthesia Services (continued)**	AAAHC Ambulatory 2009	Joint Commission 2009	Medicare/ Medicaid 2009	NCQA 2009
9—The clinical record contains documentation that the patient was discharged from the recovery phase of the operation or procedure either by the licensed independent practitioner responsible for his or her care or according to discharge criteria. (See also PC.03.01.07, EP 4)		RC 02.01.03		
10—The clinical record contains documentation of the use of approved discharge criteria that determine the patient's readiness for discharge. (See also PC.03.01.07. EP 4)		RC 02.01.03		
11—The operative documentation contains the name of the licensed independent practitioner responsible for discharge.		RC 02.01.03		
12—For ambulatory surgical centers that elect to use the Joint Commission deemed status option: The clinical record contains the discharge diagnosis.		RC 02.01.03		
Conduct a pre-procedure verification process.	10.I.S	UP 01.01.01		
(3) Pre-operative diagnostic studies (entered before surgery), if performed. (4) Findings and techniques of the operation, including a pathologist's report on all tissues removed during surgery, except those exempted by the governing body.	4.E-9 6.H, K-5 9.I 10.I.E, K, L		ASC 416.47(b)(3), (b)(4), (b)(6)	

Standards **Renal Dialysis**	AAAHC Ambulatory 2009	Joint Commission 2009	Medicare/ Medicaid 2009	NCQA 2009
Authenticated, dated reports of all examinations performed are made a part of the patient's medical record.			RD 415.2137(a)	
A radiologist authenticates all examination reports, except reports of specific procedures that may be authenticated by physicians who are not radiologists, but who have been granted privileges by the governing body or its designee to authenticate such reports.			RD 405.2137(a)	

Standards **Pathology and Laboratory**	AAAHC Ambulatory 2009	Joint Commission 2009	Medicare/ Medicaid 2009	NCQA 2009
2009 AAAHC Accreditation Handbook for Ambulatory Health Care, Chapter 12, Pathology and Medical Laboratory Services				
An accreditable organization: 1. Meets the requirements for waived tests under CLIA (part 493 of Title 42 of the Code of Federal Regulations) if it performs its own laboratory services, performs only waived tests, and has obtained a certificate of waiver, and/or 2. Has procedures for obtaining routine and emergency laboratory services from a certified laboratory in accordance with CLIA if it does not perform its own laboratory services.	12.I.A			
Pathology and medical laboratory services include performing tests in a timely manner.	12.I.C-2 12.II.C-2			
Pathology and medical laboratory services include distributing test results after completion of a test and maintaining a copy of the results.	12.I.C-3 12.II.C-3			
Pathology and medical laboratory services include performing and documenting appropriate quality control procedures, including, but not limited to, calibrating equipment periodically and validating test results.	12.I.C-4 12.II.C-4			
The organization has a policy that ensures that test results are reviewed appropriately and that documents that test results are reviewed by the ordering physician or another privileged provider.	12.I.D 12.II.D			
Established procedures are followed in obtaining, identifying, storing and transporting specimens.	12.II.G			

Standards Pathology and Laboratory (continued)	AAAHC Ambulatory 2009	Joint Commission 2009	Medicare/ Medicaid 2009	NCQA 2009
Complete descriptions are available of each test procedure performed by the laboratory, including sources of reagents, standards and calibration procedures, and information concerning the basis for the listed "normal" ranges is also available.	12.II.H			
Reports, histories and physicals, progress notes, and other patient information (such as laboratory reports, x-ray readings, operative reports, and consultations) are reviewed and incorporated into the record in a timely manner.	6.H			
The person from the organization whose name appears on the Clinical Laboratory Improvement Amendments of 1988 (CLIA '88) certificate identifies the staff responsible for performing and supervising waived testing. Note 1: Responsible staff may be employees of the organization, contracted staff, or employees of a contracted service. Note 2: Responsible staff may be identified within job descriptions or by listing job titles or individual names.		WT 02.01.01		

Standards Radiology	AAAHC Ambulatory 2009	Joint Commission 2009	Medicare/ Medicaid 2009	NCQA 2009
Reports, histories and physicals, progress notes, and other patient information (such as laboratory reports, x-ray readings, operative reports, and consultations) are reviewed and incorporated into the record in a timely manner.	6.H			
2009 AAAHC Accreditation Handbook for Ambulatory Health Care, Chapter 13, Diagnostic and Other Imaging Services				
Imaging services include interpreting images and assuring appropriate documentation in a timely manner.	13.B-2			
Imaging services include maintaining appropriate records or reports of services provided.	13.B-3			
A radiologist authenticates all examination reports, except reports of specific procedures that may be authenticated by specialist physicians or dentists who have been granted privileges by the governing body or its designee to authenticate such reports.	13.G			
Authenticated, dated reports of all examinations performed are made a part of the patient's clinical record.	13.H			
Diagnostic imaging tests are performed only upon the order of a health care professional. Such orders are accompanied by a concise statement of the reason for the examination.	13.J			
Diagnostic images are maintained in a readily accessible location for the time required by applicable laws and policies of the organization.	13.K			
A policy addresses the storage and retention of diagnostic images.	13.L			

Standards Pharmaceutical	AAAHC Ambulatory 2009	Joint Commission 2009	Medicare/ Medicaid 2009	NCQA 2009
2009 AAAHC Accreditation Handbook for Ambulatory Health Care, Chapter 11, Pharmaceutical Services				
Measures have been implemented to ensure that prescription pads are controlled and secured from unauthorized patient access, and pre-signed and/or postdated prescription pads are prohibited.	11.F			
The organization must have policies in place for safe use of injectables and single-use syringes and needles that at minimum include the CDC or comparable guidelines for safe injection practices.	11.I			
Medication orders are clear and accurate.		MM 04.01.01		

| Standards

Pharmaceutical (continued)	AAAHC Ambulatory 2009	Joint Commission 2009	Medicare/ Medicaid 2009	NCQA 2009
When a patient is referred to or transferred from one organization to another, the complete and reconciled list of medications is communicated to the next provider of service, and the communication is documented.		NPSG 08.02.01		
(a) Standard: Administration of drugs. Drugs must be prepared and administered according to established policies and acceptable standards of practice. (3) Orders given orally for drugs and biologicals must be followed by a written order, signed by the prescribing physician.	11.B-MS-3		ASC 416.48(a)(3)	

| Standards

Summary of Care	AAAHC Ambulatory 2009	Joint Commission 2009	Medicare/ Medicaid 2009	NCQA 2009
1—A summary list is initiated for the patient by his or her third visit.		RC 02.01.07		
2—The patient's summary list contains the following information: • Any significant medical diagnoses and conditions • Any significant operative and invasive procedures • Any adverse or allergic drug reactions • Any current medications, over-the-counter medications, and herbal preparations		RC 02.01.07		
3—The patient's summary list is updated whenever there is a change in diagnoses, medications, or allergies to medications, and whenever a procedure is performed.		RC 02.01.07		
4—The summary list is readily available to practitioners who need access to the information of patients who receive continuing ambulatory care services in order to provide care, treatment, or services.		RC 02.01.07		

| Standards

Dental Services	AAAHC Ambulatory 2009	Joint Commission 2009	Medicare/ Medicaid 2009	NCQA 2009
2009 AAAHC Accreditation Handbook for Ambulatory Health Care, Chapter 14, Dental Services				
An appropriate history and physical is conducted and periodically updated, which includes an assessment of the hard and soft tissues of the mouth.	14.E			
The organization develops policies and procedures related to the identification, treatment and management of pain.	14.F			
The informed consent of the patient is obtained and incorporated into the dental record prior to the procedure(s).	14.H			
Clinical records are maintained according to the requirements found in Chapter 6, Clinical Records and Health Information, of the 2009 AAAHC Accreditation Handbook for Ambulatory Health Care.	14.I			
The organization develops policies and procedures to evaluate dental laboratories to ensure that they meet the needs of the patient and adequately support the organization's clinical capabilities.	14.J			
Anesthesia provided or made available shall meet the standards contained in Chapter 9, Anesthesia Services, of the 2009 AAAHC Accreditation Handbook for Ambulatory Health Care.	14.K			
Surgical and related services provided or made available shall meet the standards contained in Chapter 10, Surgical and Related Services, of the 2009 AAAHC Accreditation Handbook for Ambulatory Health Care.	14.L			
Imaging services provided or made available shall meet the standards contained in Chapter 13, Diagnostic and Other Imaging Services, of the 2009 AAAHC Accreditation Handbook for Ambulatory Health Care.	14.M			
The organization has guidelines to address the type, frequency, and indications for diagnostic radiographs.	14.M-1			

Standards **Travel Medicine**	**AAAHC Ambulatory 2009**	**Joint Commission 2009**	**Medicare/ Medicaid 2009**	**NCQA 2009**
2009 AAAHC Accreditation Handbook for Ambulatory Health Care, Chapter 15, Other Professional and Technical Services, Subchapter II—Travel Medicine				
Travel medicine programs include clearly defined standing orders and protocols, including management of adverse reactions to immunizations.	15.II.A-2b			
Entries in a patient's clinical record include: a. Travel destination and current health status b. Immunizations given and dosage c. Medications given, quantity and date d. Preventive health education	15.II.A-4			

Standards **Behavioral Health Services**	**AAAHC Ambulatory 2009**	**Joint Commission 2009**	**Medicare/ Medicaid 2009**	**NCQA 2009**
2009 AAAHC Accreditation Handbook for Ambulatory Health Care, Chapter 17, Behavioral Services				
Behavioral health services may include referral services.	17.A-4			
An initial behavioral health history and medical history of each client is present in the clinical record.	17.F			
The clinical record is periodically updated, and may include assessment and management of: 1. Risk of harm to self or others 2. Known or potential addictive behaviors and substance abuse 3. Client self-understanding, motivation, and decision making	17.G-1 to 3			
The written and signed informed consent of the client is obtained and incorporated into the treatment plan, which may include but is not limited to procedures, therapies, medication management, and other modalities of care and treatment.	17.H			
The organization develops and adopts written policies and procedures regarding consistent client confidentiality and privacy assurances.	17.I-1			
The organization develops and adopts written policies and procedures regarding maintenance of client records according to AAAHC standards.	17.I-2			
The organization develops and adopts written policies and procedures regarding management of referrals and transfers to and from the facility.	17.I-5			

Standards **Occupational Health Services**	**AAAHC Ambulatory 2009**	**Joint Commission 2009**	**Medicare/ Medicaid 2009**	**NCQA 2009**
2009 AAAHC Accreditation Handbook for Ambulatory Health Care, Chapter 21, Occupational Health Services				
Entries in a patient's clinical record for each visit include, as appropriate, an occupational and exposure history, including essential job functions, conditions of work, and hazards of the job.	21.E-1			
Entries in a patient's clinical record for each visit include, as appropriate, the individual's current functional abilities.	21.E-2			
Entries in a patient's clinical record for each visit include, as appropriate, whether the individual is able to perform essential job functions and suggestions for accommodations or restrictions.	21.E-3			
Entries in a patient's clinical record for each visit include, as appropriate, the relationship of medical conditions or abnormal findings to workplace conditions and exposures.	21.E-4			

Standards **Occupational Health Services (continued)**	AAAHC Ambulatory 2009	Joint Commission 2009	Medicare/ Medicaid 2009	NCQA 2009
Entries in a patient's clinical record for each visit include, as appropriate, preventive counsel concerning reduction of workplace exposures and use of personal protective equipment.	21.E-5			
Entries in a patient's clinical record for each visit include, as appropriate, relevant communications concerning the patient, work activities or exposures, including those with employers, insurance carriers, union representatives, and attorneys.	21.E-6			
Organizations providing occupational health testing and ancillary service programs such as urine collection for drugs of abuse, breath alcohol content testing, blood lead determinations, audiograms, or chest x-rays ensure that these programs are administered under appropriate written protocols, which are: 1. Specific to the service provided, addressing all relevant topics such as specimen collection, handling, transportation, receipt and report of results, record management, equipment, equipment calibration and maintenance 2. Under the supervision of a licensed physician or, if allowed, another health care professional 3. Reviewed and updated periodically	21.J-1 to 3			
Organizations providing consulting services will ensure that the role and responsibilities of the consultant are clearly defined.	21.K			
Organizations providing training and educational programs will ensure that each program: 1. Has written objectives 2. Is tailored to the specific worker population and work conditions 3. Includes an evaluation process and uses the results to improve program quality	21.L-1 to 3			

Standards **Completion of Records**	AAAHC Ambulatory 2009	Joint Commission 2009	Medicare/ Medicaid 2009	NCQA 2009
1—The organization has a written policy that requires timely entry of information into the clinical record. (See also PC.01.02.03, EP 1)	6.F-3	RC 01.03.01		
2—The organization defines the time frame for completion of the clinical record.		RC 01.03.01		
3—The organization implements its policy requiring timely entry of information into the patient's clinical record. (See also PC.01.02.03, EP 2)		RC 01.03.01		

Standards **Quality Improvement Program**	AAAHC Ambulatory 2009	Joint Commission 2009	Medicare/ Medicaid 2009	NCQA 2009
2009 AAAHC Accreditation Handbook for Ambulatory Health Care, Chapter 5, Quality Management and Improvement, Subchapter II, Quality Improvement Program				
The organization develops and implements a quality improvement program that is broad in scope to address clinical, administrative and cost-of-care performance issues, as well as actual patient outcomes, i.e., results of care, including safety of patients. Characteristics of the program must include, but are not limited to:	5.II			
A written description of the program that addresses the scope of the organization's health care delivery services and how the quality improvement plan for these services is assessed	5.II.A-1			
Identification of the specific committee(s) or individuals responsible for the development, implementation, and oversight of the program.	5.II.A-2			
Participation in the program by health care professionals, one or more of whom is a physician.	5.II.A-3			
Quality improvement goals and objectives.	5.II.A-4			

Standards Quality Improvement Program (continued)	AAAHC Ambulatory 2009	Joint Commission 2009	Medicare/ Medicaid 2009	NCQA 2009
Development of processes to identify important problems or concerns that are appropriate to address for improving the quality of services provided by the organization.	5.II.A-5			
Identification of quality improvement activities such as studies, including methods for internal and external benchmarking performance, to support the goals of the program.	5.II.A-6			
Defined linkages between quality improvement activities, peer review, and the risk management program.	5.II.A-7			
Evaluation of the overall effectiveness of the program at least annually.	5.II.A-8			
Identification of processes to report findings from the quality improvement activities to the organization's governing body and throughout the organization, as appropriate.	5.II.A-9			
The organization conducts specific quality improvement activities that support the goals of the QI program. Written reports of QI activities must demonstrate that each activity includes at least the following elements:	5.II.B			
A statement of the purpose of the QI activity that includes a description of the known or suspected problem, and explains why it is significant to the organization (see Appendix D of the 2009 AAAHC Accreditation Handbook for Ambulatory Health Care for a list of potential sources of identifiable problems).	5.II.B-1			
Identification of the performance goal against which the organization will compare its current performance in the area of study.	5.II.B-2			
Description of the data that will be collected in order to determine the organization's current performance.	5.II.B-3			
Evidence of data collection.	5.II.B-4			
Data analysis that describes findings about the frequency, severity, and source(s) of the problem(s).	5.II.B-5			
A comparison of the organization's current performance in the area of study against the previously identified performance goal.	5.II.B-6			
Implementation of corrective action(s) to resolve identified problem(s).	5.II.B-7			
Re-measurement (a second round of data collection and analysis as described in AAAHC Standard 5.II.B-4-6) to objectively determine whether the corrective actions have achieved and sustained demonstrable improvement.	5.II.B-8			
If the initial corrective action(s) did not achieve and/or sustain the desired improved performance, implementation of additional corrective action(s), and continued re-measurement until the problem is resolved or is no longer relevant.	5.II.B-9			
Communication of the findings of the quality improvement activities to the governing body and throughout the organization, as appropriate, and incorporation of such findings into the organization's educational activities ("closing the QI loop").	5.II.B-10			
Results of benchmarking activities must be incorporated into other quality improvement activities of the organization.	5.II.C-2			
Pathology and medical laboratory services include performing and documenting appropriate quality control procedures, including, but not limited to, calibrating equipment periodically and validating test results.	12.I.C-4			
Health education and disease prevention programs should be included in quality management and improvement activities.	16.J			
The organization improves performance.		PI 03.01.01		
To ensure appropriate and adequate medical record documentation, the organization must take steps to assess and improve the medical recordkeeping practices of practitioners who provide primary care. The organization must conduct focused follow-up to improve medical records of primary care practitioners who perform poorly against its documentation standards. The organization can also implement general actions aimed toward improving medical records with the entire practitioner network.				QI 12B

Standards Quality Improvement Program (continued)	AAAHC Ambulatory 2009	Joint Commission 2009	Medicare/ Medicaid 2009	NCQA 2009

The organization's policies and procedures for primary care medical records reflect the following information.
 	
• All services provided directly by a practitioner who provides primary care services
• All ancillary services and diagnostic tests ordered by a practitioner
• All diagnostic and therapeutic services for which a member was referred by a practitioner, such as:
  – Home health nursing reports
  – Specialty physician reports
  – Hospital discharge reports
  – Physical therapy reports
				QI 12A

Standards Medical Record Management Policies	AAAHC Ambulatory 2009	Joint Commission 2009	Medicare/ Medicaid 2009	NCQA 2009
A designated person is in charge of clinical records. This person's responsibilities include, but are not limited to: 1. The confidentiality, security, and physical safety of records 2. The timely retrieval of individual records upon request 3. The unique identification of each patient's record 4. The supervision of the collection, processing, maintenance, storage, retrieval, and distribution of records 5. The maintenance of a predetermined, organized, and secured record format	6.E-1 to 5			
Policies concerning clinical records address the retention of active records.	6.F-1			
Policies concerning clinical records address the retirement of inactive records.	6.F-2			
Policies concerning clinical records address the timely entry of data in records.	6.F-3			
Policies concerning clinical records address the release of information contained in records.	6.F-4			
1—The organization identifies the internal and external information needed to provide safe, quality care.		IM 01.01.01		
2—The organization identifies how data and information enter, flow within, and leave the organization.	6.O	IM 01.01.01		
3—The organization uses the identified information to guide development of processes to manage information.		IM 01.01.01		
4—Staff and licensed independent practitioners, selected by the organization, participate in the assessment, selection, integration, and use of information management systems for the delivery of care, treatment, or services.	3.A-12	IM 01.01.01		
1—The organization has a written plan for managing interruptions to its information processes (paper-based, electronic, or a mix of paper-based and electronic). (See also EM 01.01.01, EP 6)		IM 01.01.03		
2—The organization's plan for managing interruptions to information processes addresses the following: Scheduled and unscheduled interruptions of electronic information systems. (See also EM.01.01.01, EP 6)		IM 01.01.03		
3—The organization's plan for managing interruptions to information processes addressing the following: Training for staff and licensed independent practitioners on alternate procedures to follow when electronic information systems are unavailable.		IM 01.01.03		
4—The organization's plan for managing interruptions to information processes addresses the following: Backup of electronic information systems. (See also EM.01.01.01, EP 6)		IM 01.01.03		

Standards **Medical Record Management Policies (continued)**	**AAAHC Ambulatory 2009**	**Joint Commission 2009**	**Medicare/ Medicaid 2009**	**NCQA 2009**
5—The organization's plan for managing interruptions to electronic information processes is tested for effectiveness according to time frames defined by the organization.		IM 01.01.03		
6—The organization implements its plan for managing interruptions to information processes to maintain access to information needed for patient care, treatment, or services.		IM 01.01.03		
1—The organization has a written policy addressing the privacy of health information. (See also RI.01.01.01, EP 7)	3.A-11	IM 02.01.01		
2—The organization implements its policy on the privacy of health information. (See also RI.01.01.01, EP 7)		IM 02.01.01		
3—The organization uses health information only for purposes as required by law and regulation or as further limited by its policy on privacy. (See also MM.01.01.01, EP 1; RI.01.01.01, EP 7)		IM 02.01.01		
4—The organization discloses health information only as authorized by the patient or as otherwise consistent with law and regulation. (See also RI.01.01.01, EP 7)	1.C	IM 02.01.01		
5—The organization monitors compliance with its policy on the privacy of health information. (See also RI.01.01.01, EP 7)	5.III.F	IM 02.01.01		
1—The organization has a written policy addressing the security of health information, including access, use, and disclosure.	3.A-11	IM 02.01.03		
2—The organization has a written policy addressing the integrity of health information against loss, damage, unauthorized alteration, unintentional change, and accidental destruction.	6.D	IM 02.01.03		
3—The organization has a written policy addressing the intentional destruction of health information.	6.F-2	IM 02.01.03		
4—The organization defines when and by whom the removal of health information is permitted. Note: Removal refers to those actions that place health information outside the organization's control.		IM 02.01.03		
5—The organization protects against unauthorized access, use, and disclosure of health information.	6.E	IM 02.01.03		
6—The organization protects health information against loss, damage, unauthorized alteration, unintentional change, and accidental destruction.	3.A-10, 11	IM 02.01.03		
7—The organization controls the intentional destruction of health information.		IM 02.01.03		
8—The organization monitors compliance with its policies on the security and integrity of health information.	5.III.F	IM 02.01.03		
1—The organization uses uniform data sets to standardize data collection throughout the organization.	3.A-12a	IM 02.02.01		
2—The organization uses standardized terminology, definitions, abbreviations, acronyms, symbols, and dose designations.	6.G	IM 02.02.01		
2—The organization's storage and retrieval systems make health information accessible when needed for patient care, treatment, or services. (See also IC.01.02.01, EP 1)	6.C	IM 02.02.03		
3—The organization disseminates data and information in useful formats within time frames that are defined by the organization and consistent with law and regulation.	3.A-7	IM 02.02.03		
1—The organization provides access to knowledge-based information resources during hours of operation.	5.I.H-1	IM 03.01.01		
1—The organization has processes to check the accuracy of health information.		IM 04.01.01		

Standards	AAAHC Ambulatory 2009	Joint Commission 2009	Medicare/ Medicaid 2009	NCQA 2009
Medical Record Management Policies (continued)				
The organization's medical record policies, procedures, and documentation standards must include the following. • Medical record content • Medical record organization • Information filed in medical records • Ease of retrieving medical records • Confidential patient information • Standards and performance goals for participating practitioners	6.D, E, G			QI 12A
The organization must distribute the medical record standards to all practitioners and appropriate staff members.				QI 12A
Security	6.E	IM 02.01.03		
Retention	6.F	RC 01.05.01		

Standards	AAAHC Ambulatory 2009	Joint Commission 2009	Medicare/ Medicaid 2009	NCQA 2009
Confidentiality of Health Records				
Patient disclosures and records are treated confidentially, and patients are given the opportunity to approve or refuse their release, except when release is required by law.	1.C			
Administrative responsibilities include maintaining the confidentiality, security and physical safety of data on patients and staff.	3.A-11			
Except when otherwise required by law, any record that contains clinical, social, financial, or other data on a patient is treated as strictly confidential and is protected from loss, tampering, alteration, destruction, and unauthorized or inadvertent disclosure.	6.D			
• Records are stored securely • Only authorized personnel have access to records • Staff receive periodic training in member information confidentiality	6.C, E 5.III.E, F			QI 12A

Standards	AAAHC Ambulatory 2009	Joint Commission 2009	Medicare/ Medicaid 2009	NCQA 2009
Health Record Documentation Standards				
Each medical record must include the following information: • History and physicals • Allergies and adverse reactions • Problem list • Medications • Documentation of clinical findings and evaluation for each visit • Preventive services/risk screening	6.E-5			QI 12A

Standards	AAAHC Ambulatory 2009	Joint Commission 2009	Medicare/ Medicaid 2009	NCQA 2009
Organized Health Record Keeping Systems/Standards for the Availability of Health Records				

Maintaining a health information system that collects, integrates, analyzes, and reports data as necessary to meet the needs of the organization.
 	
a. Characteristics of the system should include, but are not limited to:
  1. Linkage between the quality improvement program to meet performance improvement/quality indicators and quality improvement activities
  2. Ensuring accurate, timely, and complete data in a consistent manner as appropriate for the organization
  3. Maintaining collected data in a standardized format to the extent feasible and appropriate
	3.A-12			

Standards Organized Health Record Keeping Systems/Standards for the Availability of Health Records (continued)	AAAHC Ambulatory 2009	Joint Commission 2009	Medicare/ Medicaid 2009	NCQA 2009
• Medical records are organized and stored in a manner that allows easy retrieval • Medical records are stored in a secure manner that allows access by authorized personnel only	6.C			QI 12A

Standards Performance Goals to Assess the Quality of Health Record Keeping	AAAHC Ambulatory 2009	Joint Commission 2009	Medicare/ Medicaid 2009	NCQA 2009
The practitioner must meet the organization's established quantifiable performance goals for medical record keeping. NCQA does not prescribe a specific performance goal, but expects that the organization's performance goals are clearly defined in its medical record policies.				QI 12A

Standards Medical Home ("Physician" refers to the physician or the physician-directed health care team)	AAAHC Ambulatory 2009	Joint Commission 2009	Medicare/ Medicaid 2009	NCQA 2009
2009 AAAHC Accreditation Handbook for Ambulatory Health Care, Chapter 27, Medical Home				
Relationship—communication, understanding, and collaboration.	27.A			
The patient can identify his/her physician and patient care team members.	27.A-1			
The physician explains information in a manner that is easy to understand (to include AAAHC Standard 1.D).	27.A-2			
The physician listens carefully to the patient and, when appropriate, the patient's personal caregiver(s). Caregivers may include a parent, legal guardian, or person with the patients' power of attorney.	27.A-3			
The physician speaks to the patient about his/her health problems and concerns.	27.A-4			
The physician provides easy-to-understand instructions about taking care of health concerns.	27.A-5			
The physician knows important facts about the patient's health history.	27.A-6			
The physician spends sufficient time with the patient.	27.A-7			
The physician is as thorough as the patient feels is needed.	27.A-8			
The staff keeps the patient informed with regard to his/her appointment when delayed.	27.A-9			
The physician addresses specific principles to prevent illness.	27.A-10			
The physician speaks with the patient about making lifestyle changes to help prevent illness.	27.A-11			
The physician inquires as to the patient's concerns/worries/stressors.	27.A-12			
The physician inquires as to the patient's mental health status (i.e., sad/empty or depressed).	27.A-13			
The Medical Home provides services within a team framework, and that "team" provider concept has been conveyed to the patient.	27.A-14			
The family is included, as appropriate, in patient care decisions, treatment, and education.	27.A-15			
The Medical Home treats its patients with cultural sensitivity.	27.A-16			
Continuity of Care	27.B			
A significant number (more than 50%) of the Medical Home visits of any patient are with the same physician/physician team.	27.B-1			
If a consultation is ordered for the patient, it is documented in the clinical record.	27.B-2			
Referrals for services (external to the Medical Home) are documented in the clinical record.	27.B-3			

Standards **Medical Home (continued)** ("Physician" refers to the physician or the physician-directed health care team)	AAAHC Ambulatory 2009	Joint Commission 2009	Medicare/ Medicaid 2009	NCQA 2009
Consultations (medical opinions obtained from other health care professionals) are recorded in the clinical record.	27.B-4			
Referrals are disease- or procedure-specific.	27.B-5			
The results of a patient referral are recorded in the clinical record. Follow-up procedures exist, and the results of the referral are appropriately reported to the Medical Home as they are made available.	27.B-6			
Follow-up appointments are documented in the clinical record.	27.B-7			
After-hour encounters are documented in the clinical record.	27.B-8			
Missed appointments are documented in the clinical record and managed appropriately depending on the patient's care needs and diagnosis.	27.B-9			
Critical referrals, critical consultations, and critical diagnostic studies are tracked, and appropriate follow-up is made when the results are not received within a timely manner.	27.B-10			
Transition of care (e.g., pediatric to adult or adult to geriatric) is proactively planned, coordinated, and documented in the clinical record when indicated or when appropriate.	27.B-11			
Electronic data management is continually assessed as a tool for facilitating the above-mentioned standards, including consultations, referrals, and lab results.	27.B-12			
Comprehensiveness of Care	27.C			
If the Medical Home limits the population served, those limitations are disclosed to prospective patients.	27.C-1			
The Medical Home scope of service includes, but is not limited to: a. Preventive care (including surveillance and screening for special needs) b. Wellness care (healthy lifestyle issues—appropriate sleep, stress relief, etc.) c. Acute illness and injury care d. Chronic illness management e. End-of-life care	27.C-2			
Patient education and self-management resources are provided.	27.C-3			
Knowledge of community resources that support the patient's (and family's, as appropriate) needs are known by the Medical Home.	27.C-4			
The community's service limitations are known and alternate sources are coordinated by the Medical Home.	27.C-5			
Referrals are appropriate to the patient's needs. When referrals occur, the Medical Home collaborates with the specialist.	27.C-6			
The needs of the patient's personal caregiver (see definition in AAAHC Standard 27.A-3), when known, are assessed and addressed to the extent that they impact the care of the patient.	27.C-7			
Electronic data management is continually assessed as a tool for facilitating the abovementioned standards.	27.C-8			
Accessibility	27.D			
The Medical Home establishes standards in writing to support patient access, such as provider availability, information, clinical record contents, advice, routine care, and urgent care. The Medical Home's data supports that it meets those standards.	27.D-1			
Patients are routinely and continuously assessed for their perceptions about access to the Medical Home (provider availability, information, clinical record contents, advice, routine care, and urgent care).	27.D-2			
Patients are provided information about how to obtain medical care at any time, 24 hours per day, every day of the year.	27.D-3			
The Medical Home ensures on-call coverage (pre-arranged access to a clinician) when the Medical Home is not open.	27.D-4			

Standards	AAAHC Ambulatory 2009	Joint Commission 2009	Medicare/ Medicaid 2009	NCQA 2009
Medical Home (continued) ("Physician" refers to the physician or the physician-directed health care team)				
Electronic data management is continually assessed as a tool for facilitating the abovementioned standards.	27.D-5			
Quality	27.E			
Patient care is physician-directed.	27.E-1			
The Medical Home incorporates evidence-based guidelines and performance measures in delivering clinical services, including: a. Preventive care (including surveillance and screening for special needs) b. Wellness care (healthy lifestyle issues—appropriate sleep, stress relief, etc.) c. Acute illness and injury care d. Chronic illness management e. End-of-life care	27.E-2			
The Medical Home periodically assesses its use of evidence-based guidelines and performance measures to ensure that they are being used effectively and appropriately.	27.E-3			
Supervision of patient care by the Medical Home, as evidenced by: a. Medication review and update including prescription, over-the-counter, and diet supplements b. Appropriate ordering of diagnostic tests (avoidance of redundancies and unnecessary testing) c. Appropriate management of patient referrals (avoidance of unnecessary referrals)	27.E-4			
The Medical Home assesses and continuously improves the services it provides. Measurements, quality studies, data trending, and benchmarking are key tools in a quality improvement/management program.	27.E-5			
In addition to the standards presented in *2009 AAAHC Accreditation Handbook for Ambulatory Health Care,* Subchapter II, Quality Improvement Program, of Chapter 5, the Medical Home's quality improvement program should include at least one (1) study every three (3) years on each of the following topics: a. Patient/Physician Relationship b. Continuity of Care c. Comprehensiveness of Care d. Accessibility to Care e. Clinical Study	27.E-6			
Electronic data management is continually assessed as a tool for facilitating the abovementioned standards.	27.E-7			

*New Health Plan Accreditation only

Abbreviations

AAAHC Accreditation Association for Ambulatory Health Care
AMAHC Accreditation Manual for Ambulatory Health Care
ASC Ambulatory Surgery Center
HR Health Record
IM Management of Information
JC Joint Commission
MR Medical Record
NCQA National Committee for Quality Assurance
PE Assessment of Patients
PI Improving Organizational Performance

PL Pathology and Medical Laboratory Services
PT/SP Physical Therapy/Speech Pathology
QA Quality Assurance
QC Quality of Care
QI Quality Assessment and Improvement
RC Record of Care, Treatment and Services
RD Renal Dialysis
RS Radiology Services
SA Surgical and Anesthesia Services
TX Care of Patients

Appendix M

Minnesota Standard Consent Form for ROI

Instructions for Minnesota Standard Consent Form to Release Health Information

Important: Please read all instructions and information before completing and signing the form.

An incomplete form may not be accepted. Please follow the directions carefully. If you have any questions about the release of your health information or this form, please contact the organization you will list in section 3.

This standard form was developed by the Minnesota Department of Health as required by the Minnesota Health Records Act of 2007. If completed properly, this form must be accepted by the health care organization(s), specific health care facility(ies), or specific professional(s) identified in section 3.

A fee may be charged for the release of the health information.

The following are instructions for each section. Please type or print as clearly and completely as possible.

1| Include your full and complete name. If you have a suffix after your last name (Sr., Jr., III), please provide it in the "last name" blank with your last name. If you used a previous name(s), please include that information. If you know your medical record or patient identification number, please include that information. All these items are used to identify your health information and to make certain that only your information is sent.

2| If there are questions about how this form was filled out, this section gives the organization that will provide the health information permission to speak to the person listed in this section. **Completing this section is optional.**

3| In this section, state who is sending your health information. **Please be as specific as possible.** If you want to limit what is sent, you can name a specific facility, for example Main Street Clinic. Or name a specific professional, for example chiropractor John Jones. Please use the specific lines. Providing location information may help make your request more clear. Please print "All my health care providers" in this section if you want health information from all of your health care providers to be released.

4| Indicate where you would like the requested health information sent. It is best to provide a complete mailing address as not everyone will fax health information. A place has been provided to indicate a deadline for providing the health information. **Providing a date is optional.**

5| Indicate what health information you want sent. If you want to limit the health information that is sent to a particular date(s) or year(s), indicate that on the line provided.

For your protection, it is recommended that you initial instead of check the requested categories of health information. This helps prevent others from changing your form. EXAMPLE: *jh* All health information

If you select **all health information**, this will include any information about you related to mental health evaluation and treatment, concerns about drug and/or alcohol use, HIV/AIDS testing and treatment, sexually transmitted diseases and genetic information.

Important: There are certain types of health information that require special consent by law.

Chemical dependency program information comes from a program or provider that specifically assesses and treats alcohol or drug addictions and receives federal funding. This type of health information is different from notes about a conversation with your physician or therapist about alcohol or drug use. To have this type of health information sent, mark or initial on the line at the bottom of page 1.

Psychotherapy notes are kept by your psychiatrist, psychologist or other mental health professional in a separate filing system in their office and not with your other health information. **For the release of psychotherapy notes, you must complete a separate form noting only that category. You must also name the professional who will release the psychotherapy notes in section 3.**

6| Health information includes both written and oral information. If you do not want to give permission for persons in section 3 to talk with persons in section 4 about your health information, you need to indicate that in this section.

7| Please indicate the reason for releasing the health information. If you indicate marketing, please contact the organization in section 4 to determine if payment or compensation is involved. If payment or compensation to the organization is involved, indicate the amount.

8| This consent will expire one year from the date of your signature, unless you indicate an earlier date or event. Examples of an event are: "60 days after I leave the hospital," or "once the health information is sent."

9| Please sign and date this form. If you are a legally authorized representative of the patient, please sign, date and indicate your relationship to the patient. You may be asked to provide documents showing that you are the patient or the patient's legally authorized representative.

 This form was approved by the Commissioner of the Minnesota Department of Health on January 30, 2008. JAN2008

Minnesota Standard Consent Form to Release Health Information

PAGE 1 OF 2

1 Patient information

First name_____ Middle name _____ Last name _____

Patient date of birth ___ / ___ / _____ Previous name(s) _____
                         MM   DD   YYYY

Home address _____

City_____ State_____ Zip code _____

Daytime phone _____ E-mail address (optional)_____

Medical Record/patient ID number (optional)_____

2 Contact for information about how this form was filled out (optional) :

I give permission for the organization(s) listed in section 3 permission to talk to

First name_____ Last name_____ about how this form was completed,

this person can be reached at: Daytime phone _____ E-mail address (optional)_____

3 I am requesting health information be released from at least one of the following:

Organization(s) name _____

Specific health care facility or location(s) _____

Specific health care professional's name(s) _____

4 I am requesting that health information be sent to:

Organization(s) name _____

And/or person: First name _____ Last name _____

Mailing address _____

City_____ State_____ Zip code _____

Phone (optional) _____ Fax (optional) _____

Information needed by (date) ___ / ___ / _____ (optional)
                               MM   DD   YYYY

5 Information to be released

IMPORTANT: indicate only the information that you are authorizing to be released.

☐ Specific dates/years of treatment _____

☐ All health information *(see description in instructions for what is included)*

OR to only release specific portions of your health information, indicate the categories to be released:

☐ History/Physical   ☐ Mental health   ☐ HIV/AIDS testing

☐ Laboratory report   ☐ Discharge summary   ☐ Radiology report

☐ Emergency room report   ☐ Progress notes   ☐ Radiology image(s)

☐ Surgical report   ☐ Care plan   ☐ Photographs, video, digital or other images

☐ Medications   ☐ Immunizations   ☐ Billing records

☐ Other information or instructions _____

The following information requires special consent by law. Even if you indicate **all health information**, you must specifically request the following information in order for it to be released:

☐ Chemical dependency program *(see definition in instructions)*

☐ Psychotherapy notes *(this consent cannot be combined with any other; see instructions)*

This form was approved by the Commissioner of the Minnesota Department of Health on January 30, 2008.

JAN2008

Minnesota Standard Consent Form to Release Health Information

Patient's name _____

6 | **Health information includes written and oral information**

By indicating any of the categories in section 5, you are giving permission for written information to be released **and** for a person in section 3 to talk to a person in section 4 about your health information.

If you do not want to give your permission for a person in section 3 to talk to a person in section 4 about your health information, indicate that here (check mark or initials) _____

7 | **Reason(s) for releasing information**
- ☐ Patient's request
- ☐ Review patient's current care
- ☐ Treatment/continued care
- ☐ Payment
- ☐ Insurance application
- ☐ Legal
- ☐ Appeal denial of Social Security Disability income or benefits
- ☐ Marketing purposes   (payment or compensation involved?   ☐ NO   ☐ YES, amount _____)
- ☐ Other (please explain) _____

8 | I understand that by signing this form, I am requesting that the health information specified in Section 5 be sent to the third party named in section 4 above.

I may stop this consent at any time by writing to the organization(s), facility(ies) and/or professional(s) named in section 3. If the organization, facility or professional named in section 3 has already released health information based on my consent, my request to stop will not work for that health information.

I understand that when the health information specified in section 5 is sent to the third party named in section 4 above, the information could be re-disclosed by the third party that receives it and may no longer be protected by federal or state privacy laws.

I understand that if the organization named in section 4 is a health care provider they will not condition treatment, payment, enrollment or eligibility for benefits on whether I sign the consent form.

If I choose not to sign this form and the organization named in section 4 is an insurance company, my failure to sign will not impact my treatment; I may not be able to get new or different insurance; and/or I may not be able to get insurance payment for my care.

This consent will end one year from the date the form is signed unless I indicate an earlier date or event here:

Date ___ / ___ / _____ Or specific event _____
         MM   DD   YYYY

9 | **Patient's signature** _____ Date ___ / ___ / _____
                                                                              MM   DD   YYYY

Or legally authorized representative's signature_____ Date ___ / ___ / _____
                                                                                         MM   DD   YYYY

Representative's relationship to patient (parent, guardian, etc.)_____

This form was approved by the Commissioner of the Minnesota Department of Health on January 30, 2008.   JAN2008

Appendix N

Sample Policy—Disclosure of Patient PHI

ABC Medical Facility

CORPORATE POLICY

DISCLOSURE OF PATIENT PROTECTED HEALTH INFORMATION

Origination Date: September, 2003	**Policy No.: 01**
Effective Date: July, 2004; Revised: January, 2006; August, 2006; June 2007; November 2009	**Revision No.: 3**
Scope: All ABC Corporation Health Care Organizations	

Distribution:

- Administration
- Patient Care Areas
- Health Information Management Department

Purpose: To establish guidelines for the disclosure or release of patient protected health information (PHI) in compliance with federal and state regulations.

Policy Statement:

It is the policy of ABC Health Care and its affiliated entities to safeguard the privacy and security of PHI and to ensure that external disclosure of PHI is carried out through patient[1] authorization or in compliance with state and federal regulations covering treatment, payment, health care operations and/or other mandatory reporting requirements.

Federal and state regulations and statutes afford additional privacy protection for patients treated for the following conditions: 1) AODA/Substance Abuse; 2) Mental/Behavioral Health; 3) HIV. Questions with regard to disclosing patient information relating to any of these three conditions should be referred to the _____[e.g. Health Information Management (Medical Record) Department] and/or the Privacy Officer.

Patient protected health information (medical record) files, whether paper or electronic, are the property of the ABC Health Care organization and may not be removed from the organization without administrative approval.

Background:

Disclosure of patient PHI is subject to both state and federal regulations. The issue of preemption is addressed through an analysis of regulations and determining which law is more stringent. In general, a State law is "more stringent" than the HIPAA Privacy Rule if it relates to the privacy of individually identifiable health information and provides greater privacy protections for an individual's identifiable health information, or greater rights to the individual with respect to that information, than the Privacy Rule does. For the purposes of this policy, the preemption analysis has been carried out and is reflected throughout the guidance. A brief

---

[1] If a patient is unable to authorize disclosure of PHI, authorization may be completed by an individual legally authorized to act on behalf of the patient (i.e., parents, guardians, personal representatives, durable power of attorney for health care).

summary of the key regulations impacting protected health information is provided below. Consideration of these regulations was taken in the development of this policy.

Applicable State Regulations		
Federal Regulations		
42 CFR	Alcohol & Drug Abuse	Regulations impacting health care records created and maintained for alcohol and drug abuse.
45 CFR Parts 160 and 164	Standards for Privacy of Individually Identifiable Health Information (Privacy Rule)	Regulations impacting the privacy of protected health information by covered entities (providers, health plans, healthcare clearing houses).

As noted, the disclosure of PHI is subject to federal and state regulations. Due to the complexity of these regulations, as well as the different types of PHI which may be disclosed, multiple supporting policies and position statements have been developed to support this policy and disclosure practices (see "Related Policies & Position Statements").

Related Policies/Position Statements/Other Documents:
- Faxing Patient Health Information
- Clergy Access to Protected Health Information
- Accounting and Tracking Disclosures of Protected Health Information
- Facility Directory Uses and Disclosures of Protected Health Information
- Patient Right to Access, Inspect, and Copy Protected Health Information Policy
- Release of Patient Protected Health Information to the Media
- Reporting/Disclosing Patient Protected Health Information to Law Enforcement Officials
- Minors' Privacy Rights Related to Consent, Care, Treatment & Access to Protected Health Information Policy
- Research and the Use of Protected Health Information
- Authorization for the Use and Disclosure of Protected Health Information
- Charging for Copies and Summaries of Protected Health Information
- Workers' Compensation and Disclosure of Protected Health Information
- Communication of Protected Health Information with Patient Family Members, Friends, and Personal Representatives
- Adoption – Managing and Safeguarding the Privacy of Patient Protected Health Information
- Subpoenas, Court Orders, and Depositions
- Analysis of Advance Directives and Guardianship and Impact on Uses and Disclosures of Protected Health Information.
- E-Mail Communications Containing Business and Patient Protected Health Information

Attachments:
- Addendum A: Guidance – Disclosure of Patient Protected Health Information

Definitions:

<u>Designated Record Set</u>:   A "designated record set" is the group of records maintained by or for the healthcare organization that is used, in whole or in part, by or for the organization to make decisions about individuals.   The "record" within the designated record set is any item, collection, or grouping of information that contains protected health information and is maintained, collected, used or disseminated by or for the organization.

<u>Disclosure</u>:   The external release, transfer, provision of access to, or divulging in any other manner, of information outside the organization; traditionally referred to as "release."

<u>Minimum Necessary Information</u>:   That protected health information that is the minimum necessary to accomplish the intended purpose of the use, disclosure, or request. The "minimum necessary" standard applies to all protected health information whether in paper or electronic format.

<u>Protected Health Information (PHI)</u>: Individually identifiable health information that is created by or received by the organization, including demographic information that identifies an individual, or provides a reasonable basis to believe the information can be used to identify an individual, and relates to:

- Past, present or future physical or mental health or condition of an individual.
- The provision of health care to an individual.
- The past, present, or future payment for the provision of health care to an individual.

Policy:

1. ABC Health Care organizations shall disclose patient protected health information (PHI) in accordance with federal and state regulations and/or upon the authorization of the patient or the patient's legal representative (see Addendum A: Guidance – Disclosure of Patient Protected Health Information for specific information by category).

2. All disclosures of PHI shall be carried out in accordance with this policy, regardless of the location/department processing the disclosure.   Disclosure processes shall be consistently applied across all departments and business units.

3. Disclosures of PHI which may be carried out without patient authorization and in compliance with federal and state regulations include:
    A.   Treatment, payment or healthcare operations.
    B.   Public health or health oversight activities.
    C.   Use for victims of abuse, neglect, or other persons at risk.
    D.   Workers' Compensation claims processing.
    E.   Judicial and administrative proceedings.
    F.   Investigation of death by medical examiners/coroners.

4. Authorization for disclosure of PHI may be made by the (see PV-30: Authorization for the Use and Disclosure of Protected Health Information):

    A.   Patient (adult, competent).

    B.   Parent, guardian or legal custodian of a minor patient).

    C.   Legal guardian of a patient adjudged incompetent.

    D.   Personal representative, or spouse of a deceased patient. If not spouse survives a deceased patient, adult member of the deceased patient's immediately family (as defined in WI Stat 632.895(1)(d) which includes children, parents, grandparents, brothers, and sisters.

    E.   Person authorized in writing by the patient.

    F.   Health care agent as designated by the patient (e.g., durable power of attorney for healthcare).

    G.   Court-ordered temporary guardian of the patient.

5. Disclosures of PHI requested by patient authorization should be in writing and may be accomplished by completion of an authorization form or a written statement containing the key elements of an authorization. In special circumstances, disclosure of information may be requested orally (e.g., patient request by phone). If the request is made orally, verification of the requester's identity should be carried out and the disclosure documented by the person receiving and processing the request. *In some settings, such as a clinic environment, it may be appropriate to respond to a patient's request for a copy of a test result at or near the time of the encounter. The patient's request and the provision of the report should be documented in the record. As this type of request is usually made at the time of the encounter and in a face-to-face manner, documentation in the record is sufficient. A signed patient authorization may be waived at the health care provider's discretion.*

6. <u>Requirements of a Valid Authorization</u>: To be valid and in compliance with federal and state regulations, an authorization is required in writing, written in plain language, and contains the following elements:

    A. Identification of patient whose PHI is being disclosed.

    B. Identification of individual, agency, or organization to which the disclosure is to be made.

    C. Description/identification of type of information to be disclosed.

    D. Identification of provider/organization authorized to make disclosure.

    E. Purposes of the disclosure identified.

    F. Signature of the patient/ person authorized by the patient.

    G. Relationship/authority to act if authorization is signed by other than the patient.

    H. Date on which the authorization is signed.

    I. Time period identified for which authorization is effective/expiration date or event.

    J. Statement regarding right to withdraw or revoke authorization as well as information for doing so.

    K. Statement that information may be subject to redisclosure and may no longer be protected.

    L. Statement placing individual on notice of the ability or inability to condition treatment, payment or enrollment or eligibility for benefits.

    M. Statement that if the ABC Health Care organization is seeking the authorization, the patient must be given a copy of the signed authorization.

7. ABC Health Care organizations shall not honor an invalid authorization. An authorization is invalid if any of the following elements exist:

    A.   The expiration date or event has passed.

    B.   The authorization lacks any of the required elements noted above.

    C.   The authorization is not filled out properly.

    D.   The authorization contains material information that the organization knows to be false.

    E.   The authorization is known by the organization to have been revoked.

    F.   The authorization is of a type prohibited by law.

8. ABC Health Care organizations shall provide the individual a copy of the signed authorization when the ABC organization seeks the authorization.

9. Federal and state regulations require that certain disclosures of PHI be tracked in order to comply with a patient's right to request an accounting of disclosures of PHI. Guidelines have been provided to determine what requests must be tracked and accounted for (see PV-9: Accounting and Tracking Disclosures of Protected Health Information for more information).

10. ABC Health Care organizations shall provide the minimum amount of information necessary to meet the needs of the requestor. In most cases, this information may be limited to the key summary documents that are identified below. Requests for additional information should include further justification for the purpose.

    A.   Admission History & Physical.

    B.   Operative Reports.

    C.   Radiology/Diagnostic Reports.

    D.   Discharge Summaries.

E.   Other Key Organizational Documents that Reflect the Scope or Nature of the Organization (e.g., Clinic Notes, Home Health Histories, etc.).

11. **<u>Redisclosure</u>**:   ABC Health Care organizations will not redisclose protected health information obtained from other health care providers unless that information has become a permanent part of the patient's designated record set and was used in the care and treatment of the patient.

A.   Copies of information maintained in "correspondence" or "other" sections of the patient record shall not be redisclosed unless it is necessary to support the health and safety of the patient or the patient is unable to obtain the most complete and accurate copies from the originating provider.

B.   Other requests for information redisclosure shall be directed back to the originating provider.

12. ABC Health Care organizations shall provide "Certification" of copies of PHI only upon specific request.

13. ABC Health Care organizations reserve the right, as established by federal and state regulations, to assess fees for copying and/or coordinating PHI documents, files, or summaries in response to requests for disclosure of PHI (see PS-D: Charging for Copies and Summaries of Protected Health Information).

14. ABC Health Care organizational delivery methods for disclosing PHI shall include the following:

A.   Telephone.
   1.   If patient contact/verification is made, information can be disclosed by telephone.
   2.   If the patient/authorized requesting party is unable to receive the call, limited contact information may be left on the individual's answering machine.
   3.   If the purpose of the call is to leave diagnostic test results, it is recommended that the patient call the provider back; the information should not be left on an answering machine.

B.   U.S. Mail.
   1.   Information should be sealed in an envelope.
   2.   A return address should be identified on the envelope; specific department/contact information which may inadvertently identify a patient's condition (e.g., diabetic clinic) should be avoided.
   3.   The recipient's address should be verified and complete.

C.   Fax.
   1.   A completed fax coversheet should be utilized when faxing (see PV-1: Faxing Patient Health Information).
   2.   Verification of the recipient's fax number should be made.

D.   E-Mail.
   1.   E-mail communications are not generally recommended unless the organization can ensure that the privacy and the security of PHI is

safeguarded (see SE-3: E-Mail Communications Containing Business and Patient Protected Health Information).

E. Patient/Personal Representative Pick-Up.

1. Information may be made available for patient/personal representative pick up at a designated area.

2. Verification of the identity of the person picking up the information shall be made.

15. Additional guidance for determining the appropriateness of responding to requests for disclosure of patient PHI may be found with the following resources:

A. Director of Health Information Management/Medical Record Department.

B. Local Privacy Officer.

C. ABC Health Care Director of Privacy.

D. State Health Information Management Association Legal Resource Manual.

E. Organization's Legal Counsel

Responsibility for Implementation:

- Privacy Officer
- Director, Health Information Management (Medical Record) Department

Subject Matter Expert:

- Director of Privacy

Approved By:
Senior Vice President, Title   **Date:** 8/21/06

Distribution: All Departments

Key Words: Disclosure, PHI, Protected Health Information, Release

Sources: To Be Customized by State

Applicable Standards/Regulations:

- As Delineated Throughout Policy and Addendum

Disclaimer:

This information is an accurate statement of published ABC Health Care policy as of the time of printing. Permission is granted to electronically copy and to print in hard copy for internal use only. No part of this information may be reproduced, modified, or redistributed in any form or by any means, for any purposes other than those noted above. The user is advised to check for the latest version at the ABC I-Connect site before any subsequent use.

ADDENDUM A: GUIDANCE – DISCLOSURE OF PATIENT PROTECTED HEALTH INFORMATION

BREAKOUT SECTIONS:

- **FEDERAL AGENCIES**
- **MANDATORY REPORTING – STATE OF WISCONSIN**

"Requires Tracking" generally refers to a HIPAA requirement; however, in the State of Wisconsin, patient authorized disclosures require tracking as well. Limited tracking covers mandated reporting. Disclosures for purposes of treatment, payment, and healthcare operations will not be formally tracked.

DISCLOSURE TYPE	GUIDANCE	REF
Administrative Oversight ** Requires Tracking*	PHI may be accessed, used and disclosed as appropriate to facilitate administrative oversight (healthcare operations) for the organization (patient authorization not required). Examples of administrative oversight/healthcare operations include: • Accreditation, licensing and other governmental agency monitoring compliance with state and federal regulations; • Participation in medical, nursing, and ancillary healthcare professional training and education programs; • Participation in approved internal and external research projects;* • Mandatory reporting to state registries (e.g., Wisconsin Bureau of Health Information, tumor registry, birth, death, fetal demise registries/certificates, etc.);* • Compliance with internal and external quality improvement and/or peer review activities (MetaStar, National Practitioners Data Bank) • External review of medical, legal, compliance or other healthcare operations by third party business associates.	HIPAA – 45 CFR 164.501; WI Stat 146.82(2)
Admission Pre-Certification	PHI may be disclosed to the patient's insurance provider/case management agency to facilitate the pre-certification/pre-admission process, which is considered an activity related to "payment." Precautions should be taken to determine the appropriateness of mental health disclosures without specific patient authorization (e.g., nature of treatment).	HIPAA – 45 CFR 164.501

DISCLOSURE TYPE	GUIDANCE	REF
Adoption Records *Requires Tracking*	Sections 48.432 and 48.433, Wis. Stats., authorize adopted persons and individuals to request a search for their birth parents through the Adoption Records Search Program. Wisconsin law does not allow information about adoptions, birth parents, or individuals to be disclosed without making a request through the Adoption Records Search Program. Provider health records are not to be externally disclosed. All adoption search inquiries shall be referred to the Adoption Records Search Program (see PS-Q: Adoption – Managing and Safeguarding the Privacy of Patient Protected Health Information).	WI Stat 48.432, 48.433
Advance Directive Documents	Advance directive documents (living will, power of attorney) may be shared with other healthcare providers for purposes of treatment or placement without patient authorization. Requests for copies of these documents from those other than providers should be referred to the patient/patient representative.	WHIMA Legal Manual
Alcohol and Substance Abuse *May Require Tracking*	A written patient authorization is required prior to disclosure of PHI from mental health records, including treatment and rehabilitation services for all mental disorders, developmental disabilities, alcoholism and other drug abuse (AODA). Provisions are set forth by Wisconsin's State Alcohol, Drug Abuse, Developmental Disabilities and Mental Health Act (Chapter 51). Exception: Disclosure of PHI in a medical emergency to a licensed physician who has determined that the life or health of the individual is in danger and that treatment	WI Stat 51.30; WI HFS 92; 42 CFR Part 2
Ambulance Services	PHI may be disclosed to ambulance service providers involved in transporting the patient; PHI may be requested and disclosed for purposes of treatment, payment, and (with the approval of the Privacy Officer), limited healthcare operations.	HIPAA – 45 CFR 164.506; WI Stat 146.82(2)
Attorneys/Law Firms *Requires Tracking*	PHI may be disclosed to attorneys or legal counsel upon authorization by the patient/legal representative (see PS-Y: Subpoenas, Court Orders, and Depositions). Exception: Disclosure of PHI to the organization's own legal counsel for purposes of healthcare operations (e.g., medical malpractice claim review, etc.).	WI Stat – 146.82
Birth Registry/ Certificates *Requires Limited Tracking*	Required reporting under Wisconsin Statutes; patient authorization is not required. Includes births and stillbirths.	WI Stat – 69.14-15
Bureau of Health Information *Requires Limited Tracking*	Required reporting under Wisconsin Statutes; patient authorization is not required.	WI Stat – Chapter 153

DISCLOSURE TYPE	GUIDANCE	REF
Clergy	PHI may be disclosed to members of the clergy. The organization may disclose a patient's name, general condition, location within the facility, and religious affiliation to members of the clergy as long as the patient has not opted out/or informed staff otherwise. PHI may be provided only for those patients belonging to the clergy member's religious affiliation (see PV-8: Clergy Access to Protected Health Information).	HIPAA – 45 CFR 164.510(a)
Coroner *Requires Tracking*	See "Medical Examiner."	WI Stat 146.82(2)(a)18; 69.18(2); 979.01; 979.10
Correctional Institutions	PHI may be disclosed to a prisoner's healthcare provider, medical staff of a prison or jail in which a prisoner is confined, receiving institution intake staff at a prison or jail to which a prisoner is being transferred, or a person designated by a jailer to maintain prisoner health records; patient authorization is not required.	WI Stat 146.82(2)(a)21
Court Orders *Requires Tracking*	PHI may be disclosed by court order; patient authorization is not required (see PS-Y: Subpoenas, Court Orders, and Depositions).	WI Stat 146.82(a)4
Death Registry/ Certificates *Requires Limited Tracking*	Required reporting of PHI under Wisconsin Statutes; patient/legal representative authorization is not required.	WI Stat 69.18
Department of Health & Family Services *Requires Tracking*	PHI may be disclosed for purposes of investigation of threatened or suspected child abuse or neglect or suspected unborn child abuse or for purposes of prosecution of alleged child abuse or neglect. See other categories for types of information to be reported to Department of Health & Family Services (e.g., elder abuse).	WI Stat 146.82(2)(a)11

Appendix N

DISCLOSURE TYPE	GUIDANCE	REF
Department of Transportation – Unsafe Drivers *Requires Tracking*	PHI may be reported by a healthcare provider/optometrist (patient authorization not required) to the Department of Transportation if it is deemed that the patient's condition affects the patient's ability to operate a motor vehicle. **Who:** Professional providing care to the patient. **When:** As soon as reasonably possible (no statutory time period). **Where:** Department of Transportation. **What:** Patient's name and other information relevant to the patient's condition. The DOT has a "Driver Condition or Behavior Report" which can be completed by the provider (second page); the form is located at: http://www.dot.state.wi.us/drivers/forms/mv3141.pdf The provider may also submit a statement on the organization's letterhead with the name, DOB, and a brief description of the condition. The letter should be forwarded to the Wisconsin Department of Transportation; Medical Review; P.O Box 7918; Madison, WI 53707-7918. A copy of the form or other notification shall be maintained in the "Correspondence Section of the health record" – (not part of the DRS/LHR).	WI Stat 146.82(3)(a-b), 448.03(5)(b)1
Disaster Relief Agencies/ Organizations *Requires Tracking*	PHI may be disclosed to federal, state, or local government agencies engaged in disaster relief activities, as well as private disaster relief/assistance organizations, such as the Red Cross, as authorized by law or by charters, to assist in disaster relief efforts. Seek approval by Privacy Officer/administrative prior to disclosure of PHI. During national disasters, federal guidance will be issued (e.g., Hurricane Katrina).	HIPAA – 45 CFR 164.510(b)(4)
Emergency Medical Technicians	PHI may be disclosed to Emergency Medical Technicians (EMTs) providing care to a patient. PHI may be requested and disclosed for purposes of treatment, payment, and (with the approval of the Privacy Officer), limited healthcare operations.	HIPAA – 45 CFR 164.506; WI Stat 146.82(2)
Employers *Requires Tracking*	PHI may not be disclosed to an employer without patient authorization. Exception: Worker's Compensation claim in progress (See Workers Compensation).	WI Stat 146.82

DISCLOSURE TYPE	GUIDANCE	REF
Facility Directory Information	Unless the patient has objected or restricted disclosure of information provided in the facility directory, the following formation may be disclosed to those people who request information by patient name: the patient's location in the facility and/or the patient's general condition. Appropriate one-word descriptions for general condition include: Undetermined, Good, Fair, Serious, and Critical. See PV-11: Facility Directory Uses and Disclosures of Protected Health Information.	HIPAA – 45 CFR 164.510(a)
Family Members and Friends *Written Disclosures Require Tracking*	<u>Oral Communications/Requests for PHI</u>: PHI may be disclosed to a patient's family members and/or friends if it is determined that they are involved in the care of the patient, and the patient has expressed approval of sharing the health information. If it cannot be established that the family member or friend has approved access, then a written authorization from the patient is required (exceptions apply for patients treated for AODA conditions under WI Statute 51.30(4)(b)20.). <u>Copies of PHI</u>: A written patient authorization must be provided prior to disclosure of PHI documents/records. See PS-J: Communication of Protected Health Information with Patient Family Members, Friends, and Personal Representatives and PS-X: Analysis of Advance Directives and Guardianship and Impact on Uses and Disclosures of Protected Health Information.	HIPAA – 45 CFR 164.510 WI Stat 146.82 & 146.83
Faxing *May Require Tracking*	Faxing of PHI should be limited to urgent patient care and treatment purposes whenever possible. A written authorization must be obtained for any disclosure of PHI made via fax or software when not otherwise covered by treatment, payment, or healthcare operations purposes (see PV-1: Faxing Patient Health Information).	AHIMA Guidance; WI Stat 146.82
FEDERAL AGENCIES		
Armed Forces *Requires Tracking*	<u>Non-Military Personnel</u>: PHI may not be disclosed to the Armed Forces without a written authorization from the patient or a court order. <u>Active Military Personnel</u>: PHI may be provided to the individual's commanding/military officer in response to a written request. The provider may want to consider having the patient sign an authorization as well to document an "informed" process. <u>Exception</u>: Access to PHI related to mental health, AODA, and/or HIV encounters must be authorized in writing by the patient. *As clarified by Susan Manning, JD, June, 2004.*	WI Stat 146.82(2)(5)

Appendix N

DISCLOSURE TYPE	GUIDANCE	REF
Centers for Disease Control (CDC) *Requires Tracking*	PHI may be disclosed (without patient authorization) to the Centers for Disease Control when reporting mandatory communicable disease cases (rare). Reporting is generally coordinated with the Local Health Officer/Department and/or State Epidemiologist.	WI Stat 146.82
Central Intelligence Agency (CIA) *Requires Tracking*	PHI may not be disclosed to the Central Intelligence Agency without a written patient authorization or a court order.	WI Stat 146.82
Food & Drug Administration (FDA) *Requires Tracking*	Providers are required to report PHI in cases of: 1) serious illness, 2) serious injury; 3) or death of a patient or an employee that was caused by a medical device, instrument, or appliance. The reports are sent either to the FDA, or the manufacturer, or both. The determination of who to send it to is based on whether or not the event was caused by a manufacturing or design defect. Report forms are available on-line at the FDA website: (http://www.fda.gov/cdrh/mdr/mdr-general.html).	Safe Medical Devices Act of 1990
Federal Bureau of Investigation (FBI) *Requires Tracking*	PHI may not be disclosed to the Federal Bureau of Investigation without a written patient authorization or a court order.	WI Stat 146.82
Internal Revenue Service (IRS) *Requires Tracking*	PHI may not be disclosed to the Internal Revenue Service without a written patient authorization or a court order.	WI Stat 146.82
Occupational Health Safety Agency (OSHA) *Requires Tracking*	PHI may be disclosed to the Occupational Health Safety Agency for purposes of investigation (patient authorization not required).	OSHA - CFR 29
Office of Inspector General (OIG) *Requires Tracking*	PHI may be disclosed to the Office of the Inspector General (patient authorization not required) as part of an investigation process.	WI Stat 146.82
END OF FEDERAL AGENCY REPORTING SECTION		
Funeral Directors *Requires Tracking*	Limit PHI related to a deceased individual's HIV Test status may be disclosed to a funeral director for preparation of the body for burial/other disposition (authorization is not required).	WI Stat 252.15(5)(a)(7)

DISCLOSURE TYPE	GUIDANCE	REF
Guardians – Legal *Written Disclosures Require Tracking*	PHI may be disclosed to those individuals who have been made court-appointed legal guardians (patient authorization not required).	WI Stat 146.82 2)(a9.c
Healthcare Providers	PHI may be disclosed to healthcare providers involved in the care of the patient. PHI may be requested and disclosed for purposes of treatment, payment, and (with the approval of the Privacy Officer), limited healthcare operations. Health care providers may include: licensed nurse, chiropractor, dentist, physician, podiatrist, physical therapist, certified occupational therapist, occupational therapy assistant, physician assistant, respiratory care practitioner, dietician, licensed optometrist, certified acupuncturist, licensed psychologist, certified social worker, marriage and family therapist, professional counselor, licensed speech language pathologist, audiologist, partnership or corporation of any providers listed above, operational cooperative sickness plan, licensed hospice, inpatient health care facility, community-based residential facility, rural medical center.	HIPAA – 45 CFR 164.506; WI Stat 146.81(1) – 1/10/07
Health Maintenance Organizations (HMO's)	PHI may be disclosed to the patient's HMO without authorization if it can be determined that the HMO is responsible for coverage of the patient's care. Verification of HMO involvement may be confirmed by accessing the patient registration/admission information.	HIPAA – 45 CFR 164.506; WI Stat 146.82
HEDIS – Health Plan Employer Data Information Set	PHI may be disclosed to a health plan for the quality related health care operations of the health plan, if the health has or has had a relationship with the individual who is the subject of the information and the PHI requested pertains to the relationship (patient authorization not required).	HIPA – 45 CFR 164.506 C(4)
HIV/AIDS Testing, Care, & Treatment *Requires Tracking*	HIV tests results may be provided to the subject of the individual tests, or when applicable, the designated health care agent. With few exceptions, a patient authorization is required for disclosure of HIV/AIDS testing, care and treatment. For a complete listing of these exceptions (individuals/agencies), see WI Statute 252.15.	WI Stat 252.15
Hospitals	See Health Care Provider category.	HIPAA – 45 CFR 164.506; WI Stat 146.82

DISCLOSURE TYPE	GUIDANCE	REF
Insurance Companies *Requires Tracking If Not Related to Payment for Care*	PHI may be disclosed to the patient's insurer without authorization if it can be determined that the insurer is responsible for coverage of the patient's care. Verification of an insurer's involvement may be confirmed by accessing the patient registration/admission information. Precautions should be taken to determine the appropriateness of mental health disclosures without specific patient authorization (e.g., nature of treatment). Information requested from an insurer (e.g., life insurance) unrelated to coverage of a patient care encounter should not be processed without patient authorization.	HIPAA – 164.506/ WI Stat 146.82(2)
Law Enforcement Officials *Requires Tracking & Patient Authorization In Certain Circumstances*	See PV-18: Reporting/Disclosing Patient Protected Health Information to Law Enforcement Officials for complete information on disclosures to law enforcement officials involving: ▪ Accident ▪ Animal Bite ▪ Bioterrorism Threat ▪ Boating Accident ▪ Child Abuse ▪ Crime Committed on the Premise ▪ Crime Perpetrator ▪ Crime Victim ▪ Dangerous Patient ▪ Dangerous Visitor ▪ Deaths ▪ Disaster/Public Health Emergency ▪ Domestic Abuse ▪ Drug Seeking Activity ▪ Elder Abuse ▪ Emergency Situation ▪ Gunshot Wound ▪ HIV Condition/Status of Individual ▪ Hunting Accident ▪ Identity Theft ▪ Jails, Prisons, Correction Facilities ▪ Legal Blood Draw ▪ Missing Person ▪ National Security & Intelligence Activities ▪ Prisoner ▪ Sexual Assault (Rape) ▪ Suspicious Wound or Injury (Including Burns) ▪ Volunteer-Crime Victim Crisis Support Team Members	Multiple

DISCLOSURE TYPE	GUIDANCE	REF
Legal Blood Draws *Requires Tracking*	PHI may be disclosed PHI to law enforcement officials accompanying a patient for a legal blood draw. Any person operating a motor vehicle has given "implied consent" to have blood, breath, or urine tested for the presence of certain prohibited substances. Testing shall be done at the request of a law officer and shall be done by the officer or by a designated facility. A healthcare provider drawing the blood at the behest of the law enforcement official is not acting in a patient-physician or patient-nurse relationship. The provider/facility doing the test for this purpose shall report/disclose the results of the test to the officer who requested the test be performed. This does not apply to blood draws for clinical purposes. Clinical blood draw patient PHI may be reported and disclosed to law enforcement officials in response to a patient authorization or other legal process (e.g., court order.	WI Stat 343.305
Legal Counsel (Organization's) *Requires Tracking*	PHI may be disclosed to the organization's legal counsel (without patient authorization) to facilitate the organization's healthcare operations.	HIPAA – 164.510(a)
Long Term Care Ombudsman *Requires Tracking*	PHI may be disclosed to a designated representative of the long-term care ombudsman for the purpose of protecting and advocating the rights of an individual 60 years of age or older who resides in a long-term care facility.	WI Stat 146.82(2)(a)1 6, 16.009(4)

MANDATORY REPORTING – STATE OF WISCONSIN
(Patient Authorization Not Required)

Abuse, Child *Requires Tracking*	Providers are required to report and disclose patient PHI to law enforcement officials when there is reasonable cause to suspect a child (or unborn child) has been abused or neglected or reason to believe the child has been threatened with child abuse or neglect and that the abuse or neglect will occur, including any sexual intercourse or inappropriate sexual contact with a minor child. **Who:** Provider Who Has Seen the Child in Course of Duties **When:** Immediately **Where:** Responsible County Department or Police/Sheriff Dept.	WI Stat 48.981(2)(a), 48.981(2m)(d), 146.82 (2)(a)(11)
Abuse, Elder *Requires Tracking*	Providers shall report and disclose patient PHI to the county agency or other investigating agency when there is reasonable cause to suspect elder abuse, material abuse, or neglect. An "elder person" means a person who is age 60 or older or who is subject to the infirmities of aging. **Who:** Professional providing care to the patient. **When:** As soon as reasonably possible (no statutory time period). **Where:** Responsible County Agency or State Official	WI Stat 46.90(1)(s), 46.90(1)(c), 46.90(4), 146.82(2)(a)(7)

DISCLOSURE TYPE	GUIDANCE	REF
Birth & Development Outcome Report *Requires Tracking*	Providers are required to report PHI of patients with adverse neonatal outcomes occurring either at birth or in the first month following birth; includes reporting of birth weight of less than 2500 grams, a chronic condition including central nervous system hemorrhages, infection of the central nervous system which may require long term care, Apgar scores of 3 or less at five minutes following birth, or other birth defects such as structural deformities, developmental malformations, genetic, inherited, biochemical dieses or developmental disabilities. In addition, severe disabilities such sensory impairment, severe physical handicaps or developmental delays resulting from injury, infection or disease, which are chronic in nature and require long term care, must also be reported. **Who:** Responsible Healthcare Provider **When:** Within 90 days of diagnosis **Where:** Wisconsin Department of Health & Family Services	WI Stat 253.12; HFS 116
Cancer Reporting/ Registry *Requires Limited Tracking*	Hospitals, physicians and laboratories are required to report information concerning any person diagnosed as having cancer or a precancerous condition. **Who:** Healthcare Providers as Denoted Above **When:** Within 6 Months of Diagnosis/Presentation at Facility **Where:** State of Wisconsin Cancer Reporting System	WI Stat 255.04
Communicable Diseases *Requires Tracking*	Providers are required to report PHI of a person infected with a communicable disease. Wisconsin Administrative Code HFS 145 has delineated by Category (I-III) the types of diseases to be reported and the time frame in which they should be reported. The information is available in Appendix A of HFS 145. **Who:** Responsible Healthcare Provider **When:** See Information in Appendix A **Where:** Local Health Officer/Department and/or State Epidemiologist	WI Stat 252.11; HFS 145
Death of a Person With Communicable Disease *Requires Tracking*	Providers are required to report PHI of a patient who has had a communicable disease and has died. Wisconsin Administrative Code HFS 145 has delineated by Category (I-III) the types of diseases to be reported and the timeframe in which they should be reported. The information is available in Appendix A of HFS 145. **Who:** Responsible Healthcare Provider **When:** Reports Shall be Made Within 24 hours **Where:** Local Health Officer/Department and/or State Epidemiologist	WI Stat 252.05

Corporate Policy – Disclosure/Release of PHI
Page 17

DISCLOSURE TYPE	GUIDANCE	REF
Deaths, Reportable *Requires Tracking*	Providers are required to report PHI on all patient deaths in which there are unexplained, unusual or suspicious circumstances, all homicides, all suicides, all deaths following an abortion, all deaths due to poisoning, whether homicidal, suicidal, or accidental, all deaths following accidents, whether the injury is or is not the primary cause of death, when there was no physician, or accredited practitioner or bona fide religious denomination relying upon prayer or spiritual means for healing in attendance within 30 days preceding death, when a physician refuses to sign the death certificate, and when, after reasonable efforts, a physician cannot be obtained to sign the medical certification (see also section on "Medical Examiner"). **Who:** Responsible Health Care Provider **When:** Immediately **Where:** Local Law Enforcement Agency/Medical Examiner	WI Stat 979.01
Lead Poisoning/ Exposure *Requires Tracking*	Providers are required to report PHI of patients with diagnoses of lead poisoning or exposure, or any nurse, hospital administrator, director of a clinical laboratory or local health officer who has verified information of the existence of any person found or suspected to have lead poisoning or lead exposure, shall report to the Department of Public Health within 48 hours after verifying the information. **Who:** Responsible Health Care Provider **When:** Within 48 Hours After Verifying Information **Where:** Department of Public Health	WI Stat 254.13(1)
Report of Death, if by Physical Restraint, Psychotropic Drug, or Suspected Suicide *Requires Tracking*	Providers are required to report PHI of a patient death if there is reasonable cause to believe that the death was related to: - The use of physical restraints - A psychotropic medication - There is reasonable cause to believe that the death was a suicide. **Who:** Responsible Health Care Provider **When:** Immediately **Where:** Department of Health & Social Services	WI Stat 51.64

DISCLOSURE TYPE	GUIDANCE	REF
Report of Gunshot Wound or Suspicious Wounds (Including Burns) *Requires Tracking*	Providers are required to report PHI of a patient suffering from: ▪ A gunshot wound ▪ Any wound other than a gunshot would if the person has reasonable cause to believe that the wound occurred as a result of a crime ▪ Second or third degree burns to at least 5% of the patient's body ▪ A patient suffering from inhalation of superheated air ▪ Swelling of the patient's larynx ▪ A burn to the patient's respiratory tract, if the person has reasonable cause to believe that the burn occurred as a result of a crime. Reporting is not required if the patient is accompanied by a law enforcement officer at the time treatment is rendered. Gunshot/suspicious wound patient PHI may also be reported and disclosed to law enforcement officials in response to: ▪ Patient authorization; or ▪ Legal process (court order). See "Deaths" for further guidance on reporting and disclosing patient PHI when death has occurred resulting from gunshot wounds. **Who:** Responsible Health Care Provider **When:** Immediately **Where:** Local Law Enforcement Agency	WI Stat 146.995(2)
Report of HIV/ AIDS Positive Test Results *Requires Tracking*	Providers are required to report PHI if a positive, validated test result has been obtained on a patient. **Who:** Responsible Health Care Provider **When:** Immediately **Where:** Local Health Officer/Department/State Epidemiologist	WI Stat 252.15(7)(b)
Report of Sexual Exploitation by Therapist *Requires Tracking*	A therapist who has reasonable cause to suspect a patient is a victim of sexual contact with another state licensed therapist must ask the patient if he/she wants the therapist to make a report. If the patient wants the report made, they must provide a written consent to the reporter specifying whether or not they wish to be identified in the report. **Who:** Health Care Provider/Therapist **When:** Within 30 Days of the Patient's Consent to the Report **Where:** Department of Health & Social Services (Legal Counsel Should be Consulted Prior to Reporting)	WI Stat 940.22(3)

DISCLOSURE TYPE	GUIDANCE	REF
Sudden Infant Death Syndrome *Requires Tracking*	Providers are required to report PHI of a child under the age of two (2) years who has died suddenly and unexpectedly under circumstances indicating that the death may have been caused by sudden infant death syndrome. **Who:** Healthcare Provider **When:** Immediately **Where:** Medical Examiner	WI Stat 979.03
	***END OF "WISCONSIN MANDATORY REPORTING" SECTION***	
Media *Requires Tracking for PHI Shared by Authorization*	PHI may be disclosed to members of the media as follows: - In response to a request for patient-specific information as available through the facility directory (unavailable if the patient has chosen to "opt" out of the directory); see PV-11: Facility Directory Uses and Disclosures of Protected Health Information. - In response to a patient authorization for disclosure of PHI. See PV-15: Release of Patient Protected Health Information to the Media for additional guidance.	HIPAA – 45 CFR 164.510(a); WI Stat 146.82
Medical Device Reporting *Requires Tracking*	Providers are required to report PHI in cases of: 1) serious illness, 2) serious injury; 3) or death of a patient or an employee that was caused by a medical device, instrument, or appliance. The reports are sent either to the FDA, or the manufacturer, or both. The determination of who to send it to is based on whether or not the event was caused by a manufacturing or design defect. Report forms are available on-line at the FDA website: (http://www.fda.gov/cdrh/mdr/mdr-general.html).	Safe Medical Devices Act of 1990
Medical Examiner *Requires Tracking*	Providers are **required** to report to law enforcement officials and/or the medical examiner, the death of any individual who has died under any of the following circumstances: all deaths in which there are unexplained, unusual, or suspicious circumstances, homicides, suicides, deaths following an abortion, deaths due to poisoning, whether homicidal, suicidal, or accidental, deaths following accidents, whether the injury is or is not the primary cause of death, etc. (additional reporting requirements may be established through the county government process). Providers are required to disclose patient PHI to medical examiners responsible for completing a medical certificate or investigating the death.	WI Stat 146.82(2)(a)18); 69.18(2); 979.01; 979.10

DISCLOSURE TYPE	GUIDANCE	REF
Mental Health Information *May Require Tracking*	A written patient authorization is required prior to disclosure of PHI from mental health records, including treatment and rehabilitation services for all mental disorders, developmental disabilities, alcoholism and other drug abuse (AODA). Provisions are set forth by Wisconsin's State Alcohol, Drug Abuse, Developmental Disabilities and Mental Health Act (Chapter 51). Exception: Disclosure of PHI in a medical emergency to a licensed physician who has determined that the life or health of the individual is in danger and that treatment without the information could be injurious to the patient's health.	WI Statute – 51.30; HFS 92
Medical Staff Activities – Credentialing, Peer Review, Licensing, Etc.	PHI may be used and disclosed for activities related to reviewing the competence or qualifications of health care providers, evaluating performance, training and education, accreditation, certification, licensing and other related medical staff credentialing peer review, and performance improvement activities. These activities are defined as "health care operations" and do not require patient authorization prior to use and disclosure.	HIPAA – 45 CFR 164.501; WI Stat 146.82(2)(a)(1)
Minors *May Require Tracking & Special Authorization Requirements*	Due to the complexity of issues related to minors and ability to consent, care and treatment, and access to PHI, a separate policy has been developed. See PV-22: Minors' Privacy Rights Related to Consent, Care, Treatment & Access to Protected Health Information.	WI Stat 146.81(5), 51.30, 252.15,; HFS 144.03(10)
Nursing Homes	PHI may be disclosed to nursing homes to facilitate discharge placement and subsequent patient transfer and care. See also section on "Healthcare Providers."	HIPAA – 45 CFR 164.506; WI Stat 146.82(2)
Organ Procurement *Requires Tracking*	PHI may be disclosed to an organ procurement organization (authorization not required).	WI Stat – 146.82(2)(a)19; 157.06(5)(b)(1)

DISCLOSURE TYPE	GUIDANCE	REF
Patient *Requires Tracking*	The patient has the right to access, inspect and receive copies of his or her PHI maintained in the designated record. The patient shall provide a written authorization (as identified in Wisconsin law). The organization may charge a reasonable fee for copes of patient records. In some settings, such as a clinic environment, it may be appropriate to respond to a patient's request for a copy of a test result at or near the time of the encounter. The patient's request and the provision of the report should be documented in the record. As this type of request is usually made at the time of the encounter and in a face-to-face manner, documentation in the record is sufficient. A signed patient authorization may be waived at the healthcare provider's discretion.	HIPAA – 45 CFR 164.510 WI Stat 146.82 & 146.83
Personal Representative (Non-Legal Status) *Requires Tracking & Patient Authorization*	Oral Communications/Requests for PHI: PHI may be disclosed to a patient's family members and/or friends if it is determined that they are involved in the care of the patient, and the patient has expressed approval of sharing the health information. If it cannot be established that the family member or friend has approved access, then a written authorization from the patient is required (exceptions apply for patients treated for AODA conditions under WI Statute 51.30(4)(b)20). Copies of PHI: A written patient authorization must be provided prior to disclosure of PHI documents/records. See PS-J: Communication of Protected Health Information with Patient Family Members, Friends, and Personal Representatives and PS-X: Analysis of Advance Directives and Guardianship and Impact on Uses and Disclosures of Protected Health Information.	HIPAA – 45 CFR 164.510 WI Stat 146.82 & 146.83
Pharmacist/ Pharmacy	PHI may be disclosed to a pharmacist or pharmacy involved in the care of the patient. See also section on "Healthcare Providers."	HIPAA – 45 CFR 164.506; WI Stat 146.82(2)
Physicians/ Providers	PHI may be disclosed to physicians/providers involved in the care of the patient. See also section on "Healthcare Providers."	HIPAA – 45 CFR 164.506; WI Stat 146.82(2)

DISCLOSURE TYPE	GUIDANCE	REF
Power of Attorney for Health Care (Patient's) *Requires Tracking*	The patient's Power of Attorney for Health Care may request, review and/or receive copies of a PHI (without patient's authorization) upon activation of the POA-HC. Upon activation, this individual may also authorize other disclosures of the patient's PHI. Of note, this right is not extended to the patient's Power of Attorney (financial/general). See PS-X: Analysis of Advance Directives and Guardianship and Impact on Uses and Disclosures of Protected Health Information.	WI Stat 155
Protection & Advocacy Agency *Requires Tracking*	PHI may be disclosed to the Protection & Advocacy Agency or other contracted non-profit corporation for the protection and advocacy of persons with developmental disabilities or mental illness.	WI Stat 146.82(2)(a)(9) (b)
Public Health Department Reporting *Requires Tracking*	Providers are required to report PHI of a person infected with a communicable disease. Wisconsin Administrative Code HFS 145 has delineated by Category (I-III) the types of diseases to be reported and the timeframe in which they should be reported. The information is available in Appendix A of HFS 145 (see also "Communicable Diseases).	WI Stat 252.11; HFS 145
Research *May Require Tracking & Authorization*	The use of PHI for purposes of research should approved by either the organization's Institutional Research Board (IRB) or Privacy Board prior to usage. There are four ways to perform HIPAA-compliant research with PHI. They are: 1. Obtain patient authorization. 2. Obtain a waiver of authorization from the IRB or PB. 3. Use de-identified information. 4. Use a limited data set. See PV-28: Research and the Use of Protected Health Information for more detailed information.	HIPAA – 45 CFR 164.512(i); WI Stat 146.82(a)(6)
Risk Management Insurance/ Malpractice Carriers	PHI may be disclosed to the organization's risk management and insurance/malpractice carriers (without patient authorization) to facilitate the organization's healthcare operations.	HIPAA – 45 CFR 164.510(a)
Schools *Requires Tracking; May Require Authorization*	PHI may be disclosed (without patient authorization) when reporting to school district employees/agents information maintained/required in student records under state and federal regulations (i.e. immunization, vaccination status). All other disclosures of PHI to school district employees/agents require patient authorization.	WI Stat – 146.82 (2)(a)12

DISCLOSURE TYPE	GUIDANCE	REF
Subpoena/ Subpoena Duces Tecum *Requires Tracking*	Subpoenas may be issued by courts, attorneys, administrative agencies or others. Whether a subpoena is valid will depend on what authority and for what purpose the subpoena is issued. Unless there is an exception as noted below, the subpoena should include a patient authorization. PHI may be subpoenaed (subpoena duces tecum) without patient authorization only by: ▪ Court order ▪ A governmental agency performing legally authorized functions (i.e., Worker's Compensation); or ▪ Protection and advocacy agencies (i.e., investigating child abuse) If a question exists as to the validity of the subpoena, the clerk of courts or legal counsel should be contacted. Legal counsel may be engaged to attempt to "quash" (invalidate) a subpoena by motion to the court with jurisdiction over the legal matter (see PS-Y: Subpoenas, Court Orders, and Depositions).	WI Stat 146.82
Utilization Review Agency	PHI may be disclosed to the patient's insurance provider's utilization review/case management agency to facilitate pre-certification and continued stay process, which is considered an activity related to "payment." Precautions should be taken to determine the appropriateness of mental health disclosures without specific patient authorization (e.g., nature of treatment).	HIPAA – 45 CFR 164.501
Workers' Compensation *Requires Tracking*	PHI may be disclosed to a Workers' Compensation carrier if an employee has filed a claim for Workers' Compensation due to an on-the-job injury. Employees filing a Workers' Compensation claim waive all provider-patient privilege of information or results regarding any condition or complaint reasonably related to the condition that they are claiming compensation for. This includes information normally covered by WI Statutes 51.30, 146.82 and any other applicable law, but only if the information is related to the condition that the employee is seeking compensation for. Requests for information shall be made in writing (see PS-F: Workers' Compensation and Disclosure of Protected Health Information).	WI Stat 102.13 & 102.33

Appendix O

Practice Brief—Retention of Health Information (Updated)

Health information management professionals traditionally perform data and information warehousing functions (for example, purging) utilizing all media including paper, images, optical disk, computer disk, microfilm, and CD-ROM. These warehouses or resources from which to retrieve, store, and maintain data and information include, but are not limited to, application-specific databases, diagnostic biomedical devices, master patient indexes, and patient medical records and health information.

One data integrity characteristic of warehousing is relevancy of data or information. To ensure the availability of relevant data and information, appropriate retention schedules must be established. To support this requirement, the following information has been compiled. It includes AHIMA's retention recommendations (see Table 1), accreditation agency retention standards (see Table 2), federal health record retention requirements (see Table 3), and state laws or regulations pertaining to retention of health information (see Table 4).

Table 1. AHIMA's Recommended Retention Standards

Health Information	Recommended Retention Period
Diagnostic images (such as x-ray film)	5 years
Disease index	10 years
Fetal heart monitor records	10 years after the infant reaches the age of majority
Master patient/person index	Permanently
Operative index	10 years
Patient health/medical records (adults)	10 years after the most recent encounter
Patient health/medical records (minors)	Age of majority plus statute of limitations
Physician index	10 years
Register of births	Permanently
Register of deaths	Permanently
Register of surgical procedures	Permanently

Table 2. Accreditation Agency Retention Standards

Accreditation Agency	Retention Standard	Reference
Accreditation Association for Ambulatory Health Care (AAAHC)	Requires organizations to have policies that address retention of active clinical records, the retirement of inactive clinical records, and the retention of diagnostic images.	*2001 Accreditation Handbook for Ambulatory Care*
American Accreditation Healthcare Commission/ URAC	Member Protection Standard #7 states "the network shall have storage and security of confidential health information, access to hard copy and computerized confidential health information; records retention; and release of confidential health information."	*Health Network Accreditation Manual*
CARF (Rehabilitation Accreditation Commission)	Requires organizations to have policies that address record retention.	*2002 Adult Day Services Standards Manual*
	Retention periods are not specified for behavioral health. However, policy must comply with applicable state, federal, or provincial laws.	*2002 Behavioral Health Standards Manual*
	Retention periods are not specified for employment and community services.	
	Requires organizations to have policies that address retention of records and electronic records.	*2002 Assisted Living Standards Manual*
	Requires organizations to have policies that address retention of records and electronic records.	*2002 Medical Rehabilitation Standards Manual*
Community Health Accreditation Program (CHAP)	C25C—Elements 1 & 2: Records of adult patients must be retained for at least five years from the date of service and patient records for minors must be retained for seven years beyond the age of majority.	*CHAP Core Standards of Excellence*
	C27C—Element 5: The records of occupationally exposed patients must be kept for 30 years.	
Joint Commission on Accreditation of Healthcare Organizations	IM.7.1.2—The retention time of medical record information is determined by the organization based on law and regulation, and on its use for patient care, legal, research, and education activities.	*2001–2002 Comprehensive Accreditation Manual for Ambulatory Care*
	IM.7.1.2—The retention time of clinical/case record information is determined by the organization based on law and regulation, and on its use for care, legal, research, and educational activities.	*2001–2002 Comprehensive Accreditation Manual for Behavioral Care*
	IM.2.6—Data and information are retained for sufficient periods to comply with law and regulations and support member care, network management, legal documentation, research, and education.	*2001–2002 Comprehensive Accreditation Manual for Health Care Networks*
	IM.7—The organization initiates and maintains a record for every patient. Does the organization retain patient record information for the time period specified in policy and procedure and according to applicable law and regulations?	*2001–2002 Comprehensive Accreditation Manual For Home Care*
	IM.7.1.2—The hospital determines how long medical record information is retained, based on law and regulation, and the information used for patient care, legal, research, and educational purposes.	*2001–2002 Comprehensive Accreditation Manual For Hospitals*
	IM.7.1.—The retention time of medical record information is determined by law and regulation and by its use for resident care, legal, research, or educational purposes.	*2002–2003 Comprehensive Accreditation Manual for Long Term Care*
	Intent of IM.7.1.1: Medical records are retained for the period of time required by state law, or five years from the discharge date when there is no requirement in state law. For a minor, the medical record is retained for the time period defined by state law or at least three years after a resident reaches legal age as defined by state law.	
National Commission on Correctional Health Care (NCCHC)	Inactive health records are retained according to legal requirements for the jurisdiction and are reactivated if a juvenile or inmate returns to the system or facility.	*Standards For Health Services in Juvenile Detention and Confinement Facilities* (1999) *Standards for Health Services in Jails* (1996) *Standards For Health Services in Prisons* (1997)
National Committee for Quality Assurance (NCQA)	Retention periods are not specified.	

Table 3. Federal Record Retention Requirements

Type of Documentation	Retention Period	Citation/Reference
Abortions and related medical services documentation	Maintained for three years.	42 CFR 36.56 42 CFR 50.309
Ambulatory surgical services	Retention periods are not specified.	42 CFR 416.47
Clinics, rehabilitation agencies, and public health agencies as providers of outpatient physical therapy and speech-language pathology services	As determined by the respective state statute, or the statute of limitations in the state. In the absence of a state statute, five years after the date of discharge; or in the case of a minor, three years after the patient becomes of age under state law or five years after the date of discharge, whichever is longer.	42 CFR 485.721(d) 42 CFR 486.161(d)
Clinics, rural health	Six years from date of last entry and longer if required by state statute.	42 CFR 491.10(c)
Competitive medical plans (see HMOs, competitive medical plans, healthcare prepayment plans)		
Comprehensive outpatient rehabilitation facilities (CORFs)	Five years after patient discharge.	42 CFR 485.60(c)
Critical access hospitals (CAHs)	Six years from date of last entry, and longer if required by state statute, or if the records may be needed in any pending proceeding.	42 CFR 485.638(c)
Department of Veterans Affairs—Diagnostic and operation index file	Destroy monthly listing after receipt of consolidated biannual listing. Destroy consolidated biannual listing or prior equivalent 20 years after date of report.	Records Control Schedule (RCS)10-1, Section XXII—Medical Administration Service (136) (1985)
Department of Veterans Affairs—Disposition data files (PTF)	Destroy after one year and after a PTF master record has been created at the data processing center.	Records Control Schedule (RCS)10-1, Section XXII—Medical Administration Service (136) (1985)
Department of Veterans Affairs—Gains and losses file	Destroy master set after one year.	Records Control Schedule (RCS)10-1, Section XXII—Medical Administration Service (136) (1985)
Department of Veterans Affairs—Medical record or consolidated health record	Pending approval of reappraisal for destruction, 75 years from the last date of activity. *Note: All medical records of veterans are under moratorium against destruction placed by the Administrator 6/20/79 and approved by GSA/NARA (General Services Administration/National Archives and Records Administration).* This applies to medical records or consolidated health records for inpatients, ambulatory care patients, and tumor registry patients, including active records (hospital, domiciliary, nursing home units, ambulatory care, or other outpatient records), inactive records, perpetual medical records, medical records, and administrative records.	Records Control Schedule (RCS)10-1, Section XXII—Medical Administration Service (136) (1985)
Department of Veterans Affairs—Patient locator file	Destroy 50 years after last episode of care and/or only after perpetual medical record is destroyed.	Records Control Schedule (RCS)10-1, Section XXII—Medical Administration Service (136) (1985)
Department of Veterans Affairs—Register file	Destroy when no longer needed.	Records Control Schedule (RCS) 10-1, Section XXII—Medical Administration Service (136) (1985)
Department of Veterans Affairs—Tumor registry records and index cards	Live patients—destroy when 20 years old. Deceased patients or patients lost to follow up—destroy when five years old.	Records Control Schedule (RCS) 10-1, Section XXII—Medical Administration Service (136) (1985)
Device tracking (see Medical device tracking)		

(continued on next page)

Table 3. Federal Record Retention Requirements *(continued)*

Type of Documentation	Retention Period	Citation/Reference
Drug test results, students	Education records are those records that are directly related to a student and maintained by an education agency or institution or by a party acting for the agency or institution. Disclosure of education records is addressed. However, record retention periods are not specified.	34 CFR 99 Family Educational Rights and Privacy Act (20 USC §1232g)
Drug use review (DUR) (see Outpatient drug claims— Pharmacists participating in DUR program and electronic claims management system)		
End stage renal disease (ESRD) services	Not less than that determined by the state statute governing record retention or statute of limitations. In the absence of a state statute, five years from the date of discharge; or in the case of a minor, three years after the patient becomes of age under state law, whichever is longest.	42 CFR 405.2139(e)
HMOs, competitive medical plans, healthcare prepayment plans	Retention periods are not specified.	42 CFR 417
Healthcare prepayment plans (see HMOs, competitive medical plans, healthcare prepayment plans)		
Hearing aid devices, dispensers	The dispenser shall retain for three years after dispensing of a hearing aid a copy of any written statement from a physician or any written statement waiving medical evaluation.	21 CFR 801.421(d)
Home health agencies	Five years after the month the cost report to which the records apply is filed with the intermediary, unless state law stipulates a longer period of time.	42 CFR 484.48(a)
Hospice care	Retention periods are not specified.	42 CFR 418.74
Hospitals	Five years.	42 CFR 482.24(b)(1)
Hospitals—Nuclear medicine services	Report copies will be retained for five years.	42 CFR 482.53(d)
Hospitals— Radiologic services	Report copies and printouts, films, scans, and other image records will be retained for five years.	42 CFR 482.26(d)
Hospitals and other dispensers of drugs used for treatment of narcotic addicts, i.e., methadone	Three years.	21 CFR 291.505(d)(13)(ii)
Hospitals, critical access (see Critical access hospitals)		
Immunizations (see Vaccine)		
Institutional review board (IRB) for clinical devices	Two years after the latter of the following two dates: The date on which the investigation is terminated or completed, or the date that the records are no longer required for purposes of supporting a pre-market approval application or notice of completion of a product development protocol.	21 CFR 812.140(d)
IRB or institutions that review a clinical investigation documentation	Three years after completion of research.	21 CFR 56.115(b) 38 CFR 16.115(b)
Intermediate care, mentally retarded	Retention periods are not specified.	42 CFR 482.410
Investigator—Investigators in clinical devices	Two years after the latter of the following two dates: The date on which the investigation is terminated or completed, or the date that the records are no longer required for purposes of supporting a premarket approval application or notice of completion of a product development protocol.	

Table 3. Federal Record Retention Requirements *(continued)*

Type of Documentation	Retention Period	Citation/Reference
Investigator—Investigators of new drugs and antibiotic drugs for investigational use	Two years following the date a marketing application is approved for the drug for the indication for which it is being investigated. If no application is to be filed or if the application is not approved for such indication, until two years after the investigation is discontinued and the FDA is notified.	21 CFR 312.62(c)
Laboratory—immunohematology	Five years.	42 CFR 493.1777(d)(1) 42 CFR 493.1780(e)(1)
Laboratory—pathology tests	Ten years after the date of reporting.	42 CFR 493.1777(d)(2) 42 CFR 493.1780(e)(3)
Laboratory—all other records	Two years.	42 CFR 493.1777(d)(3) 42 CFR 493.1780(e)(4)
Laboratory stains and specimen blocks—histopathology, oral pathology	Stained slides—10 years from the date of examination. Specimen blocks—two years from the date of examination.	42 CFR 493.1259(b)
Long-term care facilities	As required by state law; or five years from the date of discharge when there is no requirement in state law; or for a minor, three years after a resident reaches legal age under state law.	42 CFR 483.75(l)(2)
Mammography—screening and/or diagnostic mammography services	Five years, or not less than 10 years, if no additional mammograms of the patient are performed at the facility, or longer if mandated by state or local law.	21 CFR 900.12(e)(1)(i)
Medical device tracking	Maintain such records for the useful life of each tracked device manufactured or distributed. The useful life of a device is the time a device is in use or in distribution for use.	21 CFR 821.60
Mental retardation intermediate care (see Intermediate care, mentally retarded)		
Methadone (see Hospitals and other dispensers of drugs used for treatment of narcotic addicts, i.e., methadone)		
Mine Safety and Health Administration—MSHA Form 5000-3	The mine operator shall have MSHA Form 5000-3 certifying medical fitness completed and signed by the examining physician for each member of a mine rescue team. These forms shall be kept on file at the mine rescue station for a period of one year.	30 CFR 49.7(c)
Narcotic addict treatment (see Hospitals and other dispensers of drugs used for treatment of narcotic addicts, i.e., methadone)		
Nuclear medicine services, hospitals (see Hospitals—Nuclear medicine services)		
Nursing home or skilled nursing home (see Long-term care facilities)		
Occupational Safety and Health Administration (OSHA)—employee exposure records	Employee exposure record means a record containing any of the following kinds of information: • Environmental (workplace) monitoring or measuring of a toxic substance or harmful physical agent, including personal, area, grab, wipe, or other form of sampling, as well as related collection and analytical methodologies, calculations, and other background data relevant to interpretation of the results obtained	29 CFR 1910.1020(d)(1) 29 CFR 1915.1020 29 CFR 1926.33

(continued on next page)

Table 3.   Federal Record Retention Requirements *(continued)*

Type of Documentation	Retention Period	Citation/Reference
Occupational Safety and Health Administration (OSHA)—employee exposure records (continued)	• Biological monitoring results that directly assess the absorption of a toxic substance or harmful physical agent by body systems (e.g., the level of a chemical in the blood, urine, breath, hair, fingernails) but not including results that assess the biological effect of a substance or agent or which assess an employee's use of alcohol or drugs • Material safety data sheets indicating that the material may pose a hazard to human health, or • In the absence of the above, a chemical inventory or any other record that reveals where and when used and the identity (e.g., chemical, common, or trade name) of a toxic substance or harmful physical agent Unless otherwise specified, each employee exposure record shall be preserved and maintained for at least 30 years, except that: • Background data to environmental (workplace) monitoring or measuring, such as laboratory reports and worksheets, need only be retained for one year as long as the sampling results, the collection methodology (sampling plan), a description of the analytical and mathematical methods used, and a summary of other background data relevant to interpretation of the results obtained, are retained for at least 30 years, and • Material safety data sheets and paragraph (c)(5)(iv) records concerning the identity of a substance or agent need not be retained for any specified period as long as some record of the identity (chemical name if known) of the substance or agent, where it was used, and when it was used is retained for at least 30 years; and material safety data sheets must be kept for those chemicals currently in use that are affected by the Hazard Communication Standard in accordance with 29 CFR 1910.1200(g) • Biological monitoring results designated as exposure records by specific occupational safety and health standards shall be preserved and maintained as required by the specific standard • Each analysis using exposure or medical records shall be preserved and maintained for at least 30 years	
	1, 2, dibromo-e-chloroprane (DBCP)—The employer shall maintain this record for at least 40 years or the duration of employment plus 20 years, whichever is longer.	29 CFR 1910.1044(p)(1)(iii) 29 CFR 1915.1044 29 CFR 1926.1144
	1, 3-butadiene—Retain in accordance with 29 CFR 1910.20.	29 CFR 1910.1051(m)(2)(iii) 29 CFR 1915.1051
	Acrylonitrile (vinyl cyanide)—The employer shall maintain this record for at least 40 years, or for the duration of employment plus 20 years, whichever is longer.	29 CFR 1910.1045(q)(2)(iii) 29 CFR 1915.1045 29 CFR 1926.1145
	Asbestos—Retain in accordance with 29 CFR 1910.20.	29 CFR 1910.1001(m)(3) 29 CFR 1015.1001(n)(2)(iii) 29 CFR 1926.58
	Benzene—Retain in accordance with 29 CFR 1910.20.	29 CFR 1910.1028(k)(1)(iii) 29 CFR 1915.1028 29 CFR 1926.1110

Table 3. Federal Record Retention Requirements *(continued)*

Type of Documentation	Retention Period	Citation/Reference
Occupational Safety and Health Administration (OSHA)—employee exposure records (continued)	Carcinogens—Records shall be maintained for the duration of the employee's employment. Upon termination of the employee's employment, including retirement or death, or in the event that the employer ceases business without a successor, records, or notarized true copies thereof, shall be forwarded by registered mail to the director.	29 CFR 1910.1003(g)(2) 29 CFR 1910.1004 29 CFR 1910.1006-1016 29 CFR 1915.1003-1004 29 CFR 1915.1006-1016 29 CFR 1926.1103-1104 29 CFR 1926.1106-1116
	Coke oven emissions—The employer shall maintain this record for at least 40 years or for the duration of employment plus 20 years, whichever is longer.	29 CFR 1910.1029(m)(1)(ii) 29 CFR 1926.1129
	Cotton dust—The employer shall maintain this record for at least 20 years.	29 CFR 1910.1043(k)(1)(iii)
	Ethylene oxide—Retain in accordance with 29 CFR 1910.20.	29 CFR 1910.1047(k)(2)(iii) 29 CFR 1915.1047 29 CFR 1926.1147
	Formaldehyde—Retain in accordance with 29 CFR 1910.20.	29 CFR 1910.1048(o)(5)(i) 29 CFR 1915.1048 29 CFR 1926.1148
	Hazardous materials—Retain in accordance with 29 CFR 1910.20.	29 CFR 1910.120(f)(8)(i)
	Inorganic arsenic—The employer shall maintain these monitoring records for at least 40 years or for the duration of employment plus 20 years, whichever is longer.	29 CFR 1910.1018(q)(E)(iii) 29 CFR 1915.1018 29 CFR 1926.1118
	Laboratory use of hazardous chemicals—Retain in accordance with 29 CFR 1910.20.	29 CFR 1910.1450(j)(2) 29 CFR 1915.1450
	Lead—The employer shall maintain these monitoring records for at least 40 years or for the duration of employment plus 20 years, whichever is longer.	29 CFR 1910.1025(n)(1)(iii) 29 CFR 1915.1025
	Methylene chloride—Retain in accordance with 29 CFR 1910.20.	29 CFR 1910.1052(m)(2)(iv) 29 CFR 1915.1052
	Methylenedianiline—Retain in accordance with 29 CFR 1910.20.	29 CFR 1910.1050(n)(3)(iii) 29 CFR 1915.1050 29 CFR 1926.60
OSHA—employee medical records	Employee medical record means a record concerning the health status of an employee that is made or maintained by a physician, nurse, or other healthcare personnel or technician, including: • Medical and employment questionnaires or histories (including job description and occupational exposures) • The results of medical examinations (pre-employment, pre-assignment, periodic, or episodic) and laboratory tests (including chest and other x-ray examinations taken for the purposes of establishing a baseline or detecting occupational illness, and all biological monitoring not defined as an employee exposure record) • Medical opinions, diagnoses, progress notes, and recommendations • First aid records • Descriptions of treatments and prescriptions, and • Employee medical complaints	29 CFR 1910.1020(d)(1) 29 CFR 1915.1020 29 CFR 1926.33

(continued on next page)

Table 3. Federal Record Retention Requirements *(continued)*

Type of Documentation	Retention Period	Citation/Reference
OSHA—employee medical records (continued)	Unless otherwise specified, the medical record for each employee shall be preserved and maintained for at least the duration of employment plus 30 years, except that the following types of records need not be retained for any specified period: • health insurance claims records maintained separately from the employer's medical program and its records • first aid records (not including medical histories) of one-time treatment and subsequent observation of minor scratches, cuts, burns, splinters, and the like, which do not involve medical treatment, loss of consciousness, restriction of work or motion, or transfer to another job, if made on site by a non-physician and if maintained separately from the employer's medical program and its records, and • the medical records of employees who have worked for less than one year for the employer need not be retained beyond the term of employment if they are provided to the employee upon the termination of employment	
	1, 2, dibromo-e-chloroprane (DBCP)—The employer shall maintain this record for at least 40 years or the duration of employment plus 20 years, whichever is longer.	29 CFR 1910.1044(p)(2)(iii) 29 CFR 1915.1044 29 CFR 1926.1144
	1, 3-butadiene—Retain in accordance with 29 CFR 1910.20.	29 CFR 1910. 1051(m)(4)(iii) 29 CFR 1915.1051
	Acrylonitrile (vinyl cyanide)—The employer shall maintain this record for at least 40 years, or for the duration of employment plus 20 years, whichever is longer.	29 CFR 1910.1045(q)(3)(iii) 29 CFR 1915.1045 29 CFR 1926.1145
	Asbestos—Retain in accordance with 29 CFR 1910.20.	29 CFR 1910.1001(m)(3) 29 CFR 1015.1001(n)(3)(iii) 29 CFR 1926.58
	Benzene—Retain in accordance with 29 CFR 1910.20.	29 CFR 1910.1028(k)(2)(iii) 29 CFR 1915.1028 29 CFR 1926.1110
	Blood-borne pathogens—Retain in accordance with 29 CFR 1910.20.	29 CFR 1910.1030(h)(1)(iv) 29 CFR 1915.1030
	Cadmium—Retain in accordance with 29 CFR 1910.20.	29 CFR 1910.1027(n)(3)(iii) 29 CFR 1915.1027 29 CFR 1926.1127
	Coke oven emissions—The employer shall maintain medical records for at least 40 years, or for the duration of employment plus 20 years, whichever is longer.	29 CFR 1910.1029(m)(l)(iii) 29 CFR 1926.1129
	Cotton dust—The employer shall maintain this record for at least 20 years.	29 CFR 1910.1043(k)(2)(iii)
	Dive team member—Five years.	29 CFR 1910.440 (a)(3)(i)
	Ethylene oxide—Retain in accordance with 29 CFR 1910.20.	29 CFR 1910.1047(k)(3)(iii) 29 CFR 1915.1047 29 CFR 1926.1147
	Formaldehyde—Retain in accordance with 29 CFR 1910.20.	29 CFR 1910.1048(o)(5)(ii) 29 CFR 1915.1048 29 CFR 1926.1148
	Laboratory use of hazardous chemicals—Retain in accordance with 29 CFR 1910.20.	29 CFR 1910.1450(j)(2)

Table 3. Federal Record Retention Requirements *(continued)*

Type of Documentation	Retention Period	Citation/Reference
OSHA—employee medical records (continued)	Lead—The employer shall maintain or assure that the physician maintains those medical records for at least 40 years, or for the duration of employment plus 20 years, whichever is longer.	29 CFR 1910.1025(n)(2)(iv) 29 CFR 1915.1025
	Methylene chloride—Retain in accordance with 29 CFR 1910.20.	29 CFR 1910.1052(m)(3)(iii) 29 CFR 1915.1052
	Methylenedianiline—Retain in accordance with 29 CFR 1910.20.	29 CFR 1910.1050(n)(4)(iv) 29 CFR 1915.1050 29 CFR 1926.60
	Vinyl chloride—Medical records shall be maintained for the duration of the employment of each employee plus 20 years, or 30 years, whichever is longer.	29 CFR 1910. 1017(m)(2)(C)(iii) 29 CFR 1915.1017 29 CFR 1926.1117
OSHA—employee medical removal records, lead	The employer shall maintain each medical removal record for at least the duration of an employee's employment.	29 CFR 1910.1025(n)(3)(iii) 29 CFR 1915.1025
Outpatient drug claims— Pharmacists participating in drug use review (DUR) program and electronic claims management system	Retention periods are not specified.	42 CFR 456.705 42 CFR 456.709
Outpatient physical therapy (see Clinics, rehabilitation agencies, and public health agencies as providers of outwpatient physical therapy and speech-language pathology services)		
Outpatient rehabilitation facilities, comprehensive (see Comprehensive outpatient rehabilitation facilities)		
Psychiatric hospitals	Retention period five years.	42 CFR 482.61
Public health agencies (see Clinics, rehabilitation agencies, and public health agencies as providers of outpatient physical therapy and speech-language pathology services)		
Radiologic services, hospitals (see Hospitals—Radiologic services)		
Rehabilitation agencies (see Clinics, rehabilitation agencies, and public health agencies as providers of outpatient physical therapy and speech-language pathology services)		
Renal disease (see End stage renal disease services)		
Rural health clinics (See Clinics, rural health)		
Speech-language pathology services (see Clinics, rehabilitation agencies, and public health agencies as providers of outpatient physical therapy and speech-language pathology services)		
Utilization review committee	Retention periods are not specified.	42 CFR 456.100-145

(continued on next page)

Table 3. Federal Record Retention Requirements *(continued)*

Type of Documentation	Retention Period	Citation/Reference
Vaccine	Retention periods are not specified. However, each healthcare provider who administers a vaccine set forth in the Vaccine Injury Table (42 CFR 100.3) to any person shall record, or ensure that there is recorded, in such person's permanent medical record (or in a permanent office log or file to which a legal representative shall have access upon request) with respect to each such vaccine the date of administration of the vaccine, the vaccine manufacturer and lot number of the vaccine, the name and address and, if appropriate, the title of the healthcare provider administering the vaccine, and any other identifying information on the vaccine required pursuant to regulation promulgated by the Secretary. Note: For injuries, claims can be filed within 36 months after the first symptoms appeared. In the case of death, the claim must be filed within 24 months of the death and within 48 months after the onset of the vaccine-related injury from which the death occurred. AHIMA recommends that records be retained at least through this period.	42 CFR 300aa-11 42 CFR 300aa-25
Veterans Administration (see Department of Veterans Affairs)		

CFR: Code of Federal Regulations (includes Conditions of Participation, Food and Drug Administration, Department of Health and Human Services, Health Care Financing Administration, Public Health Service, Occupational Safety and Health Administration, and other federal agencies)
USC: United States Code

Table 4. State Laws or Regulations Pertaining to Retention of Health Information

State	Summary of Law/Regulation	Citation
Alabama	Assisted living facilities and abortion/reproductive health centers must retain medical records three years.	ADPH, 420-5-4.06(1)(c) ADPH, 420-5-1.02(5)(h)
	Hospital and sleep disorders facilities must retain medical records five years.	ADPH, 420-5-7-.10 ADPH, 420-5-18-.06(8)
	Hospices, nursing facilities, and rehabilitation centers must retain medical records five years from the date of discharge or three years after the age of majority.	ADPH, 420-5-17-.18(6) ADPH, 420-5-10-.03(33) ADPH, 420-5-11-.02(6)(f)
	End stage renal disease treatment and transplant centers and ambulatory surgical treatment centers must retain medical records six years from the date of discharge or six years after the age of majority.	ADPH, 420-5-5-.02(7)(e)2 ADPH, 420-5-2-.02(6)(g)
	Birthing centers must retain medical records 20 years for adults or seven years after the age of majority for minors.	ADPH, 420-5-13.11(4)
Alaska	Unless otherwise specified by the Department of Health and Social Services, hospitals must preserve records that relate directly to the care and treatment of a patient for seven years following discharge. However, records of a patient under 19 years of age shall be kept at least two years after the patient reaches 19 or seven years following discharge of the patient, whichever is longer. X-ray film must be retained for five years.	Alaska Stat. Section 18.20.085 (1992)
	Facilities providing healthcare to Medicaid recipients must retain fiscal, patient care, and related records for three years following the year in which services were provided, unless the Department of Health and Social Services requests retention for a longer period.	Alaska Admin. Code tit. 7 Section 43.030 (Apr. 1984)
Arizona	There is no state statute specific to retention of health information. However, the statute of limitations for medical malpractice claims is two years from the time the patient discovers or should have discovered an injury. The statute of limitations for minors is two years past the age of 18. Providers must keep adult patient records for a minimum of two years and minor patient records for a minimum of two years past the age of 18 to comply with statute of limitations.	ARS 12-502 (1996) ARS 12-542 (1985) ARS 12-550 (1994)

Table 4. State Laws or Regulations Pertaining to Retention of Health Information *(continued)*

State	Summary of Law/Regulation	Citation
Arizona (continued)	Any institution that provides inpatient medical, surgical, diagnostic, nursing, custodial, or domiciliary care must retain the information necessary to complete birth, death, and fetal death registration forms, and records of disposal of remains for at least 10 years.	ARS Section 36-343 (1992)
	For licensing purposes, hospital medical records must be retrievable for a period of not less than three years, except for vital records (birth and death) and statistics, which must be retained for 10 years.	ARS Section 36-343 (1992)
	Arizona requires that duplicate lab reports be retained in the laboratory area for at least one year after the date results are reported.	Arizona Comp. Admin. Rules & Regs. Section 9-10-222 (1982)
Arkansas	All medical records shall be retained in either the original form or microfilm or other acceptable methods for ten years after the last discharge. After ten years a medical record may be destroyed provided the facility permanently maintains the information contained in the master patient index. Complete medical records of minors shall be retained for a period of two years after the age of majority.	Arkansas Regs. 0601
California	Hospitals must maintain medical records for a minimum of seven years following patient discharge, except for minors. Records of minors must be maintained for at least one year after a minor has reached age 18, but in no event for less than seven years.	California Code Regs. tit. 22 Section 70751 (c) (1993) California Code Regs. tit. 22 Section 71551(c) (1993)
	Acute psychiatric hospitals, skilled nursing facilities, intermediate care facilities, home health agencies, primary care clinics, psychology clinics, and psychiatric facilities must maintain medical records and exposed x-rays for a minimum of seven years following patient discharge, except for minors. Records of minors must be maintained for at least one year after a minor has reached age 18, but in no event for less than seven years.	California Code Regs. tit. 22 Section 73543(a) (1993) California Code Regs. tit. 22 Section 74731(a) (1993) California Code Regs. tit. 22 Section 75055(a) (1993) California Code Regs. tit. 22 Section 75343(a) (1993) California Code Regs. tit. 22 Section 77143(a) (1993)
Colorado	Hospitals must preserve medical records as originals or on microfilm for not less than 10 years after the most recent patient care use, except that records of minors must be preserved for the period of minority plus 10 years.	6 Colorado Code Regs Section 1011-1, Section 4.2 (1977)
Connecticut	Medical records, other than nurses' notes, must be kept for a minimum of 25 years after patient discharge, but may be destroyed sooner if microfilmed by a process approved by the Department of Health.	Connecticut Agencies Regs. Section 19-13-D4(b)(1979)
	Homes for the aged and rest homes must maintain information on forms approved by the state Department of Health at least 10 years following patient death or discharge.	Connecticut Agencies Regs. Section 19-13-D6(e)(1988)
Delaware	Nursing home records should be retained five years before being destroyed.	Delaware State Board of Health, Nursing Home Regs. for Skilled Care Section 810 (1986)
District of Columbia	Regulations require a medical record to be kept for not less than 10 years following the date of the patient's discharge.	DC Mun. Regs. tit. 22 Section 2216.3 (1986)
Florida	Hospital shall retain inpatient medical records, emergency room records, and outpatient/ clinical records for seven years after the last entry. X-ray films are to be retained for seven years.	General Records Schedule for Hospital Records GS4 (1997)
	Nursing homes must retain medical records a minimum of seven years after the last entry or retain until 24 years of age, whichever is longer.	Florida Admin. Code Annotated r. 59A4.118(8)(1992)
	Physicians are required to maintain records for at least seven years.	Florida Admin. Code Annotated r. 59A-3.214
	Dentists must maintain written dental records for four years after the patient is last examined or treated.	Florida Admin. Code Annotated r. 61FS 17.005
Georgia	Hospitals must preserve medical records as originals, microfilms, or other useable forms until the sixth anniversary of the patient's discharge or longer. Hospitals must keep a minor's records until the patient's 27th birthday. (This regulation was promulgated at a time when the age of majority in Georgia was 21. Since that time, the age of majority has been lowered to 18.)	Georgia Comp. Rules & Regs. r. 290-5-6-.11(1991)

(continued on next page)

Table 4. State Laws or Regulations Pertaining to Retention of Health Information *(continued)*

State	Summary of Law/Regulation	Citation
Hawaii	Healthcare medical records must be retained for a minimum of seven years after the last data entry. Medical records for minors shall be retained during the period of minority plus seven years after the minor reaches the age of majority. X-ray films, electro-encephalogram tracings, and similar imaging records shall be retained for at least seven years, after which they may be presented to the patient or destroyed. The healthcare provider or the healthcare provider's successor shall be responsible for the retention of basic information from the medical records for 25 years from the last entry, or in the case of a minor, for the duration of minority plus 25 years after reaching the age of majority. Basic information from a physician or surgeon's record includes the patient's name and birthdate, a list of dated diagnoses and intrusive treatments, and a record of all drugs prescribed or given. Basic information from a healthcare facility shall include the patient's name and birthdate, dates of admission and discharge, names of attending physicians, final diagnoses, major procedures performed, operative reports, pathology reports, and discharge summaries.	Hawaii Rev. Stat. Section 622-58
Idaho	Clinical laboratory test records and reports may be destroyed three years after the date of the test.	Idaho Code Section 39-1394 (1992)
	Long term care facilities are required to preserve records for a period of time not less than seven years. If the patient/resident is a minor, the record shall be preserved for a period of not less than seven years following his 18th birthday.	IDAPA 16.03.02203,04b
	X-ray films may be destroyed five years after the date of exposure or five years after the patient reaches the age of majority, whichever is later, if the hospital has written findings of a physician who has read such films.	Idaho Code Section 39-1394 (1992)
	Skilled nursing and intermediate care facilities must keep records not less than seven years. If the patient is a minor, the facility must preserve the records for not less than seven years following the patient's 18th birthday. Proprietary home health agencies must maintain clinical records for six years from the date of discharge or in the case of minors, three years after the patient becomes of age.	Licensing and Certification Section, Bureau of Welfare Medical Programs, Division of Welfare, Idaho Dept. of Health and Welfare, Statutes and Regs. Dealing with Medical Record Retention 5 (1992)
	Health maintenance organizations must keep medical records for six years after the termination of the enrollee's contract.	Idaho Code Section 41-3909 (1992)
Illinois	All original medical records or photographs of such records shall be preserved in accordance with a hospital policy based on American Hospital Association recommendations and legal opinion.	Illinois Admin. Rules, Title 77, Subpart L, §250.1510
	Home health agencies shall retain records for a minimum of five years beyond the last date of service provided. Agencies that are subject to the Local Records Act should note that "except as otherwise provided by law, no public record shall be disposed of by an officer or agency unless the written approval of the appropriate Local Records commission is first obtained."	50 ILCS (Illinois Compiled Statutes) 205/1
	Hospitals that produce photographs of the human anatomy by the x-ray or roentgen process on the request of licensed physicians for use by them in the diagnosis or treatment of a patient's illness or condition shall retain such photographs or films as part of their regularly maintained records for a period of five years provided that retention of said photographs or film may be by microfilm or other recognized means of minification that does not adversely affect their use for diagnostic purposes. However, if the hospital has been notified in writing by an attorney-at-law before the expiration of the five-year period that there is a litigation pending in court involving a particular x-ray or roentgen photograph in their records as possible evidence, and that the subject person of such photograph is his client, or is the person who has instituted such litigation against his client, then the hospital shall keep such photograph or film or minified copy thereof in its regular records until notified in writing by the plaintiff's attorney with the approval thereon of the defendant's attorney of record that the case in court involving such photograph has been concluded, or for a period of 12 years from the date that the x-ray photograph film was produced, whichever comes first in time.	210 ILCS (Illinois Compiled Statutes) 90/1

Table 4. State Laws or Regulations Pertaining to Retention of Health Information *(continued)*

State	Summary of Law/Regulation	Citation
Indiana	Physicians, dentists, nurses, optometrists, podiatrists, chiropractors, physical therapists, psychologists, audiologists, speech-language pathologists, home health agencies, and hospitals must maintain the original health records or microfilms of the records for at least seven years. They must maintain patient x-ray film, scans, and diagnostic images for at least five years.	IC 16-39-7-1(b)(1993) IC16-39-7-2 (b) and (d) (1993) 410 IAC 15-1.5-9 (e)
	Ambulatory outpatient surgical centers must retain medical records or microfilms for at least 25 years. Microfilms may be substituted for original records that are three years or more of age. A center may submit a request to the Licensing Council for approval to microfilm earlier.	410 IAC 15-2-8
	Comprehensive care facilities and residential care facilities must preserve medical records in the facility for a minimum of one year after discharge of the resident or in accordance with applicable federal and state laws.	410 IAC 16-2-3-13(f)(2) (1984) 410 IAC 16.2-5-8 (1984) 431 IAC 2-2-6(a)
	In facilities for the mentally ill, medical records must be retained at least 10 years after the resident leaves the program, or in the case of minors, 10 years after discharge or until the child's 23rd birthday, whichever is the longer period. Patient registers shall be maintained within the facility for the period required by statutes of limitations.	410 IAC 15-2-7 (1976)
	Any such photographic, photostatic, miniature photographic, or optical image copy or reproduction shall be deemed to be an original record for all purposes and shall be treated as an original record in all courts or administrative agencies for the purpose of its admissibility in evidence.	IC34-3-15-2 (1995)
Iowa	Hospitals must keep admission records, death records, birth records, and narcotic records. Medical records must be filed and kept in an accessible manner in the hospital in accordance with the statute of limitations.	Iowa Admin. Code r. 481-51.6(1) (1987)
	The hospital pharmacy must keep records of transactions for the control and accountability of drugs, as well as records of all medications and prescriptions dispensed.	Iowa Admin. Code r. 481-51.25(2) (135B)
	Nursing facilities must keep a resident's medical record for three years.	Iowa Admin. Code 4.441-81.9(2)
Kansas	Kansas hospitals must maintain medical records 10 years after the last discharge of the patient or one year beyond the date that patients who are minors reach their majority, whichever is longer.	Kansas Hospital Regs. 28-34-9(d)(1)
Kentucky	Hospitals must maintain inpatient and outpatient records a minimum of five years from the date of discharge, or in the case of a minor, three years after the patient reaches the age of majority under state law, whichever is longer.	902 Kentucky Admin. Regs. 20:016 Section 3(11)(a)(1991)
Louisiana	Hospitals must retain hospital records in their original, microfilmed or similarly reproduced form for a minimum of 10 years after the patient is discharged. Hospitals must retain graphic matter, images, x-ray films, and the like necessary to produce a diagnostic or therapeutic report in their original, microfilmed, or similarly reproduced form for three years from the date the patient was discharged. The hospital must retain records for a longer period when the patient's physician, the patient, or legal representative requests so in writing.	Louisiana Rev. Stat. Annotated Section 40:2144 (West 1992)
	Physicians must retain medical records in their original, microfilmed, or similarly reproduced form for a minimum of six years from the date the physician last treats the patient. Graphic matter, images, x-ray films, and the like necessary to produce a diagnostic or therapeutic report must be retained in the original, microfilmed, or similarly reproduced form for a minimum of three years from the date the patient is last treated by the physician and must be kept longer when requested in writing by the patient.	Louisiana Rev. Stat. Annotated Section 40:1299.96 (West 1992)
Maine	Hospital records shall be preserved on paper or by other electronic/optical means for a period of seven years. If the patient is a minor, the record must be retained for at least six years past the age of majority. Hospital x-ray films will be retained in the original or electronic form for five years, or in the case of a minor, five years past the age of majority. Patient logs and written x-ray report will be retained permanently.	State of Maine, Regs. for the Licensure of General and Specialty Hospitals, ch. VI: XII B.1. State of Maine, Regs. for the Licensure of General and Specialty Hospitals, ch. VI: XV.C.5.
	Maine regulations do not apply to healthcare providers other than hospitals. In particular, there is no state law or regulation covering retention of physicians' office records.	State of Maine, Regs. for the Licensure of General and Specialty Hospitals, ch. VI: XII B.

(continued on next page)

Table 4. State Laws or Regulations Pertaining to Retention of Health Information *(continued)*

State	Summary of Law/Regulation	Citation
Maryland	"Healthcare provider" means: an acupuncturist, audiologist, chiropractor, dietitian, dentist, electrologist, massage therapist, mortician, nurse, nutritionist, occupational therapist, optometrist, physical therapist, physician, podiatrist, professional counselor, psychologist, social worker, or speech-language pathologist.	Maryland Health-General Code Annotated Section 4-403
	Except for a minor patient, unless a patient is notified, a health-care provider may not destroy a medical record or laboratory or x-ray report about a patient for five years after the record or report is made. In the case of a minor patient, a medical record, or laboratory or x-ray report about a minor patient may not be destroyed until the patient attains the age of majority plus three years or for five years after the record or report is made, whichever is later, unless the parent or guardian of the minor patient is notified or if the medical care documented in the record was provided under 20-102 (c) or 20-103(c) of the Health-General Article, the minor patient is notified.	
Massachusetts	Hospitals: All hospitals and clinics licensed by the Department of Public Health or supported in whole or in part by the Commonwealth shall keep records of the treatment of cases under their care, including the medical history and nurses notes for 30 years following discharge or final treatment. Hospitals or clinics licensed by the Department of Mental Health shall maintain patient records for at least 30 years after discharge or last contact of patient.	Massachusetts Gen. Laws c. 111, s. 70 Massachusetts Gen. Laws c. 123 CMR 104
	Long term care: All clinical records of discharged patients or residents shall be completed within two weeks of discharges and filed and retained for at least five years.	Massachusetts Gen. Laws c. 105 CMR 150.013(E)
	Ambulatory services: For patients' records existing on or after January 1, 1990, the patient medical record must be maintained for a minimum of seven years from the date of the last patient encounter.	Massachusetts Gen. Laws c. 243 CMR 2.07(13)
Michigan	Nursing homes must maintain clinical records for a minimum of six years from discharge or, in the case of a minor, three years after the individual comes of age under state law, whichever is longer.	Michigan Admin. Code r. 325.21102 (1987)
	Medicaid providers must maintain records substantiating the medical necessity, appropriateness, and quality of services rendered for which a Medicaid claim is made for a period of six years.	MCL 400-111b (6) and (8)
	Clinical laboratories shall preserve original or duplicate laboratory reports at least one year.	MDPH R325.2353(1)
	Dentists must retain their records of treatment for a period of not less than 10 years after the performance of last service upon the patient.	MCL 333.16644
	Outpatient and residential substance abuse records are required to be maintained for a minimum of three years after services are discontinued.	OSAS R 325.14711(4) OSAS R. 325.14910(4)
Minnesota	Hospitals must maintain the original medical record in its entirety for a minimum of three years. The medical record may be destroyed after three years if it has been microfilmed in its entirety. The hospital governing body must approve destruction of records. After seven years, only the portion of the entire record defined by statute as the "individual permanent medical record" must be retained. For minors, the entire record must be retained for seven years past the age of majority.	Minnesota Statute 145.32, 145.30 Minnesota Rule 4642.1000
	Long term care facility medical records must be retained for a period of at least five years following discharge or death.	Minnesota Rules 4658.0470 Section 1
	Supervised living facilities are required to maintain records for three years following discharge or death.	Minnesota Rules 4665.4100, Section 4
Mississippi	Hospitals must maintain records for such period of reasonable duration as may be prescribed by the rules and regulations of the licensing authority. Such rules may provide for different retention periods for the various parts of the record or for various medical conditions and may require that the hospital make an abstract of the record. However, hospitals must retain complete medical records for a period of at least seven years for patients discharged at death, 10 years for adult patients of sound mind at the time of discharge, and for the period of minority or other disability plus seven years, but not to exceed 28 years for minors or disabled adults. If a patient dies in a hospital or within 30 days of discharge and the hospital knows or has reason to know that the patient left one or more disabled survivors who are or claim to be entitled to damages for wrongful death of the patient, the hospital must maintain the patient's record for the period of the disability	Mississippi Code Annotated Section 41-9-69 (1991)

Table 4. State Laws or Regulations Pertaining to Retention of Health Information *(continued)*

State	Summary of Law/Regulation	Citation
Mississippi (continued)	of the survivors plus seven years, but not to exceed 28 years. The facility may destroy x-ray films four years after the date of exposure provided the radiologist has documented and authenticated findings in the patient's medical record. Before x-rays or graphic data can be destroyed, the facility must notify the patient or patient's legal representative by certified letter. The patient or his representative has 60 days to request the facility retain the material for the same retention period as hospital records and the hospital must abide by such a request.	
Missouri	Hospitals must maintain medical records for a period of time not less than that required by the statute of limitations. In no event can action for damages for malpractice be commenced more than 10 years from the date of the complained of act of neglect.	19 CSR 30-20.021 (3)(D)(15) (1993)
	Special record retention rules apply to Missouri hospital districts, county hospitals, and public hospitals. Those rules are published in the Missouri Hospital District Records Manual available through the Office of the Secretary of State. Skilled nursing, intermediate care, and residential care facilities must maintain medical records for five years after the resident leaves the facility, or until the resident reaches the age of 26, whichever is longer.	RS Missouri Section 198.052.7 (1983)
	Abortion records must be retained at the abortion facility for a period of seven years from the time of discharge. Patient records for minors must be kept for seven years after discharge, or until the patient reaches age 25, whichever is longer.	RS Missouri Section 188.060 (1983); 19 C.S.R. 30-30.060(2)(D) (1990)
	Vital records (birth and death information) must be maintained for at least five years.	RS Missouri Section 193.275 (1995 Supp.)
Montana	Hospitals must retain the patient's entire medical record for at least 10 years following the patient's discharge or death, or, in the case of a patient who is a minor, for not less than 10 years following the date the patient either attains the age of majority or dies, whichever occurs earlier. After the expiration of the applicable 10-year period, the patient's medical record may be abridged to "core records." Core records should be retained permanently, but are required to be retained for an additional 10 years following the patient's discharge or death.	ARM 16.32.328 (1990)
	Diagnostic imaging film and electrodiagnostic tracings must be retained for at least five years; their interpretations must be retained for the length of time required for other medical records.	ARM 16.32.328 (1990)
	Other healthcare facilities must retain patient or resident medical records for no less than five years following the patient's or resident's discharge or death.	ARM 16.32.308 (1990)
Nebraska	Hospitals must keep medical records in original, microfilm, or other approved copy form for at least 10 years following discharge. In the case of minors, hospitals must keep the record until three years after the age of majority.	Nebraska Admin. Rules & Regs. 775-9-003.04A6 (1979)
	Intermediate care facilities must keep medical records for at least as long as the resident remains at the facility and five years thereafter, or in the case of a minor, five years after the resident reaches the age of majority.	Nebraska Admin. Rules & Regs. 175-8-003.04A3 (1987)
	Health clinics must maintain client records for not less than five years.	Nebraska Admin. Rules & Regs. 175-7-004.04 (1975)
	Substance abuse treatment centers (which includes alcohol and drug—inpatient and outpatient) rules and regulations are pending at this time due to a statute change.	Pending
	Home health agencies must retain records in retrievable form for at least five years after last discharge. The home health agency must keep records of minors at least five years after the patient reaches the age of majority.	Nebraska Admin. Rules & Regs. 175-14-006.01I (1988)
Nevada	Healthcare providers must retain health records for five years after their receipt or production.	Nevada Rev. Stat. Annotated Section 629.051 (Michie 1991)
New Hampshire	Both hospitals and health facilities must retain medical records of adults for a period of seven years from discharge. Children's records must be retained to the age of majority plus seven years.	New Hampshire Code Admin. R. Dept. of Health and Human Services Reg. 802.11, 803.06 (1986)
	X-ray film must be stored at least seven years.	New Hampshire Code Admin. R. Dept. of Health and Human Services Reg. 802.08(b)(5)(1986)

(continued on next page)

Table 4. State Laws or Regulations Pertaining to Retention of Health Information *(continued)*

State	Summary of Law/Regulation	Citation
New Jersey	Hospitals must preserve medical records for a period of not less than 10 years following the most recent discharge of the patient or until the discharged patient reaches age 23, whichever is the longer period. In addition, a discharge summary sheet shall be retained for a period of 20 years following the most recent discharge of the patient. X-ray films shall be retained for a period of five years.	N.J.A.C. Title 26 §26:8-5
New Mexico	Hospitals must retain all records that relate directly to the care and treatment of a patient for 10 years following the patient's last discharge. X-ray films may be destroyed four years after exposure. After three years, a patient may recover the x-rays.	New Mexico Stat. Annotated Section 14-6-2 (Michie 1992)
New York	Hospital: Medical records shall be retained in their original or legally reproduced form for a period of at least six years from the date of discharge or three years after the patient's age of majority (18 years), whichever is longer, or at least six years after death.	Title 10 NYCRR §405.10(a)(4)
	Long-term care facility: Clinical records shall be retained for six years from the date of discharge or death, or for residents who are minors, for three years after the resident reaches the age of majority (18).	Title 10 NYCRR §415.22(b)
	HMO: The HMO shall require and assure that the medical records of enrollees be retained for six years after the date of service rendered to enrollees or cessation of HMO operation, and in the case of a minor, for six years after majority.	Title 10 NYCRR §98.12(j)
	Clinical laboratory or blood bank: All records and reports of tests performed, including the original or duplicates of original reports received from another laboratory, shall be kept on the premises of both laboratories and shall be exhibited to representatives of the department on request. Records listed below shall be retained by the laboratory for at least the period specified. If other New York state or federal regulations or statutes require retention for different periods of time, the laboratory shall retain the appropriate record for the longest period applicable. Records shall be retained in their original form for a period of three months and may thereafter be stored on microfilm, microfiche, or other photographic record, or as magnetic tapes or other media in an electronic processing system. Such record shall be adequately protected against destruction, either by archival storage of duplicated photographic or electronic medium or by other suitable means providing equivalent protection. Records that are required to be retained for more than two years may, after two years, be stored off the immediate laboratory premises, provided they can be available to the laboratory staff or other authorized persons in the laboratory within 24 hours of a request for records. Request for tests shall be retained for the same period of time as required for the test results or seven years, whichever is less, except that referral information for cytogenetic cases shall be retained for six years. Accession records shall be retained for seven years. Records of quality control results shall be retained for two years. Preventative maintenance, service, and repair records shall be retained for as long as the instrument remains in use, except that records of monitoring of temperature-controlled spaces shall be kept for one year.	Title 10 NYCRR §58-1.11(c)
	The following types of laboratory reports shall be retained for at least the period specified: tissue pathology including exfoliative cytology—20 years; syphilis serology—negative report—two years; cytogenetics—25 years; all others— seven years. Worksheets containing instrument readings and/or personal observations upon which the outcome is based shall be retained for one year. Specimens shall be retained so as to be accessible to the laboratory within 24 hours for at least the period set forth below: blood film— other than routine—one year; blood film— routine—six months; bacteriology slide on which a diagnosis depends—one year; cytology slide showing any abnormality— seven years; cytology slide showing no abnormality—three years; tissue block—20 years; histopathology block—20 years; histopathology slide—20 years; bone marrow biopsy—20 years; cytogenetic slide—six years; photographic slide of cytogenetic karyotype—25 years; and recipient blood specimens—one week stoppered at 6°C.	Title 10 NYCRR §58-1.11(c)
North Carolina	Hospitals must maintain medical records, whether original, computer media, or microfilm for a minimum of 11 years following the discharge of an adult patient. Hospitals must maintain the medical records of minors until the patient's 30th birthday.	T10:03C:3903(1996)
	Hospice medical records must be retained for a period of not less than three years from the date of discharge of the patient, unless the patient is a minor, in which case the record must be retained until five years after the patient's 18th birthday. If a minor patient dies, as opposed to being discharged for other reasons, the minor's records must be retained at least five years after the minor's death.	T10:03T:0900 (1996)

Table 4. State Laws or Regulations Pertaining to Retention of Health Information *(continued)*

State	Summary of Law/Regulation	Citation
North Carolina (continued)	Nursing homes must maintain medical records, whether original, computer media, or microfilm for a minimum of five years following the discharge of an adult patient. Nursing homes must maintain the medical records of minors until the patient's 19th birthday and then for five years.	T10:03H:2402 (1996)
North Dakota	Hospital records must be preserved in original or any other method of preservation, such as by microfilm, for a period of at least the 10th anniversary of the date on which the patient who is the subject of the record was last treated in the hospital. If a patient was less than 18 years of age at the time of last treatment, the hospital may authorize the disposal of medical records relating to the patient on or after the date of the patient's 21st birthday or on or after the 10th anniversary of the date on which the patient was last treated, whichever is later. The hospital may not destroy medical records that relate to any matter that is involved in litigation if the hospital knows the litigation has not been finally resolved. It is the governing body's responsibility to determine which records have research, legal, or medical value and to preserve such records beyond the above-identified time frames until such time in the governing body's determination the record no longer has a research, legal, or medical value. Long term facilities must retain their records as original or any other method of preservation for 10 years after discharge or seven years after death. Records of minors must be retained for the period of minority, plus 10 years after discharge.	North Dakota Admin. Code Section 33-07-01 20 (1994)
Ohio	Maternity hospitals and homes must keep medical records of each maternity patient and infant for not less than two years. Resident records of alcoholism inpatient/emergency care facilities must be kept for at least three years after patient discharge. All facilities participating in the Title XIX program must keep medical records for the longer of seven years or six years after the fiscal audit.	Ohio Admin. Code Section 3701-7-35 (1989) Ohio Admin. Code Section 3701-55-15 (1989) Ohio Admin. Code Section 5101: 3-3-26 (1992)
Oklahoma	Healthcare facilities must retain medical records for a minimum of five years beyond the date the patient was last seen or a minimum of three years beyond the date of the patient's death.	Oklahoma Dept. of Health Reg. ch. 13, Section 13.13A
	Hospitals in which abortions are performed must keep records not less than seven years.	Oklahoma Stat. Annotated tit. 63, Section 1-739 (West 1991)
	Medicaid providers must maintain at their principal place of Medicaid business all required records for at least six years from the date of claimed provision of any goods or services to the Medicaid recipient and to make these records accessible to the attorney general for investigation concerning whether any person may have committed welfare fraud.	Oklahoma Stat. Annotated tit. 56, Section 1004 (West 1991)
Oregon	Hospital inpatient records must be preserved 10 years from last discharge.	OAR 333-505-050(1)
	Long term care records must be maintained five years from last discharge.	OAR 411-86-300(6)
	Home healthcare records must be maintained 10 years from last discharge.	OAR 333-27-060(2)
	All clinical records or photographic records not incorporated into the records, such as x-rays, EKGs, EEGs, and radiological isotope scans, shall be retained for seven years.	ORS 333-505-050(16)
	Patient delivery, death, operation registers, and the master patient index must be retained permanently. Outpatient registers for acute care facilities and emergency room registers must be retained seven years. Blood bank registers must be retained 20 years.	ORS 333-505-050(8)
Pennsylvania	Hospitals and ambulatory surgical facilities must maintain medical records—whether original, reproductions, or microfilm—for a minimum of seven years following the discharge of a patient. If the patient is a minor, records shall be kept on file until his majority and then for seven years or as long as the records of adult patients are maintained.	28 Pennsylvania Code Section 115.23 28 Pennsylvania Code Section 563.6
	Physicians shall retain medical records for at least seven years from the date of the last medical service for which a medical record entry is required. The medical record for a minor patient shall be retained until one year after the minor patient reaches majority, even if this means that the physician retains the record for a period of more than seven years.	49 Pennsylvania Code Section 16.95

(continued on next page)

Table 4. State Laws or Regulations Pertaining to Retention of Health Information *(continued)*

State	Summary of Law/Regulation	Citation
Puerto Rico	Medical records shall be conserved in their original form or in any medium that utilizes the advances of recognized technology such as microfilm, or computerized or electronic forms, among others, for a minimum of five years. The medical records of patients under 21 years of age shall be conserved until the patient (minor) reaches his/her 22nd birthday. Those medical records that because of the needs or particular interests of the health facility are retained for a period of time greater than that stated here, shall be retained for the duration of the need as expressed in writing in its internal statutes. After the five years or once the minor reaches the age of 22 or after the additional time in the cases of particular interest, the facility shall conserve for at least five additional years the following documents in their original form or in a recognized technology medium (microfilm or computerized or electronic forms, among others): • Inpatient records: Admission and discharge records, discharge summary, operative reports, pathology reports, labor room and newborn reports, and autopsy report. • Outpatient record: Problem list (summary list); clinical history and report of significant findings of the basic or clinical services such as dental, social, psychiatric, psychological, or nutritional services, adolescent or prenatal clinics, post-partum, family planning, and WIC among others; operative/procedure reports (ambulatory surgery); and pathology/cytology reports. • Emergency room record: Emergency room evaluation and procedure reports. • Mental health/physical disability records: In addition to the previously mentioned list, the following documents shall be conserved—psychological, social services, and psychiatric evaluations. • The facility may also conserve any other document it deems pertinent according to its particular needs.	Puerto Rico Health Information Regulations #99
Rhode Island	Medical records must be kept for five years following discharge of the patient. Records may be kept in either original or accurately reproduced form. Hospitals must maintain a minor's record for at least five years after the minor reaches 18 years of age.	Rhode Island General Laws Section 23-3-26 (1990) 1991 Rhode Island Acts & Resolves R23-17Hosp. 25.9
South Carolina	Hospital records must be retained for 10 years. The records of minors are retained until after the expiration of the period of election following achievement of majority prescribed by statute (one year).	South Carolina Code Regs. Section 601.7(a)(1982)
	Nursing homes must store medical records for 10 years from discharge or death.	South Carolina Code Regs. 61.13 Section 503 (1980)
South Dakota	Except for resident assessment records, a healthcare facility must retain medical records for at least 10 years after the last date of patient or resident care. Records of minors must be retained until the minor reaches the age of majority plus an additional two years or 10 years—whichever is longer.	ARSD 44:04:09:08 (1995)
	The nursing facility must retain the original resident assessment instrument together with the supporting documentation for at least six years following the date of the assessment.	ARSD 44:04:09:12 (1995)
Tennessee	Healthcare facilities are required to keep medical records as originals or reproductions for 10 years following discharge or death of the patient. In cases involving minors or patients with mental disabilities, the hospital must keep records for the period of disability or minority plus one year, or 10 years following discharge of the patient, whichever is longer.	Tennessee Code Annotated Section 68-11-305(a) (1998)
	Healthcare facilities may retire x-ray film four years after the date of exposure.	Tennessee Code Annotated Section 68-11-305 (b)(1998)
Texas	Hospitals may dispose of medical records on or after the 10th anniversary of the date on which the patient was last treated in the hospital. If the patient was under age 18 when last treated, the hosital may dispose of the records on or after the 20th birthday or on or after the 10th anniversary of the date on which the patient was last treated, whichever is later. The hospital may not destroy medical records that relate to any matter that is involved in litigation if the hospital knows the litigation has not been resolved.	Texas Health and Safety Code Section 241.103 (West 1993)
Utah	Hospitals must retain medical records for seven years after the last date of patient care, or three years after a minor reaches the age of 18, whichever is first.	Utah Admin. R. 432-100-35 (6)(a)
	Intermediate care, nursing care, and mental disease facilities must retain medical records for at least five years after the last date of resident care. The records of minors, including newborns, must be retained for three years after the minor reaches legal age, but in no case less than five years.	Utah Admin. R. 432-149-33 Utah Admin. R. 432-150-27 (2)(c) Utah Admin. R. 432-151-21

Table 4. State Laws or Regulations Pertaining to Retention of Health Information *(continued)*

State	Summary of Law/Regulation	Citation
Utah (continued)	Mental retardation facilities and small healthcare facilities must retain medical records for at least seven years after the last date of client care. Records of minors must be retained at least two years after the minor reaches age 18 or the age of majority, but in no case less than seven years.	Utah Admin. R. 432-152-30 Utah Admin. R. 432-201-28 Utah Admin. R. 432-200-28
	Limited capacity/type N residential healthcare facilities shall retain medical records for at least seven years following discharge.	Utah Admin R. 432-300-10
	Residential healthcare facilities and assisted living facilities must retain resident records for at least three years following discharge.	Utah Admin. R. 432-250-11 Utah Admin. R. 432-270-25 Utah Admin. R. 432-500-21
	Free-standing ambulatory surgical centers shall retain medical records at least seven years after the last date of patient care. Records of minors shall be retained until the minor reaches age 18 or the age of majority plus an additional three years. Birthing centers must retain medical records at least five years after the last date of patient care. Records of minors, including records of newborn infants, shall be retained for three years after the minor reaches legal age under Utah law, but in no case less than five years.	Utah Admin. R. 432-550-22
	Abortion clinics shall retain medical records for at least seven years after the last date of patient care. Records of minors shall be retained until the minor reaches age 18 or the age of majority plus an additional two years, but in no case less than seven years.	Utah Admin. R. 432-600-24
	End stage renal disease facilities must retain medical records at least seven years after the last date of patient care. Records of minors must be retained until the minor reaches the age of majority plus an additional two years, but in no case less than seven years.	Utah Admin. R. 432-650-12
	Hospices must retain medical records at least seven years after the last date of patient care.	Utah Admin. R. 432-750-12
	Home health agencies must retain medical records seven years after the last date of patient care. Records of minors must be retained until the minor reaches the age of majority plus two years, but in no case less than seven years.	Utah Admin. R. 432-700-18
Vermont	Hospitals must maintain medical records for 10 years following patient discharge.	18 VSA Section 1905 (8); 4 CVR 13140019, Section 3-946 (a)(1989)
	Residential care homes must keep residents' records on file for at least seven years after the date of discharge or death of the resident, whichever occurs first.	Residential Care Home Licensing Regs., 4 CVR 13162004, Section 5.11(c)(1993)
	Nursing homes must keep residents' records for at least six years following discharge or death.	State of Vermont Nursing Home Regs., 4 CVR 13140025 (1989)
Virginia	Hospitals and nursing homes must preserve medical records, either as originals or accurate reproductions for a minimum of five years following patient discharge, except for minors. Records of minors must be kept for at least five years after the patient reaches 18 years of age.	Virginia Reg. Regs. Hosp. & Nursing Home Licensure of and Inspection, part II Section 208 and 24.5 (1985)
Washington	Acute care medical records and master patient index (MPI) will be retained as follows: Adult patients: No less than 10 years following most recent discharge. Minors: Three years following the date upon which the minor attained the age of eighteen years or 10 years following the most recent discharge, whichever is longer. Outpatient diagnostic service reports: At least two years. Data in emergency services register: No less than 10 years following most recent discharge or only three years after last entry if hospital includes all outpatient emergency care in the MPI. Data on inpatient and outpatient registers: for at least three years.	Washington Admin. Code Section 248-318-440 RCW 70.41.190
	Physicians: No code addressing retention of records.	
	Behavioral health medical records will be retained a minimum of 10 years following most recent discharge for adults, and for minors, no less than three years following date upon which client obtained age of 18 years or five years following most recent discharge, whichever is longer.	Washington Admin. Code Section 246-322-200
	Substance abuse medical records will be retained 10 years following most recent discharge for adults, and for minors, a minimum of three years following patient's 18th birthday or 10 years following most recent discharge, whichever is longer.	Washington Admin. Code Section 246-322-200
	Rehabilitation medical records will be retained no less than five years following the resident's most recent discharge.	Washington Admin. Code Section 246-325-060

(continued on next page)

Table 4. State Laws or Regulations Pertaining to Retention of Health Information *(continued)*

State	Summary of Law/Regulation	Citation
Washington (continued)	Nursing home medical records will be retained eight years following discharge for adults, and for minors, a minimum of three years following patient's 18th birthday or 10 years following most recent discharge, whichever is longer.	RCW 18.51.300
	Hospice medical records will be retained 10 years following discharge for adults, and for minors, 10 years or until the patient attains age of 21, whichever is longer.	Washington Admin. Code Section 246-321-045
	Home health medical records will be retained three years following date of termination of services for adults and, for minors, no less than three years after attaining age of 18 or five years following discharge, whichever is longer.	Washington Admin. Code Section 246-327-165
West Virginia	Regulations for hospital licensure state that records must be preserved in the original form, microfilm, or electronic data process, without specifying a retention period, implying that retention must be permanent.	West Virginia Acts, tit. 64 West Virginia Leg. Rules, Dept. of Health; Hospital Licensure Series 12 Section 10.3.1, 10.3.1(e)(1987)
Wisconsin	Hospitals must retain medical records at least five years after discharge.	Wisconsin Admin. Code HFS 124.14(2)(c)
	Hospitals must maintain authenticated laboratory reports in the patient's medical record. Duplicate records shall be maintained by the laboratory for at least two years.	Wisconsin Admin. Code HFS 124.17(1)(f)
	Hospitals must keep copies of tracings, reports, printouts, films, scans, and other image records at least five years.	Wisconsin Admin. Code HFS 124.18(1)(e)(4) Wisconsin Statute 146.817
	Skilled nursing/long term care facilities must retain medical records five years following death or discharge. Registers of resident identification, final diagnosis, physician, and dates of admission and discharge shall be kept permanently.	Wisconsin Admin. Code HFS 132.45 (4) (f) (1-5) Wisconsin Admin. Code HFS 132.45 (4)
	Mental health records must be maintained at least seven years after treatment is completed or until minor turns 19, whichever is longer.	Wisconsin Admin. Code Alcohol, Drug Abuse, Developmental Disabilities, and Mental Health Services HFS 92.12 Wisconsin Statute Section 51.01(19)
Wyoming	Hospital administrative and discharge records, diagnoses of operations, operative reports, pathology reports, and discharge summaries must be kept permanently. Nursing histories and care plans must be kept for three years. Facilities must keep emergency care records and outpatient records for 10 years. Other medical records must be maintained for 30 years, then destroyed.	Wyoming State Archives & Historical Dept., Records Disposal Manual for Wyoming, County Hospitals (1987)

Recommendations

- Each healthcare provider should ensure that patient health information is available to meet the needs of continued patient care, legal requirements, research, education, and other legitimate uses

- Each healthcare provider should develop a retention schedule for patient health information that meets the needs of its patients, physicians, researchers, and other legitimate users, and complies with legal, regulatory, and accreditation requirements

- The retention schedule should include guidelines that specify what information should be kept, the time period for which it should be kept, and the storage medium (paper, microfilm, optical disk, magnetic tape, or other)

- Compliance documentation

   — Compliance programs should establish written policies to address the retention of all types of documentation. This documentation includes clinical and medical records, health records, claims documentation, and compliance documentation. Compliance documentation includes all records necessary to protect the integrity of the compliance process and confirm the effectiveness of the program, including employee training documentation, reports from hot lines, results of internal investigations, results of auditing and monitoring, modifications to the compliance program, and self-disclosures

— The documentation should be retained according to applicable federal and state law and regulations and must be maintained for a sufficient length of time to ensure their availability to prove compliance with laws and regulations

— The organization's legal counsel should be consulted regarding the retention of compliance documentation

- The majority of states have specific retention requirements that should be used to establish a facility's retention policy. In the absence of specific state requirements for record retention, providers should keep health information for at least the period specified by the state's statutes of limitations or for a sufficient length of time to prove compliance with laws and regulations. If the patient was a minor, the provider should retain health information until the patient reaches the age of majority (as defined by state law) plus the period of the statute of limitations, unless otherwise provided by state law. A longer retention period is prudent, since the statute may not begin until the potential plaintiff learns of the causal relationship between an injury and the care received. In addition, under the False Claims Act (31 USC 3729), claims may be brought for up to seven years after the incident; however, on occasion, the time has been extended to 10 years

- Unless longer periods of time are required by state or federal law, the American Health Information Management Association recommends that specific patient health information be retained for established minimum time periods. (See Table 1.)

Prepared by

Harry Rhodes, MBA, RHIA, Director of HIM Products and Services

originally prepared by
Donna M. Fletcher, MPA, RRA, HIM practice manager

Acknowledgments

Roberta Aiello

Jennifer Carpenter, RHIA

CSA central office coordinators, executive directors, presidents, and legislative committee officers

Sandra Fuller, MA, RHIA

Margaret Joichi, MLIS

Harry Rhodes, MBA, RHIA

Julie Welch, RHIA

Notes

This practice brief replaces an earlier practice brief published in the January 1997 *Journal of AHIMA*.

Laws addressing health information continue to evolve. Consult with legal counsel regarding recent legislation and/or the advisability of retaining records for longer periods of time.

Prior to disposing of records, review AHIMA's practice brief "Destruction of Patient Health Information," originally published in 1996, updated in the April 2000 *Journal of AHIMA*.

References

Department of Health and Human Services. *Office of Inspector General's Compliance Program Guidance for Hospitals*, February 1998. Available at OIG Releases Compliance Program Guidance for Hospitals.

Legal Issues for School-based Programs Handbook. New York, NY: Legal Action Center, 1996.

Office of the Federal Register. *Guide to Record Retention Requirements in the Code of Federal Regulations*. Washington, DC: National Archives and Records Administration, 1994.

Prophet, Sue. *Health Information Management Compliance: Model Program for Healthcare Organizations*. Chicago, IL: AHIMA, 1998.

Russo, Ruthann. *Seven Steps to HIM Compliance*. Marblehead, MA: Opus Communications, 1998.

Tomes, Jonathan P. *Healthcare Records Manual*. New York, NY: Warren Gorham LaMont, 1994.

Related AHIMA practice briefs:

- Protecting Patient Information After a Facility Closure (March 1999)
- Data Quality Management Model (June 1998)
- Destruction of Patient Health Information (January 1996—Updated April 2000)

Issued June 1999 (Updated June 2002)

Appendix P

Practice Brief—Protecting Patient Information after a Facility Closure (Updated)

Patients trust their healthcare providers to respect their privacy, maintain the confidentiality of their health information, and assure its availability for their continuing care. Providers must be concerned with the protection of health information when healthcare facilities close or medical practices dissolve.

Procedures for disposition of patient records[1] must take several factors into consideration, including:

- state laws regarding record retention and disposal, as well as statutes of limitation
- state licensing standards
- Medicare and Medicaid requirements
- federal laws governing treatment for alcohol and drug abuse (if applicable)
- guidelines issued by professional organizations
- the needs and wishes of patients

In some states, a state archive or health department will store health records from closed facilities. Generally, state regulations recommend records be transferred to another healthcare provider. If a healthcare facility or medical practice is sold to another healthcare provider, patient records may be considered assets and included in the sale of the property. If a facility closes or a practice dissolves without a sale, records should be transferred to another healthcare provider that agrees to accept the responsibility. If this is not feasible, records may be archived with a reputable commercial storage firm. Before records are transferred to an archive or another provider, patients should be notified, if possible, and given an opportunity to obtain copies of their health information. Patients may be notified of the opportunity to obtain copies by publishing a series of notices in the local newspaper. Only copies of the health records should be given to patients unless the required retention period has expired.

Editor's note: This update supplants information contained in the March 1999 and September 1996 practice briefs "Protecting Patient Information after a Facility Closure."

Background

During the course of treatment, patients share private details of their lives with physicians and other healthcare providers. Patients trust their healthcare providers to respect their privacy, maintain the confidentiality of their health information, protect the integrity of the information, and assure its availability for their continuing care. Because of this trust, healthcare providers must be concerned with the protection of health information when facilities close or medical practices dissolve.

Liability Issues

Generally, a healthcare provider remains liable for accidental or incidental disclosure of health information during or after a closure. Therefore, the provider must make appropriate plans to protect the integrity of the records and the confidentiality of the information they contain, while assuring access for continued patient care. State laws and regulations addressing facility or practice closure should be followed. These are usually available from the state department of health. If state laws and regulations are silent on how to proceed, the provider should consider several other factors, as outlined below.

Retention Issues

State Laws/Licensure Requirements

A provider is bound by applicable federal and state laws and regulations after closure, as well as during its operation. Many state health departments and licensing authorities govern healthcare facility closures and may outline to whom records should be transferred. In some states, a state archive or health department will store health records from closed facilities. More commonly, state regulations recommend records be transferred to another healthcare provider.

If records cannot be transferred to a state archive or state health department, the state's requirements for record retention for both adult and minor patients should be reviewed before a policy is formulated. *(Note: Many states require approval from the state department of health or licensing authority before any plan is implemented.)*

To minimize storage and/or transfer costs, the provider may wish to destroy records that are past the period of required retention. For example, if state law requires that records be retained for 10 years after the patient's last encounter, records that are more than 10 years old could be destroyed. If state law does not specify the length of time records must be kept, the provider must consider the state's malpractice statute of limitations for both adults and minors and assure that records are maintained for at least the period of time specified by the state's statutes of limitations. A longer retention period is prudent, since the statute may not begin to run until the potential plaintiff learns of the causal relation between an injury and the care received. If the patient was a minor, the provider should retain health information until the patient reaches the age of majority (as defined by state law) plus the period of the statute of limitations, unless otherwise provided by state law.

The provider should also contact its malpractice insurance carrier. Both the provider and the carrier must have access to patient records after the closure in the event a malpractice claim is filed.

Medicare Requirements

If the provider participates in the Medicare program, records must be kept in their original or legally reproduced form for at least five years from the date of the settlement of the claim to comply with the Medicare Conditions of Participation. Skilled Nursing Facilities and Home Care Agencies must retain their records for five years after the month the cost report was filed. (For example: Cost report for 1998 was submitted on 01/15/99 the records must be retained until 02/01/04.)

Federal Regulations re: Alcohol and Drug Abuse Treatment

If the provider has offered services pertaining to alcohol and/or drug abuse education, training, treatment, rehabilitation, or research, disposition of these records must meet requirements outlined by federal law.[2] When a program discontinues operations or is acquired by another program, this law requires the patient's written authorization for records to be transferred to the acquiring program or any other program named in the patient's authorization. If records are required by law to be kept for a specified period which does not expire until after the discontinuation or acquisition of the program and the patient has not authorized transfer of the records, these records must be sealed in envelopes or other containers and labeled as follows:

> "Records of [insert name of program] required to be maintained pursuant to [insert citation to law or regulation requiring that records be kept] until a date not later than December 31, [insert appropriate year]."

Records marked and sealed as prescribed may be held by any lawful custodian, but the custodian must follow the procedures outlined by law for disclosure. If the patient does not authorize transfer of his records to another program, they may be destroyed after the required retention period.

Recommendations from Professional Organizations

Professional organizations should be contacted for guidelines or recommendations. Such professional organizations may include local or state:

- health information management associations
- hospital associations
- medical societies

Physicians who are closing their practices may wish to contact the American Medical Association and their state licensure board for guidance.

Legal Advice

Advice from legal counsel should be sought to determine the appropriate retention period, assure compliance with state laws and regulatory agencies, and help plan for an orderly closure or transfer.

Budgeting for a Closure

Regardless of which plan of action your facility institutes to deal with the patient records, resources will need to be allocated to carry out the plan. Some of the resources that need to be budgeted for include:

- labor

- copy equipment and supplies

- postage

- telephone

- utilities

- storage boxes and supplies

- transportation costs (to storage unit)

- storage and retrieval costs for required retention period

Recommendations

As soon as a healthcare provider anticipates a facility closure or dissolution of a medical practice, the provider should begin planning for proper disposition of patient health records. The primary objective is to assure future access by patients, future healthcare providers, and other legitimate users.

The second objective should be to protect the confidentiality of the information contained in the records.

To ensure accurate information for continuing care, all health information documentation must be completed before the records are archived. This includes transcription of all dictated reports and interpretation of any diagnostic tests.

Before records are transferred to an archive or another provider, patients should be notified, if possible, and given an opportunity to obtain copies of their records. Letters and or e-mail messages may be sent to former patients, or announcements may be repeated in local newspapers and professional journals to notify patients and their physicians about the upcoming closure/practice dissolution and let them know how to access their information.

Patients should be given a reasonable amount of time (at least one month, unless a longer time period is required by state law) to request copies of their records.

Elements to consider including in the letter and/or e-mail to the patient are as follows:

- the date the facility will close

- notification of where the records will be stored and how to access them

- a release of information authorization form to be completed to receive a copy of their medical record

- notification that only written requests for copies of health information will be honored

- notification of any time limitations (submission deadlines) on the period of time during which requests will be accepted

- instructions on how to seek a new healthcare provider

The custodian of the retained records should retain a copy of the actual letter and/or e-mail sent to patients, along with the mailing list, broadcast e-mail list, post office receipt, all returned (undeliverable) envelopes, and a list of returned or undeliverable e-mails.

If the records pertain to treatment for alcohol and/or drug abuse, specific federal regulations[3] must be followed.

Closure/Dissolution with a Sale

If a healthcare facility or medical practice is sold to another healthcare provider, patient records may be considered assets and included in the sale of the property. As part of the agreement, the original provider who created the records should retain the right to access the records and obtain copies, if needed, from the new owners. In addition, if the new owner considers a sale to a third party, the original provider should retain the right to reclaim the patient records.

If the facility or medical practice is sold to a non-healthcare entity, patient records should not be included in the assets available for purchase. The provider should make arrangements to either transfer the records to an archive or another provider who agrees to accept responsibility for maintaining them.

Closure/Dissolution without a Sale

If a facility closes or a practice dissolves without a sale, arrangements should be made with another healthcare provider where patients may seek future care, unless otherwise required by state law. That provider should agree to maintain the records, permit access by authorized persons, and destroy the records when applicable time periods have expired.

Health information management professionals at the receiving facility should be familiar with record retention and destruction requirements and confidentiality concerns and have systems in place to allow patients and other legitimate users access to the information. Prior to transferring the records, a written agreement outlining terms and obligations should be executed. The original provider is responsible for assuring that records are stored safely for an appropriate length of time.

If transfer to another provider is not feasible, records may be archived with a reputable commercial storage firm. Such a firm should be considered only if it:

- has experience in handling confidential patient information

- guarantees the security and confidentiality of the records

- assures that patients and other legitimate requestors will have access to the information

If a storage firm is used, specific provisions should be negotiated and included in the written agreement. Such provisions include but are not limited to:

- agreement to keep all information confidential, disclosing only to authorized representatives of the provider or upon written authorization from the patient/legal representative

- prompt return of all embodiments of confidential information without retaining copies thereof upon the provider's request

- prohibition against selling, sharing, discussing, assigning, transferring, or otherwise disclosing confidential information with any other individuals or business entities

- prohibition against use of confidential information for any purpose other than providing mutually agreed upon services

- agreement to protect information against theft, loss, unauthorized destruction, or other unauthorized access

- return or destruction of information at the end of the mutually agreed upon retention period

- assurance that providers, patients, and other legitimate users will have access to the information

Providers may consider giving original records directly to patients, but only copies should be given to patients unless the required retention period has expired. During the required retention period, the provider may need access to the original records for the provider's own business reasons.

Regardless of the archival method used, the provider must assure that the integrity and confidentiality of the patient health records will be maintained and that the records are accessible to the patient and other legitimate users.

Acknowledgements

Assistance from the following individuals on this update is gratefully acknowledged:

Mary D. Brandt, MBA, RHIA, CHE, CHP

Jill Burrington-Brown, MS, RHIA

Alane Combs, RHIA

Michelle Dougherty, RHIA

Sue Gentilli, RHIA

Reesa Gottschalk, RHIA

Beth Hjort, RHIA, CHP

Sherri Hutchins, RHIA

Carol Quinsey, RHIA

Tracey Stanich Witherow, RHIA

Special thanks to KelliSue Montague, AHIMA executive assistant, and to all AHIMA component state associations.

Updated by

Harry Rhodes, MBA, RHIA, CHP

Originally prepared by

Mary D. Brandt, MBA, RHIA, CHE, CHP
Harry Rhodes, MBA, RHIA, CHP

Notes

1. Patient records may include paper, microfilm, optical storage, or computer-based health information, diagnostic images (such as radiology films, nuclear medicine scans, and cineangiography films), fetal monitor recordings, videotaped operative procedures, and information stored on other media.

2. *Code of Federal Regulations* 42 CFR Ch. 1 (10-1-85). [42 CFR Part 2 Subpart B, Paragraph 2.19].

3. *Ibid.*

References

American Hospital Association. *Guidelines for Managing Hospital Closures*. Report of the Ad Hoc Committee for Hospital Closures. Chicago, IL: 1990.

Centers for Medicare and Medicaid Services. Medicare/Medicaid State Operations Manual. Appendix A. *Hospitals Interpretive Guidelines and Survey Procedure*. Springfield, VA: US Department of Commerce, 1995.

Jaklevic, Mary Chris. "Hospital Closures Open Opportunities." *Modern Healthcare* 30, no. 48 (2000): 34–38.

Jaklevic, Mary Chris. "Trouble in the City." *Modern Healthcare* 31, no. 2 (2001): 52.

Lillie, Celine M. "Legal Issues in Closing a Medical Record Department," *Journal of AHIMA* 64, no. 5 (1993): 28–29.

Murer, Cherilyn, Murer, Michael, and Brick, Lyndean Lenhoff. *The Complete Legal Guide to Healthcare Records Management*. New York, NY: McGraw-Hill, 1999.

Tomes, Jonathan P. *Healthcare Records: A Practical Legal Guide*. Dubuque, IA: Kendall Hunt Publishing Company for the Healthcare Financial Management Association, 1990.

Tomes, Jonathan P. *Healthcare Records Manual*. Boston, MA: Warren Gorham Lamont, 1993.

Woodcock, Elizabeth. "Plan Ahead for a Smooth Closure of Your Practice." *American Medical News* 39, no. 28 (1996): 16.

Exhibit 1. States with Laws/Regulations/Guidelines Pertaining to Facility Closure

State	Summary of Law/Regulation	Citation
Alabama	When a hospital ceases to operate, either voluntarily or by revocation of its license, the governing body (licensee) at or prior to such action shall develop a proposed plan for the disposition of its medical records. Such plan shall be submitted for review and approval to the Division of Licensure and Certification and shall contain provision for the proper storage, safe-guarding and confidentiality, transfer, and/or dis-posal of patient medical records and x-ray files. Any center that fails to develop such plans for disposition of its records acceptable to the Division of Licensure and Certification shall dispose of its records as directed by a court or appropriate jurisdiction.	Rule 420-5-7.10 (1) Hospitals; Rule 420-5-5-.02 (7) (h) End Stage Renal Disease Treatment & Transplant Centers; Rule 420-5-2-.02 (6) (h) Ambulatory Surgical Treatment Facilities; Rule 420-5-1.02 (5) (f) Abortion and Reproductive Health Centers; Rule 420-5-18-.06 (9) Sleep Disorders Facilities
Alaska	When a hospital ceases to operate, a plan approved by the Department of Health and Social Services will outline arrangements for the immediate preservation of its records. Healthcare providers of Medicaid recipients must notify the department. Instructions will be provided by the department as to the disposition of Medicaid records. Nursing homes that cease to operate must contact the department for direction on disposition of their admission and death records.	Alaska Statutes 18.20.085 (c) 7 AAC 43.030 7 AAC 12.040(I) (2)
Arizona	If a hospital discontinues hospital services, the Department is notified in writing, not less than 30 days before hospital services are discontinued, of the location where the medical records are stored.	Arizona Administrative Code R9-10-228
Arkansas	All medical records shall be retained in either the original or microfilm or other acceptable methods for 10 years after the last discharge. After 10 years, a medical record may be destroyed provided the facility permanently maintains the information contained in the master patient index. Complete medical records of minors shall be retained for a period of two years after the age of majority. Should a facility close, the medical records shall be stored for the required retention period and shall be accessible for patient use.	Rules & Regulations for Hospitals and Related Institutions in Arkansas: Section 14: 20-21
California	Within 48 hours of ceasing to operate, the facility must notify the Department of Health of its plan for the safe preservation of medical records. Should the facility change ownership, written documentation must be provided by both the old and new licensee outlining the arrangements made for transfer of medical record custody, safe preservation of the records, and access to the information by both the new and old licensees and other authorized individuals.	Title 22, section 70751 (d) Title 22, section 70751 (e)
Colorado	When a facility closes, arrangements must be made for transfer of the medical records to a new custodian. A written memorandum of understanding or contract shall be signed by the new custodian outlining the date, location, and receipt of transfer. The written agreement will transfer responsibility for the retention and maintenance to the new custodian. If a willing custodian cannot be obtained, the facility must contact the local health department or other appropriate local government so temporary storage may be arranged. Public notice should be provided through the newspaper or general news release. Authorized parties should be given the opportunity to assume identified records.	Guidelines from Colorado Hospital Association, *Consent Manual and Guidelines for Release of Health Information,* 1996
Connecticut	A practitioner or agency should be aware of the specific requirements as to the existence and contents of the medical record and at least the legal requirement for retention of the record. The retention period applies even if the agency or individual ceases to operate.	Guideline from Connecticut Health Information Management Association
Delaware	No regulation within Delaware code.	
Florida	Facilities involved in an acquisition, merger, or closing should maintain records in accordance with state law. In a merger, the new facility should merge the old entity's active records with its records and prepare a retention schedule for the inactive records. The merger agreement should include a provision detailing who is responsible for records. Florida General Records Schedule for Hospital Records requires facilities to submit a records destruction request, form LS5E107, and obtain permission from the licensing agency before proceeding with a record destruction. Florida Administrative Code requires a licensee to notify the department of impending closure 90 days before the closure. The facility must advise the licensing agency as to the disposition of medical records.	Florida Administrative Code 59A-1.004
Hawaii	Before a healthcare provider ceases operations, immediate arrangements approved by the Department of Health shall be made to ensure the retention and preservation of its patient records. In an acquisition or merger, the succeeding providers are liable for preservation of basic information from the medical records in accordance with state law.	Title 33, section 622-58 (e)

Exhibit 1. States with Laws/Regulations/Guidelines Pertaining to Facility Closure *(continued)*

State	Summary of Law/Regulation	Citation
Idaho	Facilities should adhere to Idaho code and Idaho Practice Acts regarding maintenance and retention of patient information when a facility closes.	Idaho code 39-13941.C IDAPA 16.03.0220304b IDAPA 116.03.14360
Illinois	The licensee shall notify the Department of Public Health of the impending closure of the hospital at least 90 days prior to such closure. The hospital shall implement a policy for the preservation of patient medical records and medical staff credentialing files.	77 Illinois Administrative Code, Chapter I Section 250.120 (b), 250.1510 (e) (2), and 250.310 (a) (16)
Indiana	Upon closure, the facility must transfer the medical records (preferably in microfilmed format) to a local public health department or public hospital in the same geographic area. If the records cannot be transferred to a public health department or public hospital in the same geographic area, the records should be sent to the Board of Health.	Hospital Licensure Rules of the Indiana State Board of Health 410 IAC 15-1-9 (2)
Iowa	When a facility closes or transfers ownership, all active patients should be notified and given an opportunity to obtain copies of their records. In addition to individual notices to patients, a public notice is generally published in the newspaper of general circulation advising patients and physicians of the location of the facility's medical records and how access may be gained to them. The facility is liable for preserving the confidentiality and security of the records until ownership is assumed by another or the required retention period has expired.	Guidelines from Iowa Health Information Management Association's *Guide to Medical Record Laws,* 2001
Kansas	If a hospital discontinues operation, the hospital shall inform the licensing agency of the location of its records. A summary shall be maintained of medical records that are destroyed. This summary shall be retained on file for at least 25 years and shall include the following information: (A) the name, age and date of birth of the patient; (B) the name of the patient's nearest relative; (C) the name of the attending and consulting practitioners; (D) any surgical procedure and date, if applicable; and (E) the final diagnosis	Kansas Regulations 28-34-9a (d) (2) (3)
Kentucky	Provisions shall be made for written designation of the specific location for storage of medical records in the event the hospital ceases to operate because of disaster or for any other reason. It shall be the responsibility of the hospital to safeguard both the record and its informational content against loss, defacement, and tampering. Particular attention shall be given to protection from damage by fire and or water.	Kentucky Administrative Regulations 902 KAR 20:016 Section 3 (11) 3
Louisiana	The secretary of the Department of Health and Human Resources shall adopt rules, regulations, and minimum standards providing for the disposition of patients' medical records upon closure of a hospital. Such regulations may require submission by a hospital that is closing of a plan for disposition of patients' medical records to the secretary for approval.	Louisiana Health and Human Resources Administration Acts La, RS 40; 2109 E
Maine	No statutes exist relating to closure.	
Maryland	Should a physician practice expire, his/her representative must send a notice to the patient at the patient's last address. A notice should be published in a daily newspaper that is circulated locally for 2 consecutive weeks. Information should state the starting date the records will be transferred or destroyed and a location, date and time where medical records may be retrieved, if wanted. Only home health agencies are required by state regulations to retain medical records after the agency closes.	Code of Maryland Regulations Subtitle 4. Personal Medical Records, 4 — 403 Destruction of Records
Massachusetts	Should the ownership of a hospital, an institution for unwed mothers, or a clinic change, the new owner must maintain all medical records from the purchased facility. Should an institution permanently close, the institution will arrange for preservation of such medical records for the 30-year retention period. The facility/physician must also inform the state of the location and availability of these records.	Massachusetts Statutes 111, section 70
Minnesota	No specific statutes or regulations exist to address disposition of medical records at the time of a facility or practice closure. Statutes require hospitals to permanently retain those portions of medical records as defined by the Commissioner of Health. Physicians have a professional responsibility for the proper management of medical records, including disposition at the time of a practice closure.	Minnesota Statutes 145.30, 145.32, and 147.091 Minnesota Rule 4642.1000

(continued on next page)

Exhibit 1. **States with Laws/Regulations/Guidelines Pertaining to Facility Closure** *(continued)*

State	Summary of Law/Regulation	Citation
Mississippi	When a facility closes, it must turn over its records to any other hospital or hospitals in the vicinity that is willing to accept and retain the medical records. If no facility is available or willing to accept the medical records, then they will be promptly delivered to the licensing agency.	Mississippi Code, section 41-9-79
Missouri	New operators of nursing, convalescent, and boarding homes are required to retain the original records of residents.	Section 198.052
Montana	Montana does not have specific legislation that addresses retention of medical records upon facility closure.	
Nebraska	**Centers for the developmentally disabled:** In cases in which a center for the developmentally disabled ceases operation, all records of residents shall be transferred to the facility to which the resident moves; all other records of such center for developmentally disabled, if not specifically governed by the provisions of these regulations, shall be disposed of in accordance with center policy so long as the resident's rights of confidentiality are not violated.	Title 175, Chapter 3, 005.04A
	Assisted living facilities: When an assisted living facility ceases operation, all resident records must be transferred to the licensed healthcare facility or healthcare service to which the resident is transferred. All other resident records that have not reached the required time for destruction must be stored to assure confidentiality and the Department must be notified of the address where stored.	Title 175, Chapter 4, 4-006.12A2
	Health clinics: When a health clinic ceases operation, all medical records must be transferred as directed by the patient or authorized representative to the licensed healthcare facility or healthcare service to which the patient is transferred. All other medical records that have not reached the required time for destruction must be stored to assure confidentiality and the Department must be notified of the address where stored.	Title 175, Chapter 7, 7-006.07A3
	Hospitals: In cases in which a hospital ceases operation, all medical records of patients must be transferred as directed by the patient or authorized representative to the hospital or other healthcare facility or healthcare service to which the patient is transferred. All other medical records that have not reached the required time for destruction must be stored to assure confidentiality and the Department must be notified of the address where stored.	Title 175, Chapter 9, 9-006.07A5
	Skilled nursing facilities, nursing facilities, and intermediate care facilities: In cases in which a facility ceases operation, all records of each resident must be transferred to the healthcare facility to which the resident moves. All other resident records of a facility ceasing operation must be disposed of by shredding, burning, or other similar protective measures in order to preserve the resident's rights of confidentiality. Records or documentation of the actual fact of resident medical record destruction must be permanently maintained.	Title 175, Chapter 12, 12-006.16D
	Hospice services: Policies provide for retention even if the hospice discontinues operation.	Title 175, Chapter 16, 16-006.12D
	Substance abuse treatment centers: Prior to the dissolution of any facility, the administrator must notify the Department in writing as to the location and storage of client records.	Title 175, Chapter 18, 18-006.16B5
	Mental health centers: Prior to the dissolution of any facility, the administrator must notify the Department in writing as to the location and storage of client records.	Title 175, Chapter 19, 19-006.18B5
New Hampshire	Should an outpatient clinic, residential treatment and rehabilitation facility, or home health service cease operation, the safe preservation of the clinical records must be provided for.	Administrative Regulations He-P 806.10, He-P 807.07, and He-P 809.07
New Jersey	Before closing, the hospital's governing authority must submit a plan for record storage and service to the Department of Health.	Section 8: Section 10 NCASC 34B-7.4 (b)
New Mexico	No statutes exist relating to closure.	
New York	Retirement/death of physician and/or sale of practice: a. When physician retires, sells his/her practice, or dies, patients should be notified (usually by newspaper advertisement)—but NYS law does not mandate patient notification at this time. b. Patients may request copies sent to another physician for continued care-reasonable charges may apply. [Not recommended that original record be forwarded for legal reasons.]	NYS CRR 405.10

Exhibit 1.   States with Laws/Regulations/Guidelines Pertaining to Facility Closure *(continued)*

State	Summary of Law/Regulation	Citation
New York (continued)	c. Retired/deceased physician: arrangements should be made to have original records retained by another physician, local hospital, or other lawfully permitted agency. d. If practice is sold: ownership of records should be part of sales agreement. Physician purchasing must establish physician/patient relationship prior to accessing records or must obtain patient authorization. Area hospital/appropriate medical society should know disposition of the physician records.	
North Carolina	Hospitals: If a hospital discontinues operation, its management shall make known to the Division where its records are stored. Records are to be stored in a business offering retrieval services for at least 11 years after the closure date. Prior to destruction, public notice shall be made to permit former patients or their representatives to claim their own records. Public notice shall be in at least two forms: written notice to the former patient or their representative and display of an advertisement in a newspaper of general circulation in the area of the facility.	T10: 03C. 3903—Hospitals
	Nursing homes: (c) If a facility discontinues operation, the licensee shall make known to the division of facility services where its records are stored. Records are to be stored in a business offering retrieval services for at least 11 years after the closure date.	T10: 03H .2400—Nursing Homes
North Dakota	North Dakota hospital licensing rules require that if a hospital discontinues operation, it shall make known to the department where its records are stored. Records are to be stored in a facility offering retrieval services for at least 10 years after the closure date. Prior to destruction, public notice must be made to permit former patients or their representatives to claim their own records. Public notice must be in at least two forms, legal notice and display advertisement in a newspaper of general circulation.	North Dakota Administrative Code, section 33-07-01.1-20 (1994)
Ohio	Upon closure of a nursing home, the operator shall provide for and arrange for the retention of records and reports in a secured manner for not less than seven years. Presently, Ohio statutes do not specifically address physicians'/hospitals' responsibilities regarding the retention of medical records or procedures for transfer of such records. For physicians, American Medical Association Council of Ethical and Judicial Affairs Current Opinion 7.04 states that the physician must ensure that all medical records are transferred to another physician or entity who is held to the same standards of confidentiality and is lawfully permitted to act as the custodian of the records. The Current Opinion states further that all active patients should be notified that the physician is transferring the records and that upon the patient's written request, within a reasonable time as specified in the notice, and at a reasonable cost, the records (or copies) may be transferred to the physician or entity of the patient's choice. Legal briefs from the Ohio State Medical Association, "Medical Practice Retention and Transfer of Records" and "Medical & Billing Records: Privacy and Patient Rights," offer further guidance.	OAC 3701-17-19 (C) (1) (c)
Oklahoma	In the event of closure of a hospital, the hospital shall inform the Department of Health of the disposition of the records. Disposition shall be in a manner to protect the integrity of the information contained in the medical record. These records shall be retained and disposed of in a manner consistent with the statute of limitations.	Oklahoma Hospital Standards 310:667-19-14 (b) (4)
Oregon	If a subject healthcare facility changes ownership, all medical records in original, electronic, or microfilm form shall remain in the hospital or related institution, and it shall be the responsibility of the new owner to protect and maintain these records. If any subject healthcare facility shall be finally closed, its medical records and the registers may be delivered and turned over to any other hospital or hospitals in the vicinity willing to accept and retain the same. A hospital which closes permanently shall follow the procedure for Division and public notice regarding disposal of medical records delineated under 333-500-0060. If the hospital voluntarily discontinues operation, a multimedia press release must be initiated by the hospital, within 24 hours, notifying the public of facility closure. Such notice shall include procedure by which individuals may obtain their medical records. In addition, notification of facility closure and plan for disposal of medical records must be given to the Division.	Oregon Administrative Rules 333-70-055(13) (14) Rule 333-500-0060

(continued on next page)

Exhibit 1. States with Laws/Regulations/Guidelines Pertaining to Facility Closure *(continued)*

State	Summary of Law/Regulation	Citation
Oregon (continued)	Medical records not claimed that are beyond seven years of the last date of discharge may be destroyed. Medical records not claimed that are within seven days of the last date of discharge must be stored until they are seven years past the last date of discharge. These medical records may be thinned to include only the admission/discharge sheet (face sheet), discharge summary, history and physical, operative report(s), pathology report(s), and x-ray report(s).	
Pennsylvania	The Department of Health must be informed of the location of the stored records for the closed hospital. The storage facility chosen must provide retrieval services for five years after the closure. No records can be destroyed until after public notice, in the form of both legal notice and display advertisement, is placed in a newspaper of general circulation. Former patients or their representatives must be provided the opportunity to claim their records prior to destruction.	28 Pennsylvania Statutes, section 115.24
South Carolina	South Carolina Department of Health and Environmental Control regulations specify that hospitals and institutional general infirmaries must transfer ownership of all medical records to the new owners if the facility is sold. The facility will make arrangements for the preservation of the medical records after a closure. The department will be notified of the arrangements made to preserve the records.	Regulation 61-16 section 601.7D, Regulation 61-14 section 504.3, Regulation 61-17, Regulation 61-13
South Dakota	When a healthcare facility ceases operation, the facility must provide for safe storage and prompt retrieval of medical records and the patient indexes specified in ARSD 44:04:09:10. The healthcare facility may arrange storage of medical records with another healthcare facility of the same licensure classification, transfer medical records to another healthcare provider at the request of the patient, relinquish medical records to the patient or his parent or legal guardian, or arrange storage of remaining medical records with a third-party vendor who undertakes a storage activity.\n\nAt least 30 days before closure, the healthcare facility must notify the department (of health) in writing indicating the provisions for safe preservation of the medical records and their location and publish in the local newspaper the location and disposition arrangements of the medical record.\n\nIf the ownership of a healthcare facility is transferred, the new owner shall maintain the medical records as if there was not a change in ownership.	ARSD 44:04:09:10-11, Disposition of Medical Records Upon Closure of Facility or Transfer of Ownership
Tennessee	Should a hospital close, it must surrender the hospital records to the Department of Health and Environment. The facility must deliver the records to the department in good order and properly indexed.	Tennessee Code section 68-11-308
Texas	The licensing agency shall be notified by the closing facility of the identity of the record custodian and the location of the stored records. Should a special facility change ownership, the new owners must maintain proof of medical information required for the continued care of the residents.	Texas Hospital Licensing Standards 1-22.1.6 and 12-8.7.6
Utah	A licensee that voluntarily ceases operation shall complete the following:\n\n(a) notify the Department and the patients or their next of kin at least 30 days before the effective date of closure.\n(b) make provision for the safekeeping of records.\n\nIf a hospital ceases operation, the hospital shall make provision for secure, safe storage and prompt retrieval of all medical records, patient indexes and discharges for the period specified in R432-100-33(4)(c). The hospital may arrange for storage of medical records with another hospital, or an approved medical record storage facility, or may return patient medical records to the attending physician if the physician is still in the community.	UT Admin Code R432-2-14 General Licensing Provisions\n\nUT Admin Code R432-100-33 (4) (e) General Hospital Standards
Vermont	No statutes exist relating to closure.	
Virginia	Virginia has no regulations that address hospital closure, but nursing home closure is addressed in its Rules and Regulations for the Licensure of Nursing Homes. At closure the owners shall make provisions for the safeguarding of all medical records. Should the facility change ownership, provisions will be made for the orderly transfer of all medical records.	Rules and Regulations for the Licensure of Nursing Homes 24.7

Exhibit 1.   States with Laws/Regulations/Guidelines Pertaining to Facility Closure *(continued)*

State	Summary of Law/Regulation	Citation
Washington	When a hospital closes, it shall make arrangements for the preservation of its records in accordance with applicable state statutes and regulations. Any plan of action must first be approved by the Department of Social and Health Services. If a hospital changes ownership, the medical records, indexes, and analysis of hospital services are not to be removed from the facility and will be retained and preserved by the new owners in accordance with applicable state statutes and regulations.	Title 70 Revised Code of Washington section 70.411.90 and section 248-18-440
Wisconsin	When an independent health practitioner ceases practice or business as a healthcare provider, the healthcare provider or the personal representative of the deceased healthcare provider shall do one of the following for all patient health records: 1. Provide for the maintenance of the patient health records by a person who states, in writing, that the records will be maintained in accordance with state statutes. 2. Provide for the deletion or destruction of all or part of the patient health records. 3. Provide for maintaining some of the records and deleting or destroying some of the records. If maintaining the records, statute requires notice to be made to the patients by one of the following methods: 1. Written notice sent by first-class mail to the patient's last known address, describing where and by whom the records will be maintained. 2. Publication of a class 3 notice in a newspaper located in the county where the healthcare provider's practice was located, describing where and by whom the records will be maintained. If deleting or destroying the records, a required notice is made to the patients by one of the following methods: 1. Written notice at least 35 days prior to destroying the records, sent via first-class mail to the patient's last known address, and it must include the following: • The date when the records will be deleted or destroyed • The location, dates, and times when the records can be retrieved by the patient or their authorized representative 2. Publication of a class 3 notice in the newspaper in the county where the healthcare provider's practice was located. Must specify the date the records will be destroyed unless the records are retrieved from a particular location and by what date. This statute only applies to independent practitioners who cease practice or who die; it does not apply to residential facilities, nursing homes, hospitals, home health agencies, tuberculosis sanitariums, hospices, or local health departments.	Wisconsin Statute 146-819
Wyoming	When a publicly funded hospital or nursing home ceases operation, the records are to be transferred to the state archives. The state archives will maintain the records and abide by the established records retention schedules adopted for these institutions, destroying or maintaining the records and providing access to them.	Wyoming Statutes 9-2-401 through 9-2-419, and specifically W.S. 9-2-408.

Note: State laws addressing facility closure continue to evolve. If your state is not listed, please check with your state licensing authority.

Source: Rhodes, Harry, and Mary D. Brandt. "AHIMA Practice Brief: Protecting Patient Information after a Facility Closure" (Updated November 2003)

Appendix Q

Records Necessary for Travel

Centers for Disease Control—Travel Information

The key resource for health information related to travel is the Travelers' Health page of the Centers for Disease Control (CDC) Web site at http://www.cdc.gov/travel.

Some of the key areas discussed on the CDC Travel Information site are:

- Destinations: Health information for specific destinations
- Vaccinations
- Diseases
- Mosquito and tick protection
- Safe food and water
- Illness and injury abroad
- Travel medicine clinics
- Avian influenza and travel
- FAQs
- Traveling with children
- Special needs travelers
- Travel health tips for students studying abroad
- Traveling with pets

Healthcare Tips for Traveling Abroad

What You Need to Know in Advance of Travel

All travelers should familiarize themselves with conditions at their destination that could affect their health (high altitude or pollution, types of medical facilities, required immunizations, availability of required pharmaceuticals, and so on.).

Insurance, Medicare and Medicaid, Medical Evacuation

Obtaining medical treatment and hospital care abroad can be expensive, and medical evacuation to the United States can cost more than $50,000. Note that U.S. medical insurance is generally not accepted outside the United States, and the Social Security Medicare and Medicaid programs do not provide coverage for hospital or medical costs outside the United States.

If your insurance policy does not cover you abroad, it is a good idea to consider purchasing a short-term policy that does. Health insurance policies designed specifically to cover travel exist; many travel agents and private companies offer insurance plans that will cover health care expenses incurred overseas including emergency services such as medical evacuations.

Bringing Medications or Filling Prescriptions Abroad

A traveler with a preexisting medical problem who is traveling abroad should carry a letter from his or her attending physician that describes the medical condition and any prescription medications, including the generic names of prescribed drugs. Any medications being carried overseas should be left in their original containers and be clearly labeled. Travelers should check with the foreign embassy of the country they are visiting to make sure any required medications are not considered to be illegal narcotics.

If you wear eyeglasses, take an extra pair with you. Pack medicines and extra eyeglasses in your hand luggage so they will be available in case your checked luggage is lost. To be extra secure, pack a backup supply of medicines and an additional pair of eyeglasses in your checked luggage.

If you have allergies, reactions to certain medications, foods, or insect bites, or other unique medical problems, you should consider wearing a "medical alert" bracelet. You may also wish to carry a letter from your physician explaining required treatment should you become ill.

Traveling Abroad with Your Pet

If you are flying to a foreign country or Hawaii, be sure to find out whether your destination requires quarantines or other health requirements. For example, rules in the United Kingdom are very strict. It is essential to comply with such requirements. A full-service travel agency or pet travel service should be able to provide you with this information. You should also contact the appropriate embassy or consulate at least four weeks before the trip to verify these requirements; most countries have Web sites that can provide information about pet travel requirements, or you can find them through the http://www.aphis.usda.gov/lpa/news/2003/05/travelingpets.html. You are ultimately responsible for the required documentation that will allow your pet to complete its trip which will include the pet's medical history.

At the end of this appendix is a form that can be used to carry essential personal health information with you as you travel.

Traveling in the United States

As you travel for business or pleasure, make sure you bring along some of your health information so that you are prepared in case an event occurs that may affect your health.

Necessary information:

- Emergency contact information
- Current medications—prescription and over the counter (OTC)
- Current medical conditions
- Allergies
- Treating physician's contact information

Optional information:

- Previous conditions
- Family history

Methods to carry information:

- Access through Web site
- Portable USB drive
- Paper (for example, in a three-ring binder)
- Card in wallet

At the end of this appendix is a form that can be used to carry essential personal health information with you as you travel.

Traveler's Personal Health Record Form

The form presented here (and available on the CD that accompanies this book) can be used to carry essential personal health information with you as you travel.

TRAVELER'S PERSONAL HEALTH RECORD

Traveler's Name: _____
                Last   First   Middle

Date of Birth: ___/___/_____ **Gender:** Male ☐ Female ☐ **Weight** : _____kilos
                (mm/dd/yyyy)   *(divide pounds by 2.2)*

INSURANCE INFORMATION *(check with the insurance company to make sure it covers care abroad)*

Primary Health Insurance Carrier   Secondary Health Insurance Carrier

Name of Insured _____   Name of Insured: _____

Insurance Company _____   Insurance Company _____

Phone (___) _____   Phone (___) _____

Policy # _____ Group # _____   Policy # _____ Group # _____

PHYSICIAN INFORMATION

Primary Care Physician: _____

          Phone: (___)_____ Exchange: (___)_____

Other physician: _____

          Phone: (___)_____ Exchange: (___)_____

ALLERGIES *(Food, medication, environmental, other)*

Type of Allergy	Typical Reaction	Treatment

MEDICAL CONDITIONS CURRENTLY BEING TREATED

Condition	Date of Onset	Treatment	Treating Physician

CURRENT PRESCRIPTION MEDICATIONS

Medication	Dose	Frequency	Reason for Taking	Prescribing Physician

© 2008, Department of Health Informatics & Information Management, Saint Louis University

Traveler's Name: _____

OTHER NONPRESCRIPTION MEDICATIONS

Medication	Dose	Frequency	Reason for Taking

EMERGENCY CONTACTS

NAME	RELATIONSHIP TO TRAVELER	WORK PHONE #	HOME PHONE #	MOBILE PHONE #

IMMUNIZATIONS

Up-to-date per the regulations required by the State. ☐ Yes   ☐ No

In accordance with the recommendations by the Centers for Disease Control and Prevention and your physician if traveling outside the U.S.   ☐ Yes   ☐ No

ANCILLARY AIDS   ☐ Retainer   ☐ Glasses   ☐ Contact lenses   ☐ Glucose meter   ☐ Insulin pump   ☐ Inhaler

DIETARY RESTRICTIONS/NEEDS

Food	Amount Allowed	Reason

PHYSICAL RESTRICTIONS/NEEDS

Restriction	Activity Allowed	Reason

Other necessary information/special needs

The information contained here is accurate as of today, _____ / _____ / _____

Form completed by: _____
                         Name   Relationship to traveler

2

Source: Department of Health Informatics & Information Management, Saint Louis University.
Reprinted with permission.

Appendix R

HIM in Physician Practice Job Description

General Purpose: The HIM professional in a small physician practice plans, organizes, manages, coordinates, and controls many facets of the practice including all health information management areas.

Reports to: Administrator or Head Physician

Responsibilities:

Knowledge, Skills, and Experience

- Expertise in the management of health information standards, best practices, processes, and procedures including knowledge of medical terminology, classification systems, and vocabularies.

- Expertise in compliance; knowledge of state and federal regulations and accrediting bodies; knowledge of confidentiality, privacy and security laws; knowledge of all regulations pertaining to access and release of information.

- Experience working with health information systems and applications; specifically the EHR.

- Experience in financial management billing processes including revenue cycle management, denials management, and coding.

- Demonstrates strong computer skills using word processing, spreadsheet, and other various software applications.

- Demonstrates leadership skills ensuring timely communication of pertinent information to all staff as well as exercising initiative in decision making and problem solving.

Daily Operations

- Plans, organizes, and evaluates the processes, functions, and resources for the practice.

- Develops and maintains policies and procedures for all HIM processes within the practice including information systems.

- Manages and oversees general financial management of the practice including expenses, billing, revenue cycle management, denials management, and coding.

- Maintains compliance with all regulations (federal, state, accrediting bodies, and other external agencies).

- Collaborates with physicians and staff on the development, implementation, and management of performance targets for the practice.

- Collaborates with IT, staff, and physicians for the development, management, and progress with health information systems and applications.

- Responsible for the review and monitoring of all contracts and services outsourced to HIM vendors.

- Provides overall management to the practice as needed including but not limited to patient, staff, and physician scheduling.

Coding, Billing, and Revenue Cycle Management

- Using experienced-based knowledge, appropriately applies procedures when coding specific body systems.

- Works to prevent delays in reimbursement associated with coding and/or billing practices.

- In all areas of the revenue cycle, provides individual and group education for physicians and coders with specific focus on evaluation and management (E/M) documentation requirements, and ICD-9-CM, CPT/HCPCS coding, and specific usage of modifiers.

- Works collaboratively with physicians and staff to provide periodic reviews, focused reviews, or a complete practice compliance analysis.

- Establishes controls to capture the appropriate revenue using a mechanism to bill and collect for all services performed including, but not limited to, development of appropriate fee schedules and/or charge tickets/superbills.

Information Systems Management

- Collaborates with IT, physicians, and staff on the selection, installation, and maintenance of all systems impacting HIM.

- Develops and/or coordinates the analysis and redesign of workflow processes in conjunction to computerized clinical information systems including the electronic health record to assure efficient and optimal operations.

- Demonstrates knowledge and understanding of general IT concepts and techniques including standards, infrastructure, development, and operations for implementation and best practices.

- Researches and develops appropriate solutions to all system issues within the practice.

- Trains and educates physicians and other users on all HIM systems.

Confidentiality, Privacy, and Security

- Ensures compliance with all privacy regulations including the creation and maintenance of appropriate policies and procedures.

- Collaborates with IT to ensure all security regulations are met including the creation and maintenance of policies and procedures.

- Serves as internal consultant on health information management issues including, but not limited to, access, disclosure, and release of information.

- Provides oversight for the compliance of information systems' confidentiality, privacy, and security safeguards including access and disclosure.

- Serves as HIPAA Privacy Officer; receives and investigates reports of noncompliance and makes recommendations for disciplinary action for violations as necessary.

- Serves as security contact person; receives reports of noncompliance and collaborates with IT to investigate, report (where applicable), and make recommendations for disciplinary action for violations as necessary.

- Directs training related to patient privacy and HIPAA compliance for all staff as needed.

Compliance

- Achieves and monitors all aspects of healthcare compliance including state, federal, and accrediting agencies.

- Monitors and maintains continuing education credits for changes in legislation and accreditation standards that affect health information management principles including coding, reimbursement, documentation practices, and technology impacts; anything that affects the overall practice and make necessary changes accordingly.

- Serves as a resource for staff, physicians, and administration to obtain information or clarification on accurate and ethical coding and documentation standards, guidelines, and regulatory requirements.

- Acts as internal consultant on authorship and authentication of health record documentation as well as quality documentation practices, standardization of medical vocabularies, and use of classification systems.

Human Resources

- Staffs and manages the practice accordingly for efficient and effective operations; interviews, hires, assigns work, and evaluates the performance of subordinates.

- Plans and provides orientation training, and in-service education programs.

- Exercises fair, unbiased judgment and precise decision making in the resolution of personnel issues.

- Stimulates and motivates staff toward successful performance of duties for positive relationships with self as well as others; promotes innovation.

- Creates a supportive environment for open communication.

Qualifications:

- Bachelor's or Associate's degree in health information management or related field

- RHIA or RHIT credential required

- Minimum three to five years experience in a physician practice setting working in health information management related functions.

- Previous related operational or supervisory experience in health information management.

Glossary

Abbreviations   Shortened forms of words or phrases; in healthcare, when there is more than one meaning for an approved abbreviation, only one meaning should be used or the context in which the abbreviation is to be used should be identified.

Abuse   Provider, supplier, and practitioner practices that are inconsistent with accepted sound fiscal, business, or medical practices that directly or indirectly may result in unnecessary costs to the program, improper payment, services that fail to meet professionally recognized standards of care or are medically unnecessary, or services that directly or indirectly result in adverse patient outcomes or delays in appropriate diagnosis or treatment.

Accounts receivable (A/R)   1. Records of the payments owed to the organization by outside entities such as third-party payers and patients. 2. Department in a healthcare facility that manages the accounts owed to the facility by customers who have received services but whose payment will be made at a later date.

Accounts receivable days or aging   Calculation that begins with the total dollars in the accounts receivable. This number is divided by the sum of total gross charges divided by 365 days.

Example: Total A/R divided by (total gross charges/365 days)

A deviation from the annual calculation is to complete the calculation for a shorter period of time, such as only the past three months. The statistics utilized would only be from the most current three-month period.

Accreditation   1. A voluntary process of institutional or organizational review in which a quasi-independent body created for this purpose periodically evaluates the quality of the entity's work against preestablished written criteria. 2. A determination by an accrediting body that an eligible organization, network, program, group, or individual complies with applicable standards. 3. The act of granting approval to a healthcare organization based on whether the organization has met a set of voluntary standards developed by an accreditation agency.

Accreditation Association for Ambulatory Health Care (AAAHC)   A professional organization that offers accreditation programs for ambulatory and outpatient organizations such as single-specialty and multispecialty group practices, ambulatory surgery centers, college/university health services, and community health centers.

Accreditation coordinator The professional who oversees and ensures compliance with an accreditation process (the act of granting approval to a medical practice based on whether the practice meets a set of voluntary standards developed by an accreditation agency).

Accreditation organization A professional organization that establishes the standards against which healthcare organizations are measured and conducts periodic assessments of the performance of individual healthcare organizations and awards an organizational status based on the outcomes of the assessments.

Accreditation standards Preestablished statements of the criteria against which the performance of participating healthcare organizations will be assessed during a voluntary accreditation.

Actuarial model A statistical analysis utilized in evaluating alternative risk scenarios and probability in order to make future projections.

Acute Of short duration.

Acute subluxation Chiropractic term utilized when the patient's spinal joint condition is considered acute as with the result of a new injury. The patient's condition is expected to improve or arrest as a result of chiropractic manipulation.

Advance directive Legal written document that specifies patient preferences regarding future healthcare or the person who is authorized to make medical decisions in the event the patient is not capable of communicating his or her preferences; the patient must be competent at the time the document is prepared and signed. Living wills and durable power of attorney are both considered advance directives.

Advanced practice nurse The term being increasingly used by legislative and governing bodies to describe the collection of registered nurses who practice in the extended role beyond the normal role of basic registered nursing. Refers to nurse practitioners, clinical nurse specialists, nurse midwives, and nurse anesthetists.

Adverse event An untoward, undesirable, and usually unanticipated event that occurs in the healthcare setting (Joint Commission 2009).

Affiliated covered entity Legally-separate covered entities, affiliated by common ownership or control; for purposes of the Privacy Rule, these legally separate entities may refer to themselves as a single covered entity.

AHIMA certified professional An HIM professional who holds in good standing one of the following credentials: (1) Registered health information administrator (RHIA): An AHIMA credential awarded to individuals after completion of an AHIMA-accredited four-year program in health information management and the successful credentialing examination. The RHIA professional has demonstrated expertise in managing patient health information and health records, administering computer information systems, collecting and analyzing patient data, and using classification systems and medical terminologies. RHIAs possess comprehensive knowledge of medical, administrative management, ethical, and legal requirements and standards related to healthcare delivery, and the privacy of protected patient information; (2) Registered health information technician (RHIT): An AHIMA credential awarded to individuals after completion of an AHIMA-accredited two-year program in health information management and the successful credentialing examination. The RHIT professional has demonstrated proficiency in ensuring the quality of health records by verifying their completeness, accuracy, and proper entry into computer systems. RHITs use computer applications to assemble and analyze patient data for the purpose of improving patient care or controlling costs, as well as often specializing in coding diagnoses and procedures in patient records for reimbursement and research; (3) Certified coding specialist—physician-based (CCS-P): An AHIMA credential awarded to individuals who have demonstrated coding expertise in physician-based settings, such as group practices, by passing a certification examination; (4) Certified coding specialist (CCS): An AHIMA credential awarded to individuals who have demonstrated skill in classifying medical data from patient records, generally in the hospital setting, by passing a certification examination; (5) Certified coding associate (CCA): An AHIMA credential awarded to entry-level coders who have demonstrated skill in classifying medical data by passing a certification exam; (6) Certified in healthcare privacy (CHP): An AHIMA credential denoting advanced competency in designing, implementing, and administering comprehensive privacy protection programs in all types of healthcare organizations; requires baccalaureate or master's degree, or healthcare information management credential plus experience (this credential continues to be recognized by AHIMA but is no longer offered); (7) Certified in healthcare privacy and security (CHPS): An AHIMA credential that recognizes advanced competency in designing, implementing, and administering comprehensive privacy and security protection programs in all types of healthcare organizations; requires successful completion of the CHPS exam sponsored by AHIMA; and (8) Certified health data analyst (CHDA): An AHIMA credential awarded to individuals who demonstrate expertise in health data analysis and validation. CHDAs utilize knowledge to acquire, manage, analyze, interpret, and transform data into accurate, consistent, and timely information, while balancing the "big picture" strategic vision with day-to-day details. CHDA-credentialed professionals exhibit broad organizational knowledge and the ability to communicate with individuals and groups at multiple levels, both internal and external.

AHIMA Standard of Ethical Coding   The American Health Information Management Association's principles of professional conduct for coding professionals involved in diagnostic and/or procedural coding or other health record data abstraction.

Allowable amount   A prenegotiated or agreed-upon dollar figure accepted as payment for services between an insurer and provider.

Alphabetic filing system   A system of health record identification and storage that uses the patient's last name as the first component of identification and his or her first name and middle name or initial for further definition.

Ambulatory care   Preventive or corrective healthcare services provided on a nonresident basis in a provider's office, clinic setting, or hospital outpatient setting.

Ambulatory Care Accreditation Program   The segment of the Joint Commission's accreditation program that evaluates and accredits freestanding ambulatory care facilities.

American Chiropractic Association (ACA)   The largest professional association in the world representing doctors of chiropractic.

American College of Obstetricians and Gynecologists (ACOG)   The professional association of medical doctors specializing in obstetrics and gynecology.

American Medical Association (AMA)   The national professional membership organization for physicians that distributes scientific information to its members and the public, informs members of legislation related to health and medicine, and represents the medical profession's interests in national legislative matters; maintains and publishes the Current Procedural Terminology (CPT) coding system.

American Physical Therapy Association (APTA)   The national professional organization whose goal is to foster advancements in physical therapy practice, research, and education.

American Recovery and Reinvestment Act (ARRA)   P.L. 111-5, signed into law in February 2009, which earmarks significant funds toward health information technology and makes notable changes to the Health Insurance Portability and Accountability Act.

American Society of Anesthesiologists (ASA)   The professional association of medical doctors specializing in anesthesiology.

Ancillary services   1. Tests and procedures ordered by a physician to provide information for use in patient diagnosis or treatment. 2. Professional healthcare services such as radiology, laboratory, or physical therapy.

Ancillary systems   Applications, such as a radiology information system, used primarily to operate the clinical department and that contribute health information to an EHR.

Anesthesia report   The report that notes any preoperative medication and response to it, the anesthesia administered with dose and method of administration, the duration of administration, the patient's vital signs while under anesthesia, and any additional products given the patient during a procedure.

Appeal   1. A request for reconsideration of a denial of coverage or rejection of claim decision. 2. The next stage in the litigation process after a court has rendered a verdict; must be based on alleged errors or disputes of law rather than errors of fact.

Application service provider (ASP)   A model of health information technology acquisition where a vendor hosts software and data in its computing facility for a set monthly fee. This significantly reduces the up-front cost of acquiring hardware and software and ongoing need for IT staff.

Assessment   1. For purposes of patient or resident assessment, an objective evaluation or appraisal of an individual's health status, including acute and chronic conditions. The assessment gathers information through data, observation, and physical examination. 2. For purposes of performance improvement, the systematic collection and review of patient or resident-specific data. (Joint Commission 2009)

Attorney ad litem   A guardian appointed to represent the interests of a person with respect to a single action in litigation. A guardian ad litem is often appointed in divorce cases or in parenting time disputes to represent the interests of the minor children. A guardian ad litem is used in other family matters involving grandparents obtaining custody or grandparenting time as well as protection orders where one parent is attempting to get an order against another party with a legal connection to the mother of the child. A guardian ad litem is also appointed in cases where there has been an allegation of child abuse, child neglect, juvenile delinquency, or dependency. The guardian ad litem can be appointed by the court to represent the interests of mentally ill or disabled persons.

Attorney–client privilege   An understanding that protects communication between client and attorney.

Audit   1. A function that allows retrospective reconstruction of events, including who executed the events in question, why, and what changes were made as a result. 2. To conduct an independent review of electronic system records and activities in order to test the adequacy and effectiveness of data security and data integrity procedures. Also, to ensure compliance

Chart conversion   The process of enabling information from active patient charts to be made available in the EHR at the time of first use. Most often, chart conversion refers to scanning all or parts of the chart for viewing images in the EHR. *See also* Pre-load.

Chief complaint   A concise statement, usually stated in the patient's words, describing the symptom, problem, condition, diagnosis, physician-recommended return, or other factor that is the reason for a healthcare encounter.

Chief executive officer (CEO)   The senior manager appointed by a governing board to direct an organization's overall long-term strategic management.

Chief financial officer (CFO)   The senior manager responsible for the fiscal management of an organization.

Chief information officer (CIO)   The senior manager responsible for the overall management of information resources in an organization.

Chief medical informatics officer (CMIO)   An emerging position, typically a physician with medical informatics training who provides physician leadership and direction in the deployment of clinical applications in healthcare organizations.

Chief operating officer (COO)   An executive-level role responsible at a high level for the day-to-day operations of an organization.

Chief privacy officer   A position that (1) oversees activities related to the development, implementation, and maintenance of, and adherence to, organizational policies and procedures regarding the privacy of and access to patient-specific information and (2) ensures compliance with federal and state laws and regulations and accrediting body standards concerning the confidentiality and privacy of health-related information.

Chief security officer (CSO)   The middle manager responsible for overseeing all aspects of an organization's security plan.

Chronic   Of long duration.

Chronic subluxation   Chiropractic term utilized when the patient's spinal joint condition is considered chronic and is not expected to significantly improve or resolve with further treatment. There is, however, the expectation that continued therapy may result in some functional improvement. Once the clinical status is stabilized and the expectation is that there will be no further improvement, then additional manipulative treatment is considered maintenance therapy and is not covered.

Chronological order   A sequence according to time of occurrence where the most recent documentation is found at the end of a document or health record.

Claim   An itemized statement of healthcare services and their costs provided by a hospital, physician office, or other healthcare provider; submitted for reimbursement to the healthcare insurance plan by either the insured party or the provider.

Clinical decision support (CDS)   Functionality using sophisticated modeling, data mining, expert system technology, fuzzy logic, neural networks, visualization, and other techniques to provide context-sensitive (that is, specific to a given patient) templates, reminders, alerts, and other aids that help apply knowledge resources to the patient's care.

Clinical guidelines/protocols With clinical care plans and clinical pathways, a predetermined method of performing healthcare for a specific disease or other clinical situation based on clinical evidence that the method provides high-quality, cost-effective healthcare.

Clinical nurse specialist A registered nurse with a master's degree who provides case management skills to coordinate comprehensive health services and ensure continuity of care; evaluates client progress in attaining expected outcomes; consults with other healthcare providers to influence care of clients, effect change in symptoms, and enhance the ability of others to provide healthcare; and performs additional functions specific to the specialty areas. A certified psychiatric clinical nurse specialist may independently assess, diagnose, and therapeutically intervene in complex mental health problems using psychotherapy and other interventions.

Clinical practice standards The established criteria against which the decisions and actions of healthcare practitioners and other representatives of healthcare organizations are assessed in accordance with state and federal laws, regulations, and guidelines; the codes of ethics published by professional associations or societies; the criteria for accreditation published by accreditation agencies; or the usual and common practice of similar providers or organizations in a geographical region.

Clinical systems Applications that focus on supporting documentation, information retrieval, and knowledge generation at the point of care by providers (that is, physicians, nurses, therapists, pharmacists, and others).

Clinical trial Experimental study in which an intervention or treatment is given to one group in a clinical setting and the outcomes compared with a control or comparison group that did not have the intervention or treatment or that had a different intervention or treatment.

CMS-1450 A Medicare form used for standardized uniform billing for hospital services.

CMS-1500 The universal insurance claim form developed and approved by the American Medical Association and the Centers for Medicare and Medicaid Services. Physicians use it to bill Medicare, Medicaid, and private insurers for professional services provided.

COBRA *See* Consolidated Omnibus Budget Reconciliation Act of 1975.

Coder A professional assigned solely to the function of coding.

Coding Clinic for ICD-9-CM A publication issued quarterly by the American Hospital Association and approved by the Centers for Medicare and Medicaid Services to give coding advice and direction for ICD-9-CM.

Coding compliance plan A component of a health information management compliance plan or a corporate compliance plan modeling the OIG Program Guidance for Individual or Small Group Physician Practices that focuses on the unique regulations and guidelines with which coding professionals must comply.

Coinsurance Cost sharing in which the policy or certificate holder pays a preestablished percentage of eligible expenses after the deductible has been met; the percentage may vary by type or site of service.

Collection The part of the billing process in which payment for services performed is obtained.

Collection agency   An outsourced company that performs the collections for outstanding accounts for a fee.

Competency   The ability to perform a specific task, action, or function successfully.

Compliance   1. The process of establishing an organizational culture that promotes the prevention, detection, and resolution of instances of conduct that do not conform to federal, state, or private payer healthcare program requirements or the healthcare organization's ethical and business policies. 2. The act of adhering to official requirements. 3. Managing a coding or billing department according to the laws, regulations, and guidelines that govern it.

Compliance officer   A designated individual who monitors the compliance process at a medical practice.

Compliance plan   A process that helps an organization, such as a medical practice, accomplish its goal of providing high-quality medical care and efficiently operating a business under various laws and regulations.

Compliance program guidance   The information provided by the Office of Inspector General of the Department of Health and Human Services to help healthcare organizations develop internal controls that promote adherence to applicable federal and state guidelines.

Computerized provider order entry (CPOE)   An application that supports the entry of and associated decision making for directing patient care processes, such as ordering medications, requesting nursing services, and so forth.

Consent   1. A patient's acknowledgment that he or she understands a proposed intervention, including that intervention's risks, benefits, and alternatives. 2. A patient's up-front agreement and acknowledgment that a particular event or condition can occur with their knowledge and permission, such as treatment services, surgical procedures, or disclosure of health information.

Consolidated Omnibus Budget Reconciliation Act of 1975 (COBRA)   The federal law requiring every hospital that participates in Medicare and has an emergency room to treat any patient in an emergency condition or active labor, whether or not the patient is covered by Medicare and regardless of the patient's ability to pay; COBRA also requires employers to provide continuation benefits to specified workers and families who have been terminated but previously had healthcare insurance benefits.

Consultation report   1. A written opinion by a consultant that reflects, when appropriate, an examination of the individual and the individual's medical record(s). 2. Information given verbally by a consultant to a care provider that reflects, when appropriate, an examination of the individual. The individual's care provider usually documents those opinions in the clinical/case record.

Consumer   A person who purchases and/or uses goods or services; in healthcare, a patient, client, resident, or other recipient of healthcare services.

Consumer-directed (driven) healthcare   A form of healthcare providing greater information and decision-making control in the hands of individual consumers, frequently characterized by increased choice over how healthcare dollars are spent.

Consumer-directed (driven) healthcare plan (CDHP)   Managed care organization characterized by influencing patients and clients to select cost-efficient healthcare through the provision of information about health benefit packages and through financial incentives.

Content and records management   The management of digital and analog records using computer equipment and software. It encompasses two related organization-wide roles: content management and records management.

Continual quality improvement (CQI)   A planned and systematic process to provide confidence that work performed (that is, patient care) achieves its intended purpose and meets or exceeds the expectations of those involved (including patients, providers, health plans, and others).

Continuity of care document (CCD)   The combination of the standard data content recommended by the ASTM International standards development organization for patient referral information (that is, continuity of care record (CCR)) and the clinical document architecture (CDA) standard from Health Level Seven (HL7) to enable transmission of the information to a referring physician. Also used extensively as the desirable content to compile in a personal health record (PHR).

Contractual adjustment   The difference between what is charged by the healthcare provider and what is paid by the managed care company or other payer.

Conversion factor   A national dollar amount that Congress designates to convert relative value units to dollars; updated annually.

Copayment   Cost-sharing measure in which the policy or certificate holder pays a fixed dollar amount (flat fee) per service, supply, or procedure that is owed to the medical practice by the patient. The fixed amount that the policyholder pays may vary by type of service, such as $20 per prescription or $15 per physician office visit. Also known as a copay.

Coverage   The level of health insurance benefits provided for an individual or group health plan, often based on the amount of premium dollars paid.

Covered entity   Under HIPAA regulations, any health plan, healthcare clearinghouse, or healthcare provider that transmits specific healthcare transactions in electronic form.

CPT   *See* Current Procedural Terminology.

CPT Assistant   The official publication of the American Medical Association that addresses CPT coding issues.

Credentialing   The process of reviewing and validating the qualifications (degrees, licenses, and other credentials) of physicians and other licensed independent practitioners, for granting medical staff membership to provide patient care services.

Credit balance   Positive dollar amount posted to an account.

C-suite positions   Executive positions of an organization that begin with the letter *C*, such as chief executive officer or chief operating officer.

Current Procedural Terminology (CPT)   A comprehensive, descriptive list of terms and associated numeric and alphanumeric codes used for reporting diagnostic and therapeutic procedures, other medical services, and quality performance measures performed by physicians; published and updated annually by the American Medical Association.

Current Procedural Terminology Category I Code   A CPT code that represents a procedure or service that is consistent with contemporary medical practice and is performed by many physicians in clinical practice in multiple locations.

Current Procedural Terminology Category II Code   A CPT code the represents services and/or test results that contribute to positive health outcomes and quality patient care.

Current Procedural Terminology Category III Code   A CPT code that represents emerging technologies for which a Category I Code has yet to be established.

Customer   An internal or external recipient of services, products, or information, alternatively referred to as consumer or patient.

Database   An organized collection of data, text, references, or pictures in a standardized format, typically stored in a computer system for multiple applications.

Days in accounts receivable   The ending accounts receivable balance divided by an average day's revenues.

Deductible   The amount of cost, usually annual, that the policyholder must incur (and pay) before the insurance plan will assume liability for remaining covered expenses.

Denial   The circumstance when a bill has been accepted, but payment has been denied for any of several reasons (for example, sending the bill to the wrong insurance company, patient not having current coverage, inaccurate coding, lack of medical necessity, and so on).

Denial management   A detailed process that identifies, monitors, reports, and resolves denied claims.

Department of Justice (DOJ)   A federal agency, led by the U.S. attorney general, that enforces the law of the United States, including actions against healthcare fraud and abuse.

Designated record set   A group of records maintained by or for a covered entity that may include patient medical and billing records; the enrollment, payment, claims adjudication, and cases or medical management record systems maintained by or for a health plan; or information used, in whole or in part, to make patient care related decisions.

Diabetes educator   The designation given to an individual who has become certified in diabetes education. The individual may be a clinical psychologist, registered nurse, occupational therapist, optometrist, pharmacist, physical therapist, physician, podiatrist, dietitian, physician assistant, exercise physiologist, social worker, or a healthcare professional with a minimum of a master's degree in nutrition, health education, or specified areas of public health.

Discharge   The point at which an individual's active involvement with an organization or program ends, and the organization or program no longer maintains active responsibility for the care of the individual. In ambulatory or office-based settings where episodes of care occur even though the organization continues to maintain active responsibility for the care of the individual, discharge is the point at which any encounter or episode of care (that is, an office or clinic visit for the purpose of diagnostic evaluation or testing, procedures, treatment, therapy, or management) ends (Joint Commission 2009).

Disclosure   The release, transfer, provision of access to, or divulging in any other manner of patient health information to others outside of the organization and its workforce members.

Documentation   The recording of pertinent healthcare findings, interventions, and responses to treatment as a business record and form of communication among caregivers.

Documentation guideline (DG)   A statement that indicates what health information must be recorded to substantiate use of a particular CPT code.

Due diligence   A formal process to investigate all aspects of a product and its vendor prior to acquisition. For an EHR acquisition, this generally includes requesting a proposal, product demonstrations, site visits, reference checks, and review of corporate financial viability.

Dunning message   Written statement that is automatically printed on statements that details steps that will be taken by the practice if payment is not received.

e-Discovery   The discovery of evidence contained in electronic documents such as e-mails or electronic health records.

Electronic document management system (EDMS)   An application that enables scanned images and other forms of electronic documents, such as digital dictation and e-mail, to be indexed and retrieved electronically.

Electronic health record (EHR)   A digitized collection of information about a patient that does not necessarily meet the requirements of a valid medical record and therefore is not an electronic medical record.

Electronic registry   A system that compiles a specific set of data, usually for a specific disease (for example, diabetes mellitus, cancer), and may be used for research, public health, and/or patient-specific care planning and follow-up.

Element of performance   A specific performance expectation associated with a Joint Commission standard.

Emancipated minors   Persons (generally under 18 years of age, or the state's age of majority) who are considered by the court to be independent, self-supporting, or otherwise responsible to make their own decision.

Encounter   The professional, direct personal contact between a patient and a physician or other person who is authorized by state licensure law and, if applicable, by medical staff bylaws to order or furnish healthcare services for the diagnosis or treatment of the patient; face-to-face contact between a patient and a provider who has primary responsibility for assessing and treating the condition of the patient at a given contact and exercises independent judgment in the care of the patient.

Entity authentication   The corroboration that an entity is who it claims to be.

Episode of care   1. A period of relatively continuous medical care performed by healthcare professionals in relation to a particular clinical problem or situation. 2. One or more healthcare services given by a provider during a specific period of relatively continuous care in relation to a particular health or medical problem or situation. 3. In home health, all home care services and nonroutine medical supplies delivered to a patient during a 60-day period; the episode of care is the unit of payment under the home health prospective payment system (HHPPS).

e-Prescribing (e-Rx)   When a prescription is created/written using an electronic medium; when an actual electronic data interchange transaction is generated that transmits the prescription directly to the retail pharmacy's information system.

Evaluation and management   1. The type of inpatient and outpatient visits and consultative services reported by medical providers, inclusive of such elements as a patient history, focused examination, and medical decision making. 2. The amount of work and involvement by a medical provider, which determines the corresponding intensity and code level for each service.

Evaluation and management (E/M) codes   Current Procedural Terminology codes that describe patient encounters with healthcare professionals for assessment counseling and other routine healthcare services.

Evaluation and management (E/M) services   The history, examination, and medical decision-making services that physicians must perform in evaluating and treating patients in all healthcare settings.

Examination   The act of evaluating the body to determine the presence or absence of disease.

Explanation of Benefits   A statement issued to the insured and the healthcare provider by an insurer to explain the services provided, amounts billed, and payments made by a health plan.

Fair Debt Collections Practices Act (FDCPA)   A federal law that regulates the conduct of debt collectors and protects consumers from unreasonable collection practices and abuses.

False Claims Act   1. Legislation passed during the Civil War that prohibits contractors from making a false claim to a governmental program; used to reinforce the prevention of healthcare fraud and abuse. 2. Federal legislation stipulating that an individual may file claim (for example, against a medical practice) for up to 10 years after an incident has occurred.

Family history   A review of medical events in the patient's family, including health or cause of death of relatives, and diseases that may be hereditary or place the patient at risk.

Federal Bureau of Investigation (FBI)   An agency within the U.S. Department of Justice that investigates federal crimes, including healthcare fraud and abuse.

Federal poverty level (FPL)   The income qualification threshold established by the federal government for certain government entitlement programs.

Federal Rules of Civil Procedure   Body of rules regarding legal procedures that govern civil actions in the federal trial court system; many states have similar rules that are patterned after the federal rules (Garner 2004).

Federal Rules of Evidence   Body of rules regarding the admissibility of evidence in the federal trial court system; many states have similar rules that are patterned after the federal rules (Garner 2004).

Fee   Price assigned to a unit of medical or health service, such as a visit to a physician or a day in a hospital; may be unrelated to the actual cost of providing the service. *See also* Charge.

Fee schedule   A list of healthcare services, procedures, and supplies (usually CPT/HCPCS codes) and the charges associated with them developed by a third-party payer to represent the approved payment levels for a given insurance plan.

Financial assistance   Service provided by the practice or other agency to assist patients of low income or indigent patients in payment of healthcare services.

Fiscal intermediary (FI)   An organization that contracts with the Centers for Medicare and Medicaid Services to serve as the financial agent between providers and the federal government in the local administration of Medicare Part A or Part B claims; usually, but not necessarily, an insurance company.

Flexible spending account (FSA)   Employer- or employee-funded account used to pay eligible expenses for healthcare and dependent care on a pretax basis.

Flow chart   A graphic tool that uses standard symbols to visually display detailed information, including time and distance, of the sequential flow of work of an individual or a product as it progresses through a process.

Fraud   1. An intentional misrepresentation of facts to deceive or mislead in order to unjustly gain from another party. 2. Intentionally making a claim for payment that one knows to be false.

Free text data   Data that are narrative in nature and entered into a field without any formal or predefined structure.

General consent to treatment   A consent signed upon admission to the facility that allows the clinical staff to provide care and treatment for the resident and that usually includes the resident's agreement to pay for the services provided by the facility, to assign insurance benefits to the facility, and to allow the facility to obtain or release health records for payment purposes.

General health record documentation policy   A policy that outlines documentation practices within the facility.

Geographic practice cost index (GPCI)   An index developed by the Centers for Medicare and Medicaid Services to measure the differences in resource costs among fee schedule areas compared to the national average in the three components of the relative value unit (RVU): physician work, practice expenses, and malpractice coverage; separate GPCIs exist for each element of the RVU and are used to adjust the RVUs, which are national averages, to reflect local costs.

Global fee   The amount charged for a healthcare service that combines the physician professional component and health facility technical component into one lump charge.

Group practice   An organization of physicians who share office space and administrative support services to achieve economies of scale.

Growth chart   Document that allows the recording of height, weight, head circumference, and body mass index for newborns, infants, toddlers, and older children. Forms are in a graphic format and typically provided in a color to easily visualize the growth progression of the patient.

Guidelines   Statement of advice.

Health Care Common Procedural Coding System (HCPCS)   An alphanumeric classification system that identifies healthcare procedures, equipment, and supplies for claim submission purposes. The two levels are as follows: I, Current Procedural Terminology codes, developed by the AMA; and II, codes for equipment, supplies, and services not covered by Current Procedural Terminology codes as well as modifiers that can be used with all levels of codes, developed by CMS.

Healthcare provider   A provider of diagnostic, medical, and surgical care as well as the services or supplies related to the health of an individual and any other person or organization that issues reimbursement claims or is paid for healthcare in the normal course of business. A provider is legally responsible for the patient's diagnosis and treatment.

Health history   Record of subjective statements made by the patient.

Health information exchange (HIE)   Seamless exchange of information across disparate organizations.

Health information management (HIM)   The study of the principles and practices of acquiring, analyzing, and protecting digital and traditional medical information vital to providing quality patient care.

Health information organization (HIO)   A governance structure that formally manages health information exchange among its disparate participants.

Health Insurance Portability and Accountability Act of 1996 (HIPAA)   The legislation enacted to provide continuity of health coverage, control fraud and abuse in healthcare, reduce healthcare costs, and guarantee the security and privacy of health information; limits exclusion for pre-existing medical conditions, prohibits discrimination against employees and dependents based on health status, guarantees availability of health insurance to small employers, and guarantees renewability of insurance to all employees regardless of size; requires covered entities (most healthcare providers and organizations) to transmit healthcare claims in a specific format and to develop, implement, and comply with the standards of the Privacy Rule and the Security Rule; and mandates that covered entities apply for and utilize national identifiers in HIPAA transactions. Also known as Public Law 104-191 and the Kassebaum-Kennedy Law.

Health maintenance organization (HMO)   Entity that combines the provision of healthcare insurance and the delivery of healthcare services, characterized by: (1) organized healthcare delivery system to a geographic area, (2) set of basic and supplemental health maintenance and treatment services, (3) voluntarily enrolled members, and (4) predetermined fixed, periodic prepayments for members' coverage.

Health plan   An entity that provides or pays the cost of medical care on behalf of enrolled individuals; includes group health plans, health insurance issuers, health maintenance organizations, and other welfare benefit plans such as Medicare, Medicaid, CHAMPUS, and Indian Health Services.

Health record   1. A paper- or computer-based tool for collecting and storing information about the healthcare services provided to a patient in a single healthcare facility; also called a patient record, medical record, resident record, or client record, depending on the healthcare setting. 2. Individually identifiable data, in any medium, that are collected, processed, stored, displayed, and used by healthcare professionals; documents the care rendered to the patient and the patient's healthcare status.

Health reimbursement account (HRA)   An employer-funded account used to reimburse employees for eligible medical expenses not covered by an employer's health plan. The additional employee reimbursement is paid on a pretax basis and the employer distributions are tax-deductible.

Health savings account (HSA)   An employee- or consumer-funded account used to pay deductible and other eligible health expenses on a pretax basis.

Hearsay   An out-of-court statement that is offered in court to prove the truth of a particular matter in question. The Federal Rules of Evidence provide that hearsay is not admissible as evidence unless it meets one or more numerous exceptions (Garner 2004).

High deductible health plan (HDHP)   An insurance coverage option that offers the benefit of lower premiums in exchange for higher deductibles in comparison to coverage typical of a traditional health plan.

History   The pertinent information about a patient, including chief complaint, past and present illnesses, family history, social history, and review of body systems.

History and physical (H&P)   Information gathered about an individual using a holistic approach for the purpose of establishing a diagnosis and developing a treatment plan. The history may include information about previous illnesses, previous medical or surgical interventions and response to treatment, family health history, and social, cultural, economic, and lifestyle issues that may affect the individual's health and well being. The physical involves the physical examination of the individual's body by the following means: inspection, palpation, percussion, and auscultation (Joint Commission 2009).

History of present illness (HPI)   A chronological description of the development of the patient's present illness from the first sign and/or symptom or from the previous encounter to the present.

Hospital-based practice   A factor for designating medical practice location characterized by the use of hospital staff, equipment, and other resources in providing healthcare services rendered, and used in determining prices and amount billed for services.

Hospital information system (HIS)   Applications that capture patient demographics and insurance and help manage financial and administrative information (for example, census and billing) for a hospital.

Hybrid health record   A combination of paper and electronic records; a health record that includes both paper and electronic elements.

ICD-9-CM   A coding and classification system used in the United States to report diagnoses in all healthcare settings and inpatient procedures and services as well as morbidity and mortality information.

ICD-10-CM   The planned replacement (October 2013) for ICD-9-CM, volumes 1 and 2, developed to contain more codes and allow greater specificity.

Implied consent   The type of permission that is inferred when a patient voluntarily submits to treatment.

Improving Organization Performance   A chapter in the Joint Commission accreditation manual that provides standards for the appropriate management of sentinel events.

Incident report   A quality/performance management tool used to collect data and information about potentially compensable events (events that may result in death or serious injury).

Incident to   Services that are performed by nonphysician personnel under the direct supervision of the physician. The services must be an integral, although incidental, part of the physician's personal, professional services (CMS 2009).

Information Management   A chapter in the Joint Commission accreditation manual that provides standards for managing health information as part of the organizational plan, including areas such as policy and procedures, privacy and security practices, and storage and retrieval.

Informed consent   1. A legal term referring to a patient's right to make his or her own treatment decisions based on the knowledge of the treatment to be administered or the procedure to be performed. 2. An individual's voluntary agreement to participate in research or to undergo a diagnostic, therapeutic, or preventive medical procedure.

Insurance 1. A purchased contract (policy) according to which the purchaser (insured) is protected from loss by the insurer's agreeing to reimburse for such loss. 2. Reduction of a person's (insured's) exposure to risk by having another party (insurer) assume the risk.

Integrated delivery network (IDN) An organizational model in which there is common ownership of different care delivery settings (for example, hospital(s), physician office(s), and nursing home(s)).

Integrated health record A system of health record organization in which all the paper forms are arranged in strict chronological order and mixed with forms created by different departments.

International Classification of Diseases, ninth revision, Clinical Modification (ICD-9-CM) A coding and classification system used in the United States to report diagnoses in all healthcare settings and inpatient procedures and services as well as morbidity and mortality information.

Interoperability The ability of two disparate systems to communicate data from one to the other.

Joint Commission An independent, not-for-profit organization dedicated to improving the safety and quality of healthcare through standards development, public policy initiatives, accreditation, and certification. The Joint Commission accredits and certifies more than 15,000 healthcare organizations and programs in the United States.

Key performance indicators Areas identified for needed improvement through benchmarking and continuous quality improvement.

Legacy systems Applications that are built on older forms of technology.

Legal guardian A person who has the legal authority (and the corresponding duty) to care for the personal and property interests of another person, called a ward. Usually, a person has the status of guardian because the ward is incapable of caring for his or her own interests due to infancy, incapacity, or disability. Most countries and states have laws that designate the parents of a minor child as the legal guardians of that child, and that allow the parents to designate who shall become the child's legal guardian in the event of death or incapacitation.

Legal health record The form of a health record that is the legal business record of the organization and serves as evidence in lawsuits or other legal actions; what constitutes an organization's legal health record varies depending on how the organization defines it.

Liability 1. A legal obligation or responsibility that may have financial repercussions if not fulfilled. 2. An amount owed by an individual or organization to another individual or organization.

Licensed practical nurse The designation given to an individual who is a graduate of an approved practical nursing program and who is licensed as a practical nurse pursuant to state law.

Local coverage determination (LCD) Coverage rules, at a carrier or fiscal intermediary (FI) level, that provide information on what diagnoses justify the medical necessity of a test; LCDs vary from state to state.

Lost charge Service, procedure, or supply (including pharmaceuticals) that was provided or administered during a patient visit yet never marked on the charge slip or entered into the EHR and consequently is never billed to the payer or patient.

Managed care 1. Payment method in which the third-party payer has implemented some provisions to control the costs of healthcare while maintaining quality care. 2. Systematic merger of clinical, financial, and administrative processes to manage access, cost, and quality of healthcare.

Managed care organization (MCO) A type of healthcare organization that delivers medical care and manages all aspects of the care or the payment for care by limiting providers of care, discounting payment to providers of care, and/or limiting access to care; also known as a coordinated care organization.

Master patient index (MPI) A patient-identifying directory referencing all patients related to an organization that also serves as a link to the patient record or information, facilitates patient identification, and assists in maintaining a longitudinal patient record from birth to death.

Medical assistant An individual trained to assist medical professionals.

Medical history A record of previous information provided by a patient to his or her physician to explain the patient's chief complaint, present and past illnesses, and personal and family medical problems; includes also medications and health risk factors.

Medical home A comprehensive model of healthcare linking consumers and providers in a continuous and coordinated manner for all types of care, including preventive care, acute care, chronic care, and palliative end-of-life care.

Medical identity theft The inappropriate or unauthorized use of a person's name (and often other identifiers) to obtain or make false claims for medical services or goods; includes creation of erroneous health information in the victim's name.

Medical informatician An individual who works in the field of medical informatics (a field of information science concerned with the management of data and information used to diagnose, treat, cure, and prevent disease through the application of computers and computer technologies).

Medically Unlikely Edits (MUEs) Implemented on January 1, 2007 to adjudicate claims, the Centers for Medicare and Medicaid Services utilized MUEs to reduce the paid claims error rate for Part B claims. An MUE for a HCPCS/CPT code is the maximum units of service that a provider would report under most circumstances for a single beneficiary on a single date of service. All HCPCS/CPT codes do not have an MUE (CMS 2010a).

Medical necessity 1. The likelihood that a proposed healthcare service will have a reasonable beneficial effect on the patient's physical condition and quality of life at a specific point in his or her illness or lifetime. 2. Healthcare services and supplies that are proven or acknowledged to be effective in the diagnosis, treatment, cure, or relief of a health condition, illness, injury, disease, or its symptoms and to be consistent with the community's accepted standard of care. Under medical necessity, only those services, procedures, and patient care warranted by the patient's condition are provided. 3. The concept that procedures are only eligible for reimbursement as a covered benefit when they are performed for a specific diagnosis or specified frequency; also called the "Need to Know" principle.

Medicare Part B An optional and supplemental portion of Medicare that provides benefits for physician services, medical services, and medical supplies not covered by Medicare Part A.

Medication list Health record documentation that lists all of the medications administered to a patient.

Minimum necessary   The principle that, to the extent practical, individually identifiable health information should only be disclosed to the extent needed to support the purpose of the disclosure. Proposed health IT legislation under ARRA suggests that the covered entity respond to requests for PHI utilizing a limited data set and when a limited data set doesn't meet the need for disclosure, a covered entity can determine what needs to be disclosed based on "minimum necessary" (Rhode 2009).

MMR vaccine   An abbreviation for the combination measles, mumps, and rubella vaccine.

Modifier   A two-digit numeric code listed after a service or procedure code that indicates that a service was altered in some way from the stated CPT or HCPCS descriptor without changing the definition; also used to enhance a code narrative to describe the circumstances of each procedure or service and how it individually applies to a patient.

Multispecialty medical practice   A medical practice that contains more than one specialty of providers.

National Committee for Quality Assurance (NCQA)   A private not-for-profit accreditation organization whose mission is to evaluate and report on the quality of managed care organizations in the United States.

National Correct Coding Initiative (NCCI)   A series of coding regulations to prevent fraud and abuse in Medicare Part B claims; specifically addresses unbundling and mutually exclusive procedures.

National Coverage Determination (NCD)   National medical necessity and reimbursement regulations.

National Patient Safety Goals   Goals issued by the Joint Commission to improve patient safety in healthcare organizations nationwide.

National Provider Identifier (NPI) number   A Health Insurance Portability and Accountability Act (HIPAA) administrative simplification standard. The NPI is a unique identification number for covered healthcare providers. Covered healthcare providers and all health plans and healthcare clearinghouses will use the NPIs in the administrative and financial transactions adopted under HIPAA. The NPI is a 10-position, intelligence-free numeric identifier (10-digit number) (CMS 2010b).

Never event   A medical care error that signals deficiencies in the safety and credibility of a healthcare provider (for example, surgery on the wrong part of the body) (CMS 2006).

Nonphysician practitioner   An umbrella term used to describe a healthcare provider who meets state licensing obligations to provide specific medical services but is not a physician. Some of these practitioners include: audiologist, certified registered nurse practitioner, certified registered nurse anesthetist (CNRA), certified nurse midwife (CNM), licensed clinical social worker (LCSW), physical and occupational therapist, physician assistant (PA), and registered dietitian/nutrition professional.

Nonreviewable sentinel events   Subset of sentinel events that are not subject to review by the Joint Commission under the sentinel event policy.

No-show   Classification given to an appointment that is scheduled but the patient does not appear on the date of service.

NPO   An abbreviation meaning "nothing by mouth." Latin for *nil per os.*

Nurse practitioner (NP) A nurse with a graduate degree in advanced practice nursing. This allows him or her to provide a broad range of healthcare services, including:

- Taking the patient's history, performing a physical exam, and ordering appropriate laboratory tests and procedures, as well as diagnosing, treating, and managing acute and chronic diseases

- Providing prescriptions and coordinating referrals

- Promoting healthy activities in collaboration with the patient

Occupational therapy A treatment that uses constructive activities to help restore an individual's ability to carry out needed activities of daily living and improve or maintain functional ability.

Office of Inspector General (OIG) 1. The office through which the federal government established compliance plans for the healthcare industry. 2. A division of the Department of Health and Human Services (HHS) that investigates issues of noncompliance in the Medicare and Medicaid programs such as fraud and abuse; overseen by the Department of Justice.

Office of Inspector General Work Plan Yearly plan released by the OIG that outlines the focus for reviews and investigations in various healthcare settings.

Office of the National Coordinator for Health Information Technology (ONC) Created by presidential order; serves as the HHS Secretary's principal advisor on the development, application, and use of health information technology in an effort to improve the quality, safety, and efficiency of the nation's health through the development of an interoperable harmonized health information infrastructure.

Open enrollment The specified time period each year or upon employment in which individuals have the opportunity to review and evaluate health insurance coverage option details and make benefit selections for a future period.

Operative report A formal document that describes the events surrounding a surgical procedure or operation and identifies the principal participants in the surgery.

Orders A physician's written or verbal instructions to the other caregivers involved in a patient's care.

Organized healthcare arrangement An agreement characterized by more than one covered entity who share PHI to manage and benefit their common enterprise and are recognized by the public as a single entity.

Outguide A device used in paper-based health record systems to track the location of records removed from the file storage area; placeholder for filing and/or tracking charts removed from the storage area.

Out-of-pocket costs The dollar amounts paid by consumers upon receiving healthcare services that insurance does not pay, including copayments, deductibles, coinsurance, and alternative types of spending limits.

Paper-based health record Collection of healthcare documents on paper format, rather than electronic format.

Past, family, and/or social history (PFSH) The patient's past experience with illnesses, hospitalizations, operations, injuries, and treatments; a review of medical events in the patient's family, including diseases that may be hereditary or place the patient at risk; and an age-appropriate review of past and current activities.

Past history The patient's experience with illness, operations, injuries, treatments, current medications, allergies, immunizations, and diet.

Pathology report A type of health record or documentation that describes the results of a microscopic and macroscopic evaluation of a specimen removed or expelled during a surgical procedure.

Patient An individual who receives care, treatment, or services. For hospice providers, the patient and family are considered a single unit of care. Synonyms used by various healthcare fields include client, resident, patient and family unit, consumer, healthcare consumer, customer, and beneficiary. When appropriate, the term patient may also refer to the "legally responsible individual" (Joint Commission 2009).

Patient history questionnaire A series of structured questions to be answered by patients to provide information to clinicians about their current health status.

Payer An insurance company (for example, Blue Cross/Blue Shield) or healthcare program (for example, Medicare) that pays or reimburses healthcare providers (second party) and/or patients (first party) for the delivery of medical services.

Payer mix The percentage of revenue by individual payer.

Peer review records Documentation resulting from activities in which healthcare professionals review their peers in an effort to continually ensure high-quality care.

Personal health record (PHR) An electronic or paper health record maintained and updated by an individual for himself or herself.

Physical examination Record of the provider's assessment of the patient's current health status.

Physical therapy (PT) The field of study that focuses on the physical functioning of the patient on a physician-prescribed basis.

Physician assistant A healthcare professional licensed to practice medicine with physician supervision.

Physician-office based A factor for designating medical practice location characterized by providers assuming responsibility for practice resources in a nonfacility setting, and used in determining prices and amount billed for services.

Physician Quality Reporting Initiative (PQRI) The 2006 Tax Relief and Health Care Act (TRHCA) (P.L. 109-432) required the establishment of a physician quality reporting system, including an incentive payment for eligible professionals (EPs) who satisfactorily report data on quality measures for covered services furnished to Medicare beneficiaries during the second half of 2007 (the 2007 reporting period). CMS named this program the Physician Quality Reporting Initiative (PQRI) (CMS 2010c).

Picture archiving and communication system (PACS) An application that enables images of diagnostic studies to be stored, retrieved, and enhanced (for example, rotated, enlarged) electronically.

Place of service   A method of categorizing medical practice location and defining whether healthcare services and procedures occur in a facility or nonfacility setting; used as an element in establishing prices.

Point-of-service collections   A method to communicate amount owed and to secure payment in advance or at the time of providing services; includes payments from the uninsured as well as unmet deductibles, copayments, and coinsurance from those consumers who have insurance.

Point-of-service plan   A managed care arrangement characterized as a hybrid between an HMO and a PPO. Enrolled members must select a primary care physician (PCP) who must follow approved referral guidelines for specialist care similar to an HMO; members can also exercise an option to see an out-of-network provider.

Policies   1. Governing principles that describe how a department or an organization is supposed to handle a specific situation. 2. Binding contracts issued by a healthcare insurance company to an individual or group in which the company promises to pay for healthcare to treat illness or injury; such contracts may also be referred to as health plan agreements and evidence of coverage.

Power of attorney for healthcare   The legally recognized authority to act and make decisions on behalf of another party for healthcare-related purposes.

Practice management system (PMS)   Applications that capture patient demographics, insurance, and other financial and administrative information (for example, scheduling, billing) for ambulatory care.

Precollection   The act of collecting on outstanding accounts prior to turning accounts over to a collection company. This task may be completed in-house or may be outsourced to a collection company. Precollections performed by an outsourced company typically have lower fees than other collection protocols. Also known as soft collections.

Preferred provider organization (PPO)   A managed care arrangement based on a contractual agreement between healthcare providers (professional and/or institutional) and employers, insurance carriers, or third-party administrators to provide healthcare services to a defined population of enrollees at established fees that may or may not be a discount from usual and customary or reasonable charges.

Pre-load   Populating an EHR with selected data from active patients' records to make the EHR easier for new users to use.

Premium   Amount of money that a policyholder or certificate holder must periodically pay an insurer in return for healthcare coverage.

Preoperative evaluation   Record of examinations and diagnostic tests performed to verify a patient's candidacy for surgery.

Preregistration   The act of gathering demographic and payer information from a patient prior to the date of service. This may be completed over the telephone, via the mail, or electronically using registration forms on the practice's Web site.

Pricing transparency   The process of communicating the cost of healthcare services in advance, with the outcome of placing greater decision-making control and purchasing power into the hands of consumers.

Primary care   The continuous and comprehensive care provided at first contact with the healthcare provider in an ambulatory care setting.

Primary care provider (PCP)   Healthcare provider who provides, supervises, and coordinates the healthcare of a member; PCPs can be family and general practitioners, internists, pediatricians, and obstetricians/gynecologists; other PCPs are nurse practitioners and physician assistants.

Problem list   A list of illnesses, injuries, and other factors that affect the health of an individual patient, usually identifying the time of occurrence or identification and resolution.

Problem-oriented medical record (POMR)   A way of organizing information in a health record in which clinical problems are defined and documented individually; also called problem-oriented health record.

Professional component (PC)   1. The portion of a healthcare procedure performed by a physician. 2. A term generally used in reference to the elements of radiological procedures performed by a physician.

Progress note   The documentation of a patient's care, treatment, and therapeutic response, which is entered into the health record by each of the clinical professionals involved in a patient's care, including nurses, physicians, therapists, and social workers.

Protected health information (PHI)   Individually identifiable health information, transmitted electronically or maintained in any other form, that is created or received by a healthcare provider or any other entity subject to HIPAA requirements.

Provider   Physician, clinic, hospital, nursing home, or other healthcare entity (second party) that delivers healthcare services.

Record completion   The act of ensuring that all health information documentation is complete, including content and proper authentication.

Record of Care, Treatment, and Services   A chapter in the Joint Commission accreditation manual that provides standards for managing health information specifically addressing the clinical record itself.

Records retention period   The period of time during which records must be maintained by an organization because they are needed for operational, legal, fiscal, historical, or other purposes.

Record tracking   Maintaining information about the current location of a record.

Recovery audit contractor (RAC)   A governmental program whose goal is to identify improper payments made on claims of healthcare services provided to Medicare beneficiaries. Improper payments may be overpayments or underpayments. Overpayments can occur when healthcare providers submit claims that do not meet Medicare's coding or medical necessity policies. Underpayments can occur when healthcare providers submit claims for a simple procedure, but the medical record reveals that a more complicated procedure was actually performed. Section 302 of the Tax Relief and Health Care Act of 2006 makes the RAC Program permanent and requires the HHS Secretary to expand the program to all 50 states by no later than 2010 (CMS 2010d).

Redisclosure   The release, transfer, provision of access to, or divulging in any other manner of patient health information that was generated by an external source to others outside of the organization and its workforce members.

Registration   The act of gathering demographic and payer information from a patient at the time of service.

Registration record   The document that contains the demographic and insurance information of a patient.

Reimbursement   Compensation or repayment for healthcare services.

Relative value unit (RVU)   A number assigned to a procedure that describes its difficulty and expense in relationship to other procedures by assigning weights to such factors as personnel, time, and level of skill.

Release of information (ROI)   The process of disclosing patient-identifiable information from the health record to another party.

Remittance advice (RA)   An explanation of payments (for example, claim denials) made by third-party payers.

Request for proposal (RFP)   A type of business correspondence asking for very specific product and contract information that is often sent to a narrow list of vendors that have been preselected after a review of requests for information during the design phase of the systems development life cycle.

Reserves   1. Unused profits from a not-for-profit organization that stay in the business. 2. Dollars set aside to cover unexpected expenses, such as bad debt or revenue audit contractor recovery dollars.

Results management   The ability to process results of diagnostic studies, such as laboratory tests, into tables, trend lines, and comparisons with other data, such as vital signs.

Results review   The ability only to view results of diagnostic studies (this does not include results management).

Retail healthcare   A model of healthcare driven by basic economic forces and market competition, which aligns the specific needs of consumers (demand) with the services to satisfy those needs offered by providers and entities (supply).

Retail medical center   A business entity built around a specific target consumer (customer) segment, offering products and health services ranging from primary care to specialty care in a competitive market-driven environment, and a focus on how potential consumers view price, quality, accessibility, and convenience.

Revenue cycle   1. The process of how patient financial and health information moves into, through, and out of the medical practice, culminating with the practice receiving reimbursement for services provided. 2. The regularly repeating set of events that produce revenue.

Revenue cycle management   The supervision of all administrative and clinical functions that contribute to the capture, management, and collection of patient service revenue, with the goals of accelerated cash flow and lowered accounts receivable.

Reverse chronological order   A sequence according to the reverse time of occurrence where the most recent documentation is found at the beginning of a document or health record.

Reviewable sentinel events   Subset of sentinel events that are subject to review by the Joint Commission under the sentinel event policy.

Review of systems (ROS) An inventory of body systems obtained through a series of questions seeking to identify signs and/or symptoms the patient may be experiencing or has experienced.

Risk management The processes in place to identify, evaluate, and control risk, defined as the organization's risk of accidental financial liability.

Root cause analysis Analysis of a sentinel event from all aspects (human, procedural, machinery, material) to identify how each contributed to the occurrence of the event and to develop new systems that will prevent recurrence.

SCHIP *See* State Children's Health Insurance Program.

Secure messaging system A system that eliminates the security concerns that surround e-mail but retains the benefits of proactive, traceable, and personalized messaging.

Sentinel event An unexpected occurrence involving death or serious physical or psychological injury, or the risk thereof. Serious injury specifically includes loss of limb or function. The phrase "or risk thereof" includes any process variation for which a recurrence would carry a significant chance of serious adverse outcome. Such events are called "sentinel" because they signal the need for immediate investigation and response.

Sentinel event database Data collected and compiled by the Joint Commission pertaining to sentinel events, root cause analyses, action plans, and follow-up that have been reported by accredited healthcare organizations.

Sentinel event policy Established by the Joint Commission to guide accredited organizations in defining, responding to, and reporting sentinel events.

Serial filing system A health record identification system in which a patient receives sequential unique numerical identifiers for each encounter with, or admission to, a healthcare facility.

Serial numbering system A type of health record identification and filing system in which patients are assigned a different but unique numerical identifier for every admission.

Shared/split visit Evaluation and management visits conducted in hospitals by a nonphysician practitioner (nurse practitioner, clinical nurse specialist, certified nurse midwife, or physician assistant) and a physician employed by the same practice for the same patient on the same calendar day.

Small balance A determined dollar amount for which statements are not sent and dollars may be potentially written off.

S.M.A.R.T. goals Specific, measurable, achievable, right, and time-based statements of what an organization hopes to accomplish once an EHR has been successfully implemented.

Social history An age-appropriate review of past and current activities, including marital status; employment; use of drugs, alcohol, or tobacco; level of education; and sexual history.

Software as a service (SaaS) Similar to the ASP model of EHR acquisition in which the EHR is hosted by a vendor but is only Web-enabled, SaaS utilizes newer, Web-based software to both develop and provide the EHR application.

Solo practice A practice in which the physician is self-employed and legally the sole owner.

Source-oriented health record A way of organizing information in the health record in which sections are divided according to the source of information, such as one section for physician notes, another for laboratory results, a third for radiology results, and so forth.

Speech-language therapy A treatment intended to improve or enhance an individual's ability to communicate and/or swallow.

Spoliation Intentional destruction, alteration, or concealment of evidence.

Standard A statement that defines the performance expectations that must be in place in order for an organization to provide safe and high-quality care, treatment, and service.

Standing orders Orders that an individual provider has established as routine care for a specific diagnosis or procedure.

State Children's Health Insurance Program (SCHIP) The children's healthcare program implemented as part of the Balanced Budget Act of 1997; sometimes referred to as the Children's Health Insurance Program, or CHIP.

Statute of limitations Law that determines the period in which a legal action can be brought against a facility for injury, improper care, or breach of contract; legal limit on the time allowed for filing suit, usually measured from the time of the wrong or from the time when a reasonable person should have discovered the wrong. Proceedings brought after this time limit are subject to dismissal by the court.

Structured text data 1. Binary, computer-readable data. 2. High-level, text-based programming language, with a syntax similar to Pascal.

System build The process of configuring a system to meet specific requirements.

Technical component (TC) The portion of radiological and other procedures that is facility-based or nonphysician-based (for example, radiology films, equipment, overhead, endoscopic suites, and so on).

Telehealth/telemedicine The provision of remote healthcare, including exchange of medical information from one site to another via electronic communications to improve, maintain, or assist patients' health status.

Telephone contact record Record that documents telephone communications between the patient and his or her healthcare providers.

Terminal digit filing system A system of health record identification and filing in which the last digit or group of digits (terminal digits) in the health record number determines file placement.

Terminology asset manager Professional responsible for connecting two different terms that mean the same thing to two different users or creating digital links between one electronic terminology and another electronic terminology, such as between SNOMED CT terms and the corresponding ICD-9, HCPCS, and CPT codes (Dimick 2008).

Third-party payer An insurance company (for example, Blue Cross/Blue Shield) or healthcare program (for example, Medicare) that pays or reimburses healthcare providers (second party) and/or patients (first party) for the delivery of medical services.

Unapplied cash Payments received without specific patient and/or account numbers associated. Since the correct patient or patient account cannot be identified, the funds are posted to a separate account called an unapplied account.

Unique identifier   A type of information that refers to only one individual or organization.

Urgent care medicine   The delivery of ambulatory medical care outside of a hospital emergency department on a walk-in basis without a scheduled appointment.

Vaccination   Use of vaccines to prevent specific diseases.

Visit   A single encounter with a healthcare professional that includes all of the services supplied during the encounter.

Workflow and process redesign   The mapping of existing workflows and processes to identify opportunities for improvement. In acquiring an EHR, this helps an organization discover how the EHR will impact its operations.

Write-off   The action taken to eliminate the balance of a bill after the bill has been submitted and partial payments have been made or payment has been denied and all avenues of collecting the payment have been exhausted.

References

Centers for Medicare and Medicaid Services. 2006 (May 18). Fact sheet: Eliminating serious, preventable, and costly medical errors—never events. http://www.cms.gov/apps/media/fact_sheets.asp.

Centers for Medicare and Medicaid Services. 2009. Medicare Benefit Policy Manual, Internet Only Manual (IOM), Chapter 15, Section 60.2 Medicare Carrier Manual 2050.1.

Centers for Medicare and Medicaid Services. 2010a. Medically Unlikely Edits. http://www.cms.gov/NationalCorrectCodInitEd/08_MUE.asp.

Centers for Medicare and Medicaid Services. 2010b. National Provider Identifier Standard (NPI): Overview. http://www.cms.gov/NationalProvIdentStand.

Centers for Medicare and Medicaid Services. 2010c. Physician Quality Reporting Initiative: Overview. http://www.cms.gov/pqri.

Centers for Medicare and Medicaid Services. 2010d. Recovery Audit Contractor: Overview. http://www.cms.gov/RAC.

Dimick, C. 2008. HIM jobs of tomorrow: Eleven new and revised jobs illustrate the trends changing HIM and the opportunities that lie ahead. *Journal of AHIMA* 79(10):26–34.

Garner, B. A., ed. 2004. *Black's Law Dictionary,* 8th ed. Eagan, MN: Thompson West.

Joint Commission. 2009. *Accreditation Manual for Ambulatory Surgical Centers.* E-dition Glossary. Oakbrook Terrace, IL: Joint Commission.

Rode, D. 2009. Recovery and privacy: Why a law about the economy is the biggest thing since HIPAA. *Journal of AHIMA* 80(5): 42–44.

Answer Key
Check Your Understanding

Chapter 1

Check Your Understanding 1.1
1. c
2. c
3. b
4. d
5. b
6. c
7. d
8. c
9. d
10. c

Check Your Understanding 1.2
1. a
2. d
3. d
4. a
5. b
6. e
7. c
8. c
9. a
10. d

Chapter 2
1. c
2. d
3. b
4. a
5. c
6. b
7. d
8. a
9. d
10. a

Chapter 3
1. b
2. a
3. c
4. a
5. d
6. d
7. a
8. d
9. d
10. a

Chapter 4

1. b
2. a
3. d
4. d
5. c
6. c
7. e
8. d
9. d
10. d

Chapter 5

1. a
2. a
3. d
4. b
5. d
6. c
7. d
8. b
9. d
10. a

Chapter 6

Check Your Understanding 6.1

1. b
2. d
3. c
4. c
5. d
6. a
7. c
8. d

9. b
10. a

Check Your Understanding 6.2

1. d
2. c
3. d
4. c
5. a
6. c
7. d
8. a
9. c
10. b

Check Your Understanding 6.3

1. d
2. d
3. b
4. c
5. c
6. a
7. d
8. b
9. c
10. d

Chapter 7

Check Your Understanding 7.1

1. b
2. c
3. a
4. c
5. d

Check Your Understanding 7.2

1. b
2. b
3. d
4. c
5. a

Chapter 8

1. e
2. c
3. c
4. b
5. d
6. c
7. d
8. a
9. b
10. b
11. e
12. d

Chapter 9

Check Your Understanding 9.1

1. b
2. c
3. c
4. b
5. b

Check Your Understanding 9.2

1. b
2. b
3. a

4. c
5. b

Check Your Understanding 9.3

1. a
2. b
3. c
4. a
5. a

Chapter 10

Check Your Understanding 10.1

1. d
2. c
3. b
4. d
5. a

Check Your Understanding 10.2

1. b
2. b
3. d
4. d
5. b

Check Your Understanding 10.3

1. b
2. d
3. a

Check Your Understanding 10.4

1. d
2. b
3. d

Check Your Understanding 10.5

1. a
2. c

3. d
4. c
5. d

Chapter 11

1. b
2. c
3. d
4. a
5. d

Index